Principles and Practice of ULTRASONOGRAPHY

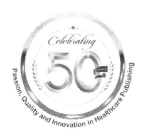

Principles and Practice of ULTRASONOGRAPHY

Third Edition

Sumeet Bhargava
MBBS DNB (Radiodiagnosis) FICRI FIMSA FIAMS FCGP MNAMS FCCP
Associate Professor
Department of Radiology and Imaging
MS Medical College and Hospital
Hapur Road, Ghaziabad, Uttar Pradesh, India

Satish K Bhargava
MD (Radiodiagnosis) MD (Radiotherapy) DMRD FICRI FIAMS FIMSA FCCP FUSI FAMS
Former Head
Department of Radiology and Imaging
University College of Medical Sciences (University of Delhi) and
Guru Teg Bahadur (GTB) Hospital
New Delhi, India
Former Head
Department of Radiology and Imaging
School of Medical Sciences and Research
Sharda Hospital, Sharda University
Greater Noida, Uttar Pradesh
Former Head
Department of Radiology and Imaging
JN Medical College
Aligarh Muslim University
Aligarh, Uttar Pradesh, India

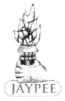

JAYPEE BROTHERS MEDICAL PUBLISHERS
The Health Sciences Publisher
New Delhi | London

Jaypee Brothers Medical Publishers (P) Ltd

Headquarters
Jaypee Brothers Medical Publishers (P) Ltd
4838/24, Ansari Road, Daryaganj
New Delhi 110 002, India
Phone: +91-11-43574357
Fax: +91-11-43574314
E-mail: jaypee@jaypeebrothers.com

Overseas Offices
JP Medical Ltd
83 Victoria Street, London
SW1H 0HW (UK)
Phone: +44 20 3170 8910
Fax: +44 (0)20 3008 6180
E-mail: info@jpmedpub.com

Website: www.jaypeebrothers.com
Website: www.jaypeedigital.com

© 2021, Jaypee Brothers Medical Publishers

The views and opinions expressed in this book are solely those of the original contributor(s)/author(s) and do not necessarily represent those of editor(s) of the book.

All rights reserved. No part of this publication may be reproduced, stored or transmitted in any form or by any means, electronic, mechanical, photocopying, recording or otherwise, without the prior permission in writing of the publishers.

All brand names and product names used in this book are trade names, service marks, trademarks or registered trademarks of their respective owners. The publisher is not associated with any product or vendor mentioned in this book.

Medical knowledge and practice change constantly. This book is designed to provide accurate, authoritative information about the subject matter in question. However, readers are advised to check the most current information available on procedures included and check information from the manufacturer of each product to be administered, to verify the recommended dose, formula, method and duration of administration, adverse effects and contraindications. It is the responsibility of the practitioner to take all appropriate safety precautions. Neither the publisher nor the author(s)/editor(s) assume any liability for any injury and/or damage to persons or property arising from or related to use of material in this book.

This book is sold on the understanding that the publisher is not engaged in providing professional medical services. If such advice or services are required, the services of a competent medical professional should be sought.

Every effort has been made where necessary to contact holders of copyright to obtain permission to reproduce copyright material. If any have been inadvertently overlooked, the publisher will be pleased to make the necessary arrangements at the first opportunity. The **CD/DVD-ROM** (if any) provided in the sealed envelope with this book is complimentary and free of cost. **Not meant for sale.**

Inquiries for bulk sales may be solicited at: jaypee@jaypeebrothers.com

Principles and Practice of Ultrasonography

First Edition: 2002

Second Edition: 2010

Third Edition: **2021**

ISBN 978-93-90020-82-9

Printed at Replika Press Pvt. Ltd.

Dedicated to
My loving late Parents Shri Jagannath Bhargava and Mrs Brahma Devi Bhargava,
My late loving Wife Kalpana and My son Dr Sumeet Bhargava, whose inspiration and sacrifice
has made it possible to bring out this book

Satish K Bhargava

Contributors

A Verma MD (Radiodiagnosis)
Resident Medical Officer
Arpana Hospital
Karnal, Haryana, India

Amit Sahu MBBS DNB (Radiodiagnosis)
Consultant
Department of Radiology
Max Superspeciality Hospital
Saket, New Delhi, India

Atul Luthra MBBS MD DNB
Diplomate, National Board of Medicine
Consultant, Physician and Cardiologist
New Delhi, India

Chander Mohan MD (Radiodiagnosis)
Senior Consultant
Interventional Radiology and HOD Radiology
BL Kapoor Memorial Hospital
New Delhi, India

Poonam Narang MD (Radiodiagnosis)
Professor
Department of Radiology
Maulana Azad Medical College and
Associated GB Pant Hospital
New Delhi, India

Rajul Rastogi MD (Radiodiagnosis)
Associate Professor
Department of Radiology
Teerthanker Mahaveer (TM) Medical College
Moradabad, Uttar Pradesh, India

Satish K Bhargava
MD (Radiodiagnosis) MD (Radiotherapy) DMRD FICRI FIAMS
FIMSA FCCP FUSI FAMS
Former Head, Department of Radiology and Imaging
University College of Medical Sciences (University of Delhi)
and Guru Teg Bahadur (GTB) Hospital
New Delhi, India
Former Head, Department of Radiology and Imaging
School of Medical Sciences and Research
Sharda Hospital, Sharda University
Greater Noida, Uttar Pradesh
Former Head, Department of Radiology and Imaging
JN Medical College
Aligarh Muslim University
Aligarh, Uttar Pradesh, India

Shuchi Bhatt MD (Radiodiagnosis) MNAMS FICR
Head, Department of Radiology and Imaging
University College of Medical Sciences
(Delhi University) and GTB Hospital
New Delhi, India

Sudhanshu Bankata MD (Radiodiagnosis)
Executive Director (CEO)
Batra Hospital and Medical Research Center
New Delhi, India

Sumeet Bhargava
MBBS DNB (Radiodiagnosis) FICRI FIMSA FIAMS FCGP
MNAMS FCCP
Associate Professor
Department of Radiology and Imaging
MS Medical College and Hospital
Hapur Road, Ghaziabad, Uttar Pradesh, India

Preface to the Third Edition

With the more and more extensive utilization of the Ultrasonography in various systems of the human body, and with ever increase demand of the book due to advancement in technology, it is essential to upgrade the book with addition of new chapters on elastography and musculoskeletal ultrasonography, replacement and addition of few important illustrations, I am sure that book will definitely be more useful to Radiologists, Obstetricians and Gynecologists, Physicians and Residents in their day to day practice.

Sumeet Bhargava
Satish K Bhargava

Preface to the First Edition

Introduction of ultrasound was a boon to the medical field, due to its noninvasive and non-ionizing nature leading to constantly growing interest in the application of ultrasound as a diagnostic modality. Its easy acceptability in the developing countries is also because of its wide availability and low cost.

Ultrasound is a stethoscope of a radiologist to look into the intriguing pathological conditions and provide useful information to the clinician for better patient care. However, this technology is very much operator-dependent and thus a thorough understanding of standard scanning technique and knowledge of the sonographic anatomy is essential for optimum results. Thus we embarked on the monumental task of providing a basic book on clinical diagnostic ultrasound. The main feature of this book is extensive coverage and easy comprehension. The book has gone deeply into normal sonographic anatomy and the basic technique of performing ultrasound. The book beautifully covers sonography of the abdomen and superficial parts. A special effort has been made to include a large number of illustrations and scans to provide a clear impression of the sonographic appearance of normal and pathologic lesions. Obstetric ultrasound has also been covered in the text. A chapter on Doppler has been included in order to provide the basic knowledge of the subject. Introduction to interventions and latest advancement in ultrasound emphasises its importance in therapeutics.

I am sure that this book will be of great help to the budding radiologists and the technologists and help them in optimum utilization of this extremely useful modality and this in turn will bring laurels to the professions.

Satish K Bhargava

Acknowledgments

We are grateful to our colleagues and friends who gave timely support and stood behind us in our joint endeavor of bringing out this book, which was required keeping in view the fact that no such book is available in an Indian perspective and wide acceptability of this imaging modality for the diagnosis and staging of the disease.

We are especially thankful to Shri Jitendar P Vij (Group Chairman), Mr Ankit Vij (Managing Director), Mr MS Mani (Group President), Ms Chetna Malhotra Vohra (Associate Director—Content Strategy), Ms Pooja Bhandari (Production Head), Ms Nedup Denka Bhutia (Development Editor) and the publishing staff at Jaypee Brothers Medical Publishers (P) Ltd, New Delhi, India, for their work in completing this book successfully.

Contents

1. **Historical Perspective of Ultrasound** — 1
   Satish K Bhargava

2. **Nature of Ultrasound** — 4
   Satish K Bhargava, Amit Sahu

3. **Interaction of Ultrasound with Matter** — 8
   Satish K Bhargava, Sumeet Bhargava

4. **Transducer** — 12
   Satish K Bhargava, Sumeet Bhargava

5. **Basic Ultrasound Instrumentation** — 20
   Satish K Bhargava, Amit Sahu

6. **Real Time Ultrasound** — 30
   Satish K Bhargava, Amit Sahu, Sumeet Bhargava

7. **Ultrasound Artifacts, Biological Effects of Ultrasound, Image Quality, and Instrumentation** — 37
   Satish K Bhargava, Sumeet Bhargava

8. **Scanning Techniques in Sonography** — 51
   Satish K Bhargava, Rajul Rastogi, Sumeet Bhargava

9. **Basic Sonographic Anatomy** — 63
   Sumeet Bhargava, Rajul Rastogi

10. **Abdomen: Hepatobiliary System and Spleen** — 130
    Sumeet Bhargava, Shuchi Bhatt, Amit Sahu

11. **Abdomen: Pancreas** — 158
    Shuchi Bhatt, Rajul Rastogi, Sumeet Bhargava

12. **Abdomen: Gastrointestinal Tract** — 164
    Satish K Bhargava, Sumeet Bhargava

13. **Abdomen: The Urinary Tract** — 172
    Sumeet Bhargava, Shuchi Bhatt, Satish K Bhargava

14. **Abdomen: Adrenal Glands** — 193
    Satish K Bhargava, Sumeet Bhargava, Rajul Rastogi

15. **Abdomen: The Retroperitoneum** — 196
    Rajul Rastogi, Amit Sahu, Shuchi Bhatt, Sumeet Bhargava

16. **Abdomen: The Peritoneum** — 202
    Sumeet Bhargava, Rajul Rastogi, Amit Sahu

17. **Abdomen: The Uterus and Adnexa** — 209
    Shuchi Bhatt, Rajul Rastogi, Sumeet Bhargava

18. **Pediatric Abdomen** — 224
    Satish K Bhargava, Sumeet Bhargava

19. **Intracranial Sonography** — 236
    Sudhanshu Bankata, Sumeet Bhargava, Satish K Bhargava

20. **Eye and Orbit** — 243
    Satish K Bhargava, Rajul Rastogi, Sumeet Bhargava

21. Thyroid *Sumeet Bhargava, Satish K Bhargava, Amit Sahu*	**250**
22. Small Part Ultrasound *Satish K Bhargava, Sumeet Bhargava, Rajul Rastogi, Shuchi Bhatt*	**253**
23. Ultrasound Examination of the Peripheral Arteries *Satish K Bhargava, Rajul Rastogi, Sumeet Bhargava*	**277**
24. Intraoperative and Laparoscopic Sonography *Satish K Bhargava, Sumeet Bhargava, Rajul Rastogi*	**293**
25. Intravascular Ultrasound: Current Concepts *Chander Mohan, Rajul Rastogi, A Verma*	**301**
26. Perendoscopic Ultrasound *Sumeet Bhargava, Satish K Bhargava, Rajul Rastogi*	**310**
27. Contrast Agents for Ultrasound *Sumeet Bhargava, Satish K Bhargava*	**314**
28. Normal Ultrasound Measurements *Satish K Bhargava, Sumeet Bhargava, Amit Sahu*	**318**
29. Obstetric Ultrasound *Satish K Bhargava, Rajul Rastogi, Sumeet Bhargava*	**331**
30. Interventional Radiology *Poonam Narang*	**378**
31. Color Doppler *Shuchi Bhatt, Rajul Rastogi, Sumeet Bhargava, Satish K Bhargava*	**383**
32. Basics of Echo *Atul Luthra*	**405**
33. Elastography *Amit Sahu, Sumeet Bhargava*	**421**
34. Musculoskeletal Ultrasonography *Amit Sahu, Sumeet Bhargava*	**423**
Index	*443*

CHAPTER 1

Historical Perspective of Ultrasound

Majority of the people approaching ultrasound for the first time assume that this is one of the newer imaging techniques. Certainly, ultrasound has only achieved wide clinical use since 1970. But medical use of ultrasound came about shortly after close of World War II. These were based on fundamental research into the principle of sound and its interaction with different material which took place centuries back.

The piezoelectric effect, upon which the generation and detection of ultrasound signal depends, was noted by Pierre and Jacques Curie in 1880.

The principle of pulse echo technique for detection of underwater bodies were already under investigation prior to the First World War and were given considerable impetus by the need to detect submarines during world war. The first major attempt at a practical application was made in the unsuccessful search for the sunken Titanic in the North Atlantic in 1912. Other early attempts at applying ultrasound met with same fate.

The physical principles on which our modern diagnostic techniques rely therefore probably owe their origin to Chilowsky and Paul Langevin who produced their early publication in 1916. Their work was on the basis for SONAR (Sound Navigation and Ranging), the first important successful application of ultrasound.

It was this pulse echo distance ranging technique which became the basis for modern diagnostic medical sonography.

The medical potential was not appreciated in early post First World War period. However, technological development occurred with small portable pulse echosystem that were developed for detecting flaws in manufactured structures.

Although it was these new flaw detectors which generated the greatest interest and several workers dedicated themselves to the detection and evaluation of biological effects.

Wood, Loomis and Johnson were probably the earliest researchers and they published their result on the bioeffect of this newly discovered form of energy in 1927 and 1929, respectively.

In view of destructive effect in both solid material and biological systems, both industrial and biological applications for these properties were soon investigated.

Lym and Putnam focused ultrasound in water bath and induced massive cerebral lesions in experimental animals by insonating them with focused 1 MHz ultrasound. Attempts were made to develop ultrasound as an alternative to radiotherapy, but the technology for beam manipulation and for interaction of the ultrasound generators with the patients was inadequate and early clinical results showed more destruction of normal tissue than with the currently available X-ray radiotherapeutic technique. In the late 30s and early 40s, SY Sokolov and Firestone took out patients on ultrasound device used for detecting metal flaws.

Karl Dussik and his brother Friederick decided to use ultrasound as an alternative source of transmitted energy in systems. In their first apparatus sound was transmitted from a single crystal which was mechanically scanned across the area of interest and transmitted signal received by a second transducer on the far side of area under investigation. They are known to have been working with this apparatus in the mid and late 1930s and published some early clinical results in the late 1940s.

Their first publications showed transmission ultrasonograms of the human head in which ventricular system appeared to be represented. Several other groups also published transmission image of head in 1950 and 1951.

However, it was late discovered that transmission ultrasonogram of the head from which the brain had been removed and replaced with saline were indistinguishable from the ultrasound already published. Clearly the apparent image of the ventricular system was due merely to varying attenuation of the transmitted ultrasound by alteration in the thickness of the lateral skull wall.

In 1949, Ludwig and Struthes used pulse echo-ultrasound as medical imaging technique to detect gallstones and foreign bodies in soft tissues.

One problem of the all the early ultrasound system was the difficulties of conducting the transmitted sound into the patient and echo-out. Thus the early pulse echosystem required total immersion of the subject in a water tank in which the scanning apparatus was also submerged.

Using such a system Howry and Bliss built a scanner based on up turned gun tunnel from a war time bomber; then clinical results were of high quality.

In 1950, Howry and Bliss produced first cross-sectional ultrasound image. In 1957, Howry and Homes assembled the first compound scanner consisting of water-filled tank in which patient was immersed surrounded by track in which transducer was moved in a series of compound motions and published their cross-sectional image of improved quality. The echoes were displaced on phosphor screens and photographed.

Wild and Reid published their work on direct contact scanner showing images of muscles of forearm and later of breast tissue. They reported 90% accuracy in differentiating benign from malignant lesions.

Mid 1950s, Saw proliferation of wider clinical application of diagnostic ultrasound. Baum developed an ophthalmic scanner.

He subsequently repeated the sonographic visualization of intraocular and orbital tumors, foreign bodies and retinal detachments.

Luksell applied the principle of industrial flaw detector to human skull and detected cerebral midline echo. Luksell and Turner were fortunate in choosing an appropriate anatomical target for their system and they laid the foundation of mid line echoencephalography. This field of investigation was further developed in Europe by Gordon, Lek Shell in Sweden and Kaizen and colleagues in Germany.

This technique was subsequently widely used in accident and emergency and in neurology department until the advent of CT scanner in the late 1970s.

Howry and other with their compound scanner produced good quality image but requirement of total immersion of the patient in water was clinically unacceptable. Tom Brown in late 1950s produced a mechanical contact compound scanner. However, image formation time was excessively long but image quality was good and rapidly gain clinical acceptance. Donald made a new apparatus on the basis of this produced direct contact manually operated scanner and applied in obstetrics and gynecology which gave a foundation of medical diagnostic ultrasound imaging as we know it today. Donald described two techniques still in use—coupling the transducer to the patient with mineral oil and using a full urinary bladder as a sonic window through which to visualize deep pelvic structures. He published a correlation of fetal biparietal diameter with gestational age.

Holm also developed a contact compound scanner which was in regular clinical use by the mid 1960s. Both Brown and Holmes scanner had ultrasound transducer mounted on an arm attached to a substantial rectilinear frame. Thereafter, Wells produced probably the first of hinged arm scanner which rapidly became the main configuration for manually operated compound static scanners until their demise at the hand of automated real-time system in early 1980s.

The display system of very early experimental scanners all used conventional cathode ray oscilloscopes with open shutter photography to store the image. These system produced images with the equivalent of what we call a gray scale display. The development of scanner proceeded over the ensuing years. The bistable storage oscilloscope was introduced in order to improve the case of both scanning and photography. The price paid for this development was the display of low level echoes disappeared and resulting ultrasound images contained information only from organ boundaries and strong reflectors. Kossoff developed (1970s) a complex water bath scanner which produced excellent high resolution images with good dynamic range display on a non-storage oscilloscope. It was probably his work which stimulated the equipment manufacturers to reintroduce gray scale image display and this was greatly facilitated by the development of television scan converter tube. This was a vacuum tube device somewhat similar to conventional cathode ray tube in which the image could be written on to a target in a random fashion during scanning and then read from the target as a conventional cathode ray tube. This device became readily available for inclusion in commercial scanners from about 1974 onwards. This revolutionized the ability of ultrasound to detect and display low echoes from soft tissue structures. Limitation of this scan converter was its average useful life which was very short and with electronic technology digital scan converter was developed in 1976. These systems were rapidly improved to give image resolution of greater than 512×512 pixels as the wide gray scan range.

The origin of real-time ultrasound imaging system lie in the late 1960s and early 1970s. Bom pioneered the development of linear array transducer as his first system having 20 elements giving 20 lines of information in the image. Sonar was simultaneously developing the phased array transducer. Both linear array and phased array scanner was practically demonstrated for its use in cardiac and abdominal injuries.

Prime clinical application of linear array real-time was in obstetrics while the scanner proved more satisfactory for cardiac and upper abdominal and pelvic imaging. The problem of small field of view with linear scanner was overcome in early 1980s by the introduction of curvilinear transducer. This design gave a very substantial improvement in image quality from these systems.

Siemens at the same time introduced mechanical real-time scanner called videoson. This system incorporated transducer mounted on a rotating wheel in front of parabolic mirror and produced good real-time images.

In early 1970s, a number of groups attempted to develop more compact real-time mechanical scanner. Their invention fell into two major groups, the rotating spinners and oscillating wobblers.

McDicken (1974) published his initial work and subsequent development in this field has led to refinement incorporated in many rotating mechanical sector scanner. The wobblers have also undergone simultaneous further development and are currently the most popular mechanical real-time sector scanner.

One of the main reason for continued popularity of mechanical sector scan systems is the symmetrical beam focusing which can be achieved with a single crystal element and suitable lenses. The main disadvantage of mechanical system has been that the focusing depth is fixed for any one crystal configuration.

In mid 1970s, annular array transducers were introduced which permitted beam focusing at any depth.

In 1980s, intracavitary mechanical rotating scanner were produced.

At the same time Doppler ultrasound were being developed. The fundamental work in this field was done by Kallnus in 1954. The detection of fetal heart movement by Doppler ultrasound was described by Callagan in 1964 and principle was rapidly developed for detection of blood flow within accessible superficial vessels throughout the body. Continuous wave Doppler system was used. The major problem of this system was the inability to produce any form of image of the vessel or determine from what depth or from how many vessels the Doppler signals were being received. In early 1970s, pulsed Doppler system was employed which could permit measurement of depth within the patient from which echoes were arising. These systems suffered from the problem of extremely slow image production.

In mid 1970s to early 1980s, a duplex system was introduced in which a high resolution conventional real-time imaging scanner was linked to a pulsed doppler device. These systems were popular for evaluation of carotid circulation. The major limitation of this system lays in its inability of real-time imaging system to detect all plaque and thrombus reliably, especially fresh thrombus within a vessel.

This problem was overcome in late 1980s by Doppler color flow mapping. This technique became possible as a consequence of continuing development in rapid parallel computer signal processing.

Continuous rate of growth of improving image qualities and introducing new technological development continues unabated at present time which is making ultrasound a dynamic and essential part of imaging system in radiology department/hospital.

CHAPTER 2

Nature of Ultrasound

Ultrasound can be defined as the sound waves beyond the ordinary limits of hearing. Therefore, simply US are high frequency sound waves. Ultrasound is a form of mechanical energy which can be characterized as a wave phenomenon. An ultrasound wave is similar to an X-ray as both are wave transmitting energy. However, there are number of basic differences between electromagnetic radiation and ultrasound. The important difference is X-rays can pass through a vacuum. However, ultrasound requires a medium for propagation as it travels poorly through air thus requiring an airless contact with the body during examination. This explains the need to use mineral oil or jelly as a coupling agent to body areas being examined. The velocity of sound depends on the nature of medium. Electromagnetic radiation is transverse in nature however ultrasound is a longitudinal wave. When sound is generated as in case of high frequency speaker, molecules of air are alternatively compressed and decompressed (rarefaction) by mechanical action of speaker cone. The sound is transmitted from speaker to the listener by the air molecules, but the air molecules themselves do not move that distance. The alternate compression and rarefaction created by motion of speaker cone produce alternate to and fro motion that is passed from molecule to molecule. This to and fro movement of air molecules is along the direction of sound wave and therefore, these waves are called longitudinal waves.

Similarly, when ultrasound pulses are directed into a medium, it causes the particle in the medium to vibrate parallel to the direction of wave propagation. The vibration affects an adjoining particle in an elastic fashion and that particle then affects the next adjoining particle and so on **(Fig. 2.1)**.

This process of transmitted vibration from particle to particle leads to the propagation of the ultrasound wave through the medium. The most important vibration is back and forth motion along the longitudinal axis of the beam. The longitudinal wave contains area of rarefaction where particle are spread apart (Low pressure) and area of compression where particle are close together (High pressures). Length of wave or wavelength is the distance between two-band of compression or rarefaction and is represented by λ. Once the sound wave has been generated it continues in its original direction until it is reflected, refracted or absorbed.

FREQUENCY AND SPEED OF SOUND

The generalized wave equation is as follows:
$$\text{Velocity} = \text{Frequency} \times \text{Wavelength} (\lambda)$$

Wavelength is the distance between one cycle and the onset of the next cycle where one cycle represents combination of one compression and one rarefaction though sound is actually a series of compressions and rarefactions.

This equation applies to all wave phenomena. However with electromagnetic radiation the velocity is constant and energy is directly related to frequency and inversely related to Wavelength.

When equation applies to sound the velocity is variable the frequency is the tone or pitch and amplitude is the intensity or loudness **(Fig. 2.2)**.

Frequency is defined as number of oscillation (cycles) per second **(Fig. 2.2)**. In modern physics, the term Hertz (Hz) is used to describe the number of oscillation per second. Audible sound lies in the range of 20 Hz to 20,000 Hz. Frequency above this range is called ultrasound but diagnostic ultrasound is concerned safely with frequencies in the range of 2 MHz to 10 MHz, the catheter based endoluminal source extend to 50 MHz. The attenuation of ultrasound beam energy and quality of image are strong function of frequency.

SPEED OF SOUND

Propagation speed is the distance traveled per unit time. The sound speed is very much dependent on medium of propagation whereas frequency is independent of the medium and does not change significantly.

Table 2.1 shows velocity of sound in some common material. In biological tissue speed is close to 1540 meters per second but in bone is above 3000 meter per second. The speed of propagation is unaffected by either the power of the sound or its frequency.

The velocity of sound is determined by the rate at which wave energy is transmitted through the medium which

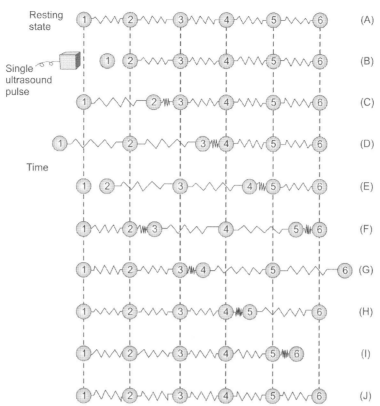

Fig. 2.1: Particle interaction. This is a schematic representation of how six hypothetical particles interact under the effect of a single ultrasound pulse. Line (A) represents the resting state and each successive line (B), (C), (D), (E), (F), (G), (H), (I), (J) represents the positions of the particles at regular intervals of time. In line (B), a single ultrasound pulse is emitted which affects particle (1). Line (C) represents the effect of particle (2) on particle (3), etc. until a resting state is again achieved in line (J). Note how each particle moves in both directions from its resting state under the effect of the ultrasound pulse.

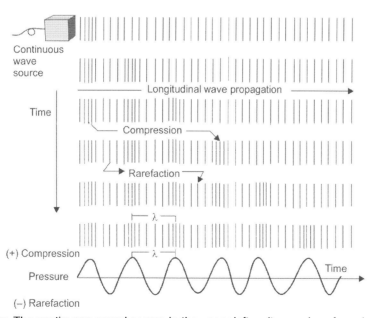

Fig. 2.2: Wave propagation. The continuous sound source in the upper left emits a series of regular ultrasound pulses, which creates areas of compression and rarefaction. If one plots pressure within the transmitting medium versus time, then a sinusoidal curve (bottom) is generated with increased pressure corresponding to the periods of compression and decreased pressure corresponding to areas of rarefaction. The wavelength (λ) is equal to the length of one complete cycle which includes a band of rarefaction and compression.

TABLE 2.1: Velocity of ultrasound in various materials.

Materials	Velocity (m/sec)
Air	330
Lung	1,160
Fat	1,450
Human soft tissue	1,540
Brain	1,541
Liver	1,549
Kidney	1,561
Blood	1,570
Fetal head	1,580
Muscle	1,585
Adult skull	4,080

depends on the density and compressibility of the medium. It should be emphasized that a medium must be present in order for sound to propagate. The medium must also be elastic; that is, the medium must have the ability to deform temporarily and their reform to its original shape.

DENSITY

Velocity of sound in the medium is inversely proportional to the square root of the density of the medium ρ; that is, the higher the density, slower the velocity of sound.

$$V_s \propto 1/\sqrt{\rho}$$

Where V_s is velocity of sound ρ is density of the medium.

However, on the basis of density alone, one would expect sound (ultrasound) to have greater velocity in air (low density) than in bone (higher density) compressibility.

The velocity is also inversely proportional to square root of the compressibility of the medium K

$$V_s \propto 1/\sqrt{K}$$

Compressibility indicates the fractional decrease in volume when pressure is applied to the material.

The easier a medium is to compress, higher the compressibility. Dense materials such as bone are difficult to reduce in volume. Hence, denser material has low compressibility.

This low compressibility predicts a high velocity of sound in bone. In contrast air has high compressibility and therefore velocity of sound would be low.

Combining compressibility and density into one equation the velocity of sound of a particular medium is determined by

$$V_s = 1/\sqrt{K\rho}$$

If density could be increased without affecting compressibility then speed of sound would decrease. However, compressibility and densities of a particular substance are interdependent, a change in density is coupled with larger and opposing change in compressibility. But since compressibility varies more rapidly, this parameter becomes a dominant factor.

Overall effect is summarized by—as the density increases speed also increases. Compressibility is key factor in determining the velocity because bone is less compressible then air and therefore velocity of sound in bone is 4080 m/sec whereas velocity of sound in air is 330 m/sec.

In another example, water has density of 1 g/cc and mercury has density 13.6 g/cc. On the bases of density alone, water would have a velocity of sound 13.6 times faster than mercury. But the compressibility of water is 13.4 times higher than mercury which tends to cancel the density effect. The velocities of water and mercury are similar. In fact all liquids tend to transmit ultrasound at same velocity.

In general because the compressibility is low, denser medium have greater velocities than do less dense media. The average velocity of ultrasound in tissue is 1540 m/sec. A slight dependence on the temperature of the medium and on the frequency is exhibited. The velocity of ultrasound waves in water at 20°C is 1480 m/sec if temperature of water is increased to 37°C the velocity became 1520 m/sec.

The velocity of sound for ultrasound remains constant for a particular medium.

INTENSITY, POWER AND DECIBELS

Intensity of the ultrasound beam is a measure of amount of energy flowing through a unit cross-sectional area at each second. Intensity is expressed in mixed unit of watt per centimeter square or milliwatts per centimeter square.

Pressure amplitude—sound energy that causes particle displacement to occurs in propagation medium and can be described either as a pressure difference, P or as pressure amplitude.

Intensity of ultrasound beam is proportional to pressure amplitude

$$I \propto P^2$$

Where, P is pressure amplitude

Intensity of beam also decreases exponentially with distance

$$I = I_0 \exp(-\mu x)$$

Where, I is intensity at the point of interest

I_0 is original intensity

μ = intensity attenuation coefficient

x = distance traversed by beam

Power—is the measure of total energy transmitted per unit time summed over entire area of cross-section of the beam.

$$\text{Power} = \text{Intensity} \times \text{Area}$$

This is why the unit of intensity is expressed as mw/cm². Average ultrasonic intensity in diagnostic ultrasound is in the range of 0.1 to 10 mw/cm².

Although absolute value of power and intensity of ultrasound beam is important when considering the biological effect of diagnostic ultrasound or therapeutic ultrasound but their absolute values are difficult to measure. This is particularly true of pulsed diagnostic beam. A more useful method of determining the reduction in power or intensity of the beam is to make relative measurement that compare the intensity or power at one reference point with that at another point in the beam.

When the range of intensities is large instead of impairing the intensities themselves, it is simpler to compare the logarithm of intensities.

The unit used to express relative intensity is the decibel (dB). A dB is defined by the equation

Where, $dB = 10 \log_{10} (I/I_0)$

I is intensity at the point of interest.

I_0 is original intensity or reference intensity.

For example, let us assume that intensity at a point was reduced to half the original and at second point the intensity is 1/10,000 of the original. Converting thus into decibel.

For point 1 $dB = 10 \log (I_0/2/I_0)$
$= 10 \log_{10} (0.5)$
$= -3.01$

For point 2 $dB = 10 \log_{10} \dfrac{1}{10,000} = -40 \text{ dB}$

The comparison of ratio for both points shows that intensity is in range of 2 to 10,000 whereas, a range of only –3 to –40 dB units expresses this same relation (–ve) shows that intensity of beam decreased from reference point to point of intensities.

A second advantage of decibel notation is that dB along the beam path are additive.

Relative amplitudes are also expressed in dB. However, because intensity and pressure are related to each other, there is slight change in the relationship between dB and amplitude.

$$dB = 20 \log_{10} A_1/A_2$$

Where, A_1 is the amplitude at point of interest;

A_2 is the amplitude at reference point.

3
CHAPTER

Interaction of Ultrasound with Matter

Ultrasound wave is generated by a transducer and is then directed into the patient body to interact with tissue in accordance with the characteristics of targeted tissue.

The results of these interactions are recorded for diagnosis in the form of ultrasound wave incident on a transducer. There are three possible interactions take place: reflection, refraction, and absorption.

REFLECTION

Reflection is the return of incident ultrasound energy as an echo directly back to the transducer when interacting at a boundary with normal incidence. Reflection occurs at the interface between two dissimilar materials **(Fig. 3.1)**. The percentage of beam reflected at tissue interfaces depends on (i) tissue's acoustic impedance and (ii) beams angle of incidence.

The reflection of ultrasound pulses by the structure within the patient's body is the interaction that creates ultrasound imaging.

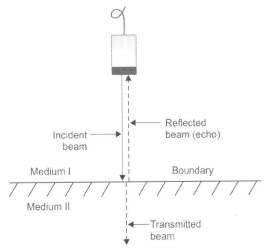

Fig. 3.1: Specular echo. The figure represents what happens when an ultrasound beam interacts with an acoustic boundary (i.e., where medium I and medium II have different acoustic impedances). Note that under these circumstances, the beam strikes the boundary at a 90° angle. This results in an undeviated transmitted beam and a reflected beam, which is called a specular echo.

Acoustic Impedance

Acoustic impedance is the characteristics of a material related to density and elastic properties.

The product of density and velocity of propagation is called acoustic impedance.

$$Z = \rho.V_s$$

This is a measure of resistance to sound passing through the medium. Acoustic impedance is measured in rays, where the fundamental unit is g/cm^2 sec. **Table 3.1** list the acoustic impedance of tissue commonly encountered in the patients. High density materials give rise to high sound speed and therefore high acoustic impedance. Similarly, low densities materials such as gases have low acoustic impedances. If the acoustic impedance is same in one medium as in other then sound is readily transmitted from one medium to other.

Amount of reflection is determined by the difference in acoustic impedance of two tissues. Greater the difference, greater the percentage reflected.

TABLE 3.1: Impedance of various materials.

Materials	Acoustic impedance (Rayls—g/cm^2 Sec × 10^{-5})
Air	0.0004
Fat	1.38
Castor oil	1.4
Water (50° C)	1.54
Brain	1.58
Blood	1.61
Kidney	1.62
Liver	1.65
Muscle	1.70
Lens of eye	1.84
Piezoelectric polymers	4.0
Skull (bone)	7.8
Quartz	15.2
Mercury	19.7
PZT-5A	29.3
PZT-4	30.0
Brass	38.0

Angle of Reflection

The angle of reflection of the sound beam is equal to angle of incidence of sound beam (**Fig. 3.4**).

These angles are defined relative to a line drawn perpendicular to surface of interface.

Amount of reflection is determined by angle of incidence. Higher the angle of incidence, less the amount of reflected sound.

In medical ultrasound in which the same transducer is used both to transmit and receive ultrasound, almost no reflected sound will be detected if ultrasound strikes the patient's surface at angle more than 3° from perpendicular.

Hence, to obtain maximum detection of reflected signal, the transducer must be oriented so that the generated sound beam strikes the interface perpendicularly. Sound is reflected at interface regard less of thickness of the material from which it is reflected.

Hence, reflection of ultrasound arises as result of difference in acoustic impedance.

When a sound beam strikes a smooth interface that is perpendicular to the beam, the amount of reflection is given by

$$R = \frac{(Z_1 - Z_2)^2}{(Z_2 + Z_1)^2} \times 100$$

R = Percent of beam reflective
Z_1 = Acoustic impedance of beam 1
Z_2 = Acoustic impedance of beam 2.

Reflection at different tissue interface is shown in **Table 3.2**. When ultrasound pulse interacts with interface the pulse is divided into two, and one pulse the echo is reflected back towards transducer and other penetrate into other material as shown in **Figure 3.2**.

The brightness of structure in an ultrasound image depends on the strength of the reflection or echo.

It is also possible to calculate the amount of transmission of a sound beam that strikes a smooth interface perpendicular to the beam. The equation is

$$T = \frac{4Z_1 Z_2 \times 100}{(Z_1 + Z_2)^2}$$

T = Percentage of beam transmitted
Z_1 = Acoustic impedance of medium 1
Z_2 = Acoustic impedance of medium 2.

If the acoustic impedance is small, the magnitude of reflected wave is small. Because same device transmits and receives the sound, maximum detection of reflected echo

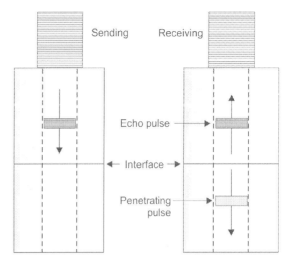

Fig. 3.2: Transducer.

occurs when sound beam strikes the interface with normal incidence.

If the acoustic impedance is large such as bone compared with soft tissue, a large fraction of ultrasound beam is reflected; little of the transmitted beam penetrates the structure behind the bone and most of the incidents beam return to the detector. Consequently, for examination involving the head, ultrasound is restricted to relatively simple noninvasive study.

The same effect would occur if structure such as liver is evaluated. One has to be careful to avoid aiming the ultrasound beam through a rib. To visualize the liver, which is largely positioned under the ribs, one must either look through intercostal spaces (between the ribs) or under the ribs and back up at the liver.

All the tissue-air interfaces using the acoustic impedance listed in **Table 3.2**, the formula for fraction of sound intensity reflected yields that nearly total reflection occurs even if the thickness of air layer is extremely small.

This explains the inability of ultrasound to penetrate the air filled structure such as lung and air filled bowel.

An acoustic window is a conduit of tissue that provides an acoustic impedance matter to allow ultrasound transmission through structure such as lung. This is why lung must be avoided when studying the heart.

Total reflection at air-tissue interface also explains the requirement of having an air-free contact between patient's body and ultrasound source. This is accomplished by using a coupling gel or mineral to eliminate air pocket that could attenuate or reflect the ultrasound beam.

The acoustic impedance difference at fat-soft tissue interface produce relatively strong echo compared with parenchyma. Reflection from fat-soft tissue interface is primarily responsible for organ outlines seen in imaging.

Suppose a phantom consists of tissue of more than one tissue as shown in **Figure 3.3A**. The objective is to determine the percentage of incident beam that return to the transducer from each interface. Let us suppose there are only four interfaces.

TABLE 3.2: Percent reflection at different interface.

	Percent reflection
Soft-tissue-air	99.9
Soft-tissue-lung	52.0
Soft-tissue-bone	43.0
Fat-liver	0.79
Soft-tissue-fat	1.1
Crystal-tissue	19
Caster oil-soft tissue	0.43

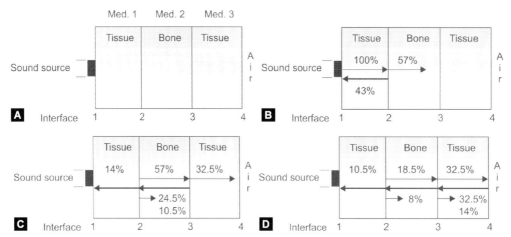

Figs. 3.3A to D: Reflections from multiple interfaces illustrated by a tissue-bone-tissue phantom: (A) Composition of tissue-bone tissue phantom; (B) Reflection and transmission from interface 2 (tissue-bone); (C) Reflection and transmission from interface 3 (bone-tissue); (D) Reflection and transmission from tissue-air interface.

- Assume that 100% of ultrasound beam enter the phantom and beam is reduced exclusively by reflection.
- Absorption is ignored.
- Interface 2 produces 43% of beam reflected at first tissue-bone interface and subsequently detected. The rest 57% of beam are transmitted into bone **(Fig. 3.3B)** at the next interface (bone tissue). Interface 3, there are 43% reflection of incident beam (57%), resulting in 24.5% of the original beam being reflected back towards the transducer and 32.5% (57% of 57%) being transmitted toward interface 4. The reflected beam from interface 3 on the return towards the transducer must interact at bone-tissue interface 2. This produces a 43% reflection away from the transducer and a 57% transmission towards the transducer. Thus only 14% of the original beam (57% of 24.5%) reaches the transducer from interface 3 **(Fig. 3.3C)**. Interface 4, tissue-air interface at the back of phantom cause 100% of the 32.5% transmission into medium 3 to be reflected back towards the transducer. This results in 18.5% of the original beam being transmitted into medium 2. At the next bone tissue interface 43% is reflected and 57% is transmitted into medium towards the sound source.

The echo from interface 4 is 10.5% of the original beam **(Fig. 3.3D)**.

Refraction

Refraction occurs when sound waves meet a tissue interface boundary at an angle other than 90°.

Refraction is the change in direction of transmitted ultrasound energy that occurs at a boundary interface. The bending of sound waves by refraction requires a nonperpendicular incidence of beam and different propagational speed of two adjacent tissues **(Fig. 3.4)**.

The change in direction results from a wave length change in second medium to accommodate a change in speed. Refraction of sound waves obeys Snell's law of optics.

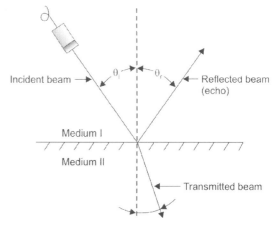

Fig. 3.4: Snell's law. This figure represents what happens when an ultrasound beam strikes a boundary obliquely. Medium I and medium II have different acoustic impedances. The velocity of sound (V_s) in medium I and II are V_{si} and V_{st} respectively. Note that the angle of incidence (q_i) equals the angle of reflection (q_r). Also note that since V_{si} is greater than V_{st}, the angle of the transmitted beam (θ_t), or angle of refraction, is less than the angle of incidence (θ_r).

Snell's law is given by
$$\frac{\sin \theta_i}{\sin \theta_r} = \frac{V_{si}}{V_{st}}$$

Where θ_i = Incident angle
θ_r = Transmitted angle
V_{si} = Velocity of sound in incident medium
V_{st} = Velocity of sound in transmitted medium
θ_i and θ_2 are defined with respect to a line drawn perpendicular to the interface.

As indicated by Snell's law the amount of deviation from expected straight line path changes with the angle of incidence and with the velocities in associated medium.

This does not generally present any difficulty in diagnostic ultrasound because velocity of sound in soft tissue is relatively constant.

Although refraction is not a major problem in diagnostic ultrasound under certain condition the bending of sound beam causes artifacts in diagnostic image. The formation of image is predicted on assumption that ultrasound beam always travels in straight line through tissues.

Absorption

Absorption is the only process where by sound energy is dissipated in a medium. All other mode of interactions (reflection, refraction, and scattering) reduce intensity by redirecting beam. However, in absorption process ultrasonic energy is transformed into other form of energy principally heat.

This is responsible for medical application of therapeutic ultrasound. The absorption of an ultrasound beam is related to the frequency of the beam, the viscosity of the medium and relaxation time of the medium.

Relaxation Time

The relaxation time describes the rate at which molecules return to their original position after being displaced by a force. If a substance has a short relaxation time, the molecules return to their original position before the next compression of waves arrives. However, if the medium has a long relaxation time, molecules may be moving back towards their original position as wave crest strikes them. Hence, more energy is required to stop and then reverse the direction of the molecules, thereby producing more heat.

Viscosity

High viscosity provides greater resistance to flow of molecules in medium. For example, a low viscosity fluid such as water flows more freely than does the more viscous maple syrup. The frictional force must be overcome by vibrating molecules and thus more heat is produced in maple syrup.

Frequency

The frequency also affects the absorption in relation to both viscosity and relaxation time. If the frequency is increased the molecules must move more often thereby generating more heat from the drag caused by friction. As frequency is increased less time is available for molecules to recover during relaxation process. Molecules remain in motion and more energy is needed to stop and redirect the molecules again producing more absorption. Rate of absorption is directly proportional to frequency.

Attenuation

Attenuation includes the contribution of reflection, scattering as well as absorption. Attenuation is reflection characterized by attenuation coefficient in unit of dB/cm

TABLE 3.3: Absorption coefficients of biologic materials.

Materials	Absorption coefficients (dB/cm)
Lung	41
Skull-bone	20
Air	12
Muscle	3.3
Kidney	1.0
Liver	0.94
Brain	0.85
Blood	0.18
Water	0.0022

which is measure of log relative intensity loss per unit centimeter of travel.

An approximate rule of thumb is attenuation coefficient of 0.5–1 dB/cm/MHz. Attenuation of ultrasound beam follow exponential law

$$A = A_o \exp(-\mu x)$$

Where 'μ' is attenuation of coefficient and
  x = distance traversed by beam
  A = amplitude of beam at a distance
  A_o = original amplitude of beam.

The attenuation coefficients at 1 MHz for various tissues are presented **(Table 3.3)**. The value in the table must be multiplied by the frequency of operation to determine the appropriate coefficient. Half value for soft tissue (Thickness of tissue necessary to attenuate the intensity by 50%) occurs when intensity drops by 3 dB.

Table 3.3 shows water is very good conductor of ultrasound. Water within the body, forms window (such as cysts and the bladder) through which underlying structures can be easily imaged. Lung has much higher attenuation rate than either air or soft tissue. This is because the small pockets of air in alveoli are very effective in scattering ultrasound energy. Because of this, normal lung structure is extremely difficult to penetrate with ultrasound. Bone has relatively high attenuation rate. Bone in effect shields some part of the body against easy access by ultrasound.

Scattering

Another component of attenuation is scattering. This type of scatter is also known as nonspecular reflection and responsible for providing the internal texture of organ in the image. The scattering occurs because the interfaces are smaller than diameter of sound beam.

For long wavelength sound waves, the tissue boundary may appear smooth. For shorter wave length bumpy feature at tissue interface are more pronounced. This bumpy surface provides a multiple of nonperpendicular surface from which reflection occurs in all different direction causing a loss of intensity.

A specular reflector represents an expensive smooth boundary relative to wavelength of incident beam while a nonspecular reflector represents a bumpy surface.

CHAPTER 4

Transducer

Ultrasound is generated by the part of ultrasound instrument known as the transducer.

In general term, a transducer is anything that converts one form of energy into another form.

In case of diagnostic ultrasound the transducer converts electric energy to mechanical sonic energy and vice versa.

TRANSDUCER CONSTRUCTION

The schematic diagram of an ultrasound transducer is shown in **Figure 4.1**.

The most important component is a thin (0.5 mm approximately) piezoelectric crystal element located near the face of transducer. The front and back face of crystal are coated with a thin conducting film to ensure good contact with two electrodes that will supply electric field to excite the crystal or produce deformity in crystal.

The surfaces of crystals are placed with gold or silver electrodes. The outside electrode is grounded to protect the patient from electric shock and its outer surface is coated with water tight electrical insulator.

The baking material occupies the space immediately behind the crystal. The purpose is to dampen or absorb sound wave that is in backward direction.

Since transducer is sensitive to strong electromagnetic interference, which contributes to noise level. High noise levels prohibit the detection of weak echoes. To reduce the electromagnetic interference, a radiofrequency shield composed of hollow metallic cylinder is placed around the crystal and baking material. The radiofrequency shield is electronically grounded to the front surface of electrode surface.

An acoustic insulator of a rubber or cork coats the inner surface of radiofrequency shield to prevent sound beam passing into the housing and to prevent reverberation. Some transducers have a facing material which lies in front of the crystal and comes in contact with the patient. This is called quarter wave matching layer. This form of special transducer design allows increased efficiency in coupling the ultrasonic energy to the patient which provide improved propagation of sound into the patients and increased sensations to returning echo.

Electric signals are transmitted through a connector on the back of the transducer to each face of the piezoelectric crystal. The connector couples the transducer to scanner arm.

GENERATION AND DETECTION OF ULTRASOUND

Piezoelectric crystal construction of such device relies on a phenomenon first studied by Pierre and Marie Curie before the turn of century and known as piezoelectric effect. The effect is found in certain crystalline materials that have dipole on each molecule. These dipolar molecules are having positive at one end and negative at other end as shown in **Figure 4.2**.

In normal crystalline lattice structure these dipole cannot migrate and they are randomly oriented (**Fig. 4.3**).

When the material is heated above a temperature called the Curie temperature, the dipolar molecules are released to move freely. Now when a pair of charged plate placed across the material heated above Curie temperature the negative region of each molecules align towards positive plate and the positive region of each molecules points towards negative plate.

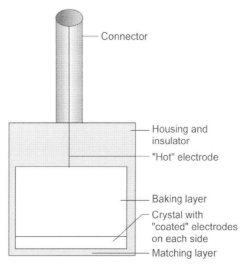

Fig. 4.1: Diagram of unfocused transducer construction.

If the material is then cooled down below Curie temperature while the charged plates are still applied, the molecules will maintain this orientation **(Fig. 4.4)**.

Since the material is cooled down below the Curie temperature the aligned charge plates are removed with at altering the configuration of the dipole.

This molecular arrangement of the dipolar molecules gives the piezoelectric material a unique property. Now the conducting plates are placed on the opposite face of crystal. Which are located on the crystal faces adjacent to positions the original alignment electrode **(Fig. 4.5)**.

Figure 4.6 is showing normal thickness of crystal with no application of electric field. When voltage is applied to the conducting plates, the molecules twist to align with the electric field thereby thickening the crystal **(Fig. 4.7)**. If polarity is

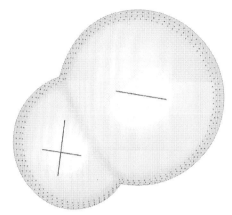

Fig. 4.2: Molecular dipole showing regions of net positive and negative charge on the molecule.

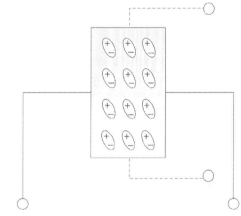

Fig. 4.5: Excitation of electrodes on the crystal—placement of excitation electrodes following removal of alignment of electrodes.

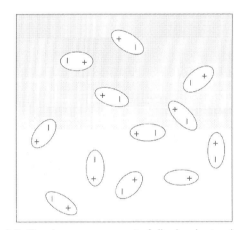

Fig. 4.3: Random arrangement of dipoles (natural state).

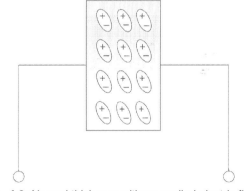

Fig. 4.6: Normal thickness with no applied electric field.

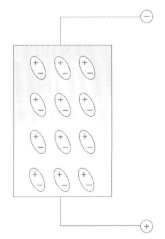

Fig. 4.4: Alignment of electrodes on the crystal. Alignment of dipoles with an externally applied electric field.

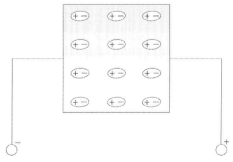

Fig. 4.7: Expansion of crystal caused by movement of dipoles trying to align with the applied electric field. The polarity is reversed from that depicted in Figure 4.6.

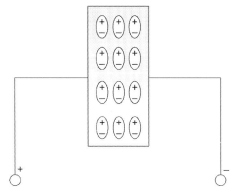

Fig. 4.8: Crystal response to voltage applied across the excitation electrodes—contraction of crystal caused by movement of dipoles trying to align with applied electric field.

removed on the plate then molecules turn back in opposite direction creating a decrease in thickness of crystal **(Fig. 4.8)**. The illustration shows a considerable change in thickness for clarity but change in thickness is actually a few microns.

This frequent reviving of electric field causes expansion and contraction of the crystal which create mechanical vibration.

By placing expanding and contracting crystal on the body. Ultrasound waves are generated and passed into the body.

The converse of piezoelectric effect allows an ultrasonic beam to be generated by transducer if the applied electric field is of appropriate frequency. The baking block dampen the vibration to unable the transducer for its other function which is to detect returning echo.

Piezoelectric effect enables the same transducer to receive an ultrasound waves returning from interaction with tissue interfaces in the body that strikes the crystal causing a physical compression of crystal element. This compression forces the tiny dipoles to change their orientation which induces a voltage between electrodes. These are signal that are processed and ultimately displayed.

MATERIAL

Piezoelectric materials are both naturally occurring and man made. An example of natural piezoelectric crystal is quartz crystal. Ultrasound application use a man made piezoelectric element such as ceramic crystal component piezoelectric having mixture of lead zirconate titanate (PZT)* and epoxy.

The advantage of PZT is that they can be shaped into any configuration like rectangular planer or concave. But disadvantage is that they are brittle and may be damaged if dropped or if heated above Curie temperature (328–365°C). Composite crystals have advantage over PZT crystal as they have lower acoustic impedance to that of tissue. They have a broad band width so that transducer can operate at different frequency. They appear to be more sensitive than that of static PZT.

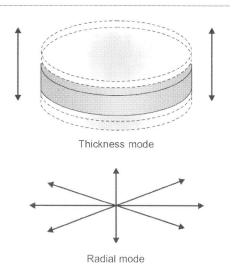

Fig. 4.9: Modes of vibration of a piezoelectric crystal.

Piezoelectric crystals are designed to vibrate in thickness mode or radial mode **(Fig. 4.9)**. Medical crystals are designed to vibrate in a less or extents in the radial mode.

Frequency

The frequency of a transducer is determined by the mechanical properties and shape of the crystal. Transducer frequency for medical imaging typically range from 2 MHz to 10 MHz with 2, 3, 5, 7.5 and 10 MHz frequency being most common.

A transducer is designed to be maximally sensitive to contain natural frequency. The thickness of a piezoelectric crystal determines its natural frequency called its resonant frequency.

The natural frequency is the one that produces internal wavelength than are twice the thickness of the crystal.

The crystal is designed so that its thickness is equal to exactly half the wavelength of ultrasound to be produced by the transducer. The crystal is made to resonate at the frequency determined by its thickness.

The frequency that corresponds half of wave length is called fundamental resonant frequency of transducer. For example 5 MHz piezoelectric crystal will have a thickness of 0.4 mm thickness by applying the formula

$$\lambda = V_s / \nu$$

where V_s is velocity of sound in PZT which is 4000 m/sec
ν = frequency in cycle/sec.

Hence, for higher frequencies the crystal thickness is smaller. Reason of being thickness of crystal half of wavelength of sound waves is that ultrasound waves originates in crystal produces wave that is transmitted back and forth without destructive interference.

To illustrate this consider a crystal suspended in air is struck with a voltage pulse, ultrasound wave are generated multiple wave front are formed; forward from the front face, backward into the crystal from face, and directed into crystal

---

*PZT is a registered trade name of PZT material from the Clevite Corporation

from back face and away from the crystal originating at the back face (**Figs. 4.10A to C**).

These waves undergo constructive and destructive interference within the crystal, depending on the crystal thickness. The ultrasound moves from one face of crystal to other, undergoing reflection between the two crystalline surfaces. The crystal has a natural vibration frequency that is related to the distance between these two surfaces. To have a constructive interference so that a single wave moves back and forth across the crystal, the distance from one surface to the other must be equal to half of wavelength.

A crystal can be forced to vibrate at frequency of any alternating voltage but intensity of this sound will be much less than it would be for a comparable voltage of the crystal at natural frequency.

In medical ultrasound the transducer is driven at natural frequency. A special circuitry is used to generate an oscillating voltage of PZT wave form that is applied to electrodes frequency of which must match on the natural frequency of crystal.

To change the frequency of ultrasound requires change of itself.

BAKING LAYER AND Q FACTOR OF TRANSDUCER

In diagnostic ultrasound the transducer sends out a short burst of ultrasound (preferable 2–3 points) followed by a period of silence in order to listen for returning echo before another burst of ultrasound is sent. This is called pulse echo system (**Fig. 4.11**).

The baking material in this case should absorb the backward directed ultrasound energy and eliminate any echo that could potentially return to the transducer from the housing assembly.

The baking material also serves as a damping device to restrict the time of vibration and keep the ultrasound pulse short.

Spatial Pulse Length (SPL)
– No. of cycles in the pulse wavelength
SPL = λn
Where n = no. of cycles in pulse.

Assume that a 3 MHz transducer produces a pulse that is 3 cycles in duration. Then:

$$\lambda = \frac{V_S}{\nu} = \frac{1540 \text{ m/sec}}{3 \times 10^6 \text{ c/sec}}$$

λ = 0.513 mm
since n = 3
SPL = λn = (0.513 mm) (3) = 1.54 mm.

SPL influences the scanner's ability to depict spatial details. Axial resolution is the ability to differentiate as separate image of two objects that are placed very close to one another along the direction of propagation. To improve the axial resolution a pulse of short duration is desirable or spatial pulse length should be shorter. To do this, number of cycles must be reduced or frequency must be increased.

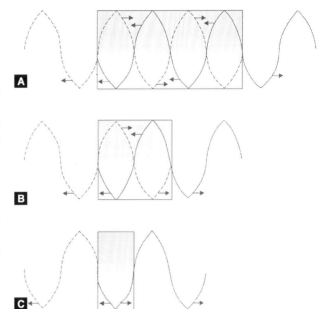

Figs. 4.10A to C: Determination of crystal thickness using superposition of waves. Waves generated at the back of the crystal (—). Waves generated from the front of the crystal (—). Arrows indicate direction of wave motion. (A) Crystal thickness greater than one wavelength produces destructive interference if the thickness is not an odd integer multiple of one half wavelength; (B) Complete destructive interference occurs when the crystal thickness is equal to one wavelength; (C) Complete constructive interference occurs when the crystal thickness is equal to one half wavelength or odd multiples one half wavelength.

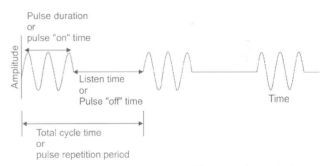

Fig. 4.11: Pulsed wave output used for scanning technique that required depth in formation.

A baking layer is incorporated to quench the vibration and to shorten the sonic pulse. The ideal baking layer should direct maximum energy from crystal to baking layer. Baking blocks generally made up of combination of tungsten with rubber powder in epoxy resin. The ratio of tungsten to epoxy resin is chosen to satisfy the impedance requirement and rubber powder is used to increase the attenuation of sound in baking block.

Q Factor

Theoretically, when the crystal is excited by electric pulse, it would vibrate at only one particular frequency. However, imperfections in manufacturing process of crystal and effect from damping the vibration of crystal no longer emit only one frequency but produce a frequency spectrum.

The range of frequencies emitted by transducer is called bandwidth. The bandwidth of transducer influences the imaging channel elements. Most transducers have wide bandwidth.

Bandwidth is related with Q factor as

Q factor = Center frequency to bandwidth.

Q factor refers to the purity of sound and length of time for which the sound persists.

High Q crystal produce a heavy pure sound made of narrow range of frequency (small bandwidth) and therefore will be more efficient transducer.

Whereas low Q transducer produces wide range of frequencies (wide bandwidth) and will be more efficient receiver. Ring down is used often as synchronous term describe the damping of crystal vibration.

Ring Down Time

It is the interval of time between initiation of wave and complete cessation of vibrations. Imaging application using pulsed ultrasound require a low Q transducer for good axial resolution since the length of ultrasound beam is equal to number of cycles of vibration.

In **Figures 4.12A and B** an example of a high Q and low Q ultrasound pulse demonstrate the relationship to SPL. This Q factor can be controlled by altering the characteristics of baking block of transducer.

Matching Layer (Quarter Wave Matching)

The matching layer optimizes the transmission of sound energy into the patients by providing a medium that is intermediate in acoustic properties to that of a piezoelectric crystal and the tissue of the patients.

Actually the acoustic impedance of transducer to the object scanner is an important factor that affects the sensitivity.

The sensitivity is the ability of ultrasound system to distinguish small objects with nearly the same acoustic properties at specific location in the medium.

The matching layer between crystal and tissue partially eliminate the acoustic impedance mismatching between crystal and tissue.

The mineral oil between the transducer and patients' skin is an effective way of transmitting maximum energy from transducer to the patient. Matching layer should have suitable thickness and characteristic impedance.

Thickness of matching layer should have one forth the wavelength of sound in matching layers. In addition the impedance of matching must be about mean of impedance on each side of layers **(Fig. 4.13A)**.

$$Z \text{ matching layer} = \sqrt{Z \text{ crystal} \times Z_S \text{ of tissue}}$$

For example, impedance of about 6.8×10^6 kg/m^2/sec is required for the matching layer between PZT ~ 4 (2 = 3 × 10^7 kg/m^2/sec) and water (2 = 1.54 × 10^6 kg/m2/sec). Such layer could be manufactured using a mixture of aluminium powder and epoxy resin. Additional improvement in performance can be achieved by using multiple matching layers on the faces of transducer **(Fig. 4.13B)**.

The multiple matching layers alter the frequency distribution towards a broader bandwidth. Increased bandwidth enhances the sensitivity of transducer which results in improved image quality. The axial resolution is enhanced because the larger bandwidth normally means a shorter spatial pulse length.

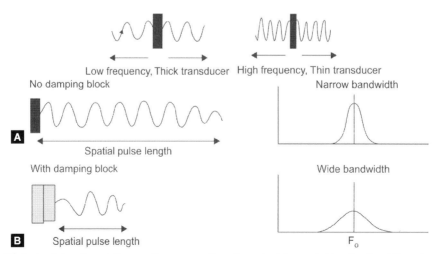

Figs. 4.12A and B: (A) A short duration voltage spike causes the piezoelectric crystal to vibrate at its natural frequency f_o which is determined by the thickness of the transducer equal to ½ l; (B) Effect of damping block on the frequency spectrum. Without a damping block, the crystal vibrates over a large number of cycles, resulting in a large spatial pulse length with a narrow bandwidth and high Q factor. To achieve a short spatial pulse length, a damping block limits the number of vibration cycles and increases the frequency bandwidth of the pulse, an adjunct in a low Q factor.

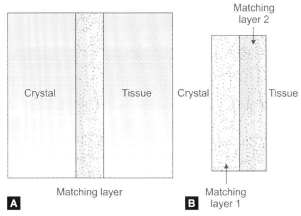

Figs. 4.13A and B: (A) Matching layer (facing material) between crystal and tissue. The objective is to reduce the depth between crystal tissues; (B) Multiple matching layers between crystal and tissue. The objective is to transfer nearly 100 percent of the generated acoustic signal into tissue, that is, minimize the impedance mismatch between crystal and tissue.

Characteristics of an Ultrasound Beam

The major factors that limits the ultrasound imaging is the blurring associated with the diameter which is also width of ultrasound beam. This is an important characteristic of an ultrasound pulse. A second major factor is the number of line of sight per field of view.

Let us talk about characteristic of beam. The diameter of pulse layers as it moves along the beam path. Now let us see how pulse dimension affects an image detail.

Lateral Resolution

Lateral resolution describes the ability to resolve two objects adjacent to each other that is perpendicular to the beam axis.

It also describes the ability of ultrasound beam to detect single small object across the width of beam.

Lateral resolution is determined by the diameter of ultrasound pulse or beamwidth, at the time it interacts with the object creating the echo. Decreasing the beamwidth improve lateral resolution by allowing object close together to be resolved and by providing a more accurate presentation of small objects.

A single object smaller than the beamwidth produces an image the entire time it is with the beam. A small beamwidth enables small object to become distinguishable.

The width of ultrasound beam is determined by characteristic of transducer such as size of element and focusing. We will see later how these facts affect the beamwidth.

Axial Resolution

It is defined as the ability of the system to distinguish as separate image of two objects that are close to each other along the direction of beam. This is determined by length of ultrasound pulse. This is in turn determined by characteristic of the transducer, primarily the frequency and damping.

Best possible axial resolution is the spatial pulse length divided by 2. Since SPL is inversely related to frequency. High frequency having short SPL produces less blurring along the axis of ultrasound beam. But as frequency is increased absorption of ultrasound also increases and therefore selection of frequency for a specific clinical situation is compromised between image detail and depth.

Axial resolution can also be explained in other way, i.e., when the distance between two objects is short compared to SPL the object will be blurred together and not resolved or imaged as a separate object.

About damping characters of sound a low Q has a broad bandwidth and has low SPL. Therefore, short low Q transducer (easily damped) will have better axial resolution. A high Q transducer has a long pulse length and a narrow bandwidth produce low axial resolution. Focusing of transducer create a region of high intensity and this greater sensitivity within focal zone. This process of focusing the beam actually lengthens the pulse, thereby deteriorating the axial resolution. This effect is normally limited.

To Summarize

Axial resolution depends on:
- SPL
- Frequency of transducer
- Q factor (damping character)

Lateral resolution depends on:
- Beamwidth, frequency of beam which is turn depends on depth or size of crystal and focusing of ultrasound beam.

Transducer Focusing

Transducer can be designed to produce either an unfocused transducer or focused beam as shown in Figures 4.14A and B.

A focused beam is desirable for most imaging application because it produces pulse of small diameter which in turn gives better visibility of details in the image. The best details will be obtained for structures within focal zone. The distance between the transducer and focal zone is focal length. We will see about focused transducer in details in later section of this chapter.

Unfocused Transducer

An unfocused transducer produce a beam with two distinct region as shown in **Figures 4.14 and 4.15** one is called near field or Freshnel zone and other is far field or Fraunhofer zone.

In near field ultrasound pulse maintain a relatively constant diameter that can be used for imaging.

In near field beam has constant diameter that is determined by diameter of transducer.

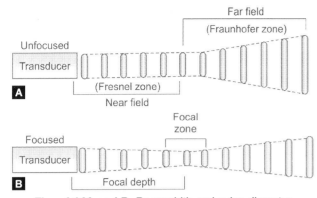

Figs. 4.14A and B: Beamwidth and pulse diameter characteristics of both unfocused and focused transducers.

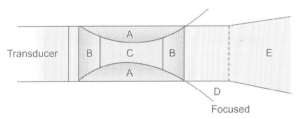

Fig. 4.15: Lateral resolution for focused versus nonfocused transducer. A. Near field of nonfocused transducer. B, C. Regions of better lateral resolution for focused transducer, in which C is the focal zone or narrowest area. D. Diverging "far field" of focused transducer with rapidly deteriorating lateral resolution. E. Far field for nonfocused transducer indicating area of better lateral resolution compared to the focused transducer.

The length of near field is related to the diameter D, of the transducer and the wavelength λ of ultrasound by

Near field length (NFL) = $\dfrac{D^2}{4\lambda}$.

Hence, for a given transducer size length of near field is proportional to frequency.

Another characteristic of the near field is that the intensity along the beam axis is not constant. It oscillates between maximum and zero several times, between the transducer surface and the boundary, between the near and far field. This is because of interference pattern created by sound waves from transducer surface.

Lateral resolution is best at the end of near field and therefore strongly dependent on depth. Axial resolution is independent of depth.

Far Field

The far field also known a Fraunhofer zone is characterized by diverging, conical shaped ultrasound beam of diminishing intensity.

Lateral resolution decreases rapidly in the depth as beam begin to diverge in far field.

The angle of divergence for the far field is calculated by

Diverging angle (degree) = $\dfrac{70\lambda}{D}$.

Hence, divergence is decreased by increasing frequency. The major advantage of high frequency is that the beam is less divergent and generally produces less blurring and better details.

Focusing

Lateral resolution can be increased by focusing the transducer crystal **(Fig. 4.15)**. Focusing limit is useful near field depth because beam diverges rapidly beyond the focal zone.

Focal zone is defined as that region in which intensity corresponds to within 3 dB of the maximum intensity along the transducer axis.

Focal zone is closer to the focal transducer than nonfocused near field depth assuming that the transducers are of equal diameter and frequency.

Axial resolution may be somewhat worse for focused beam as explained earlier. Transducer can be focused in two ways with either a curved piezoelectric crystal or with an acoustic lens **(Fig. 4.16)**.

The most common form of focusing for transducer with frequencies of less than 5 MHz is that of using a curved crystal **(Fig. 4.17)** or with an internal focusing method **(Fig. 4.18)**.

For frequencies above 5 MHz, the external focusing methods are normally used because crystal becomes extremely thin. Thin crystals are difficult to form into curved

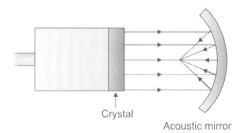

Fig. 4.16: Acoustic mirror.

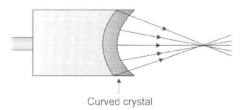

Fig. 4.17: Focusing transducer—curved crystal.

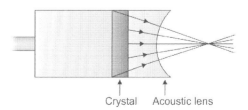

Fig. 4.18: Acoustic lens.

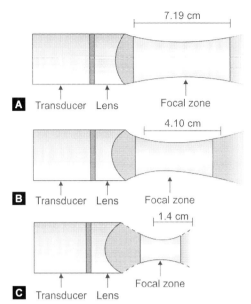

Figs. 4.19A to C: Strength of focusing—the beamwidth decreases. The focal zone moves closed to the face of transducer and intensity increases in the focal zone. FS in the focusing is made stronger (A) weak or long focusing (B) medium focusing (C) strong or short focusing.

shapes of proper uniformity and thickness without breaking them **(Fig. 4.18)**.

Lens material are usually polystyrene or an epoxy resin propagate sound at a greater velocity than body that tissues so the sound is refracted or bent towards a point in space.

Knowing the radius of curvature of the lens and velocity of the sound in lens material and body tissue, the exact focal point can be calculated. A close approximation of focal length is the diameter of curvature of lens.

Real-time ultrasound scanning systems employ electronic focusing method. The distance from front face of transducers to the focal point is called focal length F.

The degree of focusing can be changed to vary focal length by increasing in the radius of curvature of crystal or lens **(Figs. 4.19A to C)**.

This allows transducer with same frequency to be made with focal zone at different depth depending on the degree of focusing. The focal zone for weak focus (long focus transducer) is 7–19 cm. Medium focused transducer have a focal zone of 4–10 cm and strong focused transducer (Short focus transducer) have a focal zone of 1–4 cm. As the degree of focusing became stronger, beamwidth is made narrower but the focal zone is drawn closer to the face of transducer.

CHAPTER 5

Basic Ultrasound Instrumentation

Understanding ultrasound image requires knowledge of sound propagation, production, and interaction characteristics as explained in earlier chapter.

Images are created using pulse echo mode format of ultrasound production and detection. A number of basic components comprise the ultrasound system; the pulse generator, transducer, amplifier, scan converter, image memory, image display, recording system, and control panel **(Figs. 5.1A and B)**.

In medical diagnostic ultrasound the primary interest is the detection of the reflected echoes (specular and nonspecular) from various interfaces in the body.

There are three basic requirements: generation of ultrasound beam, reception, and amplification of returning echo and finally processing of signal for display. All types of ultrasound securing equipment have same basic features.

Changes in the reception and the processing analysis and display of returning echo signals differentiate one scanning mode from another.

Any discussion of ultrasound instrumentation must include the basic a mode scanner from which all other scanning systems are derived by incorporating various modification.

We would like to go into this step by step as mentioned earlier.

GENERATION OF ULTRASOUND BEAM

The first requirement of an ultrasound scanner is that a sound wave at ultrasonic frequencies must be generated.

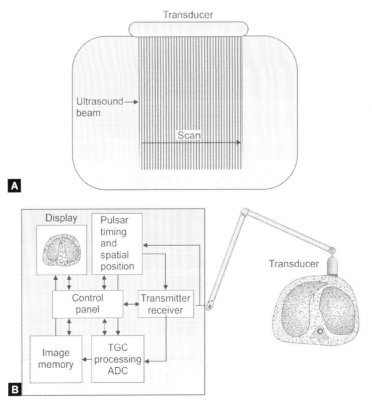

Figs. 5.1A and B: The basic components of a diagnostic ultrasound imaging system.

The primary objectives are to produce unidirectional beam, a beam of uniform intensity, and a beam of limited dimension so that a good spatial resolution is obtained.

The transducer assembly transmits a pulse ultrasonic beam into the patient's body. The beam undergoes various interactions and when interface is encountered a fraction of ultrasonic beam is reflected back towards the transducer. The transducer acting as a receiver mode, then a transmitter connects the ultrasound wave (returning echo) to an electronic signal that is processed and displayed.

Reception and Amplification

In pulse echo mode of transducer operation, a brief pulse of ultrasound is created by an extremely short 1–2 μ sec voltage spike applied to electrode of transducer crystal element. The ultrasound pulse that is generated by the transducer is typically 2–3 cycles long. After the ring down time where vibration of crystal has stopped, transducer is detecting returning echoes over a period of time up to 1000 μ sec. As the ultrasound waves strikes various interfaces in the body, some of the energy is transmitted and some is reflected in accordance with the reflective formula. The reflective echo returns toward the transducer. These pressure waves strikes the crystal and induce a radiofrequency signal via the piezoelectric effect **(Fig. 5.2)**. The microvolt or millivolt radiofrequency signal is amplified to 1–10 volt for display purpose. Combination of linear, exponential and variable amplification can be used.

One of the problems that must be considered is the attenuation of the ultrasonic beam with depth. Equally reflective interface produce different signal levels depending on their relative distance from transducer. It is often advantageous to display reflectors of similar size, shape and equal reflection coefficient with equal signal strength or brightness levels. Exponential amplification is used to correct the signal for attenuation known as time gain compensation.

Assume that a phantom is composed of alternating layer of water and gelatin **(Fig. 5.3)** that are very similar in acoustic impedance. Each layer is 1 cm thick. A small fraction of incident beam is reflected at each interface in the phantom. Because of attenuation these displays show exponentially decreasing peaks **(Fig. 5.4A)** rather than peak of equal amplitude. To compensate for this attenuation time gain compensation (TGC), depth gain compensation or swept gain control is used to increase the signal in the time or depth **(Fig. 5.4B)**.

Greater the depth of the signal, greater is the degree of amplification.

The amplification could be a reverse exponential function because the signal decreases exponentially **(Fig. 5.4C)**. If the liver is scanned with TGC, then all

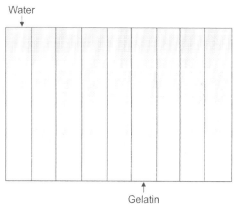

Fig. 5.3: Phantom composed of alternating layers of equal thick water and gelatin.

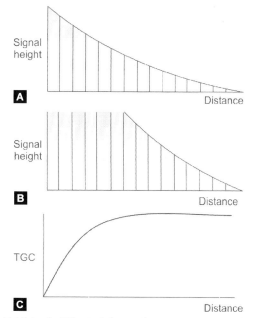

Figs. 5.4A to C: Effect of time gain compensation. (A) Signal amplitude versus depth without TGC; (B) Signal amplitude versus depth with TGC; (C) Reverse exponential TGC used to obtain signal levels in (B).

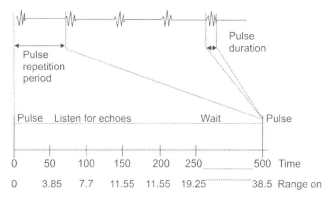

Fig. 5.2: The pulse-echo timing of data acquisition depicts the initial pulse occurring in a very short span (the pulse duration) and the remained of the time listening for echoes before the next pulse (the pulse repetition period).

echoes should be nearly of the same amplitude unless an abnormality is present or vessels are observed. Different tissues have varying rates of attenuation. Also, the frequency response of the attenuation rate depends on the tissue type. Most diagnostic ultrasound unit includes a combination of TGC controls **(Fig. 5.5A)**. The near gain or mean gain adjust the level at which the initial signal is amplified. The delay regulates the depth at which the TGC begins. The slope of TGC indicates the amount of compensation that is applied with depth. Some ultrasound units have a completely variable gain control, permitting a particular area of interest to be enhanced beyond that provided by TGC. The far gain represents the maximum amount that signal can be amplified. In this zone signals are amplified by constant amount but they exhibit an exponential decrease because of attenuation **(Fig. 5.5B)**.

The variable TGC control permits adjustable compensation for different frequency transducer allowing greater amplification when high frequencies are used. The sonographer must be more aware of the function of different controls.

A scan in with selectable TGC control can produce poor quality images when operated by an inexperienced individual. Automation of the TGC control provides more consistent image, but they are often poorer in over all quality.

SIGNAL PROCESSING

The radiofrequency (RF) signal induced in the transducer by returning echoes could be amplified and then displayed but it would appears to be similar to the acoustic pulse sent out **(Figs. 5.6A and B)**. If numerous interfaces are present the interpretation of the received signal become very confusing. For viewing ease, the goal is to process the signal before displaying it. The processing lowers the information content but at the same time, facilitate the association of final output with physical structure. The normal processing procedure involves rectification after the signal has been amplified and has gone TGC amplification **(Figs. 5.7A and B)**.

Alternatively, the negative components of RF can be eliminated rather than rectified. The peaks of the RF waves are electronically surrounded resulting in a video signal that could be further amplified for display purposes **(Figs. 5.8A to C)**.

Enveloping is often referred to as demodulation in diagnostic ultrasound and is generally accomplished by signal through a circuit with a slow time response. The overall outline of the pulse is retained but internal fast oscillations are lost.

Usually the areas under the video signal are electronically measured. Determination of the area is called integration. This area is then represented as a spike for A mode scanning or a dot for other scanning technique **(Figs. 5.9A and B)**.

An increase in the amplitude of induced RF signal results in a larger area under the curve and therefore increase in height of the spikes or brightness of the dot.

A reject control may be added that permit elimination of peaks below (or above) a certain level **(Figs. 5.10)**.

Most ultrasound units also include the output or gain control. This normally adjusts the voltage spikes to the transducer to produce an acoustic pulse or higher intensity,

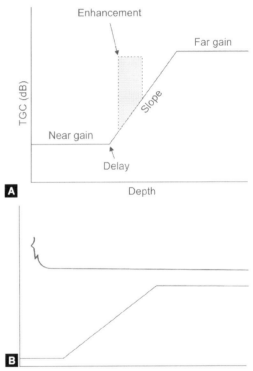

Figs. 5.5A and B: Time gain compensation. (A) Possible control adjustments for TGC; (B) Instrument display of TGC slope with no enhancement (upper curve).

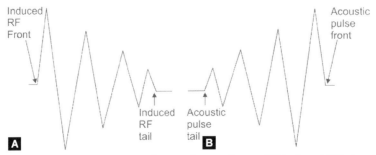

Figs. 5.6A and B: Comparison of radiofrequency and acoustic waveforms. (A) Induced RF signal in crystal; (B) Acoustic wave.

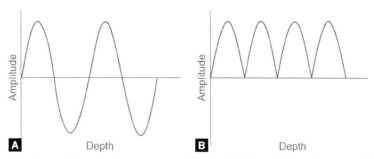

Figs. 5.7A and B: Rectification: (A) Incident sound wave induces RF signal in receiver circuit from crystal response; (B) Rectified signal in which the negative components are flipped to become positive.

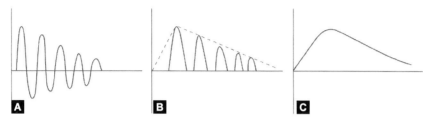

Figs. 5.8A to C: (A) Induced RF; (B) Enveloping—electronic surrounding of peaks; (C) Resultant video signals.

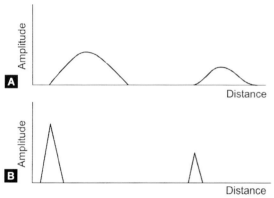

Figs. 5.9A and B: Integration: (A) video-signals; (B) area under video-signals represented as spikes.

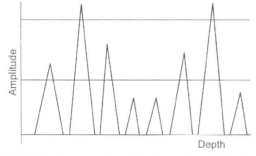

Fig. 5.10: Reject processing. The three signals in the range between the lower level and upper level (shaded area) are processed and ultimately displayed, the others are discarded and are not displayed.

resulting in the reception of a stronger echo. Frequently the control is adjustable in 3dB (50%) in increment.

Higher the intensity levels increases the exposure to the patients.

Some gains control only, adjusts the amplification of recorded signal, and have no effect on the intensity of generated ultrasound beam.

Intensity and control are also available on the display device to manipulate the presentation of scan data. The dynamic range which is a measure of range of signal amplitude that can be identified and can be handled by various components of ultrasound system needs to be considered **(Fig. 5.11)**. Echo amplitude may be as much as 100 dB to 150 dB below the original intensity sent into the body depending on the depth and frequency of transducer.

TGC and amplification process reduce the dynamic range to about 80 dB. Depending on the processing method and storage system the dynamic range may be reduced to 20–40 dB. The recording device reduces the useful range even further to 10 to 20 dB.

DISPLAY

A cathode ray tube (CRT) is the simple output device used for display purposes **(Fig. 5.12)**. For simplest scanning system, a voltage on the X deflection plates of CRT moves the time base sweep across the display at a constant rate. The rate of the movement of time base sweep must correlate with the speed of ultrasound in tissue. The electron beam must advance the equivalent of 1 cm on the distance scanner every 13 μ sec. The beginning of the sweep is initiated by a pulse from master synchronizer. As the electron beam sweep across the display the signal detected for each interface is amplified and sent to the deflection plate of CRT to control the position of electron beam in the vertical direction on the screen. Because the time duration of induced signal is short, the voltage on Y plate return to zero and electron beam moves back to the baseline **(Fig. 5.13)**. The electron beam is again

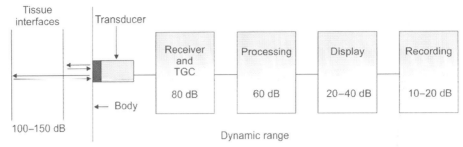

Fig. 5.11: Dynamic range associated with the various components of the ultrasonic system.

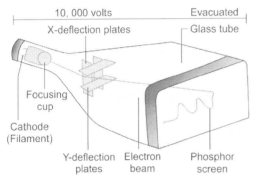

Fig. 5.12: Diagram of the principle components of a cathode ray tube.

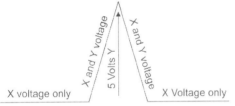

Fig. 5.13: Trace of a single interface, when X voltage corresponds to the time base sweep (1 cm every 13 ms) and the Y voltage is constant except when an interface is encountered.

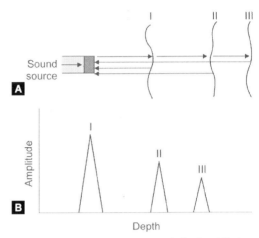

Figs. 5.14A and B: A mode scan and display (A) A mode of three interfaces (I, II, III); (B) Corresponding A mode display of the three interfaces.

deflected in the vertical direction when the next interface is encountered and sent to the display system.

This occurs for each line of sight, which defines the direction of sampling.

As long as the transducer is directed along the same line of sight, the display signal remains unchanged because the scan is repeated many times each second. The sampling rate is equal to PRF. If the transducer is positioned towards a new line of sight the scan once again is displayed at the rate of PRF.

Static Imaging—Principles of Instrumentation

Ultrasonic information received by the transducer crystal and converted into an electric signal can be displayed on ultrasound instruments in a variety of ways. The information is displayed on a screen on the instrument, usually a storage CRT.

Different types of medical imaging equipment have different types of display and types of display will vary from manufacture to manufactures.

Each mode of display has a different appearance and different clinical application.

Mode Display System

Mode scanning refers to amplitude mode scanning. This technique is based on echo ranging principle. The term amplitude in this case refers to the strengths of detected echo signal. This mode displays the magnitude of the signal as a spike in one dimension versus depth or time of signal in other dimension.

An increase in the strength of signal gives rise to an increase in the height of the spikes. **Figures 5.14A and B** show three different interfaces as three separate spikes. Interface I generate a larger signal than does either interface II or interface III. This variation in signal strength is the result of percentage of reflection from the different interface and the attenuation of the beam as the ultrasound wave travels to and from the respective interfaces. Strong reflector far away from the transducer may produce greater amplitude signal than weak reflectors located nearer to the transducer.

A mode displays now seldom used except where very accurate length measurement are required for example in

CHAPTER 5: Basic Ultrasound Instrumentation

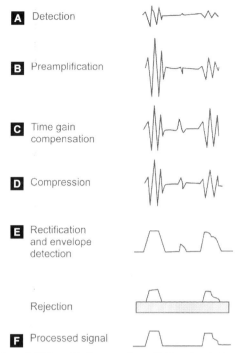

Figs. 5.15A to F: Processing of US pulse in body.

echo encephalography for detection of mid line shift and for localization of foreign bodies in the eye or measuring the length of the globe of the eye. There is a type of A-mode biopsy transducer that is useful for directing the needle puncture of cystic masses.

This transducer has a hole with cutter through which needle can be directed into the body to a specific depth as determined from the A-mode scan. Some ultrasonographers like to use the A-mode information to help characterize the internal structure of the organ or masses.

Image acquisition and processing of the A mode data in modern ultrasound instrument occur in following major step.
1. *The clock:* In A mode scanning, the master synchronizer initiates the scanning process by commanding the transmitter to send a voltage pulse to the transducer. In its simplest form, this is an oscillator produces a series of brief pulse with a PRF of approximately (1–5 kHz).
2. *Transmitter:* Upon receipt of timing pulses from clock the transmitter generates a very brief electric pulse. This pulse is passed to the transducer where crystal is excited and generates ultrasound wave frequency which is determined by the physical characteristic of transducer.

This US pulse generated by the transducer is typically 2–3 cycles long. These ultrasound pulses are sent to patient body. After a ring down time when vibration of crystal has stopped transducer in detecting returning echo over a period of time up to 1000 μ sec. Coincidence master synchronizers also send a command to receiver to activate the clock to measure the elapsed time from transmission of ultrasound pulse to the reception of echo. This term determines the depth of interface from the face of the transducer assuring a velocity of 1540 m/sec when the transducer and receiver are initiated, the master synchronizer send a command to display to begin moving electron beam across the screen of CRT. The sweep rate corresponds to 1 cm every 13 μ sec.

As ultrasonic pulse progress away from transducers the part of energy is reflected at each interface encountered along the beam path.
3. *Detection:* As echo strikes the transducer causes the mechanical deformation of piezoelectric crystal and is converted to a radiofrequency electronic signal as shown in **Figure 5.15A**.
4. *Preamplification:* Preamplification of electronic signal into a more useful range of voltages is necessary to appropriate signal processing **(Fig. 5.15B)**.
5. *Time grain compensation:* The echoes returning from beep within a patient are much weaker than those from more superficial structures. This is due to attenuation of the ultrasound pulse and echoes within the patient and if no action was taken to compensate for this, the echoes from distant structures would be so feeble as to be undetectable within the ultrasound image.

Hence, time gain compensation (TGC) compensates for the attenuation of the ultrasound with time (travel distance). TGC (also known by TVG-Time varied gain) is a user adjustable amplification that can be changed to meet the needs of the specific application. The ideal TGC curve makes all equally reflective boundaries equal in signal amplitude regardless of the depth of the boundary **(Fig. 5.15C)**. TGC wave works by increasing the amplification factor of the signal as a function of time. Variations in amplitude are thus indicative of the acoustic impedance. Differences between tissue boundaries are very important criteria for images.
6. *Compression:* Compressing of the time compensated signal is accomplished using logarithmic amplification to reduce large dynamic range of echo amplitude. Small signals are made larger and larger signal are made smaller.

This step provides a convenient scale for display of amplitude variation on the limited gray scale range of the monitor **(Fig. 5.15D)**.
7. *Rectification, demodulation, and envelop detecting:* First of all RF signals are rectified as shown in **Figure 5.15E**. Then RF signal is eliminated leaving only envelope.

This permits sampling and digitalization of echo amplitude free of variation induced by sinusoidal nature of wave form.
8. *Rejection:* Rejection level adjust the threshold of signal amplitudes that are allowed to pass to digitalization

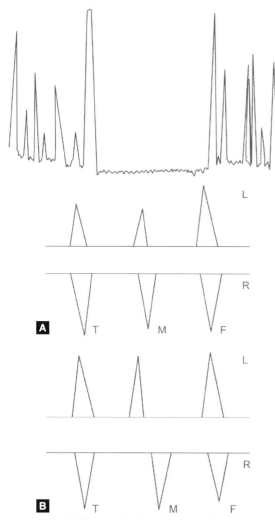

Figs. 5.16A and B: The display in A mode.

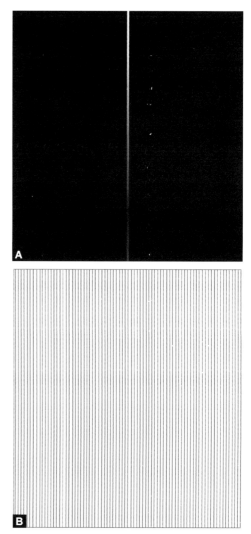

Figs. 5.17A and B: B mode display.

and display system (**Fig. 5.15F**). This removes a significant amount of undesirable low level noise generated from scatter sound or electronic.

9. *Video amplifier:* Prior to display the demodulated signal is increased in strength by a straight forward low frequency video amplifier.

10. *Display:* In the simplest of A mode machine the display takes the form of an X-Y oscilloscope. The timing signal is fed to the oscilloscope X plate and amplitude information to Y plate of CRT. The resultant display is shown in **Figures 5.16A and B**. The distance between the structures giving rise to echoes seen in the display can be measured with greatest accuracy by reference to distance makers on the X axis.

A-mode data acquisition methods are intrinsic to all other modes used in diagnostic ultrasound.

M MODE (MOTION MODE)

M mode is very similar to the A mode display except that its brightness modulated and X-axis is moved up or down the display screen during examination.

The remainder of the major components of dedicated M mode system are the same as those for an A mode system. Dedicated M modes are now essentially obsolete. Their main use was exclusively in echocardiography but this area of diagnostic ultrasound now invariably also incorporates real time B mode imaging and Doppler. Dedicated echocardiography scanners normally incorporate M mode, B mode, and Doppler facilities within a single machine. The display system of a dedicated M mode scanner is normally a simple X-Y oscilloscope very similar to that used in A mode system. The display is however brightness modulated and X axis information is swept vertically upon the screen to produce a graphic trace of any structure moving along the long axis of the ultrasound beam.

In B mode imaging the amplitude of signal is represented by brightness of dot. The position of dot represents the depth of interface from the face of transducer (**Fig. 5.17A**).

Compound B mode scanning demonstrates the acoustic impedance variation of tissue in a two-dimensional display (2D) display where by multiple sets of dots are combined to delineate the echo pattern from internal structure within the body.

To create 2D display, transducer is scanned along the patient from different direction. The superposition of multiple scan line creates 2D image.

The direction of ultrasound beam is determined by the time elapsed from initiation pulse.

The simplest way to think the B scan image is the sum of many B mode time of sight that occurs in one place. This is shown in **Figure 5.17B**. The generation of an accurate B scan image requires amplitude of various echoes, the distance from the transducer face at which these echoes are reflected and position of B mode line of sight will be recorded by the machine.

Therefore, to generate a B scan image, machine must have a way of detecting the location of transducer on the patient body at a particular time that the B mode line of sight information is recorded. The sum of many lines of sight creates a B scan image.

EARLY B MODE SCANNER

Early B mode scanners were made with a single transducer mounted on an articulating arm with angular position encodes to determine the direction of ultrasound beam path. Using ADC brightness modulated data the beam is converted to a change pattern on the storage matrix. An image was built up by repeated pulsating and position change of transducer. 2D change pattern on storage matrix was used to create a video display system.

Articulate arm scanners are manually operated with either a linear, sector or compound scan motion. The linear motion limits the echo from boundaries that are only perpendicular to the direction of the beam. Sector scan display is achieved by a rocking motion of the transducer in a fixed position. A pie-shaped sector image is a display compound scan that uses a combination of translation and sector scan motion to ensure that all tissues boundaries are perpendicular to the beam at least one during the build up of the image.

Image acquisition and display in B mode system.

The following steps are involved in the component of standard unit as shown in **Figure 5.18**.

Transmitter: The ultrasonic pulses are generated by exciting the crystal with brief electric pulse as explained in A mode system.

The purpose of transmitter is to emit the short electric shell which excites the crystal. The PRF is 0.5-2.5 kHz. Most machines have a PRF of about 1 kHz.

Receiver: The generated ultrasound pulses are sent into patient and returning echo deform in the crystal which generate RF signal. These are amplified using TGC and demodulated by a Receiver as explained in earlier section.

These signals are then changed to a form that is suitable for transmission to scan converter.

These signals contain echo amplitude information.

SCAN LINE COORDINATE DATA

In order for the echoes received by the transducer to be displayed in the correct position in the final image information has to be collected from transducer assembly concerning the direction in which the sound pulse was transmitted into the patients. In other words, position and direction of transducer must be known all time. This positional information is generated from articulate scanning arm of machine as shown in **Figure 5.19A to F**.

At each of the hinged articulation of scanning arm, there are special electronic devices which measure the angle of articulation. These devices are called potentiometer. By knowing these angles, machine can quickly calculate the direction in which transducer is aimed and position of transducer on the patient.

The scan arms are rigid and permit scanning only in one plane.

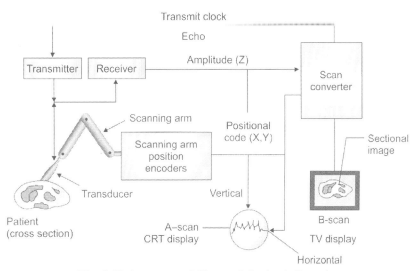

Fig. 5.18: Image acquisition and display in B mode.

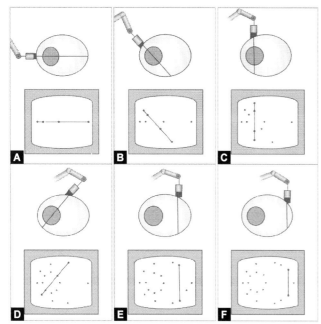

Figs. 5.19A to F: B-scan. The series of boxes (A to F) depict how a two-dimensional B scan image is generated. In box A, we see the transducer viewing a test object. On the TV screen below, four dots are recorded presenting the B mode image of the four reflectors that the transducer "sees." The line on the TV screen would not appear; it is used only to illustrate the line of sight of the transducer. Boxes B to F show the recording of other B mode lines of sight by the transducer. With enough views of the test object eventually a complete B scan image of the test object will be generated.

These potentiometers provide positional information similar to the X and Y coordinates on a graph.

To determine the distance from transducer to echo's point of origin, the time in which each echo returns up to the crystal must be accurately determined. Now two essential portions of ultrasound echo are the amplitude and the position at which echo originates.

These two pieces of information is combined in scan converter.

Scan Converter

It is a memory device which integrates the positional information and echo amplitude information into a format that can be used to produce an image. In other words, a scan converter takes information in one format and converts it into information in another format that results in B scan image.

Original B scan ultrasound equipment was termed bistable equipment. In this type of equipment position and amplitude information was fed into a storage oscilloscope. Image was generated on phosphor screen of storage oscilloscope and then photographed for permanent copy. Major limitation was storage phosphor either off or on resulting either white dot from an echo or no dot. Hence, these were only two shades of image—black or white **(Fig. 5.20)**.

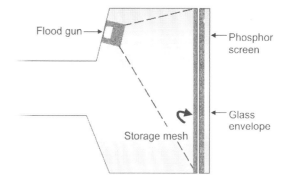

Fig. 5.20: Storage CRT. Interfaces are recorded on the storage mesh as positively charged regions. Electrons from electron flood guns are accelerated through these areas and strike and phosphor screen producing a visible image.

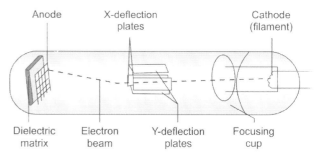

Fig. 5.21: Analog scan converter. Note similarity to the cathode ray tube discussed in Chapter 2.

The ultrasound amplitude information from the crystal can contain as much as 90 dB of dynamic range. This oscilloscope screen was capable of displaying only 20 dB of dynamic range or less and within this range it could display a single line of intersecting dots.

Thus, the system was capable of displaying echoes only above a certain predetermined threshold of amplitude. These echo generated below that threshold would not be displayed.

ANALOG SCAN CONVERTER

The storage oscilloscopes were replaced by analog scan converter. A schematic representation of an analog scan converter is shown in **Figure 5.21**.

An analog converter is specially designed vacuum tube contain on electron gun which fixes a thin electron beam towards a target.

The largest is a 1000 × 1000 matrix of 10 µ silicon oxide element.

The electron beam is directed by a series of deflection coils located outside the tube aimed at the target.

Following the path of sound beam in the patients, electron beam strikes the target and leaves a small electric charge on each of the silicon oxide element. The amount of electric charge is proportional to the amplitude of the echo generated from that corresponding spot within the patient. The location of the charge corresponds to the location from which the echo was generated. An electric image of varying electric charges is produced on silicon oxide screen that corresponds to amplitude and location of the echoes from within the patient's body. To convert this electric image to a visible image, the target screen is scanned again in a horizontal fashion by the electron beam. This time the various changes on silicon oxide target screen cause the electron beam to fluctuate in proportion to amount of change. In other words, first electron beam produces an electric image by causing the tiny element in the target to store a very small electric charge.

The second electron beam then reads the electron charges converting this information into a fluctuating electric signal which can then be sent to TV screen and displayed as an image.

Thus, positional and echo amplitude information provided from the position encoder and receiver portions of units, respectively go to scan converter where things are converted into an electric image on the scan converted tube target.

The information on the target is then converted to a video signal which can be displayed on a standard TV screen.

Advantage of Analog Scan Converter

1. This type of image production provides much more sophisticated type of gray scale processing than bistable image.
2. The analog scan converters give much greater flexibility in image presentation and allow gray scale images to be generated on all types of static imaging equipment.
3. Gray scale images provide more information about internal characteristic of structure then do bistable image. This is due to ability of scan converter to display varying amplitude of echoes at various shades of gray.

Disadvantage of Analog Scan Converter

1. All CRT tends to have their performance altered by temperature and age. There is a gradual drift of gray scale and focus capabilities of scan converter tube. As an analog scan converter tube deteriorates the image tends to look blurred and more bistable.
2. Constant alternating between "writing" the information on the target screen and the "reading" of this information causes the image to flicker while it is being generated.

Digital Scan Converter

It is also a memory device. However, instead of scan converter tube, the XY position and echo amplitude information is stored in a solid state semiconductor device.

This provides stable performance compared with analog scan converter. The information in memory is stored in a digital format which allows more sophisticated signal processing. Digital scan also allow flicker-free scanning and writing capabilities sufficient to allow real-time imaging. Essentially all modern gray scale ultrasound equipment is now manufactured with simple scan converter instead of an analog scan converter. The improved stability and reliability of a digital scan converters compared with analog scan converter results in overall improved performance.

Advantage of Digital Scan Converter over Direct View CRT

1. Reading the image on a routine TV monitor allow use of numerous accessories and an additional image control.
2. Computer data processing option is available.
3. Gray scale display is available.
4. Zoom display is available.
5. More than one image can be stored.
6. Resolution is better.
7. Prolong viewing does not degrade the image.

Display

All modern ultrasound imaging system employ a conventional TV monitor for display of final image. The information is read from image memory directly in the format of a TV image, which must then be amplified by the video amplifier before being displayed.

The large majority of scanner uses a wide dynamic range of black and white TV monitor but some more modern system make use of color overlays for different purposes, especially Doppler and final display unit in these system is a color monitor.

6

CHAPTER

Real Time Ultrasound

INTRODUCTION

2D ultrasound imaging is performed with either static B mode gray scale unit or real time gray scale scanner. In real time scanning the displayed image is continuously and rapidly updated with new scan data as beam swept repeatedly throughout the field of view. Rate at which information is displayed can be 30 or more frames per second. Since frame rate is faster, it allows movement to be followed.

For the past twenty years, the primary ultrasonic imaging modality has been static contact B scanning. However, for past ten years there has been tremendous increase in the use of real time ultrasound equipment and now real time ultrasound have technique that has almost totally replaced static B mode grayscale imaging. The increase use of real time imaging is the result of advances in transducer technology, miniaturization of electronics through the development of digital circuitry, advances in computer software and improved focusing.

Principle of Real Time Imaging

In static B mode grayscale imaging transducer is placed over the area of interest. It is placed at starting position and information is recorded along a single line of sight. All echoes from this single pulse are assumed to be originated from reflection along this line of sight. The amplitude of each signal is represented by brightness of dot. To build up a 2D image, transducer is manually moved by the sonographer to a different position or orientation to acquire information along a new line of sight. The previous line of sight data is retained on the display. The image thus is created by obtaining a large number of lines of sight over 10–20 second period of time. The resolution of the image is improved as the number of lines of sight is increased **(Figs. 6.1A to C)**. Static scanning depends on the object not moving because line of sight are acquired at different time and then combine to form a single image. Real time ultrasound imaging requires the acquisition of data in a very rapid fashion to give perception of motion.

The ultrasonic beam is swept through area of interest in a repetitive automated fashion. Instead of creating a single image with multiple lines of sight, multiple images are formed and each image composed of multiple lines of sight.

Ultrasound beam is first directed along one line of sight and after the echo is received, the beam is automatically moved to a new line of sight. A single image is formed by sweeping the sound beam through entire regions. This process is repeated to produce successive image of region.

As motion becomes more rapid within field of view (FOV), a faster frame rate is necessary to display the structure without jerkiness.

The maximum PRF or frame rate (FR) is limited by speed of ultrasound in tissue.

$$\text{Maximum FR} = \frac{V_s}{2dN} = \frac{V_s}{N} = \text{PRF}$$

Where V_s is velocity of sound in medium
d   = Depth of interest
N   = Number of lines of sight or vertical lines per field of view (also known as line density)
PRF = Pulse repetition frequency.

This indicates that visualizing deep structure will requires a slower frame rate (PRF). High frame rate is desirable, however, when imaging fast moving structure such as heart. High frequency is desirable to improve image quality, but more lines/frames require a lower number of frame/sec.

Conventional B mode scanner operates at a PRF between 200 and 2000 pulse per second. Real time scanner

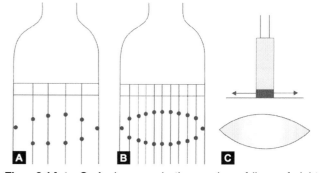

Figs. 6.1A to C: An increase in the number of lines of sight improves spatial resolution. (A) Transducer with few lines of sight; (B) Transducer with many lines of sight; (C) Compound B-mode scan with "infinite" lines of sight.

TABLE 6.1: Frame rate versus depth and the number of lines of sight.

Depth (cm)	25 LS*	Frame rate 50 LS	100 LS	200 LS
5	616	308	154	77
10	308	154	77	38
15	205	103	51	26
20	154	77	38	19
25	123	61	30	15
30	103	51	25	12

*LS indicates lines of sight

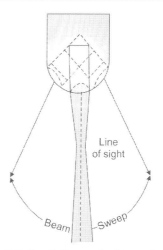

Fig. 6.2: Oscillating contact transducer.

usually have a much higher PRF (as high as 5000 pulses/second) to preserve spatial resolution.

Table 6.1 demonstrates the relation between number of lines of sight, depth of penetration and frame rate. The manufacture of real time ultrasound equipment sets the frame rate based on field of view, depth of interest and number of lines of sight required for desired image.

Instrumentation

The most classification of real time imaging system is based on the method by which ultrasound beam is swept through the region of interest. There are two major classes of scanner for producing real time ultrasound images. They are known as (i) mechanical scanner, (ii) electronic real time scanner.

Mechanical Scanner

Mechanical real time system uses one or more piezoelectric crystal attached to a stepping motor which moves the crystal to various locations. The changing position of crystal allows scan data to be collected from multiple lines of sight. Mechanical motion of crystal restricts the acquisition rate to 30 or 40 frames per second. These scanners may be of either contact scanner or liquid path scanner. Contact scanners are those in which transducer makes physical contact with the patient. Mechanical scanners are further classified into Wobbler type or rotating wheel type and spinner type or oscillating type.

All produce an image with sector formats usually encompassing an arc between 45° and 90°. The disadvantage of sector scanner is that scan format is relatively fixed for any transducer.

Wobbler or Oscillating Transducer (Contact Scanner)

In this group of scanner a single crystal is mounted on pivot within housing. A range of mechanical devices including reciprocating mechanism, linear motors and relatively simple electromagnets are used to swing the crystal through an arc.

The general design is shown in the **Figure 6.2**.

Here, the crystal vibrate or wobble back and forth during data collection. The angle through which the transducer is oscillated varies according to particular clinical application. However, most systems do not energies the crystal throughout the entire arc. The prime reason for this is the need to decelerate the crystal at the end of each sweep and then to accelerate it again in the reverse direction.

During this period the spacing between scan lines would become more cramped than in the remainder of the image and it is therefore useful to oscillate the crystal through a slightly larger angle than that used for imaging.

For example, if a 90° image angle is required the transducer is oscillated through an angle of 110° allowing 10° at each end of arc for deceleration and acceleration process.

Because the oscillating contact scanner touches the patient skin both operator and patient skin feel vibration and they were uncomfortable for patient and operator.

Working

When crystal is at extreme left position data collection is initiated. At this point the crystal is excited and ultrasound beam is directed along the line of sight. A fraction of beam energy is reflected at various interface reflected along the ultrasound path. After a time interval equal to the time required for the ultrasound wave to travel to the maximum depth of interest and return to the transducer (13 μ sec/centimeter) crystal is moved by stepping motor to a new position and excited again for new line of sight. This sequence is repeated until the last line of sight is collected for one image.

The time required to collect one image depicting information from a depth of 10 cm and 200 lines of sight is 26 m sec. This process is repeated for the next image.

$$FR = \frac{1540 \text{ m/sec}}{2(0.1 \text{ m})(200 \text{ L/frame})} = 38 \text{ frame/sec}$$

A sector shaped image is produced. The angle of Wobbler can be varied from 15°–60° and frame rate is generally between 15 and 30 frames/sec. In cardiac FR is in excess of 30/sec is used.

Advantage of Wobbler

- Cable conducting signal to and from the crystal can be permanently fixed to the crystal faces but of course need to incorporate a flexible component to permit crystal movement.
- The relatively simple construction of Wobbler scanner permits the manufacture to produce extremely small and light transducer. With small transducer scanning in tight areas between ribs and in other difficult reach area is possible.

Disadvantage

- The main theoretical disadvantage of Wobbler is the restriction of attainable FR. In cardiac application FR in excess of 30/sec may be required and vibration set-up by the more complex mechanical oscillating system prevents high FR from being attained.
- Their life is relatively short due to wear and tear and failure of mechanical components.

Despite this it has proved possible to manufacture reliable devices capable of producing very high quality images.

Spinner or Rotating Wheel Transducer

In this system scanning is achieved by a rotating wheel with several (3 or 4) ultrasound crystal mounted on its periphery. The general principle of construction of this transducer is shown in **Figure 6.3**. Rotating wheel is mounted within a housing.

The technique of acquiring the echo data is very similar to the vibrating sector scanner. When the crystal is positioned at the extreme left crystal is excited and the ultrasound beam probes interfaces along that line of sight.

The wheel then moves and crystal is excited for the next line of sight when the crystal moves to extreme right, the last line of sight is collected for one frame. The neighboring crystal on rotating wheel is then in position at the extreme left to begin the acquisition for the next frame.

It can be seen if there are four crystals mounted on a wheel, four 90° scans are performed during a single revolution of wheel.

Advantage

They can be used to achieve very fast frame rates without undue mechanical vibration.

Disadvantage

Major disadvantage is the requirement for a slip ring or commuter devices with brushes to conduct the transmitted and received electronic signal to and fro from ultrasound crystal.

Another type of mechanical scanner is the liquid bath scanner in which crystals are placed in liquid bath (usually a water and alcohol mixture) **(Fig. 6.4)**.

The liquid bath reduces reverberation from shallow structure and allows for strongly focused, large diameter transducer to be used to improve the resolution at desired depth. Liquid bath transducers are larger and bulkier than those with the contact scanner and are more difficult to apply to small areas, irregular shaped area or between ribs. Frame rate is also reduced because the liquid bath must be traversed twice by ultrasound beam.

Generally, mechanical system is less expensive and easier to operate than electronic real time scanner.

Electronic Scanner

In this group of scanner there is no mechanical moving compartment and ultrasound beam is scanned through the imaging plane by purely electronic mean.

Electronic real time scanners are classified into linear array and phased array or steered array.

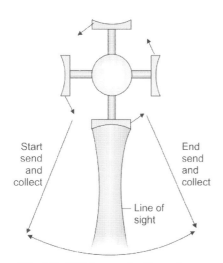

Fig. 6.3: Rotating contact transducer.

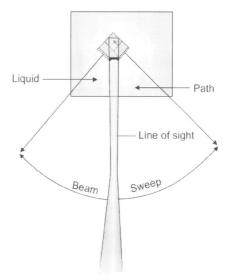

Fig. 6.4: Oscillating (liquid bath) nonreflecting transducer.

Linear Array

Linear array transducer produces rectangular scan format. They can be straight or curved also.

General purpose linear array transducer comprises a strip of piezoelectric material approximately 1.5–2.0 cm in width and 10–12 cm in length. This is divided into large number of small strip typically up to 600 in a modern transducer. Linear array transducer may be of three types:
1. Sequential linear array.
2. Segmental array.
3. Sequential and segmental.

In our example we will assume an assembly of 64 transducers.

Sequential Linear Array

Each crystal of 64 in group acts individually to produce an ultrasonic beam and then to receive the returning echoes for data collection along area line of sight. Crystals are activated in sequential fashion one after the other in the row to form the individual lines of sight **(Fig. 6.5)**.

Since physical dimension of crystal determines the width of ultrasound beam. Linear arrays are composed by many small crystals along a row. Hence, small crystal in sequential array produces a short near field and rapidly diverting far field. Hence, lateral resolution of image is poor.

Segmental Array

By simultaneously stimulating a group of crystal in the linear array, the crystal act in continuation to produce a deeper near field and less diverting far field compared with a single crystal acting alone. However, this segmental linear array creates fewer lines of sight for the same given area which did not produce satisfactory image. In this example, we observe **(Fig. 6.6)** 64 individual crystals are fired in a group of 4 so only 16 lines will be there instead of 64.

Sequential Segmental Linear Array

Combination of large diameter crystal and high line of density is required for best image resolution **(Figs. 6.7A to F)**. Slow excitation sequence for the first 16 crystal of 64

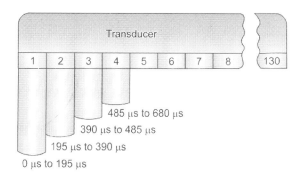

Fig. 6.5: Solid-state realtime transducer—sequential linear array.

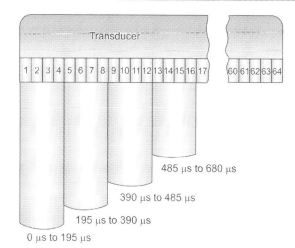

Fig. 6.6: Solid-state real-time transducer—segmental linear array.

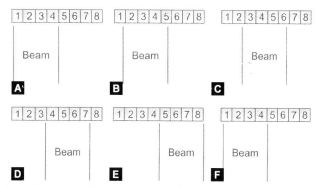

Figs. 6.7A to F: A linear sequenced array (side view). A voltage pulse is applied simultaneously to all elements in a small group: first to elements 1 through 4 (for example) as a group (A), then to elements 2 through 5 (B), and so on across the transducer assembly (C through E). The process is then repeated (F).

crystal linear array. The number of lines of sight is increased by firing crystal 1–4 cm then firing crystal 2 through 5.

In an array of 64 crystal element four crystals are fired at a time and each group was off set by one crystal a total of 61 lines of sight are acquired. Hence, a group of four will increase width of ultrasound beam and more lines of sight have produced good temporal resolution and good spatial resolution.

However, additional adjustments in focusing are necessary to narrow the beam width further so the spatial resolution is optimized. Focusing will be discussed later.

It is important to realize that in practice the beam width is considerably wider than a single element and majority of structures identified within the image inevitably occurs in two or more adjacent scan lines.

Hence, the width of FOV is constrained to be slightly less than over all length of the transducer and FOV is necessarily rectangular in shape. In fact it was found to be disadvantage, particularly in late pregnancy and abdominal imaging and curvilinear array was therefore introduced **(Fig. 6.8)**. The general construction and mode of operation is similar to the

Principles and Practice of Ultrasonography

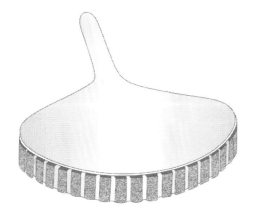

Fig. 6.8: Curved array.

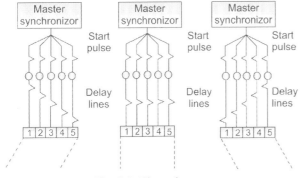

Fig. 6.9: Phased array.

linear array except that the surface of transducer is rather shorter in over all length and is curved. This gives rise to smaller area of contact with the patient and sector format to the image with the width of the FOV increasing with depth from surface. This overcomes many of the limitation of straight linear array transducer.

Phased Array

With phased array or steered array a sector scan is obtained but transducer does not move while the scan is generated. Ultrasound beam is caused to sweep back and forth across the patient by using electronically controlled steering and focusing.

The structure of phased array transducer is similar to the linear array except that the length is limited to 2-3 cm and number of element is 40-128.

In phased array each element is controlled in dependently and can be fired in rapid sequence. The principle of phased array transducer has been shown in **Figure 6.9**.

Element one is fired first and generated pulse passes a significant distance into the tissue. Shortly after firing of element one, element two is energized, and subsequently the other elements are fired in sequence across the face of transducer. Therefore, all the crystals are excited nearly at the same time to generate the ultrasonic beam. This is in contrast to linear array in which crystals are fired in group. The entire array produce one line of sight each time the crystal is excited.

The direction of beam is changed electronically by altering the excitation sequence to the crystal elements.

Steering the beam throughout the FOV allows for data collection along different line of sight. This steering is achieved by choosing appropriate delay time between stimulation of individual element of transducer.

Time delay associated with beam steering is larger than the micro second time interval to acquire data along the each line of sight.

A further enhancement of beam control used in multi-element transducer is the ability to focus the beam by sophisticated control of the variation in the delay interval between energizing of individual transducer element.

The scan format is sector with its apex at the center of array.

The ultrasound beam is caused to sweep through sector angle at a rate fast enough to form a real time image. A similar echopattern is introduced into the receiver signal, which causes the transducer to be sensitive only to echo returning along the same path as transmitted beam.

Rectangular Array

The crystals for phased array are also designed in rectangular or annular format. Rectangular phased array is composed of a matrix of crystal embedded in a plastic polymer. Rectangular phased array the electronically focused in two dimension along both direction of crystal matrix. Mechanical focusing is needed.

Electronic focusing in both dimensions is applied simultaneously, but steering is controlled in only one direction at a time. However, without moving the transducer, the beam can be steered to obtain a different plane such as sagittal rather than transducer **(Fig. 6.10)**.

Annular Array

One of major limitation of linear and phased array transducer is in their inability to control the beam with in

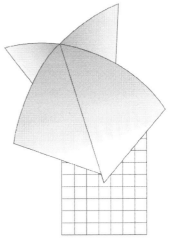

Fig. 6.10: Rectangular array showing matrix of crystals and orthogonal plane steering of rectangular array.

the orthogonal plane. The annular array has been devised in an attempt to overcome this limitation.

The annular array transducer is composed of a circular crystal usually measuring 3-4 cm in diameter, which is divided into several concentric acoustically isolated ring **(Figs. 6.11A and B)**. The number of ring is in the range of 5–8.

The mode of operation is similar to that used in phased array; the outer ring energized first and remaining rings being energized progressively towards the center.

The result is to generate a curved disc of sound within the patient.

The individual compartment of the disc travel at right angle to themselves and, therefore as the disc propagate down through the tissue it becomes progressively smaller until the focal point is reached beyond it then increase in diameter.

Electronic Focusing Technique

In mechanical scanner when a single crystal is used the beam shape is determined by physical shape of the transducer and may be modified by the presence of acoustic lenses mounted on the front of transducer as explained in focusing section earlier in Chapter 4.

So, in mechanical focusing method, beam is narrowed in width direction which is achieved by curving the crystal or by placing an acoustic lens in front of crystal.

In electronic transducer sequence of firing a group of crystal then firing the next group of crystal prohibit the mechanical focusing of the ultrasound beam in length direction.

The changing position dictate different focusing requirement for the crystal. Phased array transducers are most modern. Linear array transducers are electronically focused in the length direction which creates a narrow beam.

This is achieved by energizing the outer element in the group first and employing small variable delays between energizing of adjacent elements until the central element is energized last.

As with beam steering the individual pulses transmitted from each element combine to form a wave front which is in this circumstance is curved **(Figs. 6.12A and B)**.

The individual position of this wave front travels at right angles to themselves and thus causes to focus at the center of curvature of the wave front. The distance of this focal point from transducer is determined by degree of curvature of wave front, which itself is determined by the delay between the firing of individual crystal.

Figures 6.13A to C show the production of beam with a short focus by virtue of relatively large delays between the firing of adjacent elements, whereas in **Figure 6.13B**. The focus is longer because the delay is shorter.

The major advantage of this form of focusing is that it permits the equipment operator to ensure that the beam width is as narrow as possible at the depth of interest for each particular examination. The disadvantage is that if the beam is focused very near to the surface it will be unacceptable inside throughout the rest of FOV and it is not possible to focus the beam at more than one depth simultaneously.

A solution of this problem is swept transmit focus. This function permits simultaneous focusing at several depths.

In practice, when this function is selected a beam is initially generated with a very short focus and echoes are collected from proximal few centimeter of tissue path.

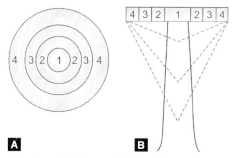

Figs. 6.11A and B: Annular array.

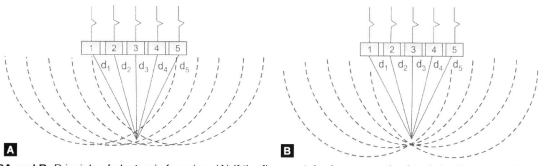

Figs. 6.12A and B: Principle of electronic focusing. (A) If the five crystals shown are stimulated simultaneously the wave fronts do not arrive at the target at the same time because the distances d_1, d_2, d_3, d_4, and d_5 are not equal; (B) Transmit delay lines are used to excite the crystals at slightly different times (nanosecond time delays between firing). The wave fronts arrive at exactly the same time at the target point resulting in focused beam. Crystals 1 and 5 are stimulated first, then 2 and 4, and finally crystal 3. Changing the time delays allows other "points" to become the center of focus.

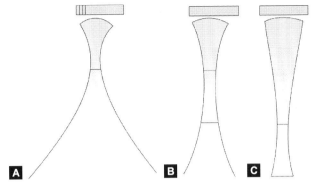

Figs. 6.13A to C: (A) The use of multiple focal zones; (B) The use of multiple focal zones; (C) The use of multiple focal zones.

As soon as the echoes from the distal part of this focal zone have been collected the receiver is switched off and all echoes returning from more distance are ignored. After sufficient time has been allowed a second pulse is generated focused at center of initially off receiver while echoes from relative wide beam passing through 'A' are received by the transducer.

The receiver is then switched on again to receive echoes from B and is switched off once those from most distant part of this focal zone are received.

This process is repeated with progressively larger focal length over three or four separate focal zones. The overall result is to obtain a single line of information in which the effective beam width is minimal throughout the entire depth.

CHAPTER 7

Ultrasound Artifacts, Biological Effects of Ultrasound, Image Quality, and Instrumentation

ULTRASOUND ARTIFACTS

Preparation for upper abdomen a six hours fast is generally recommended though not absolutely essential. At the same time prolonged fasting may increase the amount of intestinal gas as a result of aerophagy and may impair visualization. The rational behind fasting in fact is to obtain the distension of gallbladder rather than reduce amount of intestinal gases. In diabetics it is recommended that feeds be taken as fluids rather than solids.

Another advantage of fasting is that occasionally a food and fluid filled bowel loop may be mistaken for an intra-abdominal mass and stomach full of fluid may obscure pancreas. In infants it is often useful to scan the patient during the feed to ensure a quiet and immobile patient. Attempts to absorb gases by activated charcoal have generally been disappointing.

Pelvic Scanning

The instructions generally given are to drink five to six glasses of fluids about one hour preceding the scanning. Though this is variable, generally more fluid is required in the morning because of relative dehydration due to an overnight sleep than for bookings in the afternoon.

Filling the bladder has several advantages. It provides an acoustic window, straightens the axis of the uterus and demonstrates the relationship of uterine fundus to ovaries, it is useful in documenting bladder emptying to remove back pressure on kidneys, to demonstrate pelvic mass in contiguity, to avoid confusion between large pelvic cyst and urinary bladder and to visualize side walls of pelvis.

However, overfull bladder may disturb pelvic anatomy, may make gestational sac appear irregular and flattened. Produces a falsely elongated cervix and a falsely low lying placenta, the use of fluid insufflations in the rectum has been recommended to differentiate bowel from masses and to ascertain their position in pouch of Douglas or rectovesical pouch.

Transducer Selection (Figs. 7.1 to 7.6)

There are significant advantages of small faced sector transducer because small footprint with wide field of view

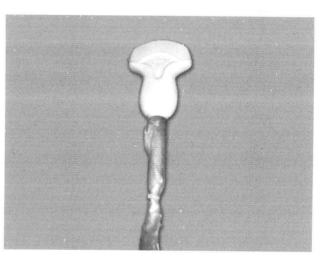

Fig. 7.1: A curvilinear probe with cable.

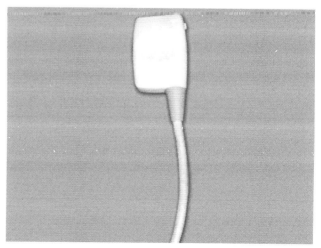

Fig. 7.2: A linear probe with cable for high resolution USG.

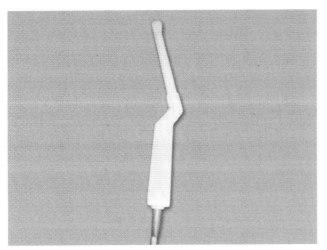

Fig. 7.3: An end firing endocavitary probe with cable for high resolution transvaginal and transrectal USG.

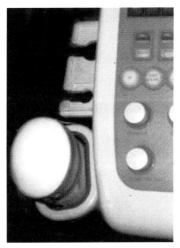

Fig. 7.6: A convex volume probe with cable (top view) for 3D live or 4D US.

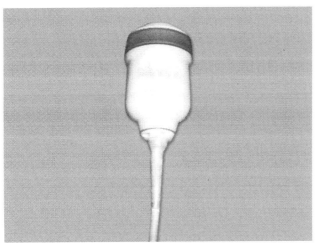

Fig. 7.4: A convex volume probe with cable for 3D live or 4D US.

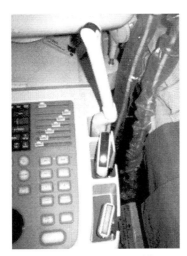

Fig. 7.5: A endocavitary, curvilinear and linear volume probe (top view) from above downwards.

provides good access in areas with limited acoustic window especially in the intercostal spaces, subxiphoid region, and low in pelvis (without completely filling the bladder) linear array is less suitable for intercostal scanning though field of view in the near zone is much more extensive than sector transducer, which makes them suitable for scanning the muscles of anterior abdominal wall, small parts scanning and superficial intra-abdominal organs like gallbladder. Micro convex transducers suffer from the same limitation of the field of view in the near zone as sector transducers.

Selection of transducers for a particular working depth is important but electronic focusing available in phased and linear arrays and annular mechanical sector transducers have made it somewhat less critical. With fixed focus transducers, it is important to rightly choose the frequency as well as focal zone at the desired depth. Simple rule to follow is—the highest frequency possible should be used that allows for adequate penetration to area of interest at low to medium power levels.

For obstetrics ultrasound use 3.5 or 5.0 MHz linear or convex focused of 7–9 cm. The 5.00 MHz transducer is best during early pregnancy: The 3.5 MHz is better for later pregnancy for general purpose, i.e., upper abdomen of adults, to pelvis as well as obstetrics, a sector or convex transducer of 3.5 MHz focused of 7–9 cm is best suitable while for pediatric 5.0 MHz with a focus of about 5–7 cm is needed. In neonatal brain, adult testis, neck 7.5 MHz focused at 4–5 cm will be required (**Figs. 7.7A to C**).

The use of standoff is useful. This achieves the same effect as using transducers with a shorter focus since it displaces the probe from the skin surface.

Patient position: supine position is standard since it allows for the muscle relaxation and flattens the abdomen. With real time ultrasound patient can be examined supine, standing or even sitting.

Right and left decubitus raising alternatively right and left sides cause descent of liver and the spleen into

CHAPTER 7: Ultrasound Artifacts, Biological Effects of Ultrasound, Image Quality, and Instrumentation

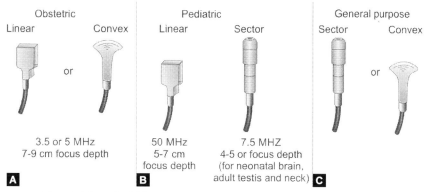

Figs. 7.7A to C: Different types of transducers with their application.

the abdomen to allow the scanning of kidneys and retroperitoneum, and also displaces the free fluid to most dependable positions. The other recommendations are left posterior oblique position for gallbladder and visualization of liver, gallbladder, and pancreas in upright position. Prone position is helpful to visualize kidneys more so during interventional procedures. Pleural fluid is best seen in the sitting position. Small children are often best examined in their mothers' arms.

Modified axial scan planes, angling the transducer superiorly to visualize hepatic veins and caudal to visualize pancreas otherwise obscured by gases through left liver lobe is another available option. The coronal plane to scan kidneys must take into account the more anteriorly placed lower poles compared to upper poles. Deliberate compression of abdomen by the transducer is valuable to displace bases and visualize inflamed appendix and associated periappendiceal fluid. Compression is used in the evaluation of bowel itself to differentiate fluid filled bowel from bowel thickening.

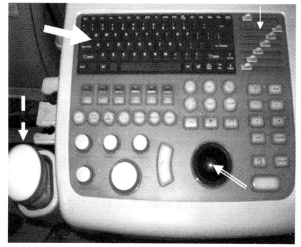

Fig. 7.8: The control panel of the US machine: Keyboard (thick arrow); probe in probe stand (broken arrow); track-ball (double line arrow) and time gain compensation (TGC) control (thin small arrow).

Optimum Use of Controls (Figs. 7.8 and 7.9)

Serial steps are as follows:
1. Check the contrast, bright nets, and focusing. Also hard copy devices at the start of the day.
2. Set time gain compensation (TGC) setting **(Fig. 7.10)** to use minimum power consistent with diagnostic image.
3. Distal part of image should provide the clue to the minimum acoustic power level to be used.
4. Near gain levels **(Figs. 7.11 to 7.13)** are to be set by TGC, sliders.
5. Then, one can set sliders for medium and superficial thickness regions.
6. Alternatively, one may set near gains next followed by TGC delay.
7. For M mode scanning set TGC to emphasize group of echoes from heart valves.
8. The TGC is now ready for low magnification settings. Zoom or scroll should be applied now if needed.

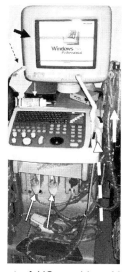

Fig. 7.9: Major part of US machine: Monitor (thick black arrow); lamp (dotted black arrow); jelly tube in jelly tube socket (small white arrow); probes in ports (thin, long white arrows), transducers in probe sockets (broken white arrow) and probe cables in cable stand (thick white arrow).

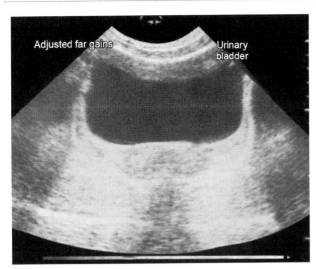

Fig. 7.10: Corrected TGC setting shows an anechoic urinary bladder.

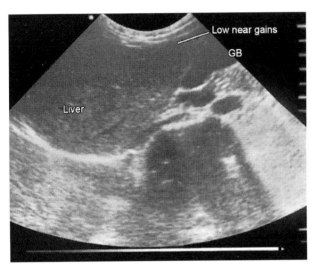

Fig. 7.11: Anterior part of liver appears dark due to low near gains.

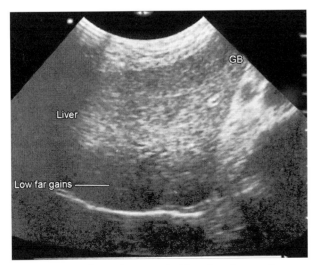

Fig. 7.12: Posterior aspect of liver is not seen due to low far gain.

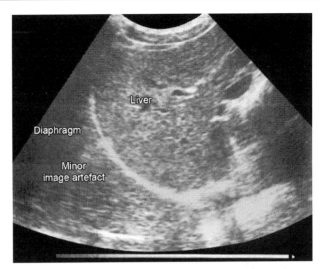

Fig. 7.13: Mirror image of the liver is seen above the diaphragm.

9. Now spatial resolution is optimized by dynamic focusing and edge enhancement.
10. If required frame rate is changed for moving structures or for optimizing spatial resolution.

Artifact in Ultrasound Imaging

All the noise can be either random or structured. Random noise can be due to random voltage fluctuations at low level which when amplified may appear fluctuating, moving pattern of gray spots resembling snow storm. This form of noise being random in nature can be reduced in the scanner by 'frame averaging' or 'persistence' which is basically a process of temporal smoothing.

Noise can also be produced by electric interference whether random or intermittent and usually forms a patterned signals in the form of flashes or bars and when structured is known as clutter. This may coincide with switching of nearby motor or diathermy unit. The other sources of such noise can be interference from scan head motor, faulty connections and improperly soldered joints.

Scattering and specular interfaces: Scattered echoes are echoes arising from very small regions (corresponding in to size to ultrasound wavelength 0.1–1.0 mm) accompanied with a change in the impedance. The amount of energy returning to transducer from each scatterer is very small and may be too feeble to be even recorded. But when a series of such scatterers form an array in the beam, for example, from surface of renal tubules and liver lobule they either sum or subtract to give rise to the pattern known as speckle. The ultrasound pattern of the structure bears little resemblance to real tissue structure or texture as it is convolution of structure by ultrasound beam itself.

When the reflecting surface is flat, all the reflected energy gets picked up by the transducer and signals are stronger even though strongly directional. Intensity falls off at angles less than 90°. Fortunately, few if any tissue

CHAPTER 7: Ultrasound Artifacts, Biological Effects of Ultrasound, Image Quality, and Instrumentation

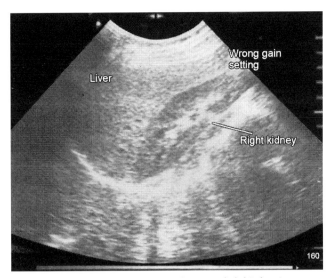

Fig. 7.14: Image is appearing very bright due to improper gain setting.

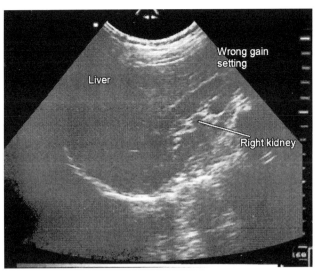

Fig. 7.16: Image is appearing dark due to improper gain setting.

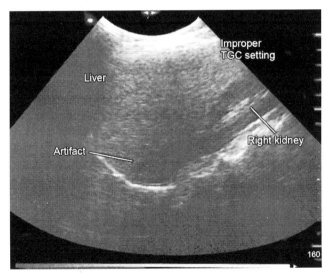

Fig. 7.15: Deeper structures not properly visualized due to improper TGC setting.

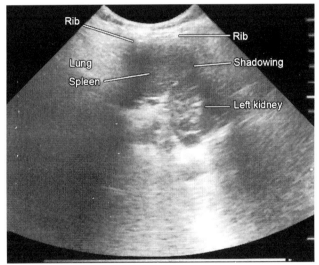

Fig. 7.17: Shadows from overlying gases hindering visualization of posterior structures.

interfaces are mirror smooth and because beam widths. In practice most interfaces are detectable up to angles greater than 60° and echoes are not just when there is tilting in excess of 90°. However, beyond certain angles flat surfaces might not be imaged and account for artifacts such as apparent communication between aorta and IVC when they are close together or invisibility of superior surface of urinary bladder in ascites from certain angles.

Shadowing and Enhancement

These are not true artifacts since they provide useful diagnostic information about the tissues. Shadowing occurs when a focus in the tissues has higher attenuation, resulting in inappropriate time. Gain compensation (TGC) **(Figs. 7.14 to 7.16)** which causes tissue deep to the focus, depicted as less reflective than it actually is. This dark band is known as acoustic shadowing the counterpart of the same is distal enhancement which is the result of over correction of time-gain compensation distal to anechoic structure. The degree of shadowing and enhancement depends upon difference in attenuation from surrounding structures and the length of traverse of beam.

Shadowing **(Figs. 7.17 to 7.19)** can also be produced by an extremely efficient reflector because very little of energy penetrates to insonate the deeper tissues. An efficient reflector may not be very echogenic because only a small proportion (1–20%) of attenuation is by reflection. Examples of strong echoes associated with enhancement are crystalline bile or pyonephrosis.

Shadowing can also be produced from the edges of the curved surfaces such as vessels, fetal skull and the cyst wall. The reasons could be two-fold: (i) ultrasound beam is dispersed as it gets reflected from the curved

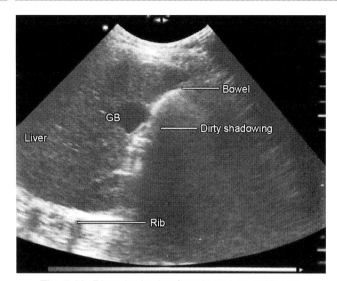

Fig. 7.18: Dirty shadowing from bowel gas with non-visualization of deeper structures.

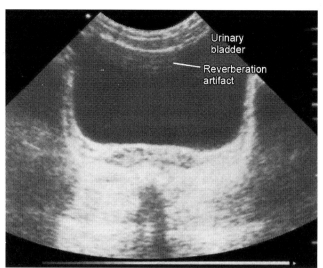

Fig. 7.20: Echoes seen in the anterior portion of the urinary bladder due to reverberation artefacts.

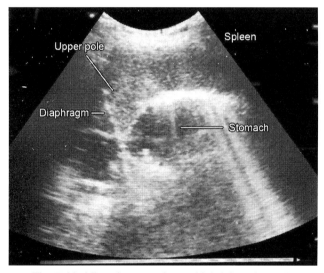

Fig. 7.19: Mirror image spleen with bright echogenic diaphragm.

surface because of leading edge of the beam strikes at an angle different than the trailing edge. The beam thus gets dispersed through a larger region resulting in weaker returning echoes. Also the beam gets focused in tissues deeper, because of velocity differences, (ii) the second explanation is that at the edge of curved surfaces beam passes through three to four times as much tissue than at other places and is thereby attenuated to a greater degree.

Refractive or edge shadowing is discussed above does not carry the same significance at the bulk-shadowing. The examples are the vessel wall in the renal sinus.

Reverberation Artifacts

Multiple echoes are more likely to be produced when surfaces are close together and when intervening tissue is a low-attenuation medium for example fluid. This is because of the fact that path lengths of multiple echoes being longer they are projected deeper and consequently get weaker and weaker.

An example of repeat echo is the mirror image artifact (**Fig. 7.13**) produced when a repeat image of a structure gets projected on the other side of the reflector which may be the diaphragm. A liver nodule or even a normal structure in the liver can appear within the lung. Actually the lung/pleura complex rather than lung itself or diaphragm acts as the reflector surface. This cause diagnostic problem but sometimes gives useful diagnostic clue about the presence of a liver cyst peripherally in the liver which may otherwise get unnoticed. An example of diagnostic problem created by such an artifact is the appearance of a mass in the region of sigmoid which is nothing but a repeat echo of bladder itself (**Figs. 7.20 and 7.21**), projected behind in the region of sigmoid.

Multiple echoes known as reverberations get produced when two strong reflectors are parallel to other. The common example being a gas bubble or stone parallel to skin surface where skin/transducer interface forms the second reflecting surface. Ultrasound gets reflected back to the transducer but a proportion gets re-reflected back into tissues and gets projected behind the real echo. When the space between reflectors is less the echoes may even merge to form a band and individual components may be difficult to detect. This produces what is known as comet-tail artifact because of very reflective object. With a bright streak, examples are foreign bodies such as surgical clips, IUCD's, catheters, bullets or shrapnel or fluid filled cavities in the wall of gallbladder such as Aschoff. Rockitansky sinuses seen in adenomyomatosis and also foamy collections of gas bubbles in the abdomen.

Artifacts because of velocity errors: Velocity of ultrasound though generally assumed to be, is not constant within tissues. For example, fat conducts ultrasounds some 10–15% more slowly than soft tissues. Prosthetic materials conduct

CHAPTER 7: Ultrasound Artifacts, Biological Effects of Ultrasound, Image Quality, and Instrumentation

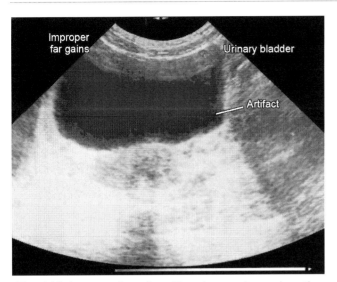

Fig. 7.21: Improper far gain setting shows echoes along the posterior wall.

velocity at very much lower level. Every 13 m sec. Delay in echoes means a 1 cm depth in the final image. Hence, deeper structures appear to be spuriously deeper. This though does not limit the lateral resolution as it is by the scanning action of the transducer. However, in ophthalmic scanning this lack of precision can be crucial. The section of retina imaged through the lens which conducts ultrasounds at 1620 ms/sec appears to be deeper and behind and is known as the Baum's bump.

Ultrasound beam when it crosses two regions of different velocity deviates from its straight path. Since the scanner only assumes a straight path, reflectors away from sources are projected to the side of their true position, since the beam crossing wedge shaped space around recti get refracted the deeper pelvic structures appear to be stretched laterally. The gestational sac may even appear to be duplicated, in extreme cases.

The artifactual displacement disappears when scanning is done from the center of rectus muscle instead of sideways. Also, this artifact is not seen when scanning laterally. Also, it is less common in epigastrium because of lesser amount of fat.

The ability and the ease with which the ultrasound waves get focused depend in the differences in the velocity in the tissues through which the waves propagate. That is why some individuals are called bad subjects for the ultrasound where this defocusing effect on account of differences in velocity results in significant degradation of lateral resolution. These effects get accentuated for the linear array transducers with wide scan head than for small scan head sector transducers, even while examining the same obese patient.

The renal ultrasound beam shape falls short of desired thin beam configuration, the typical beam shape is composed of a region of disturbance immediately underneath the scan head, then a near zone (Fresnel zone) that progressively narrows to a fine focus followed by a far zone over which it diverges (Fraunhofer zone). Not only that there are low energy beams directed at an angle from the main beam, known as side lobes.

Ultrasound energy is concentrated along the line of focusing and falls off in Gaussian distribution on either side of the line. While weak reflectors are best visualized when they are in the line of beam, strong reflectors even if they are off-axis get visualized and appear as what is known as beam width artifacts, these are seen of cigar shaped smears or streaks, which increases the apparent width of these strong reflectors. These beam width artifacts occur where a gassy or bony structure lies adjacent to a fluid space. The beam width artifacts also have tendency to fill in the echo-free fluid spaces like ducts, etc.

These beam width artifacts also occur in the orthogonal, tissue plane. With annular array transducers beam is symmetrical whereas with linear array transducers beam is wider across the slice thickness. The orthogonal beam width artifacts are analogous to slice thickness artifacts seen in the CT scanning. They are typically seen as echo-poor bands or lines within the echo free spaces. They (orthogonal beam width artifact) are more difficult to visualize because offending reflector is not visualized within the image.

The profile of beam is complicated by the presence of side lobes and grating lobes for the array transducers. These side lobes are misdirected. Aberrant lines of ultrasound energy in off. Axis regions when the transducer is in the receive mode. They are the result of beam focusing mechanisms whether by applied lenses or by curving the transducer face. These consist of ill-defined beams 20° away from the main beam and are much weaker (say by 40 dB or so).

Grating lobes are similar lobes seen in array transducers and are more discrete and powerful. They are less marked when array elements are small and numerous. If a strong reflector or even a gas bubble or bone surface lies in the position of grating lobe its echo will be depicted in the line of main beam giving rise to convex shaped streak known as "Chinese hat artifact," these artifacts are consistent on rescanning, may be visualized in the image and may occur in the orthogonal plane.

Artifacts in the Doppler imaging: Usually as beam vessel angle approaches 90°. No useful Doppler signal is recorded, though occasionally there is sufficient radial flow during pulsatile expansion in systole and bidirectional signal may be recorded but such waveforms are quite valueless.

Aliasing: Any Doppler-shift frequency greater than half the PRF is perceived by the equipment as in the opposite direction. Very often the peak systolic component of waveform appears on the wrong side of the waveform. The shifting of baseline downwards when studying arteries with high velocities often masks this artifact, which may go unrecognized if one was to just look at the waveforms.

As the PRF is increased to overcome aliasing the range ambiguities appear because of two echoes being received close together, and echoes are mistaken as coming from the superficial structures. Other approaches to overcome aliasing are to reduce insonation frequency and to reduce insonation angle.

Artifacts because of time sampling: There is limit beyond which pulse-repetition frequency cannot be increased. This limit depends upon the penetration required and the speed of traverse of ultrasound. If the echoes are sent too seen before previous echo sent is received by transducer it results in the incorrect appreciation of the depth of second echo which appears very close together. Thus, flickering objects are seen in the near field and their depth gets changed by changing the PRF or changing the scale. Properly adjusted scanners usually do not have this artifact. The limited frame rate can affect the depiction of motion of structures such as the heart valves resulting in apparent jerky, cartoon like motion and in some cases the motion can be even slow or reversed in direction.

ARTIFACTS BECAUSE OF SAMPLE VOLUME SIZE AND POSITION

Undersampling: If range gate is significantly less wide than vessel being studied it may fail to estimate the flow velocities because of failure to sample the velocities lying at the periphery of the vessel. Most array scanners permit the operator the choice to vary the gate. But some scanners do have the provision for a fixed range gate at a depth resulting in undersampling.

Another cause of undersampling could be due to vessel motion during Doppler interrogation. Such translocation of vessels, for example, is seen during cardiac pulsations, superior mesenteric artery and umbilical arteries. Occurring during systole it may only result in significant loss of signal information during systole. However, during diastole it may be read as absence of diastolic flow and may lead to inappropriate diagnostic, clinical decisions. Hence, while sampling umbilical arteries wide-gate use is recommended.

Movement of a vein containing coarse vorter flow can lead to bizarre, confusing tracing.

On the other hand, if gate is too wide for particular vessel there is likelihood of the tracing being modified by superimposition of flow from another vessel coming within the range of the gate this oversampling as it is called, may cause some confusion and on the other hand may provide some diagnostically useful information regarding umbilical or renal veins or hepatic circulation.

Problems in velocity calculation: If beam vessel angle is less than, 45° a 5° error results in an error of 10% in velocity measurements. For angles greater than 45° margin of error is quite great up to 35% at 70°. In some scanners though velocities is calculated assuming an angle of 0° and the information recording is not indicated further some errors can be introduced by even manual method of taking the tracing. If the waveform is incomplete because of inadequate gain or sensitivity, error may be introduced.

Errors in volume flow calculation: Volume flow is calculated by multiplying time averaged mean velocity with vessel cross section area. Velocity calculation may suffer from an error of at least 50%. Further, there may be errors even in the calculation of one division, i.e., diameter which gets squared when area is calculated. For arteries possible sources of error in this regard are:

- The diameter of artery varies as much as 10% over the cardiac cycle and this gets squared to 20% as cross-sectional area is calculated.
- Vessel diameter if calculated from CVI image leads to over estimation of diameter because of spillover effect of color.

For veins: The calculation of cross-sectional area is problematic since few if any veins are circular in cross-section. Further, cross-sectional measurements taken at RT angles do not allow for estimation of flow velocity in the same section. This becomes further complicated when a tributary joins adjacent to the site/sites of measurement.

Measurement of instantaneous mean velocity and time averaged mean velocity also suffers from certain limitations because of the way it is computed. For these, sometimes mean peak value is taken and is multiplied by a constant factor such as 0.6 or 0.7 assuming profile to be same through out cardiac cycle. Alternatively either mode velocity is chosen or the highest frequency at certain arbitary predetermined power or decibel level less than peak value. This may vary as much as –3, –6, –9 or even –12 dB levels less than peak value, typically the results may vary by as much as 50%.

Distortion of velocity profile resulting in coarse vorter within vessel may lead to significant velocity errors. For example, at the junction of right and left portal vein which is at 45° angle to the long axis of vessel.

Errors in Waveform Analysis

Significance of heart rate on estimation of RI values cannot be over estimated. The onset of systole encroaches upon diastole at fast heart rates. It is possible to compensate for this by extrapolating the diastolic deceleration to normal standard cardiac period. Changes in fetal circulation are possibly attributable partly on changes in the heart rate.

Another source of error in calculating PI is due to continuous forward flow and diastolic value to be picked up is in end diastole. It is important to know the method of calculation of indices by scanner so that ones own standards can be calculated. Vessel movement during sampling may further corrupt PI or RI values.

Shape of waveforms may get further affected by circulatory factors up-stream, down-stream factors, cardiac function, aortic valve function, proximal and distal stenosis and state of collateral circulation.

Spectral information: Under sampling of range of frequencies present in the waveform can be because of eccentric placement of range gate in the vessel.

The other sources of error can be due to low frequency, high amplitude signals produced in the pulsating arterial wall, which appears as the wall thump in the Doppler tracings. These low frequency signals can be removed by the 'high pass filters' which selectively remove low frequency components in the tracings but this filter also removes true low frequencies and spectrum then reveals an apparent increase in velocities.

Another source of error can be due to Doppler interrogation of veins at high filter settings which may partially or even totally reject the useful and real flow. Further one should never forget that any moving tissue can give rise to Doppler shift.

Mirror image artifact is an artificial signal on the other side of baseline along with the signal being sought. Causes of its formation are:
- Inadequacies in the scanners electronics.
- Too high a Doppler gain.
- Too small beam/vessel angle—which may lead to radial flow during systolic expansion of the vessel.
- Presence of branch vessel included in the range gate.

This artifact must be differentiated from the true flow reversal.

Artifacts in color flow imaging: Some of the pulses in most of color flow systems are used to produce the gray scale information and remainder are used for color Doppler flow. Thus, effective PRF gets lower than imaging PRF and aliasing limit becomes lower too. As a result even moderate velocities in the arteries give rise to aliasing. Aliasing appears as mosaic of colors almost indistinguishable from the true reversal. The distinguishing feature is that color changes abruptly from blue to red without an intervening black area. Aliasing also results when high velocity flow is imaged using a low velocity scale.

Color flow imaging has relatively poor spatial resolution compared with grey scale imaging. Color picture elements are larger in size than grey scale imaging elements. Also, Doppler pulses are longer than imaging pulses. These factors lower the axial as well as azimuthal resolution. The overestimation of vessel diameter on color flow image though around 1 mm only can be of the order of 100%. Further averaging of images over few frames leads to further overestimation of vessel diameter.

Beam/Vessel Artifact

It is produced because part of blood flow in the vessel may be towards and part of it opposed to the transducer.

Color mirror image artifact: With strong specular reflector such as bladder wall or diaphragm, mirror image artifact similar to 2 D scanning may occur.

Frame rate artifact: Because frame rate becomes very low when scanning the very deep vessel, confusing flow pattern may be seen.

Biological Effect of Ultrasound Safety Considerations

Physical effects of ultrasound can be divided into two groups: Thermal and nonthermal. Heating is mainly due to attenuation of sound as it passes through tissues. Nonthermal mechanisms can generate heat as well.

Nonthermal mechanisms can result in application of radiation forces (nonionizing) both at microscopic and macroscopic level resulting in exerted pressure and torque. Acoustic fields can also cause induced motion or flow of fluids known as streaming.

Acoustic cavitation is action of fields which generates bubbles which undergo volume pulsation and collapse in response to acoustic field. Other results of this activity are free radicles generation, microstreaming around bubble and mechanical action from bubble collapse.

Thermal Effects

Ultrasound produces heat through attenuation, which causes loss of penetration and inability to image deeper tissues. Some of energy transferred to tissues is back scattered. Energy is also lost by absorption along the path of propagation. Factors controlling tissue heating include: Spatial focusing, frequency of ultrasound, duration of exposure, and tissue type.

Safety considerations have become more widespread since the use of diagnostic ultrasound has become more prevalent. This being more so for the obstetrics and neonatology, because the most sensitive targets exposed to ultrasound are the embryo or fetus.

The majority of the studies reported involve the interaction of therapeutic ultrasound with biological systems and very few with the diagnostic exposures.

Therapeutic ultrasound uses continuous or tone burst exposures while diagnostic ultrasound uses short pulses. There is some overlap in the amount of acoustic power emitted during a pulse even through for therapy devices time average intensity parameters are lower, while therapy devices induce biological changes albeit beneficial, it is not known whether same could be true with the diagnostic ultrasounds.

Very few measurements of the temperature changes induced by diagnostic uses have been made. Some workers have reported biologically insignificant temperature rise in vitro following pulse exposure in diagnostic range in liver (time average peak intensity $\simeq$ 183 watts/cm^2) using 3.3 MHz frequency while 1.9° temperature rise while using Doppler ultrasound for one minute (time average peak intensity ~190 w/cm^2) higher temperatures have been recorded at the bone surface. In fact using Doppler ultrasound as above a temperature rise of as much as 4.7°C was recorded on the surface of mature bone with overlying muscle layer of 8 mm, in vitro. The greatest rise being when the beam meets the bone surface at right angle, with noncalcified fetal bones the temperature rise is less likely.

Some data are available on the effect of above normal temperature of the fetus or embryo although effects of hyperthermia on human fetus or embryo are not known. Although other mammalian species seem to be susceptible to temperature rise during pregnancy.

The factors determining the effect of hyperthermia depend upon the stage of embryonic or fetal development, quantum of temperatures rise and the duration. The hyperthermia-induced death though possible at any stage is most likely to occur even before implantation. This happens by induced delay in the development of embryo or by the change in the environment that is uterine secretions/nutrients. The result is either embryonic death if it does not overcome hyperthermia to develop normally.

Abortion as a result of hyperthermia is well known. The factors responsible for this are increased uterine activity and severe cellular damage.

Hyperthermia is known to induce teratogenic effect in a number of species viz. rats, sheep, pigs, and mice, etc. For this temperature elevation should occur during a crucial stage of organogenesis. The central nervous system seems to be most susceptible and the defects produced can be microphthalmia, neural tube defects, microcephaly, and microencephaly.

The temperature rises of the order of 1.5–2.5°C above normal can produce resorption, death, abortion, or teratogenesis. It is known from experimental studies that early embryos are more likely to have lethal effects than late embryos and when cell proliferation is most intense the sensitivity raises further.

The central nervous system is most sensitive organs though in adults too, proliferative tissues for example testes and bone marrow are at risk.

Further, it is thought on the basis of these studies that if embryo or fetus is effected by less than 1° temperature rise adverse effects outcome is less likely and scanning can proceed as long as desired, however, this is for the hyperthermia effecting whole fetus. Effects of selective heating of different regions of fetus as with Doppler ultrasounds have not been studied.

It seems overall thermal considerations do not adversely effect the safety in pulse echo scanning while for Doppler ultrasound the caution that needs to be exercised is that examination should be kept as short as possible.

All the above mentioned sequence of events requires that either stabilized microscopic gas bubbles or nucleation sites exist in the tissue. The bubbles are known to exist and enlarge in the tissues under the influence of therapeutic ultrasound. While it is not so definitely known about nucleation sites in tissues, it seems that certain tissues have in abundance than others and in different individuals increasing thereby the likelihood of cavitation because of different gaseous content.

The cavitations induced by diagnostic ultrasound pulses have not been described in the mammalian tissues.

The biological effects of cavitation are not well-understood. The tissue surrounding the site of cavitation may be completely disrupted and cell lysis may occur.

Biological Effects of Cavitation

Cavitation refers to the activity of microscopic gas bubbles (gas bodies) under the influence of the ultrasonic field. Size of the bubble and the characteristics of ultrasonic field determine the behavior of the bubble and the outcome, there being a particular bubble diameter for a frequency for which bubble becomes resonant. These bubbles then grow bigger, and undergo explosion resulting in large temperatures and sheering stresses, under the influence of powerful acoustic field. For lesser amplitudes of acoustic field small bubbles are produced which may oscillate and may have streaming motion or they may grow bigger and then collapse. Large bubbles may oscillate, may disintegrate, thus producing a population of small bubbles.

Only a few microns around and bubbles may oscillate framing streaming pattern.

In fluids the shearing stress may cause the cells in the vicinity to be lysed, whereas in more structured tissue the movements and bubble oscillation is considerably dampened. Perhaps the greatest hazard is from the cavitation event occurring in the amniotic or body fluid close to developing embryo causing cell lysis and irreparable tissue damage. This may also occur in blood plasma though thrombus formation is not known.

Biological effects from other mechanisms: There may be nonlinear propagation effects of diagnostic ultrasound about the biological effect of which, nothing is known at present.

Epidemiological studies that have been done, concern birth weight, fetal anomalies, neurological effects, childhood cancers and effect on hearing in children. None of these studies have provided any conclusive evidence of ultrasound induced abnormality. One isolated study not supported by others refers to incidence of low birth weight. Thus epidemiological data do not suggest the incidence of harmful effect of ultrasound in utero, though sample sizes used were small, but not even a few cases have been recorded considering widespread use of ultrasounds over years and years. No epidemiological data, whatsoever, is available on effects of Doppler ultrasound.

Methods to Minimize the Harmful Effects

Thermal effects are more when the acoustic output, intensity, exposure time and ultrasound frequency is increased. Also, when time average intensity is increased especially by increasing pulse repetition, frequency, the thermal effects increase. For cavitation crucial factors are peak negative pressure, pulse length, pulse repetition frequency and exposure time. Increase in exposure output and the time increases the probability of thermal and cavitation effects. Increasing the transducer frequency increases thermal effects while it decreases likelihood of cavitation.

Guidelines

- Set machine on default output settings.
- Keep the time for which transducer is in contact to minimum.
- Keep acoustic output at the minimum consistent with good results.

IMAGE QUALITY

Instrumentation

Orientation of Image

On longitudinal scan, the head of the patient should be on left side while the leg side on right side of the screen. Sometimes during screening on transverse images, the image pattern is reversed on screen, hence, it is imperative to check the transverse scan by putting image of one end of the transducer and screening. If the image does not appear as it should be, then rotate the transducer by 180° and check again **(Figs. 7.22 and 7.23)**.

- Before taking image the transducer should have enough coupling agent to make its movement continuous and gradual.
- The image should be predominantly black, if white there is a switch to change or call the engineer.

Coupling Agents

No air should be between transducers and skin as it acts as a barrier to ultrasound waves and gets reflected. The basic ingredients of coupling agents are:

- Carbomer—a synthetic high molecular weight polymer of acrylic acid cross-linked with allyl sucrose and containing 56–68% of carboxylic acid groups. It is white fluffy, acidic, hydroscopic powder with slight charactcristic odor.

  Neutralized with alkali hydroxides or amines: it is very soluble in water, alcohol, and glycerol.

  There are three carbomers. The most suitable is carbomer 940, which forms a clear gel in aqueous and

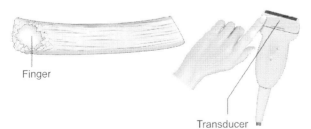

Fig. 7.22: The transducer should produce the image on the same side of the monitor. Rotate transducer to 180°, if the image is on the wrong side.

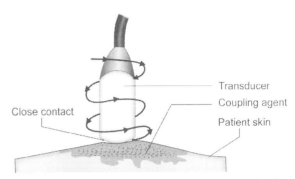

Fig. 7.23: Ultrasound transducer in contact with body.

nonaqueous vehicles. If carbomer 940 is not available, carbomer 934 or 941 can be used.

- EDTA (edetic acid) a white crystalline powder, very slightly soluble in water but soluble in solutions of alkali hydroxides.
- Propylene glycol—a colorless, odorless, viscous hydroscopic liquid with slight sweet taste. Density = 1.035-1.037 gm/mL.
- Theolamine (Triethanolamine)—a mixture of bases containing not less than 80% of triethanolamine with diethanolamine and small amounts of ethanolamine. It forms a clear colorless or slightly yellow odorless, viscous hydroscopic liquid. Density = 1.12-1.13 gm/mL.

Formula : The amounts are as follows:

Carbomer	:	10.0 g
EDTA	:	0.25 g
Propylene glycol	:	750 g (> 24 mL)
Theolamine	:	12.5 g (11.2 mL)
Distilled water	:	up to 500 g (500 mL)

Preparation

- Mix EDTA with 400 g (400 mL) of water, ones it is dissolved in dipropylene glycol
- Add carbomer and stir with high speed stirrer
- Wait till a gel is formed and no more bubbles are observed
- Add water to make it 500 mL of gel.

Spatial resolution is defined as the ability to see small structures separately along the beam (axial) as well as across (in lateral) dimension. High contrast resolution is ability to distinguish between different tissues without noise or artifacts. Good contrast resolution at sufficient depth requires sufficient sensitivity which in turn depends upon various techniques/strategies, viz. image smoothening, edge enhancement, dynamic focusing, aperture control, and apodisation. To achieve all this, analog image is first digitalized so that it can be suitably pre and post-processed. This image processing keeps to a minimum the structured noise which is because of video-lines, scan lines, etc. caused by the process of scanning.

Resolution is defined in 3 planes axial resolution, lateral resolution and vertical resolution. Axial resolution is basically a depth resolution depends on the length of ultrasound pulse and is typically 3 mm for 5 MHz. In contrast width of beam determines the lateral resolution. Unlike the former, lateral resolution changes with the depth. Vertical or azimuthal resolution, in the direction perpendicular to the plane of transducer is a function of the thickness of slice and is fixed.

Image smoothening on an average a linear array contains about 125 ultrasound lines and is around 10 cm in length. There are about 512 pixels across to accommodate this information. Thus, only one out of 4 pixels contains echo information. Unless filled these empty pixels will leave the gaps between the lines on the image. The solution lies on filling the empty pixels with some precalculated value which must take into account the graded transition from one value to next.

With sector transducers because of directional nature of information some pixels may not be touched by the line of scan or vector, while others may be crossed diagonally or just at the corners, because of which voltage value assigned to pixel may be low, high or a weighted beam of the same. To erase the drop outs, the size of pixels themselves may vary over the image, for example, from square to oblong. Also, along the scan lines direction the pixels may be arranged so that they fall along the scan line. Still another strategy could be moving nine-point average smoothening technique which involves replacing the value of a pixel by another value which is the average of its own value and other eight surrounding values.

Axial resolution in general is limited by the half the pulse length and the lateral resolution equals the width of the beam. However, the achieved resolution is better than theoretical limits. This is because the image of the organs filters out the sparkle pattern contained in the tissue texture because of small echostructures lying close together and interfering with each other. Thus texture as seen in ultrasound does not relate to real texture because of elimination of coherent radiation speckle.

It is important from the diagnostic standpoint also to remove the speckle because otherwise pathological vs normal change in reflectivity may not be discerned. The smoothing out of the speckle pattern leaves the general brightness of organ unaffected. The speckle is smoothed between subsequent similar frame which get tissue and speckle moving because of motion by cardiovascular action, muscular action or even probe movement.

However, when detailed study of architecture is required or subsequent frames are vastly different because of rapid movement this smoothening (frame averaging) does not help and needs to be switched off.

Typically, this averaging is achieved over nine frames. There is pixel by pixel subtraction over every ninth frame, all of which are stored separately in memory. The result of subtraction is used to overwrite every subsequent frame. The number of the frame used for subtraction as well as weightage of most recent versus previous frames may vary as per the different strategies adopted.

Zoom which is sometimes confused with simple magnification is of two types: (i) read zoom and (ii) write zoom.

In read zoom or magnification, only a part of computer memory containing pixels is used which themselves get enlarged. This enlargement of pixel size at larger magnification gives rise to obvious grainy images.

In write zoom on the other hand frequency of sampling of data in each pixel is made very fast so that one pixel contains many samples. If now scale is changed to enlarge the pixel contains only one value while the size of pixel remains the same. Thus, obviating the grainy image.

However, with zoom factor there may be large gaps in the scan line which need to be covered either by image smoothening processes or in the more modern technologies by insertion of more scan lines.

Image Recording

While eye can discern large number (256) shades of grey the film can respond to fewer number of shades. Hence, there is some loss of visual grey shades when image is transferred from screen to the hard copy film. Hence, it requires a compression of contrast in the ultrasound image before it is copied. This is achieved by a process called gamma correction. Where in each shade of grey is assigned a voltage value before being fed in the digital scan converter. This chart of values so to say undergoes an electronic look up to generate compression of contrast. Thus, simultaneously one image is generated for viewing and another for storage. In effect, this result in changing the displayed shade assigned to particular echo amplitude.

Post-processing may enable the contrast and also brightness levels to be changed from the storage data. Assuming half the echo information to be due to the actual change in reflectivity and not due to augmentation by TGC it would appear that strongest reflector is 300 times as strong as the weakest one. This echo information is compressed before display however actual pattern of compression varies according to the needs of diagnostic situation, for example where shape, form or outline of organ is to be emphasized in display exponential form of compression is desired. For demonstrating and emphasizing small changes in echogenicity logarithmic post-processing is suitable. For enhancing mid-range echoes sigmoid curve is chosen, and for imaging format. Reverse compression is most effective.

Signal preprocessing: Before storage is performed various examples of preprocessing are: (i) automatic gain control, (ii) edge enhancement and, (iii) rapid frequency digitization.

TGC—means deliberate compensation for attenuation of ultrasound signals so that echoes frame deeper structures appear as reflective as those from the superficial structures. However, very low echo structures such as fluid spaces confuse the system resulting in application of TGC and consequently the artifacts for which manual correction of TGC is required.

Process of TGC application requires smoothening of the rapid fluctuation in echo amplitudes. This pattern is then inverted and averaged with original echo amplitude.

Radiofrequency digitization: The returned signal from a structure is a radio frequency signal. It is digitized to video frequency signal by application of frequency specific radio frequency amplifier which produces a smooth envelope around the radio frequency signal. This results in easier handling of video frequency signal by computer then of RF signal. However, this leaves a trail around the signal producing distortion. This is avoided by direct digitization of radio frequency signal which is then stored and subsequently post-processed.

Edge enhancement is the process by which upstroke of each echo is emphasized, depending on the degree of enhancement required a voltage proportional to leading edge of echo is generated and added back to original voltage waveform, this results strong reflections for even closely spaced reflectors.

Measurements and Accuracy of Measurements

In general for the measurement the calipers on the screen which are controlled by joystick of trackball give the best results.

There is an element of imprecision in these measurements. The boundary of any given structure is bound to be at least one pixel wide, which means an inaccuracy of plus or minus diagonal width of one pixel at low magnification.

Thus, an increment of 0.1 mm may be actually 0.3 mm. At zoom image and for high frequency probes higher frequency is possible.

Digital Control

It is important to know exactly where the returning echo has originated in the tissues. An echo from one side of the beam may be displayed on the other side. Thereby degrading the lateral resolution.

The other problem refers to the grating lobes which produce artifacts from the strong reflectors present in off-axis region. These grating lobes limit the maximum amplification factor which should otherwise be as high as possible.

Thus, there is provision to provide controllable delays both for transmitted and received signals, which can be manipulated to "focus on send" as well as "focus on receive" signals.

Focusing single element mechanical transducers have weakly focused lenses which improve image in focal region but degrade it beyond.

The answer lies in electronic triggering and focusing by providing delay to outer elements compared to inner central ones. Often it is required to focus at multiple depths and obtaining image in strips at serial depths and obtaining a composites image. While beam is focused at particular depth, the echoes beyond focal depth are discarded using the electronic array, transducers do not require focusing of beam by lenses instead beam is steered electronically by utilizing the principle of interference by sequentially triggering the elements after controllable delay which determines the location and orientation of emerging wavefront relative to the transducer. The direction of travel of beam is at right angles to the wavefront. It appears as if the array transducers can bend the beam at will through a synthetic aperture.

Array transducers are made of a number of multiple elements connected by its own electronic circuitry to the pulse transmitter, attenuation and delay on input side and amplifier and variable delay on output side. Each element with its circuitry is known as channels. The channels in turn are connected to the computer range gate. This result in better image but frame rate is slowed down making it difficult to track moving structures. Also, total energy transferred to patient is increased.

The different elements in the array transducers receive returning echoes from a particular depth at different time delay resulting in artifactual high voltage signal. This can be offset by computer synchronization of calculated expected delay which is adjusted for each element. Resulting in "focus in receive" effect where echoes coming from an on the axis target to different elements are synchronized and preferentially amplified. Since the delay for the various distances is presumed to be calculated in on axis direction only, off axis target fail to synchronize and are ignored-resulting in effective focusing.

The annular array transducers have further advantage that focusing is possible both in the scanning as well as orthogonal planes, shape of beam being conical rather than wedge shaped. Annular arrays have weaker grating lobes and have potential for better spatial resolution, because they produce weaker grating lobes.

The width of beam at focus determines the lateral resolving power and is given as wavelength times the focal length divided by the aperture. The term of number is the focal length divided by aperture. Ideally beam width should be twice the wavelength. Hence, focused at 20 cm the aperture should be 10 cm wide. This can be possible only by electronic focusing in receive mode. This electronic focusing is also helpful for achieving zoom function. Also electronic focusing aperture can be varied for different depths—dynamic focusing, as more and more elements are recruited for focusing deeper and deeper.

Apodisation is the process to overcome the grating lobes' effect. The elements in outer edges of transducer are energized lesser than central elements. Something is achieved by amplifying echoes in channels of outer elements less than central elements.

Besides the digitization techniques to improve the image parameters like resolution, the other variables which affect the quality of image are those relating to the construction of the probe, for example damping provided improves resolution at the cost of sensitivity. Higher number of channels improve the performance but makes the transducer cable bulky.

The frequency of transducer is governed by the thickness of its piezoelectric crystal. Higher the frequency, thinner is the ultrasound generating element or crystal. Now multifrequency probes are available where it is possible to drive the probe at a frequency different than its resonant frequency.

The high frequency probes provide better lateral and axial resolution because narrower beams can result from decreased wavelength. Decreased beam width provides improved lateral resolution. Since pulse length also decreases at high frequency, the number of cycles in the pulse remaining the same, the axial resolution also improves. Usually axial resolution is half the pulse length.

The sensitivity of the ultrasound system is related to it's frequency, damping material, quarter wave matching and it's aperture. In a multifrequency probe though frequency quoted is the one at which power is maximum. The central frequency of the transducer tends to drop as the ultrasounds get attenuated deeper and deeper in the tissues. This requires correction by application and returning by radiofrequency amplifier set for lower frequencies. This allows higher amplification factor to be used resulting in better sensitivity of the system.

Ultrasound pulse must contain as few cycles as possible to improve axial resolution. This requires damping by a backing block with behind crystal with optimum mechanical characteristics. But efficient damping makes transducer rather insensitive.

Reverberation artifacts are produced when about 80% of returned ultrasound energy is not absorbed by transducer and gets reflected back in tissues. This can be overcome by more efficient transmission of energy back in transducer by quarter wave matching technique. Here, transducer is coated with a material, the impedance of which is the geometric mean of impedance of tissues and that of material and the thickness in the one quarter of the wavelength used.

Reverberation can also be tackled by using multiple matching layer transducers having a series of materials having a range of graded acoustic impedance rather than a single material with required impedance. Still another technique is the use of materials for transducer construction, having acoustic impedance matched to the soft-tissues. Though, such materials have good receiving characteristics, they are inefficient in producing ultrasound pulses.

Large aperture probes also improve the sensitivity because they collect more ultrasound energy.

There is another source of stationary noise, which appears immediately beyond the transducers because of sideways vibrations of transducer element. The transducer element vibrates not only across its width to produce useful beam but also sideways. These are eliminated by slicing of transducer crystal into number of thinner elements which are connected electronically, technique known as "sub-dicing", by sub-dicing frequency of sideway pulse becomes higher than wanted pulse and can get eliminated by tuning the amplifier.

Another consideration for scanning is the footprint of transducer, which must be smallest for cardiac work and

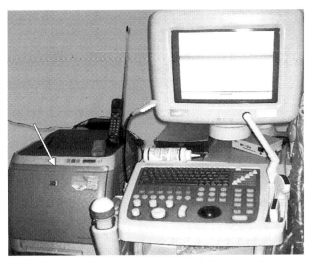

Fig. 7.24: US unit with printer (white arrow).

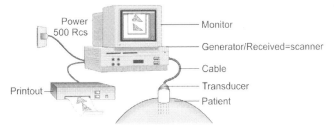

Fig. 7.25: An ultrasound unit.

relatively large for superficial soft tissues where linear or curvilinear array is preferable over sector scan.

Intracavitary probes: Need of these probes arises because external approach is limited by the reflection of sound at air/soft tissue inter faces, scattering and absorption of sound in soft tissues and refraction of sound by angulated soft tissue, muscle/fat interfaces. Intraoperative probes too like intracavitary probes provide high resolution. Besides they have small footprint and not too bulky cable.

Ultrasound Scanning (Fig. 7.24)

Room must be adequate size to accommodate scanner, couch, chair, small table, and desk and also allow trolley to be wheeled in and it be transferred to couch. Room must be kept dry and free from dust. Wall may be of any color and material as no radiation hazard from diagnostic ultrasound machine.

There should be facility for washing hands and drinking water preferably in room and should be toilet facility near by. Couch should be clean and firm but soft. It should be possible to lift one end. It should have good wheels.

Voltage should be adequate, i.e., 220 V at 5A°. If there is too much fluctuation, should always be used with voltage stabilizer.

There should be adequate ventilation and lightening preferably with dimmer switch. Bright light should be screened or contained off as it is not possible to see the image in bright light as shown in **Figure 7.25**.

CHAPTER 8

Scanning Techniques in Sonography

In this chapter the techniques of ultrasound scanning in various organs will be discussed:
- Adults
  - Abdomen—(i) liver, spleen, gallbladder and bile ducts, pancreas, gastrointestinal tract, urinary tract, prostate, adrenals, retroperitoneum, peritoneum, diaphragm abdominal wall, and (ii) gynecological and obstetric ultrasound.
  - Thorax—pleural space, mediastinum.
  - Small parts–eye and orbit, salivary glands, thyroid gland, breast, scrotum, and penis.
  - Joints and tendons—rotator cuff, elbow, wrist, and knee.
- Children
  - Abdomen
  - Brain
  - Spinal canal
  - Hip joint

Adult Abdomen

Liver

Ideally the patient should fast for a minimum of six hours before the examination so that bowel gas is limited.

Liver is examined in both supine **(Fig. 8.1A)** and RAO **(Fig. 8.1B)** positions if the patient can move or be moved. An intercostal approach **(Fig. 8.1C)** is very useful in patients in whom the liver does not extend below the right costal margin; for this a transducer with a small scanning face is used. Deep inspiration enables examination of the dome of the liver **(Fig. 8.1D)**.

Spleen

No specific patient preparation is required since the spleen is a superficial structure; a 5 MHz transducer is recommended. Sector or curvilinear transducers can be used.

The patient is supine and the transducer is placed in the coronal plane of section posteriorly **(Fig. 8.2A)** in one of the intercostal spaces. Inspiration depresses the left dome of diaphragm and spleen inferiorly so that they can be visualized. The plane of section is then swept anteriorly and posteriorly to view the entire spleen.

Often a more posterior approach can be used to visualize the spleen, by turning the patient to his right side by 45°– 90° **(Figs. 8.2B and C)**.

An oblique plane of section along an intercostal space **(Fig. 8.2D)** can be used to avoid obscuration by rib shadowing.

A transverse plane from a lateral intercostal approach may help localize a lesion within the anterior or posterior part of spleen.

If the spleen is enlarged or if there is a mass in the left upper quadrant of abdomen, the spleen may be visualized from an anterior approach. If the left lobe of liver is enlarged, we may be able to see the spleen through it.

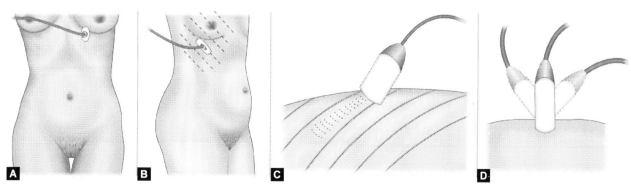

Figs. 8.1A to D: (A) Angle transducer; (B) Left side down; (C) Intercostal; and (D) Slow tracking movement of transducer in all planes.

Gallbladder

Cholecystosonography should be performed in a patient fasting overnight for 8–12 hours to ensure adequate physiological distension of the gallbladder. Physiologic contraction of the gallbladder may be misinterpreted as a pathological, small and thick-walled gallbladder.

In most patients a 3.5 MHz transducer is used, while in thin patients or in those with an anteriorly placed gallbladder a 5 MHz transducer would provide better resolution. A sector transducer is better than linear array because the former is smaller and can be easily positioned in the intercostal spaces.

Extreme obesity or overlying bowel loops may prevent a satisfactory examination of gallbladder.

Patient is in supine **(Fig. 8.3A)** or in a left oblique position **(Fig. 8.3B)**. Scanning is done through a subcostal **(Fig. 8.3C)** or sometimes a lower intercostal approach **(Fig. 8.3D)**. Optimal images can be obtained if patient suspends respiration after a deep inspiratory effort. Occasionally patient has to be scanned in erect **(Fig. 8.3E)** or prone position to demonstrate mobility of calculi.

A thorough examination of the gallbladder (GB) is possible in 5–10 min but the technique must be meticulous to prevent missing small calculi. Special attention should be directed to the dependant region of GB, which is the neck and cystic duct in most patients.

Extrahepatic Bile Duct

Common bile duct (CBD) is most commonly examined by parasagittal scans **(Fig. 8.4)** with the patient in supine LPO (left posterior oblique) position. But this position is not satisfactory to visualize the distal CBD which is obscured by gas-filled duodenum.

So first the distal CBD should be examined with patient in erect right posterior oblique (RPO) position, and rely more on transverse scans than parasagittal scans. The erect RPO position minimizes gas in the antrum and duodenum whereas the transverse scan plane maximizes the ability to trace the course of intrapancreatic bile duct. If overlying bowel gas obscures this region, the patient should be given 400–500 mL water to drink, placed in a right lateral decubitus position for 2–3 min and rescanned in erect RPO position.

Examination of distal CBD should be followed by examination of proximal CBD.

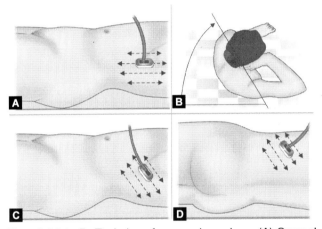

Figs. 8.2A to D: Technique for scanning spleen. (A) Coronal plane; (B) Right side down; (C) Posterior approach; and (D) Intercostal scanning.

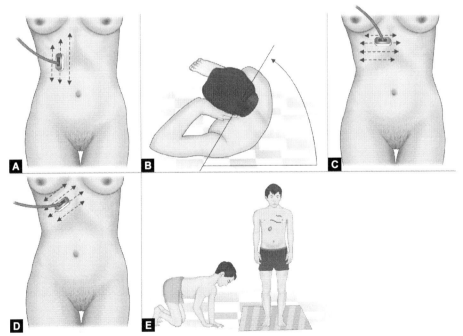

Figs. 8.3A to E: (A) Supine; (B) Left oblique position longitudinal; (C) Subcostal; (D) Lower intercostal; and (E) Erect.

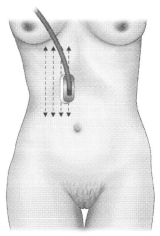

Fig. 8.4: Parasagittal scan.

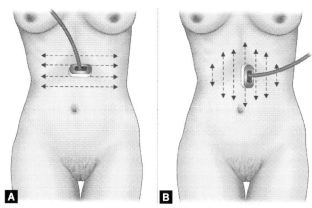

Figs. 8.5A and B: (A) Transverse; and (B) Sagittal.

In most patients examination of extrahepatic bile ducts can be completed in 5–10 min. In difficult cases the study may take as long as 15–30 min.

Pancreas

A minimum fasting of six hours is required for ultrasound examination of the pancreas. This decreases the gaseous distention of the upper GI tract which can interfere with visualization of the pancreas.

Sonographic examination of the pancreas should begin with the patient in erect position. This displaces the gas-filled colon away from the pancreas and causes the liver to move down providing an acoustic window to the pancreas. The erect position is most effective if used in the beginning of the examination because aerophagia caused by deep inspirations during examination fills the stomach with gas.

Transverse scans are made in the midline below the xiphisternum **(Fig. 8.5A)** and vascular landmarks used to identify region of pancreas. The probe may need to be oblique to visualize the entire gland. From the level of longitudinal view of splenic vein, if the transducer is angled cephalad and caudal, the entire pancreas can usually be adequately scanned.

For sagittal scans **(Fig. 8.5B)** the probe is placed in the midline below the xiphisternum and the pancreas is localized by identifying the splenoportal confluence. Tilting the probe towards right or left is more effective than lateral movement.

With a left coronal view, using the left kidney as an acoustic window, the tail of pancreas may be identified anterior to left kidney. In some thin patients, the tail of pancreas can be seen through the spleen, from a left intercostal approach using a coronal plane.

Supine, oblique, and decubitus positions may be required to displace gas-containing loops of intestine. Also, suspended inspiration, expiration or Valsalva maneuver may be helpful in examination of pancreas.

If all the above methods are unsuccessful, distending the stomach with water may allow pancreatic visualization.

Patient is made to drink a large volume of water (500 mL) through a straw to minimize air swallowing. The fluid-filled stomach causes displacement of intragastric gas and acts as a balloon displacing colon and small bowel gas inferiorly.

Gastrointestinal Tract

Patient should be fasting. The pelvis is scanned with the bladder full and after it is emptied because a full bladder may displace bowel loops.

The entire abdomen is surveyed with a 3.5 or 5 MHz linear, convex linear and sometimes sector probe **(Figs. 8.6A to C)**.

Compression sonography is performed in the regions of interest by applying slow, gentle increase in pressure of compression. Normal gut loops will be compressed and displaced away while thickened, abnormal or obstructed noncompressible loops will remain unchanged. Patients with peritonitis or even local tenderness will tolerate graded compression, but may have pain if scanning is rapid and uneven.

Occasionally to establish gastric origin of intraluminal or intramural gastric masses, oral fluid may be given during sonography.

Fluid enema may also aid sonography. Appendix is evaluated with a 7.5 MHz linear array probe with graded compression over the right iliac fossa.

Urinary Tract

Kidney No specific preparation is required for renal imaging. Visualization of renal vessels is optimum with patient fasting.

3 to 5 MHz transducer may be used depending on patient habitus.

Kidneys should be scanned in at least two planes **(Figs. 8.7A and B)**. Patient position may be supine, posterior oblique, and decubitus **(Fig. 8.7C)** or prone **(Figs. 8.7D and E)**. Occasionally intercostal scanning, or scanning in upright position and in varying phases of respiration may be required.

Renal morphology and respiratory excursion should be assessed.

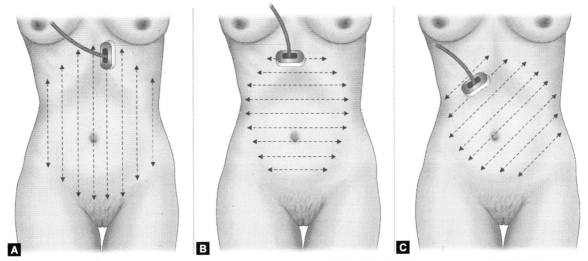

Figs. 8.6A to C: Scanning of abdomen in different plane. (A) Sagittal; (B) Transverse; and (C) Oblique.

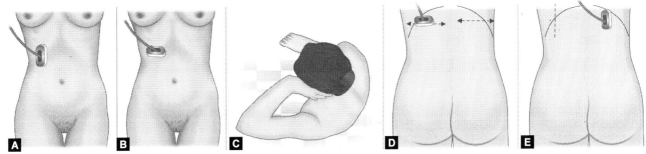

Figs. 8.7A to E: (A and B) Patient holds breath in during scanning; (C) Left decubitus; and (D and E) Prone position.

Ureters proximal ureters are best seen in coronal oblique view using the kidneys as acoustic window. Distal ureter is visualized, if dilated, using urine-filled urinary bladder as a window.

Urinary bladder: It is best evaluated when moderately full **(Figs. 8.8A and B)**. If several cystic masses are seen in the pelvis, to confirm which of the cystic structures is the bladder voiding or insertion of a urethral catheter is useful. UB is also evaluated for residual urine volume after voiding.

Prostate Gland

Transrectal ultrasound (TRUS)

Before scanning, a self-administered enema is routinely used. Per-rectal examination is performed prior to insertion of probe to detect any abnormality of prostate and exclude any rectal abnormality which may interfere with the scan.

Transrectal probes of 5–8 MHz have been developed to perform ultrasound of the prostate. Many probes require a water bath between the crystal and rectal mucosa to decrease near-field artifact and allow better visualization of the peripheral zone which may be very near to the rectal wall. Air bubbles should be eliminated from this system to prevent artifacts.

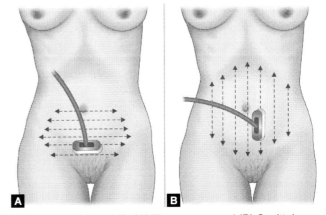

Figs. 8.8A and B: (A) Transverse; and (B) Sagittal.

Probes are covered with condom during examination. In patients who have allergy to latex condoms, alternate covers should be used.

Patient is placed in left lateral decubitus or lithotomy position. Following adequate lubrication probe is gently inserted into the rectum and balloon inflated with water, if necessary.

A systematic approach is necessary when examining the prostate. Begin in the transverse or semi-coronal plane to

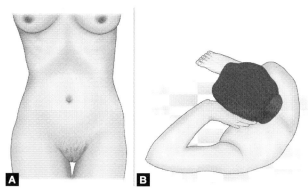

Figs. 8.9A and B: Adrenal (suprarenal) gland (A) Supine position; and (B) Lateral decubitus position.

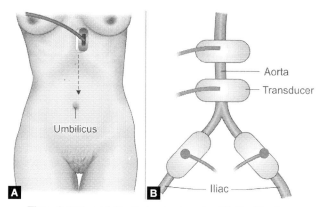

Figs. 8.10A and B: Abdominal aorta. (A) Positioning; (B) Parasagittal scan.

identify the seminal vesicles. Then examine the base of the prostate with demonstration of the central zone, transition zone and periurethral glandular area. The urethra and ejaculatory ducts may be identified. In the sagittal plane, rotating from right to left will assess glandular asymmetry and confirm any suspicious abnormality seen on axial or coronal imaging.

After use, the probe should be soaked in an antiseptic solution, e.g., glutaraldehyde. Manufacturer's instructions should be followed regarding depth of insertion of probe into the solution.

Adrenal Glands

Fasting for 6–8 hours is preferred as it helps to decrease bowel gas 3 to 3.5 MHz transducer is used. Sector transducers provide better access through the intercostal space while linear transducer may be useful in examining large masses. Patient is examined in supine **(Fig. 8.9A)** and lateral decubitus positions **(Fig. 8.9B)** in both transverse and longitudinal planes.

For evaluation of right adrenal an intercostal approach through the liver in the mid or anterior axillary line is best. Scanning in the left lateral decubitus position or anteriorly through the liver may also be useful.

The left adrenal is best examined from an intercostal approach along posterior axillary line or even farther posteriorly using spleen as a window. Right lateral decubitus or right posterior oblique positions may also be helpful. If the left adrenal is obscured by bowel gas, scanning may be done anteriorly using fluid-filled stomach as a window.

It is important to identify the echogenic retroperitoneal fat stripe of the anterior pararenal + perirenal spaces on a longitudinal scan. Anterior displacement of this stripe denotes a retroperitoneal mass, while posterior or inferior displacement suggests a hepatic or subhepatic pathology. Further, a wedge-shaped anterior displacement suggests a mass of suprarenal rather than renal origin.

Retroperitoneum

Patient fasts for 6–8 hours to decrease bowel gas which may interfere with visualization of retroperitoneum. Obesity may also cause suboptimal visualization of aorta, 3.5 MHz linear probe is used. If the patient is thin a 5 MHz transducer may be used.

Initially patient is examined in supine position. Coronal or near-coronal scans using kidney and posterior musculature as acoustic window can give excellent images in patients in whom bowel gas obscures the retroperitoneum in supine position. IVC may be seen in left lateral decubitus position also **(Fig. 8.10A)**. Changes in patient position and return to the region after other parts of the abdomen have been examined, may yield better results.

Abdominal aorta and IVC should be examined from diaphragm to iliac bifurcation at umbilicus in parasagittal **(Fig. 8.10B)** and transverse planes. The IVC is frequently not visualized beyond inferior margin of liver.

Peritoneum

No patient preparation is required. For scanning 3.5 or 5 MHz sector transducer is used. If a superficial lesion is detected a higher frequency linear probe may offer better visualization.

Patient is scanned in supine position. Decubitus scans may help to differentiate loculated and free fluid collections. When examining a collection with air-fluid level, it may be helpful to scan from a posterior approach, through the fluid-filled dependent portion, to prevent scanning through air which reflects sound waves.

Abdominal Wall

No patient preparation is required.
A high frequency linear probe is used. Skin is out of focus even with high frequency transducers. So stand-off techniques are used, e.g., flotation pads, polymer blocks and silicone elastomer blocks commercially available. These substances can stand unsupported and minimize artifacts.

To examine the abdominal wall, after removing dressings, an adhesive plastic membrane is applied over surgical wounds. This sterile adhesive prevents contamination of the wound by the transducer and vice versa. Pressure over wounds and other tender areas should be gentle.

Diaphragm

It is scanned with patient supine or sitting, in quiet respiration. Coughing or sniffing tests may be used to assess diaphragmatic motion.

Uterus and Adnexa

Transabdominal Sonography

Patient should have a distended urinary bladder which provides an acoustic window to the pelvic organs and displaces bowel loops out of the pelvis. Urinary bladder is considered ideally filled when it covers the entire fundus of uterus. Over distention may distort the anatomy by compression and also push pelvic organs beyond focal zone of the transducer.

3.5 MHz probe is generally satisfactory. Imaging is performed in the sagittal **(Fig. 8.11A)** and transverse planes **(Fig. 8.11B)**. Somewhat oblique angulations may be necessary to visualize the entire uterus and cervix. Adnexae can be scanned obliquely from contralateral side **(Fig. 8.11C)**, although usually visualization is possible by scanning directly over the adnexa.

This technique has limitations in patients who are not able to hold urine adequately, in obese patients and patients with retroverted uterus.

Transvaginal Sonography (TVS)

A preliminary transabdominal scan should be performed prior to the transvaginal scan for an overview of urinary bladder, uterus, ovaries, and adnexa. Urinary bladder must be empty to bring the pelvic organs into focal zone of transvaginal transducer.

Transducers for TVS range from 5.0–7.5 MHz frequency.

Patient is supine with knees gently flexed and hips elevated slightly on a pillow. Transducers is prepared with ultrasound gel and then covered with a condom which is lubricated externally **(Fig. 8.11D)** with gentle rotation and angulations of the transducer, both sagittal and coronal scans are obtained. Slight anterior angulation will bring the fundus of anteverted uterus into view. To visualize the cervix the transducer must be pulled slightly out away from the external OS. Extreme angulation may be required to visualize the entire adnexal and cul-de-sac.

Disadvantage of TVS is its limited field of view which makes examination of large masses difficult; and superiorly placed ovaries may not be visualized **(Fig. 8.11E)**.

TVS is used to supplement transabdominal sonography.

Obstetric Ultrasound

Linear array real time scanner is used to allow significant image width to achieve head and body measurements with minimal distortion. Because of increased detail of the image sector real time scanners are also being widely used but the main disadvantage is the limited field of view.

Patient is required to have a full bladder for evaluation of early pregnancy, to move the bowel loops out of the pelvis. In later pregnancy full bladder may be required for detailed evaluation of the lower uterine segment or better imaging of fetal structures in the caudal portion of uterus. Patient is supine and her abdomen is coated with coupling gel **(Fig. 8.12)**.

A series of longitudinal scans are obtained with the probe placed at the pubic bone and moved cephalad while angling to remain perpendicular to the structures being visualized. After a midline sagittal scan, a series of sagittal scans moving from right side of uterus to left in small intervals is recorded. Then, transverse scans are obtained beginning at the pubic bone in small increments, up to the fundus. The transducer should be perpendicular to the uterine surface with each scan. Then random scans of fetal head and body are made for measurement of diameter or circumference and pertinent small sector scans are made in any region of interest. Fetal heart rate, movement and breathing are quickly assessed.

THORAX

Pleural Space

Direct approach: A high frequency 5 MHz linear transducer is applied to the chest wall with the probe perpendicular to intercostal spaces **(Fig. 8.13)**. Sector probes have a narrow view in near field, so are unsatisfactory for examining pleural space by applying directly to the chest wall.

Abdominal approach: The lower reaches of the pleural space are effectively examined by the use of a lower frequency (3.5 MHz) sector probe directed superiorly from the abdomen. Liver and spleen provide sonographic window to the thorax.

MEDIASTINUM

- Suprasternal approach provides sonographic access to upper mediastinum.

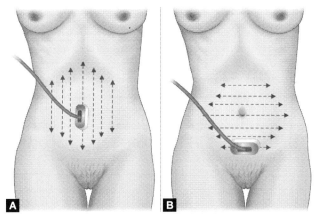

Figs. 8.11A and B: (A) Sagittal plane; and (B) Transverse plane.

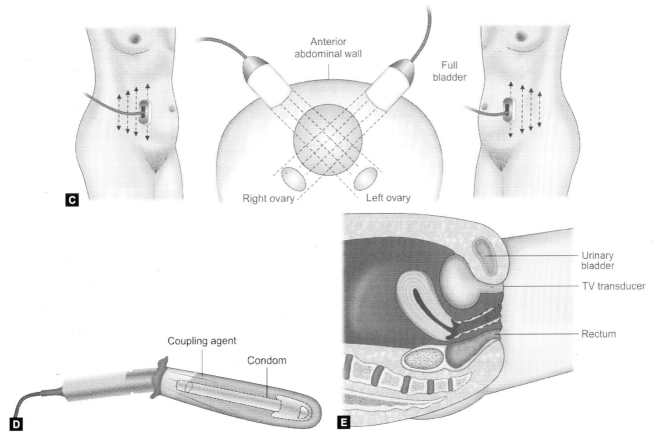

Figs. 8.11C to E: (C) Oblique scan; (D) Endovaginal transducer with cover and coupling agent; (E) Transvaginal sonography.

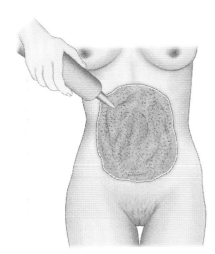

Fig. 8.12: Supine position.

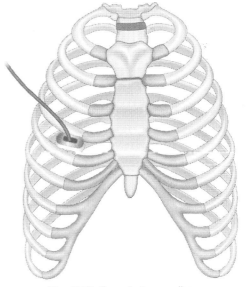

Fig. 8.13: Scan between ribs.

Patient is supine with a pillow beneath the shoulders and neck extended. Probe is placed at the base of the neck and angled behind the manubrium. Oblique, sagittal, and coronal images can be obtained.
- Parasagittal scanning of mediastinum is carried out by placing patient in appropriate lateral decubitus position. Gravity enlarges the sonographic window by swinging the mediastinum downwards. Ascending aorta, anterior mediastinum and subcarinal regions are best evaluated from a right parasternal approach with patient lying with right side down. The pulmonary trunk and left side of anterior mediastinum are scanned with left parasternal approach with patient is left lateral decubitus position.
- Posterior paravertebral approach is used to scan posterior mediastinal masses.

- Lesions near the diaphragm may be scanned from abdomen, through the liver.
- Large masses displace lung and may be scanned directly through intercostal spaces.

Eye and Orbit

2 D scanning of eye is carried out using a short focus 7.5 or 10 MHz real time small parts probe.

Patient is supine to give stability to the head. Examination is routinely carried out by the 'contact' method in which the probe is placed directly on a closed eyelid with an intervening coupling gel. Some probes require direct contact with a typically anesthetized eyeball. A 'water bath' method is useful for viewing anterior structures. Image the globe with the eye static in primary (straight ahead) position and then during rapid eye movements with the patient deviating the eyes to the right and left side and in all directions of gaze. Following an ocular excursion, movements may continue for 1 sec approximately.

Contact method is suitable for orbital scanning using 5–10 MHz transducer. Horizontal scanning is more readily carried out than scanning in the vertical plane.

SALIVARY GLANDS

Parotid Gland

It is evaluated with a high frequency linear small parts transducer with or without a stand-off pad, in the axial and coronal planes.

For axial images the transducer should be placed perpendicular to the ear, with its superior margin touching the lobule. The parotid gland is seen as an echogenic homogeneous mass located just beneath the skin surface. Coronal images are obtained by placing the transducer just anterior and parallel to the ear. The probe is then angled anteriorly and posteriorly.

Submandibular Glands

It is best scanned from a submental position with the transducer angled in both sagittal and coronal plane. The position of Wharton's duct can be seen by asking patients to move their tongue. This reveals the plane between mylohyoid and hyoglossus, where the duct runs.

Sublingual Glands

They are difficult to see sonographically.

Thyroid Gland

The 7.5 to 10 MHz linear array transducers are preferred as they provide a high resolution and wide field of view near the face of the transducer.

Patient is in supine with neck extended. A small pad may be placed under the shoulder to provide better exposure of the neck in patients with a short neck. The examiner sits at the head of the table usually and can steady the probe by resting the elbow or forearm on the table next to patient's head.

Thyroid must be examined thoroughly in transverse and longitudinal planes from upper pole to lower pole including isthmus. The lower pole of thyroid can be scanned easily by asking the patient to swallow, which raises the gland momentarily in the neck. The examination should also be extended laterally to include the region of carotid artery and jugular vein in order to identify any enlarged cervical lymph nodes.

In addition to recording images on film, a diagrammatic representation of the neck, mapping the location of any abnormal findings is also kept as permanent record for follow-up studies.

Breast

Hand-held ultrasound transducers are preferred over automated scanners as the former can perform the examination more rapidly, can better characterize a known mass and can more easily allow interventional procedures. Dynamically focused phased array, linear array and annular array transducers of 5 to 7.5 MHz are available. Standard-sized transducers and small intraoperative probes are both appropriate for breast sonography. High frequency mechanical sector probes are also suitable for breast ultrasound. The use of an offset acoustic pad often improves resolution of near-field lesions.

Adequate sonographic penetration is assured if underlying pectoral muscles and ribs are visualized.

Patient is in a supine oblique position in which bulk of breast tissue falls to contralateral side. The shoulder and torso of the side to be examined are elevated by a wedge to minimize thickness of upper outer quadrant breast tissue. The ipsilateral arm is elevated and flexed at the elbow with hand resting comfortably under the neck. Contralateral arm remains at the patient's side.

For imaging areas other than upper outer quadrant, place the patient supine with arms at her sides or behind her head.

An entire quadrant is scanned in transverse and sagittal planes. Suspected abnormality should be viewed orthogonally so that a pseudomass will not be misinterpreted as a true lesion. For example a fat lobule and fibroadenoma may resemble each other on one view but when the probe is rotated through 90°, the fat lobule appears elongated rather than rounded.

Nipple-areolar complex examination requires special technique. The air gaps between the irregular skin surface and transducer face; and fibrous elements in the nipple, produce posterior acoustic shadowing which obscure the retroareolar region. This region may be examined by placing the probe next to the nipple and angling towards retroareolar area.

If a palpable abnormality has to be examined the patient should assume that position in which the lesion is felt-sitting or standing, and locate the area with her fingers. Then this region can be scanned.

Sonographic evaluation of multiple lesions may be confusing as a lesion may be counted more than once if seen from different angles and location. Try to isolate a lesion manually, pushing it outside the scanning field.

If there is uncertainty in correlating sonographic with mammographic or palpatory findings, a small radiopaque marker can be placed on the skin overlying the lesion and this area can be restudied sonographically.

SCROTUM

Thorough history and palpation of scrotal contents should precede the sonographic examination. Patient is asked to localize painful sites and palpable nodules. This is useful during examination by sonographer.

7.5 or 10 MHz transducer is commonly used. If greater penetration is needed in a patient with marked scrotal swelling a 3.5 or 5 MHz probe may be used.

Scrotum is elevated with a towel draped over the thighs and penis is placed on the patient's abdomen and covered with a towel. Alternatively, the scrotal sac may be supported by examiner's hand.

Both testes are examined in transverse and sagittal planes. If possible, obtain a transverse scan demonstrating both testes for comparison. Additional views may be obtained when necessary in coronal and oblique planes. In suspicion of varicoceles the scan should be performed with valsalva maneuver as well as in standing position.

PENIS

7.5 to 10 MHz linear array transducer is used. Patient is supine with penis lying on anterior abdominal wall.

Transducer is placed on ventral surface of penis scanning transversely from glans down to base of penis. Longitudinal evaluation should be obtained from ventral surface. Penile urethra is optimally visualized by distending it with viscous lidocaine gel using a tapered tip syringe inserted into the urethral meatus. A distal penile clamp is applied to maintain distention of penile urethra.

Rotator Cuff

High resolution linear array 7 MHz transducers are preferred for examination of the shoulder.

Patient is seated on a revolving stool which allows easy positioning during scanning. Sonographer is also seated on a stool with wheels to enhance his mobility during examination.

Both shoulders are examined starting with the normal or less affected side.

The examination begins with a transverse image of the bicipital groove which serves as a landmark to distinguish subscapularis from supraspinatus. The groove appears as a concavity in the bright echoes of the bony surface of humerus. The tendon of long head of biceps is seen as a hypoechoic oval structure in the bicipital groove. This view is important to detect even small amounts of intra-articular fluid surrounding the biceps tendon.

The probe is then moved proximally along the humerus to visualize the subscapularis tendon as a band of medium-level echoes deep to the subdeltoid bursa. The subdeltoid bursa is seen as a thin convex echogenic line when scanning is done parallel to the axis of subscapularis. Passive internal and external rotation may be helpful in assessing the integrity of subscapularis. Turning the probe by 90° and scanning perpendicular to axis of subscapularis may be helpful in patients with chronic anterior dislocation.

The supraspinatous tendon is scanned perpendicular to its axis (transversely) by moving the probe laterally and posteriorly. The sonographic window is narrower so careful transducer positioning is essential. The supraspinatous tendon is seen as a band of medium level echoes deep to subdeltoid bursa and superficial to bony surface of greater tuberosity. It is essential to demonstrate the critical zone (i.e., the portion of the tendon that begins approximately 1 cm posterolateral to the biceps tendon), which is most susceptible to injury. Failure to visualize this area may cause a false negative result.

By moving the transducer posteriorly, in a plane parallel to dorsal spine of scapula, the infraspinatous tendon is visualized as a beak-shaped soft tissue structure which attaches to the posterior aspect of greater tuberosity. Passive internal and external rotation is helpful in examination. At this level a portion of the glenoid labrum is seen as a hyperechoic triangular structure.

By moving the transducer distally on the humerus the teres minor is seen as a trapezoid structure, differentiated from the infraspinatus by its oblique internal echoes. Although this muscle is rarely torn very small intra-articular effusions may be best visualized at this level. Its visualization also ensures that the complete infraspinatous has been scanned.

The probe is then moved anteriorly and turned by 90° to view the biceps tendon parallel to its long axis. If the transducer is not parallel to the biceps tendon, parts of it will appear hypoechoic artifactually.

The probe is then moved posteriorly so that the supraspinatus tendon is viewed parallel to its axis. The tendon appears as a beak-shaped structure of medium-level echoes extending from under the acromion, which casts an acoustic shadow to its attachment along the greater tuberosity. The bright, linear echoes from subdeltoid bursa identify the superficial margin of supraspinatous tendon. Passive abduction-adduction is helpful in assessing the integrity of supraspinatous tendon. By placing the patient's arm behind his back and scanning parallel and perpendicular to supraspinatous fibers, tendons obscured by the acromion may be visualized. Small tears and effusions may be accentuated with this maneuver.

Tendons

Linear array electronic transducers of 7.5 to 10 MHz provide exquisite results because of their wider field of view and better near field resolution, for tendon sonography.

The combination of longitudinal and transverse scans provides a three-dimensional approach to the tendon. Scanning the contralateral normal region can be available reference for normal anatomy. Tendons should be examined at rest and during active and passive flexion/extension. Performing palpation under real time sonography can also be useful.

If the transducer is not parallel to the surface of the tendon, obliquity of the ultrasound beam can cause an artifactual hypoechogenicity of the tendon. Changing the position of the probe or suppressing the curvature of the tendon through muscle contraction, clears this artifact.

Elbow (Figs. 8.14A to G)

With the elbow flexed at 90°, the tendon of triceps brachii is readily identified on coronal and transverse scans. The common tendons of the flexor and extensor muscles of forearm arising from medial and lateral epicondyle respectively are also best demonstrated with the elbow flexed at this angle.

Wrist

In the carpal tunnel, the echogenic flexor tendons of the fingers are surrounded by the hypoechoic ulnar bursa and are best seen when the wrist is moderately flexed.

Knee

Because both the quadriceps and patellar tendons may be slightly concave anteriorly when the knee is extended and at rest, scans should be obtained during contraction of the quadriceps muscle or with knee flexed, which straightens the tendons and eliminates artifacts.

Collateral ligaments and cruciate ligaments are not well delineated on sonography.

Pediatric Abdomen

In an infant 7.5 MHz transducers and in a child 5.0 MHz transducers are used. Different types of transducers are used for different parts of the body, e.g., linear, convex, or sector transducers. No special preparation is necessary except for a period of fasting in children with jaundice or when gallbladder pathology is suspected.

Pediatric patients vary in their ability to hold still for a sufficient period of time for scanning. So infants under three months of age can be fed during examination and immobilized with wraps. From three months to three years of age children may require sedation. This can be done in the ultrasound department and the child monitored during the procedure and also examined before being sent home. Children more than three years of age can be distracted or entertained during the examination by watching videotapes on a VCR or playing with toys. Parents should always be allowed to accompany children as they can act as a very valuable restraining device.

For examination of the urinary bladder in a young child who is not toilet trained yet, the scanning has to be timed with bladder filling. Child is given fluids to drink in the department and the bladder checked frequently, as the patient may fill and void suddenly.

For examination of pediatric pelvis in children who are unable to maintain a full bladder, it may be necessary to catheterize an empty bladder and fill it with sterile water.

Gastroesophageal junction can be visualized in longitudinal plane images with patient supine or right lateral decubitus position. Gastroesophageal reflux can be demonstrated when echogenic fluid (i.e., fluid mixed with air bubbles) is regurgitated into the retrocardiac portion of esophagus. However, this is usually assessed with other imaging modalities or endoscopy.

Appendix is imaged with a 7.5 MHz linear array transducer. For evaluation of acute appendicitis ask the patient where the abdominal pain is located and thereafter imaging is performed over this area with uniform graded compression.

Pediatric Brain

5 MHz rotating or mechanical sector scanners having a good sector angle of about 120° are used for adequate sound penetration of a large infant's head. Good skin-to-transducer coupling can be achieved by an acoustic coupling gel. A stand-off pad can be useful in evaluating superficial abnormalities, e.g., subdural hemorrhage.

The anterior fontanelle is suitable for scanning until 12-14 months. Through this acoustic window scans are obtained in the coronal and sagittal planes. Axial scans were used in the past for accurate measurement of ventricular dimensions. Cranial scanning using posterior and posterolateral fontanelles and foramen magnum have been described.

Every attempt should be made to maintain body temperature in premature infants during cranial sonography including use of warmed coupling gel. Hand washing and cleaning of probe head with alcohol is important to avoid spread of infection to the child. The probe is held firmly between thumb and index finger and hand should rest on infant's head for stability.

For coronal scans the probe is placed transversely across the anterior fontanelle and the sound beam is made to sweep anterior to posterior through the entire brain. Take care to maintain symmetry of image of each half of brain and skull. At least six standard frozen coronal images must be made. The most anterior cut should be at or just anterior to frontal horns in the frontal cortex. The second cut contains frontal horns and bifurcation of internal carotid into middle and anterior cerebral arteries. The third cut should be

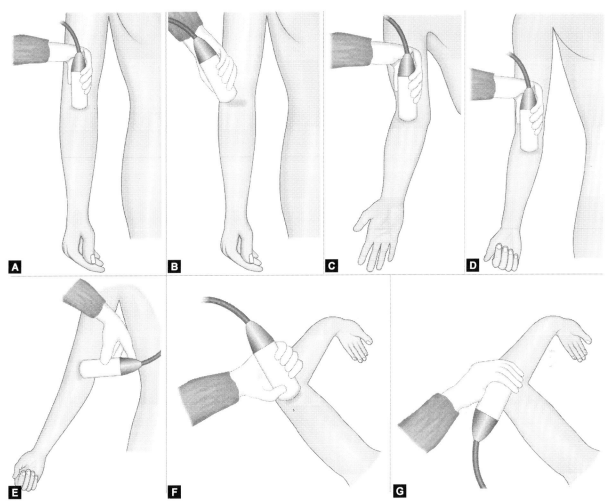

Figs. 8.14A to G: (A) Anterior longitudinal view—lateral aspect of elbow. This plane allows the visualization of radiohumeral articulation and capitulum. Diagram shows neutral position of hand and transducer is aligned with radiohumeral articulation along lateral aspects of elbow; (B) Shows slight obliquity necessary to align transducer a long axis of common extensor muscle group of forearm. Note that hand remains neutrally positioned to show tendinous origin of common forearm extensor muscle group from lateral epicondyle; (C) This plane is useful for evaluation of radioulnar articulation and for watching supination and pronation of proximal radius. Drawing shows transverse orientation of transducer so that side of image on viewer left is assigned for lateral aspect of elbow joint. Hand is supinated; (D) Anterior longitudinal view used for visualization of ulnohumeral articulation and coronoid process of ulna. Drawing shows transducer aligned longitudinally along long axis of ulna to visualize ulnohumeral articulation. Hand is supinated; (E) Anterior anteromedial longitudinal sonogram. This view is designed to visualize common tendon from which forearm flexor muscle group arise. Drawing shows that with hand in supination, transducer is slightly oblique to match long axis of common forearm flexor muscle group arising from common tendon attached to medial epicondyle; (F) Posterior midline longitudinal sonogram. This plane is useful in evaluating distal humerus and displacement of post fat-pad indicating fluid in joint. Drawing shows that for posterior scanning, arm is elevated 180° next to patient's head and elbow flexed 90° transducer should be oriented so that proximal portion of arm is oriented to viewers left on image; (G) Posterior superior transducer with sonogram. This view is useful in identifying fluid in joint and displacement of fat pad. Epicondylar injuries may also be detected. Drawing shows that arm remains in same position and transducer is oriented transversely at level of post-fat pad in olecranon fossae of distal humerus.

through the sylvian fissures and brainstem. The next cut is through the quadrigeminal cistern. The fifth cut should be through the posterior trigones. The most posterior cut should be behind the trigone in the occipital cortex.

The sagittal images are obtained by placing the probe longitudinally across the anterior fontanelle and then angling to each side by 10° and 20°.

Pediatric Spinal Canal

5 or 7.5 MHz linear array transducer is used for progressing along the longitudinal axis of the spinal canal in the sagittal plane. Sometimes a 10 MHz linear array probe may be needed.

Patient is prone or in a lateral decubitus position for scanning. Patient should be placed prone over a pillow to flex the thoracolumbar spine and separate the spinous processes. This widens the acoustic window to the spinal canal. Head may be elevated slightly to help distend the caudal end of thecal sac.

Neonates and young infants are studied from the midline between the spinous processes because their posterior vertebral elements are unossified. A broad, longitudinal view of the spinal canal over several segments is obtained and by using a split screen and combining the two aligned half screens, and gets a long panoramic longitudinal view.

In older infants and children, the transducer is placed slightly lateral and parallel to the spinous processes. From this parasagittal position the probe is directed medially into the spinal canal. Access is limited to interlaminar spaces which gives a more segmented view of the spinal canal. Yet it is adequately informative in children up to 10 years age.

Sometimes a sonographer may have a problem in correctly judging the depth, i.e., he may look either too shallowly or too deeply. In such cases it is helpful to start scanning over the sacrum where the spinal canal is easily found and then follow the spinal canal in a cephalad direction.

Pediatric Hip (Fig. 8.15)

For infants up to three months of age 7.5 MHz transducer is used. A 5 MHz transducer is generally required between three and seven months of age. Sonographic examinations are currently performed with real time linear array transducers.

For examination the child lies supine with feet towards the sonographer. When examining the left hip, the sonographer grasps the infant's left leg with the left hand and the probe is held in the right hand. When the right hip is examined, it is recommended that the sonographer hold the probe in the left hand and use the right hand to manipulate the child's right leg. This technique may be found awkward initially.

No sedation is required. Infants may be fed before examination; parents can hold the infant's arms or head and talk to the infant; toys may be used for attracting their attention. Upper body remains clothed, the infant remains diapered with only the side being examined exposed.

In dynamic hip sonography the stability of the hip is determined through motion and application of stress in a manner analogous to the "Barlow and Ortolani clinical maneuvers."

Transverse/neutral view: The transducer is directed horizontally into the acetabulum from the lateral aspect

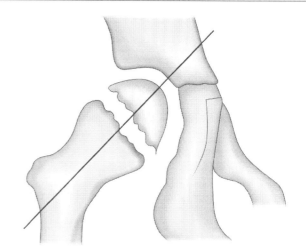

Fig. 8.15: Sonographic scan plane along with neck of femur for detecting joint effusion in hip joint.

of the hip. The plane of interest is one that passes through the femoral head into the acetabulum at the center of the triradiate cartilage. The sonogram resembles the components of a flower. The femoral head represents the flower and the echoes from ischium posteriorly and pubis anteriorly, forms the leaves at its base. Acoustic shadowing from ossific nucleus of femoral head should not be mistaken for triradiate cartilage because there are no echoes in the gap. The sonographer must angle the plane of the transducer above or below the nucleus to identify the triradiate cartilage.

Transverse/flexion view: From the previous position this view is obtained by flexing the femur 90° and transducer maintained in a horizontal orientation posterolateral to the hip. In the normal hip a 'U-configuration' is produced by the metaphysis (anterior) and ischium (posterior) around the femoral head.

Coronal/flexion view: The hip is maintained in a 90° flexion and the transducer is moved to a coronal plane with respect to acetabulum by simply rotating the transducer 90° from transverse/flexion view. A normal hip gives a 'ball on a spoon' appearance in the correct plane. The femoral head represents the ball, the acetabulum forms the bowl of the spoon and the iliac line is the handle.

To detect hip joint effusion the patient is examined supine with hips in neutral position without flexion, if possible. The hip is scanned in a ventral, oblique plane along the long axis of femoral neck.

9

CHAPTER

Basic Sonographic Anatomy

LIVER

The liver is best examined, with a 3.5 MHz or 5 MHz transducer ideally after six hours fast. With patient in supine and right anterior oblique (RAO) positions sagittal, transverse, coronal, and subcostal views are required for a complete examination.

The liver lies in the right upper quadrant of the abdomen, with its upper border approximately at the level of 5th intercostal space in the midclavicular line and lower border extending to or slightly below the costal margin.

The Glisson's capsule, a thin connective tissue layer, surrounds the entire liver and it is thickest around the porta hepatis and the inferior vena cava (IVC). At the porta hepatis, the main portal main hepatic artery and the common bile duct are contained within the hepatoduodenal ligament. A part of the posterosuperior surface of the liver is not covered with peritoneum and is called the bare area.

The liver parenchyma has a homogeneous echotexture, interrupted by the portal veins and its branches which are seen as linear tubular structures with echogenic walls. The liver is hypoechoic compared to spleen and isoechoic or hyperechoic compared to the renal cortex.

The liver is divided functionally into three lobes **(Figs. 9.1A to D)** based on its arterial and portal supply. The right lobe is separated from the left by the main lobar fissure which passes through the gallbladder fossa to the inferior vena cava. The caudate lobe is situated on the posterior aspect of the liver, and appears to be a finger like extension from posterosuperior aspect of the right lobe. The inferior vena cava lies posterior to the caudate lobe and the ligamentum venosum separates it anteriorly from the left lobe. The right lobe is further divided into anterior and posterior segments by the right inter segmental fissure, the left intersegmental fissure divides the left lobe into medial and lateral segments.

Three major hepatic veins, with thin, imperceptible walls drain blood from the liver into the IVC. Besides these, a number of small accessory hepatic veins drain directly into the IVC, including separate veins from the caudate lobe **(Figs. 9.2 to 9.17)**.

The major hepatic veins course between the lobes and segments but are visualized only when scanning the superior liver. The middle hepatic vein courses within the main lobar fissure and separates the anterior segment of the right lobe from the medial segment of the left. The right hepatic vein runs

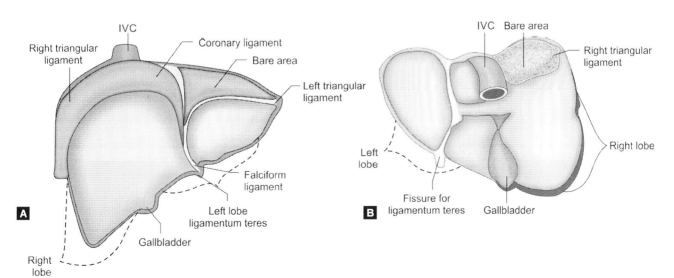

Figs. 9.1A and B: Diagram of (A) anterior, and (B) posterior surfaces of the liver (IVC: inferior vena cava).

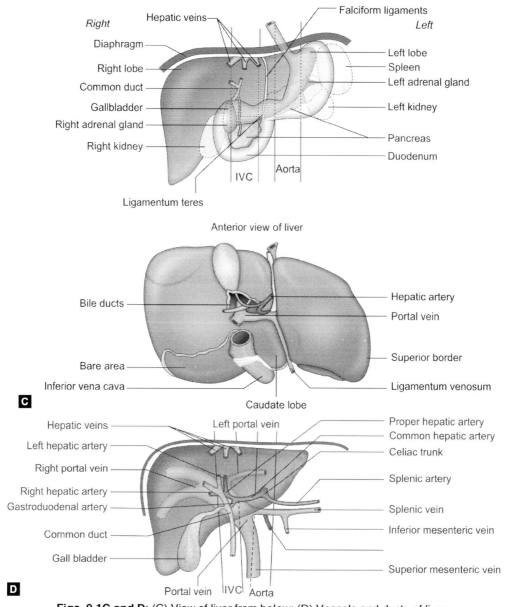

Figs. 9.1C and D: (C) View of liver from below; (D) Vessels and ducts of liver.

within the right intersegmental fissure and divides the right lobe into anterior and posterior segments. The main portal vein divides into the right and left portal veins, their major branches (anterior and posterior) of the right and medial and lateral of the left portal vein run centrally within the respective segments. The left intersegmental fissure, separating the medial and lateral segments of the left lobe, can be divided into three parts. The left hepatic vein forms the cranial one-third boundary, the ascending portion of left portal vein forms the middle third and the fissure for ligamentum teres acts as the caudal third division of the left lobe.

Couinaud's anatomy is another way of dividing the liver into eight surgically relevant segments. Each segment has its own blood supply, lymphatics and biliary drainage. The three major hepatic veins divide the liver longitudinally into four sections, each of which further divided transversely by an imaginary plane through the right main and left main portal pedicle segment I is the caudate lobe, II and III are the left superior and inferior lateral segments, respectively. The superior and inferior medial segments represent segment IVa and IVb. The right lobe consists of segments V and VI located caudal to the transverse plane (the traditional anteroinferior and posteroinferior right lobe segments) and segments VII and VIII which are cephalad representing the traditional posterosuperior and anterosuperior subsegments, respectively. The caudate lobe may receive blood supply from right and left portal veins and in contrast to the other segments, hepatic veins from the caudate lobe drain directly into the IVC.

Size of the liver correlates with gender, age, height, weight, and body surface area, it increases with height and body surface area and decreases with age. The normal

CHAPTER 9: Basic Sonographic Anatomy

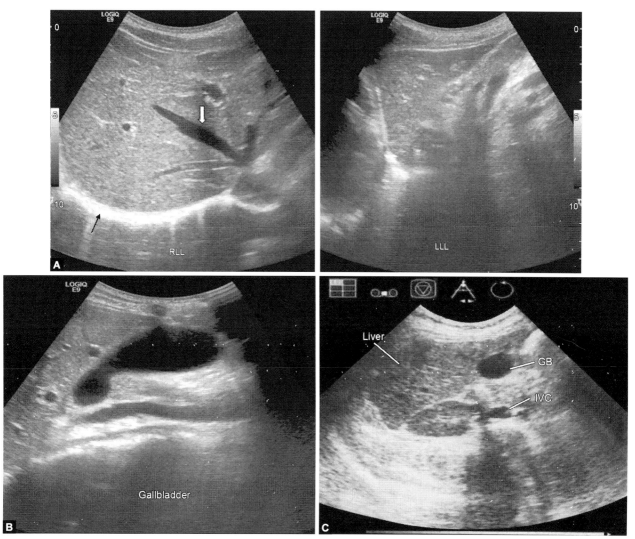

Figs. 9.2A to C: (A) Transverse section showing right (RLL) and sagittal section showing left (LLL) lobe of liver along with diaphragm (black arrow) and middle hepatic vein (white arrow). (B and C) Transverse section of liver, gallbladder (GB), and right kidney are shown in the subcostal view.

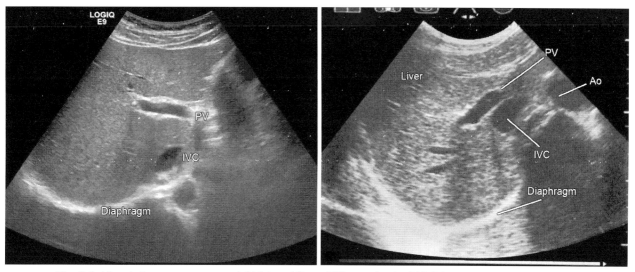

Fig. 9.3: Liver in transverse scan—right lobe of liver. (PV: portal vein; IVC: inferior vena cava; Ao: aorta)

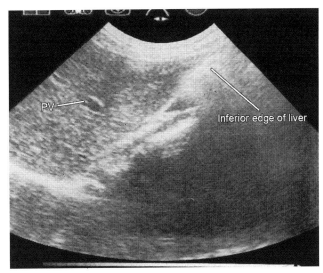

Fig. 9.4: The sharp inferior edge of the right lobe of liver in longitudinal section.

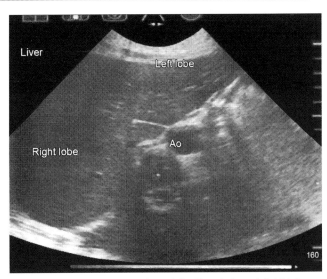

Fig. 9.6: Transverse section of the liver left and right lobes are well seen.

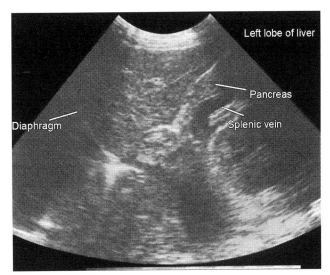

Fig. 9.5: Sagittal scan taken from the epigastrium showing the left lobe of the liver, the diaphragm is seen as a thin echogenic line, the gastroesophageal junction is also seen.

mean longitudinal (craniocaudal) diameter of the liver in the right midclavicular line is 10.5 ± 1.5 cm and the mean midclavicular AP diameter is 8.1 ± 1.9 cm. In most patients measurement of liver length suffices, but in heavy or asthenic people AP diameter, should be measured to avoid under or over estimation of liver size. AP measurement of the caudate lobe is less than one-third of the AP measurement of the overlying left lobe in normal people.

Variations

- Reidel's lobe is a tongue like extension of the inferior tip of right lobe, frequently found in women.
- Agenesis—of an entire lobe or segment, with compensatory hypertrophy of the remaining lobes.

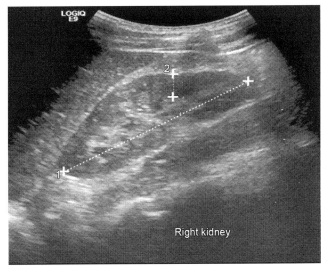

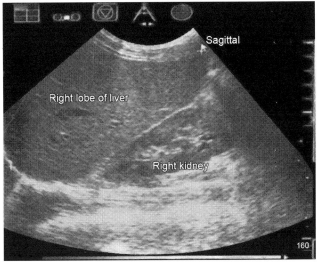

Fig. 9.7: Longitudinal dimension of right lobe of liver as seen in this subcostal scan at the mid clavicular line.

CHAPTER 9: Basic Sonographic Anatomy

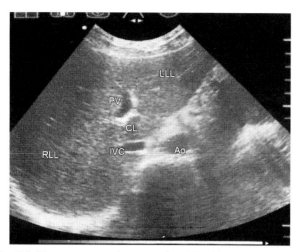

Fig. 9.8: Transverse section—caudate lobe (CL) is seen limited medially by ligamentum venosum, posteriorly by IVC, and laterally by an imaginary line joining the IVC to the main portal vein. (Ao: aorta; LLL: left lobe of liver; RLL: right lobe of liver)

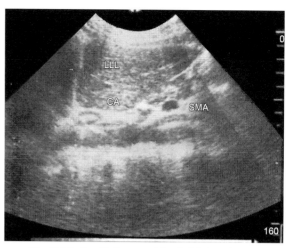

Fig. 9.10: Sagittal scan of the left lobe of liver.

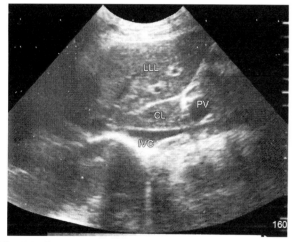

Fig. 9.9: Sagittal scan of the caudate lobe. Caudate lobe is anterior to the IVC.

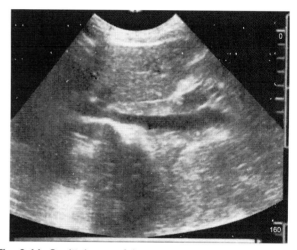

Fig. 9.11: Sagittal scan of the caudate lobe seen posterior to the left lobe of liver.

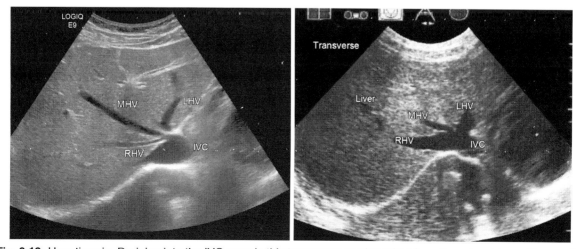

Fig. 9.12: Hepatic vein. Draining into the IVC seen in this transverse section taken from the epigastrium with superior angulation. (IVC: inferior vena cava; LHV: left hepatic vein; MHV: middle hepatic vein; RHV: right hepatic vein).

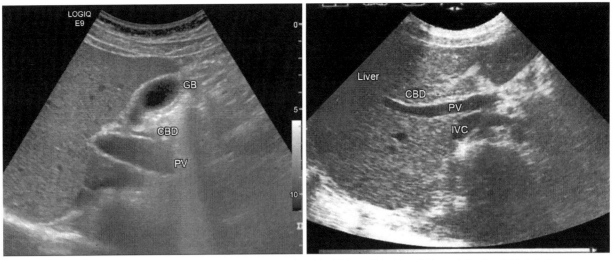

Fig. 9.13: Sagittal view of portal vein and common bile duct (CBD). (GB: gallbladder; PV: portal vein; IVC: inferior vena cava).

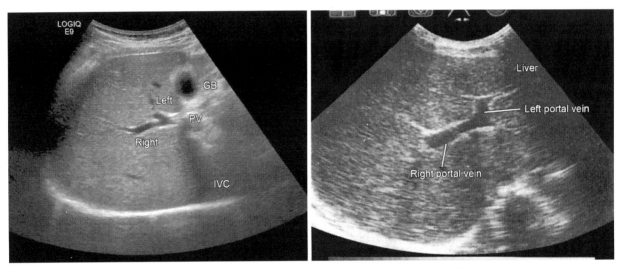

Fig. 9.14: Porta hepatis showing right and left main portal vein.

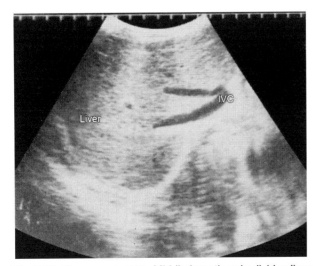

Fig. 9.15: Transverse scan. Middle hepatic vein divides liver into right and left lobes.

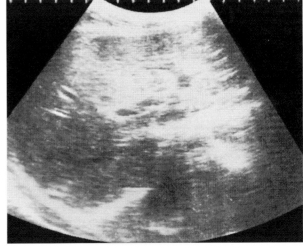

Fig. 9.16: Oblique scan of porta dividing into right and left portal veins.

- Anomalous position—in situ inversus totalis the liver found in the left hypochondrium. In congenital diaphragmatic hernia and omphalocele varying amounts of liver may herniate into the thorax or outside the abdominal cavity.
- Diaphragmatic slips may produce sonographic pseudomasses if the liver is not carefully examined in both sagittal and transverse planes. An inferior accessory hepatic fissure may extend inferiorly from the right portal vein to the inferior surface of the right lobe of liver.
- The falciform ligament may be visualized in the transverse scan as a bright rounded echogenic structure in the left lobe of liver. It is seen to elongate in the longitudinal direction and appears triangular in shape due to its attachment to the liver and anterior abdominal wall.

The Gallbladder and Bile Ducts (Fig. 9.18)

Examination of the gallbladder requires an overnight fast of 8–12 hours to ensure adequate gallbladder distention. In most patients a 3.5 MHz transducer is required, however, a 5 MHz transducer will provide a better resolution in thin patients or in those with anteriorly placed gallbladder. The scans are performed with patient in supine or in left posterior oblique position from a lower intercostal or a subcostal approach. The gallbladder lies in a fossa on the undersurface of the right lobe of liver. The anatomic position of the gallbladder fundus is very variable, but the neck of gallbladder bears a fixed anatomic relationship to the main lobar fissure and the right portal vein. In 70% of patients a thin linear echogenic line, thought to represent a part of the interlobar hepatic fissure is seen connecting the gallbladder neck to the right or main portal vein **(Figs. 9.19 to 9.24)**.

The gallbladder consists of neck or infundibulum body and fundus and is very variable in size and shape. In general if its AP diameter is >3 cm, transverse diameter >5 cm, and length >10 cm, or it loses its ovoid shape and becomes rounded. It is likely to be overdistended. However, if its transverse diameter is <2 cm despite adequate fasting it is likely to be contracted. Normal gallbladder wall is seen as a pencil thin echogenic line less than 3 mm thick. As bile contains no particulate matter, the gallbladder lumen is normally echo-free. The gallbladder is typically oval, but in a few patients a Phrygian cap deformity is present, in which the fundus appears to be folded on the body. Sometimes a fold may be seen between the neck and body of the gallbladder and is known as a junctional fold.

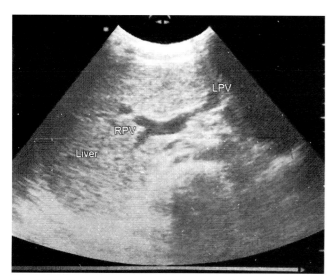

Fig. 9.17: Transverse scan—bifurcation of main portal vein into left and right branches. (LPV: left portal vein; RPV: right portal vein).

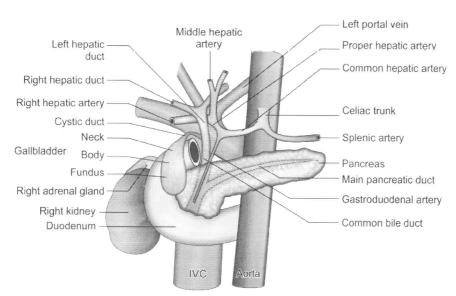

Fig. 9.18: Location and anatomy of the gallbladder and biliary tract.

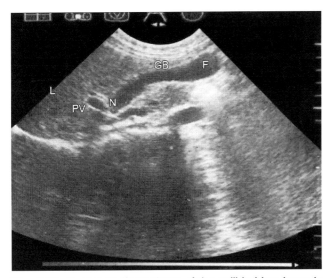

Fig. 9.19: Normal pyriform shape of the gallbladder shown in sagittal scan. Neck, body and fundus of the gallbladder are seen.

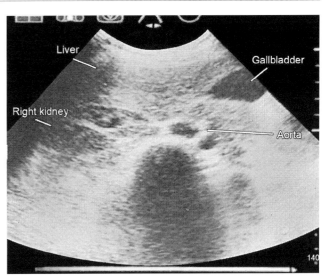

Fig. 9.21: Right kidney (RK) and gallbladder (GB) seen in transverse section.

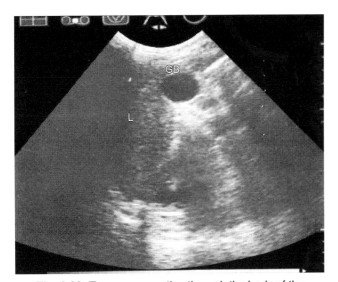

Fig. 9.20: Transverse section through the body of the gallbladder seen as a well defined circular anechoic structure.

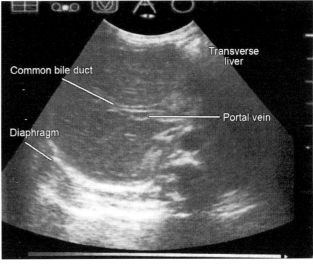

Fig. 9.22: CBD and PV as seen in a longitudinal scan.

Biliary Ducts

To minimize obscuration by overlying bowel gas, the distal common bile duct (CBD) should be examined initially. For this the patient should lie in the right lateral decubitus or in an erect right posterior oblique (RPO) position and transverse scans are obtained. In these positions there is minimal gas in the antrum and duodenum and the transverse scan plane maximizes the ability to trace the course of the intrapancreatic distal duct. If overlying bowel gas obscures the region despite exertion or gentle pressure over the pancreatic head, the patient should be given water to drink and placed in right lateral decubitus position for 2–3 minutes and rescanned. Proximal CBD is better visualized in the parasagittal plane, with patient in supine or left posterior oblique (LPO) positions.

Bile drains from the liver via the intrahepatic bile ducts which run in the portal tracts along the portal vein radicles and branches of hepatic artery. These ducts are normally too small to be sonographically visible. They anastomose to form the right and left hepatic ducts, each of which measure up to 2 mm in diameter. At the porta hepatis the right and left hepatic ducts join to form the common hepatic duct which is approximately 3 cm in length and is joined by the cystic duct to form the CBD. The common hepatic duct (CHD) and CBD are identified by their position in the porta, anterior to the portal vein and to the right of the hepatic artery. The walls of the CBD are thinner and less bright than those of the portal vein.

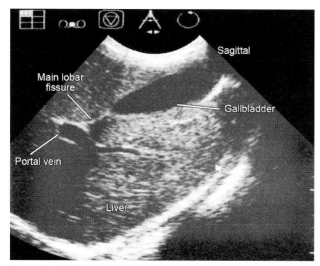

Fig. 9.23: Main lobar fissure seen as a thin echogenic line from the portal vein to the neck of the gallbladder. This landmark is used to locate the gallbladder.

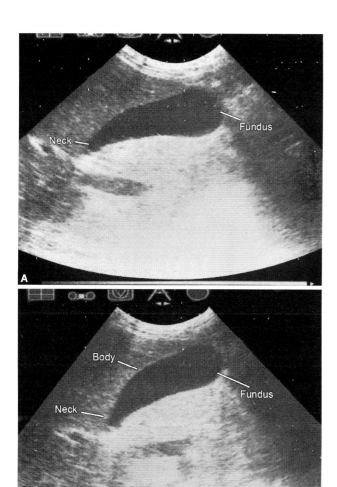

Figs. 9.24A and B: Sagittal scan of gallbladder showing the normal pyriform shape.

The maximum caliber of nondilated CHD is 4 mm and that of CBD is 7 mm. In elderly patients and those with previous hepatobiliary surgery, 10 mm is considered the upper normal CBD diameter. The diameter of CBD should be measured as distal as possible. The normal cystic duct lies posterior to the CBD, is slightly less than 2 mm in diameter and is seen in 50% of patients. Ultrasound tends to underestimate the caliber of bile ducts by 1.5–2 mm because of infilling due to the beam width artifact that causes the echogenic walls to appear thickened and to spread into the lumen. After its union with the cystic duct, the CBD descends within the hepatoduodenal ligament, anterior to the main portal vein and to the right of the hepatic artery, and travels caudally, behind the first part of duodenum. Distally it lies in a deep groove on the posterior aspect of the head of the pancreas, often completely surrounded by the pancreatic tissue. The distal end of CBD passes laterally accompanying the pancreatic duct into the second part of the duodenum and opens at the ampulla of Vater, situated on the medial wall of the duodenal lumen.

PANCREAS

Sonographic examination should begin with patient in the erect position oblique-transverse scans, (left side of probe is cranial) are taken below the xiphoid in the midline and the transducer is angled cephalad and caudal from the level of the longitudinal view of the splenic vein. Sagittal scanning is initiated in the midline below the xiphoid, the portal-splenic confluence helps in identifying the pancreas and the probe is tilted sideways to visualize the entire gland. The left kidney is used as an acoustic window to visualize the tail of the pancreas anterior to its upper pole by a left coronal view.

When the erect position fails to demonstrate the gland, the patient is given 2–3 glasses of water and placed in supine position. The fluid filled stomach provides an acoustic window, causes movement of the intragastric gas and displaces the colon and small bowel inferiorly **(Figs. 9.25A and B)**.

The pancreas is a nonencapsulated, retroperitoneal organ lying obliquely in the upper abdomen, In the anterior perirenal space between the duodenal loop and the splenic hilum over a length of 12.5 to 15 cm. The head, uncinate process, neck, body and tail constitute the different parts of the gland. The normal pancreas has homogeneous echotexture iso to hyperechoic to the liver and smooth contour. With aging and obesity it becomes more echogenic due to fatty infiltration. Size of the pancreas decreases with an advancing age. Head of pancreas measures 2.2–2.5 cm in AP diameter and 2.2 ± 0.2 cm in the craniocaudal direction. The body measures 1.8–2.1 cm in AP dimension. The pancreatic duct is seen as a single linear structure or double parallel lines measures up to 3 mm in diameter in the head, 2.1 mm in the body and 1.6 mm in the tail. Although 2–2.5 mm diameter is regarded upper limit of normal, the pancreatic duct is considered normal as long as its walls are parallel and it can be seen along its whole length to the duodenum.

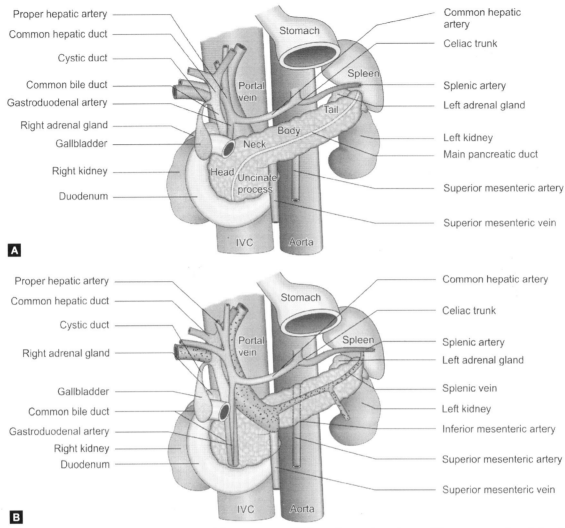

Figs. 9.25A and B: (A) Location and anatomy of the pancreas; (B) Location and anatomy of the pancreas in relation to portal venous system.

Relations (Figs. 9.26 to 9.30)

Head: In the transverse plane, the gastroduodenal artery anteriorly and the common bile duct posteriorly are seen in cross-section in the superior aspect of the head. The IVC lies posterior to the pancreatic head. In its inferior aspect the medial portion of the head tapers to form the uncinate process.

Neck, body and tail: The pancreatic neck lies between head and body anterior to the portal venous confluence. The left lateral border of the vertebral column masks the plane of demarcation between the pancreatic body and tail. In the transverse plane the celiac axis is seen cephalad to the body of pancreas. At the level of the neck, the confluence of splenic and superior mesenteric veins is seen posterior to the pancreas. More laterally the splenic vein runs posterior to the body and tail. The aorta lies posterior to the proximal body and the left renal vein courses between the superior mesenteric artery and aorta posteriorly, to drain into the IVC. The tail of pancreas lies anterior to the upper pole of left kidney and left renal vessels. Stomach may be visualized anterior to the pancreas.

In the sagittal plane, the neck is seen anterior to the superior mesenteric vein (SMV) and the uncinate process is seen posterior to it. A longitudinal view of the aorta is identified, with the body of the pancreas situated between the celiac axis and superior mesenteric artery (SMA). The stomach lies anterior to the body and tail. The splenic vein is seen posteriorly in cross section, whereas the splenic artery is seen cephalad in cross section.

SPLEEN (FIG. 9.31)

Spleen is the predominant organ in the left upper quadrant, bounded by the left hemidiaphragm. It is usually examined with a 3.5 MHz transducer, with patient in supine or RPO position. As the long axis of spleen is in line of the tenth rib, oblique coronal scans are obtained through one of the lower left intercostal spaces. The plane of section should then be

CHAPTER 9: Basic Sonographic Anatomy

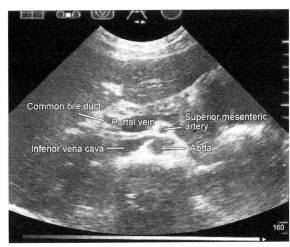

Fig. 9.26: Transverse section of pancreas.

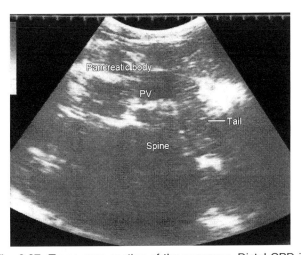

Fig. 9.27: Transverse section of the pancreas. Distal CBD is also seen inferolaterally to the head of the pancreas. Neck of the pancreas is anterior to the superior mesenteric artery (SMA). The superior mesenteric artery is seen posterior to the splenic vein and anterior to the aorta in the transverse section.

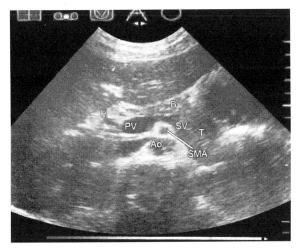

Fig. 9.28: Transverse scan of pancreas showing head (H), body (B) and tail (T). (PV: portal vein; SV: splenic vein; Ao: Aorta)

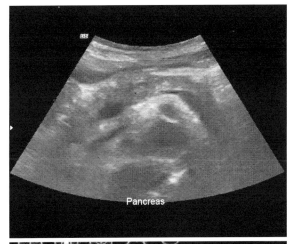

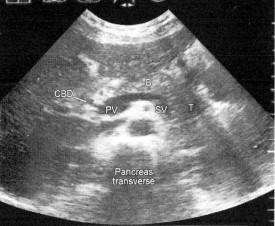

Fig. 9.29: Normal dimension of pancreatic head and body are seen.

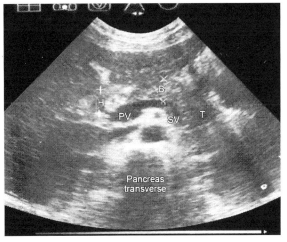

Fig. 9.30: The distal end of CBD seen in the head of pancreas.

swept posteriorly and anteriorly to view the entire volume of the spleen, with patient in various degrees of inspiration (**Figs. 9.32 to 9.37**).

The spleen is surrounded by the diaphragm posteriorly, superiorly, and laterally. The left lobe of liver, when enlarged

Principles and Practice of Ultrasonography

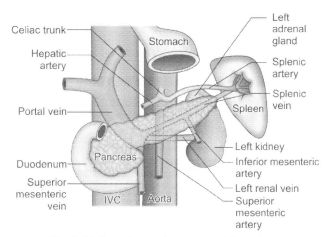

Fig. 9.31: Location and anatomy of the spleen.

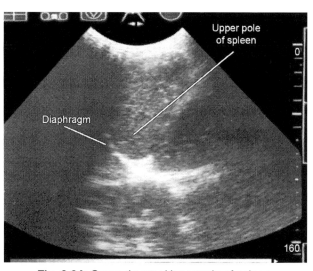

Fig. 9.34: Coronal scan: Upper pole of spleen.

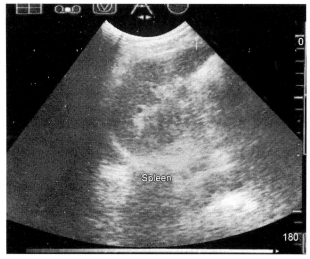

Fig. 9.32: Sagittal scan of the spleen showing the longitudinal diameter.

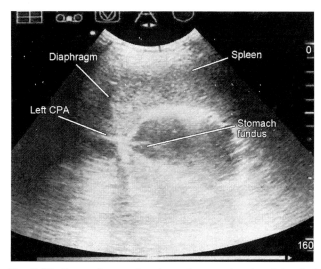

Fig. 9.35: Coronal scan showing spleen and water distended stomach. (CPA: caudal pancreatic artery)

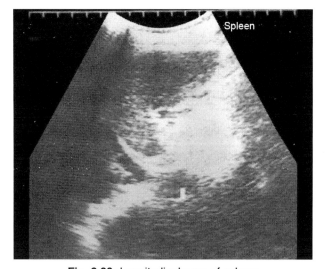

Fig. 9.33: Longitudinal scan of spleen.

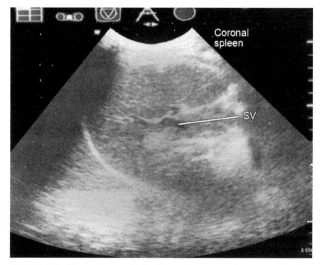

Fig. 9.36: Superior and inferior pole are well seen, splenic vein (SV) is seen at the splenic hilum.

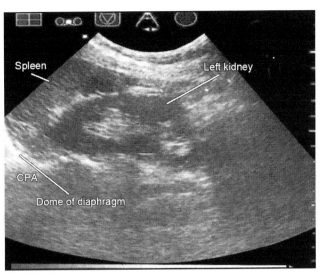

Fig. 9.37: Spleen seen in relation to the left kidney. Left costophrenic angle (CPA) is also seen through a sagittal scan from the posterior axillary line.

may extend into the left upper quadrant, anterior to the spleen. The fundus of stomach and lesser sac are anterior and medial to the splenic hilum. The tail of pancreas lies posterior to gastric fundus and lesser sac and reaches up to the splenic hilum, in close relation to the splenic vein and artery. The left kidney lies inferior and medial to the spleen.

The spleen has a variable shape, but most are convex superolaterally and concave inferomedially. The splenic hilum is located at the center of inferomedial surface and the splenic vein can often be easily demonstrated here. Normal splenic vein measures less than 1 cm in diameter. Spleen is a solid organ with homogeneous intermediate to low level echoes with no bright intraparenchymal echogenic streaks. The splenic capsule is too thin to be visualized sonographically.

The average adult spleen measures 12 cm in length, 7 cm in breadth and 3.4 cm in thickness.

Splenic volumetric index

$$\frac{height \times breadth \times width}{27}$$

= 8 – 34 in normal people

Size of the spleen, decreases with advancing age and varies in accordance with the nutritional status of the body.

Congenital Anomalies

- Accessory spleens—usually located at the splenic hilum, but may also be found in the left lower quadrant of the abdomen. They are homogenous, round or oval in shape and rarely more than 4 cm in diameter. They are isoechoic to the spleen and tend to hypertrophy in postsplenectomy patients.
- Polysplenia—is a syndrome characterized by multiple individual splenunculi and a tendency for normally asymmetrical organs to occur symmetrically (double liver, situs ambiguous)
- Asplenia is a rare anomaly and may be associated with congenital immune deficiency.
- Ectopic/wandering spleen is also rare. Seen in women of reproductive age it remains asymptomatic unless torsion occurs. When it produces chronic disabling symptoms they are mistaken for a variety of digestive disturbances. Ultrasound reveals the typical comma shaped enlarged spleen of coarse hypoechoic texture due to infarction and splenic congestion. The demonstration of an abdominal or pelvic mass with asplenia should suggest splenic torsion.
- A common congenital anomaly is a pronounced posterior location of the spleen, even posterior to the left kidney.

GASTROINTESTINAL TRACT

Technique: Patient lies supine and comes after an overnight fast and with full bladder. A 3.5 MHz and/or sometimes a 5 MHz transducer is used to look for any obvious masses or 'gut signature'. Pelvis is scanned both before and after the bladder is emptied. Areas that need detailed analyses are visualized using 5 MHz transducer, using compressions sonography technique. Slow graded pressure is applied, normal gut is compressible and gas pockets get displaced from the region of interest. Thickened abnormal bowel loops and/or obstructed noncompressible loops remain unchanged. Patients with local tenderness or peritoneal irritation comply well with the slow gentle increase in pressure of compression sonography. Doppler evaluation helps to differentiate inflammatory from ischemia gut wall thickening by showing absence or minimal blood flow in ischaemia and readily detected color Doppler flow and a RI < 0.6 in inflammation. Color Doppler also helps in differentiating thick inflamed gut wall from sympathetic wall thickening due to adjacent inflammatory focus.

Normal Sonographic Anatomy (Figs. 9.38 to 9.41)

The gut is a continuous hollow tube comprising of four concentric layers from lumen outwards they are: (i) mucosa—which consists of an epithelial lining, loose connective tissue, or lamina propria, and muscularis mucosa; (ii) submucosa; (iii) muscularis propria—with inner circular and outer longitudinal fibres and (iv) serosa or adventitia. These layers produce a characteristic appearance—gut signature on sonography **(Fig. 9.46)** and up to five concentric alternately echogenic and hypoechoic layers may be visualized. The 1st and 3rd and 5th layers are echogenic and correspond to the superficial mucosa and luminal contents, submucosa, and serosa. The 2nd and 4th layers are hypoechoic and correspond to the lamina propria and muscularis mucosa and the muscularis propria. In routine sonogram, the gut may have a bull' eye appearance in a cross section with a central echogenic area corresponding to the intraluminal contents and mucosa and a hypoechoic rim comprising of all the rest of the gut walls. Thus, the quality of scan and resolution of the transducer determines the degree of layer differentiation.

The thickness of normal gut wall is 3 mm in distended and 5 mm in the nondistended state. The content, diameter and motor activity of the gut must be noted. Peristalsis is usually seen in the stomach and small bowel. Activity may be increased in mechanical obstruction and inflammatory bowel disease and it is decreased in paralytic ileus.

Esophagus: The lower end of esophagus and GE junction are seen lying anterior to the aorta and inferior to the

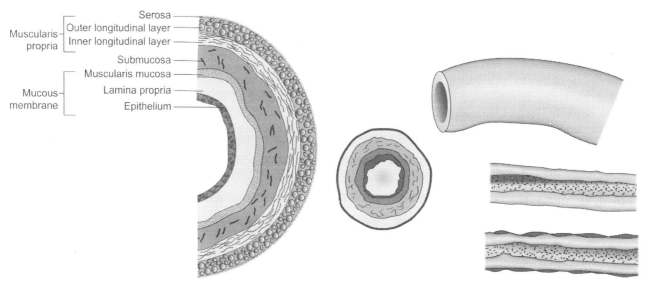

Fig. 9.38: Schematic depiction of the histologic layers of the gut wall.

Fig. 9.39: Gut signature, schematic. Top figure is a loop of gut. Bottom left is a cross-sectional and bottom right longitudinal representation of the five layers seen on a sonographic image.

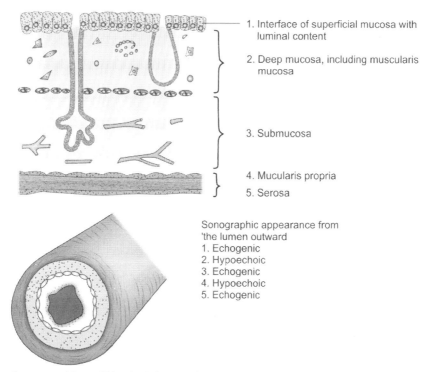

Fig. 9.40: Correlation of sonographic and histologic layers of the gut wall. Top schematic shows histologic layers of the gut wall which correspond with the sonographic layering. Bottom schematic shows gut in cross section with documented layer echogenicity as it relates to the histologic image shown above.

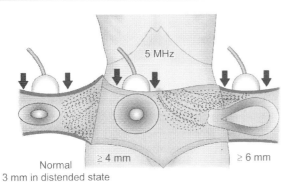

Fig. 9.41: Compression sonography, schematic depiction. (1) normal gut is compressed. (2) abnormally thickened gut or, (3) an obstructed loop such as that seen in acute appendicitis will be noncompressible.

diaphragm. The left lobe of liver forms the window for visualizing the esophagus in the sagittal and transverse planes **(Figs. 9.42 to 9.49)**.

Stomach is seen as a fluid or gas filled structure with thick walls. The stomach cavity can be well evaluated after patient takes 2–3 glasses of water.

Small and large bowel: Normal and small bowel loops show uniformly thick walls, peristaltic activity with changing caliber and mobility. Valvulae conniventes in the jejunum help to differentiate them from the featureless ileal loops. The ascending and descending colons are fixed in both flanks and can be easily evaluated for any mass or wall thickening. The transverse colon has a variable location, but a lesion within it will lie close to the anterior abdominal wall and will be movable up and down rather than side to side.

Appendix (Fig. 9.50)

A 5 MHz or 7.5 MHz transducer is used to examine the right lower quadrant using the specific technique of compression sonography. Normal appendix is difficult to visualize, it appears as an easily compressible, mobile finger like structure with the 3 mm thick uniform wall and a total diameter of 6 mm. In cross section it produces the normal 'gut signature'.

The Abdominal Wall (Figs. 9.51A and B)

The abdominal wall is visualized using high frequency 5 MHz or 7.5 MHz transducers and stand-off floatation pads.

The abdominal cavity is enclosed by a laminated abdominal wall, which is divided into anterior, anterolateral and posterior parts. From the outermost layer, working in, the wall includes the skin, superficial fascia, subcutaneous fat, the muscle layer, the fascia transversalis and a layer of intraperitoneal fat. The normal epidermis is 1–4 mm thick and highly echogenic. The subcutaneous has variable thickness and mixed echogenicity with fat lobules appearing relatively echopoor. The muscles of the anterior abdominal wall are all paired and consist of three layers of sheet like

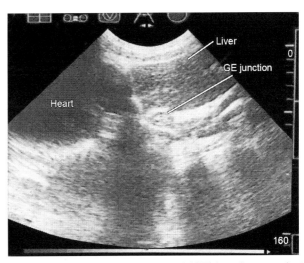

Fig. 9.42: Normal gastroesophageal (GE) junction seen just below the diaphragm.

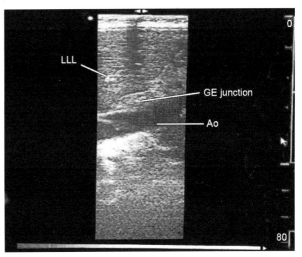

Fig. 9.43: Gastroesophageal (GE) junction seen posterior to the left lobe of liver (LLL) and anterior to the aorta (Ao).

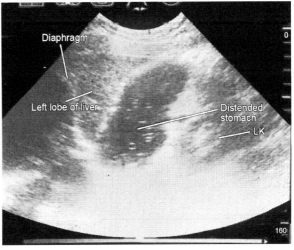

Fig. 9.44: Water distended stomach as seen from epigastric approach.

Principles and Practice of Ultrasonography

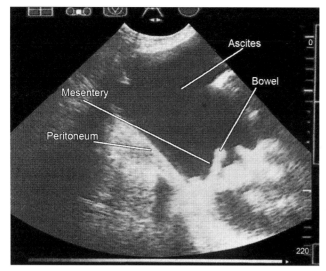

Fig. 9.45: Normal mesentery is visualized next to bowel in a case of ascites.

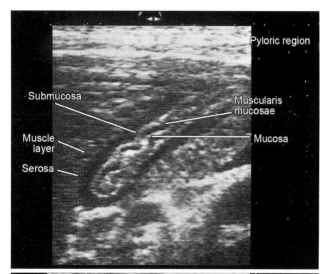

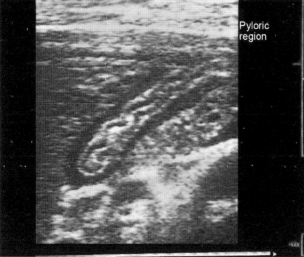

Fig. 9.46: Sagittal scan of pylorus showing the normal gut signature.

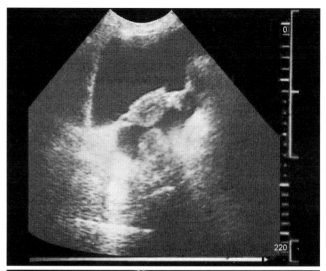

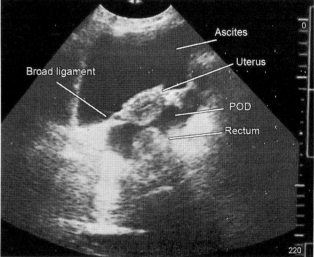

Fig. 9.47: Fluid is seen in pouch of Douglas (POD) behind the uterus. Echogenic broad ligament are seen extending from the uterus to the lateral pelvic wall.

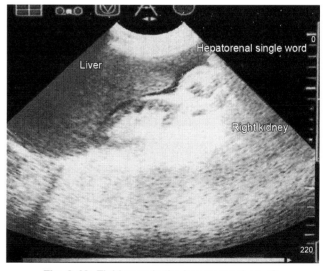

Fig. 9.48: Fluid seen in the hepatorenal pouch.

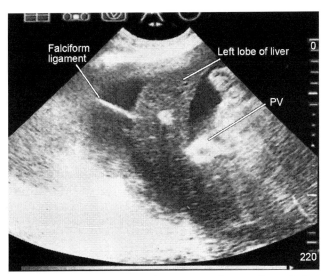

Fig. 9.49: Falciform ligament is seen as a dense echogenic line extending from the surface of liver to anterior abdominal wall.

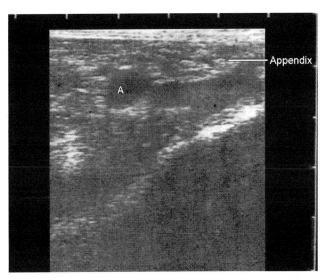

Fig. 9.50: Normal appendix, a blind tubular structure arising from the caecum showing gut signature.

muscle—external and internal oblique and transverses abdominis muscle and a fourth paired midline strap muscle—the rectus abdominis.

The rectus abdominis originates from the symphysis pubis and pubic crest and inserts into the costal cartilage of 5th, 6th, 7th ribs. It is ensheathed in the rectus sheath derived from the aponeurosis of the sheet muscles. The muscle layer appears hypoechoic and high resolution probes show individual muscle bundles having fairly uniform texture and orientation muscles of the back are thicker and thus more difficult to visualize. The extraperitoneal fat and peritoneum appears as an echogenic line below the muscle layer (Fig. 9.52).

Diaphragm (Figs. 9.53 to 9.55)

The muscles of the diaphragm appear as a thin hypoechoic band. The liver/spleen diaphragm interface appears as a thin echogenic line. The lung-diaphragm interface appears as a thicker echogenic band. Sometimes the mirror image artifact of the liver diaphragm interface is seen cephalad to the lung-diaphragm interface as another thin echogenic line. Diaphragmatic slips are the normal prominent muscular insertions that may appear as focal round, oval or triangular echogenic masses and may be mistaken for focal liver/peritoneal lesions. However, on scanning in long axis they elongate and become large in inspiration. The diaphragmatic crura are seen as thin hypoechoic bands anterior to the upper abdominal aorta and posterior to the IVC. They also become thicker on deep inspiration.

RETROPERITONEUM

The retroperitoneum is a posterior abdominal area posterior to the parietal peritoneum and anterior to the fascia transversalis, limited by the diaphragm cranially

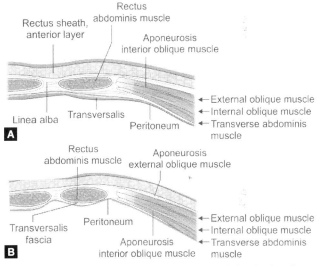

Figs. 9.51A and B: Scheme of anterior abdominal wall; (A) Above arcuate line; and (B) Below arcuate line.

and the pelvic brim caudally. Two layers of renal fascia that are occasionally identified by sonography divide the retroperitoneal potential space, coronally into three separate compartments. The anterior pararenal space lies between the posterior parietal peritoneum and anterior perirenal fascia. It contains the ascending and descending colon, the second, third, and fourth parts of duodenum, the pancreas, IVC, aorta, proximal superior mesenteric vessels and the hepatic and splenic vessels (Fig. 9.56).

The posterior pararenal spaces (Fig. 9.57) lies between the posterior perirenal fascia and the fascia covering the quadrants lumborum and psoas muscles. It contains only fat and communicates with the properitoneal space anterolaterally with posterior pelvis caudally and with the anterior pararenal space near the pelvic brim. The perirenal space lies between the two layers of perirenal fascia and contain the kidney, adrenal gland and proximal ureter and perirenal fat **(Figs. 9.58 to 9.68)**.

The retrofascial space contains the psoas and quadratus lumborum muscle. The quadratus lumborum muscles appears as a hypoechoic roughly quadrilateral shaped structure on either side, and is wider cranially. It arises from the medial part of twelfth rib, attaches to the vertebral transverse processes and inserts into the iliac crest and the iliolumbar ligament.

The psoas muscle is seen by scanning coronally through the flank. The caudal part of the muscle is usually seen in the transverse plane. The muscle originates from the lumbar vertebrae and their transverse process and inserts into the lesser trochanter of femur. They appear hypoechoic with vertically oriented fibres and caudally have an echogenic central tendon.

The diaphragmatic crura are linear muscular portions of the diaphragm that border the aortic hiatus and attach to the lateral aspects of the lumbar vertebrae. They are usually hypoechoic, surrounded by echogenic tissue. The right crux is bigger, longer and more lobular and this more easily identified.

Aorta **(Fig. 9.69)**: It is seen as a pulsatile, hypoechoic tubular structure with echogenic walls, just to the left of the midline, closely related to the anterior surface of the lumbar vertebrae. It enters the abdomen through the aortic hiatus at the level of D_{12} vertebrae, where its lumen measures 2.5 cm in diameter and gradually tapers to 1 cm at its bifurcation at the level of L_4 vertebrae. With age it normally increases in diameter by up to 25% and may measure up to 3.7 cm in diameter in a 75-year-old. It bifurcates into common iliac arteries, which are about 5 cm long and measure up to 1.5 cm in diameter in men and 1.2 cm in women.

The main aortic branches seen on ultrasound are the celiac artery, the paired renal arteries, the superior mesenteric artery, and the common iliac arteries. Other aortic branches not usually identified include the paired inferior diaphragmatic, the paired middle adrenal arteries and the paired gonadal arteries, the inferior mesenteric and the paired first to fourth lumbar arteries.

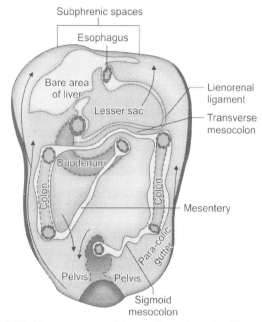

Fig. 9.52: The anatomy of the peritoneal cavity. The arrows indicate the common routes of spread for intraperitoneal disease processes.

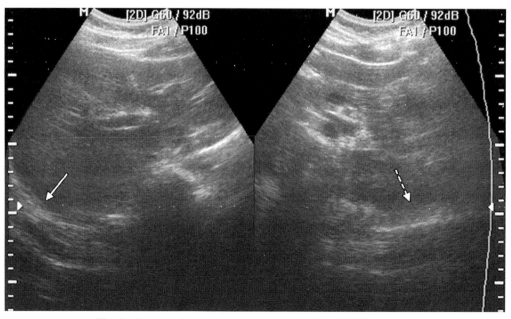

Fig. 9.53: Right dome (white arrow), Left dome (broken arrow).

CHAPTER 9: Basic Sonographic Anatomy

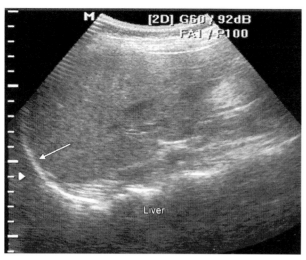

Fig. 9.54: Right dome (white arrow).

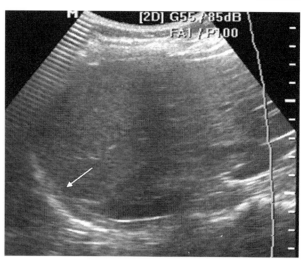

Fig. 9.55: Left dome (white arrow).

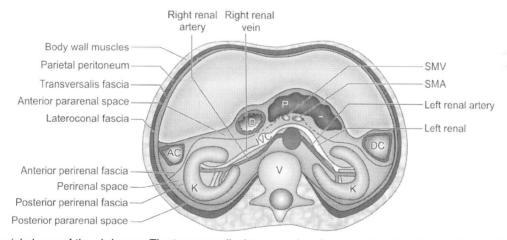

Fig. 9.56: Fascial planes of the abdomen. The transversalis, lateroconal and perirenal fascia determine the localization of fluid collections and infections in the renal areas. (AC: ascending colon; DC: descending colon; D: duodenum; IVC: inferior vena cava; K: kidney; SMA: superior mesenteric artery; SMV: superior mesenteric vein; P: pancreas; V: vertebral body).

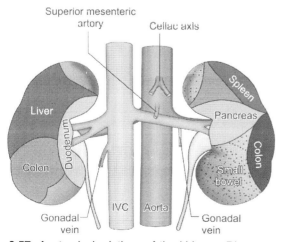

Fig. 9.57: Anatomical relations of the kidneys. Diagrammatic representation indicating the major anatomical structures which are related to the kidneys.

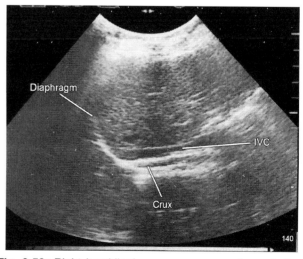

Fig. 9.58: Right hemidiaphragm seen as a echogenic line. The crux of the diaphragm is seen posterior to the IVC in this longitudinal section.

Principles and Practice of Ultrasonography

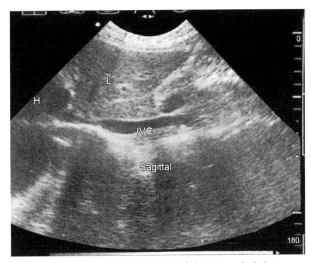

Fig. 9.59: Longitudinal section of thorax and abdomen showing IVC entering the heart.

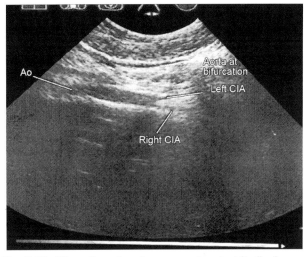

Fig. 9.62: Bifurcation of aorta as seen in a longitudinal scan. (Ao: aorta; CIA: common iliac artery).

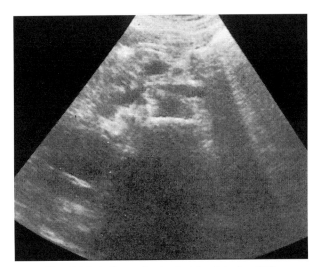

Fig. 9.60: Left renal vein draining into the IVC.

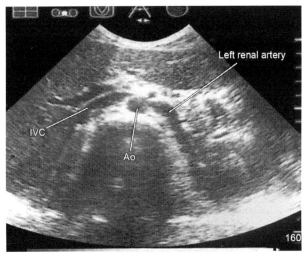

Fig. 9.63: Transverse scan—showing IVC and aorta with left renal artery.

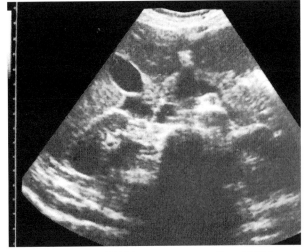

Fig. 9.61: Aorta and IVC in transverse section. SMA is seen anterior to the aorta.

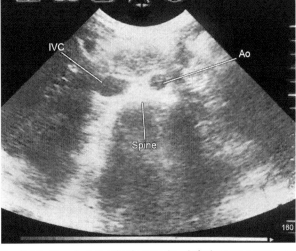

Fig. 9.64: Great abdominal vessels—Inferior vena cava and aorta seen in transverse section.

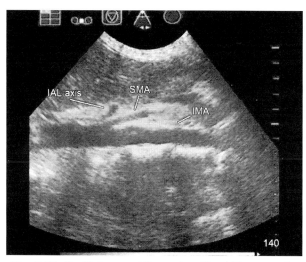

Fig. 9.65: Sagittal scan of the aorta with midline vessels.

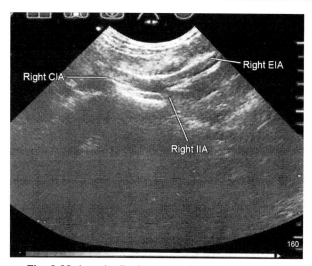

Fig. 9.68: Longitudinal section of right common iliac artery (CIA), external and internal iliac artery (IIA).

INFERIOR VENA CAVA (FIG. 9.70)

It is formed by the paired, common iliac veins on the anterior surface of L_5 vertebral body and lies anteriorly and slightly to the right of the spine. It appears as an anechoic tubular structure with thin walls and gradually increases in caliber cranially. Except for its intrahepatic position the vein is inconsistently seen as it is intermittently flat or oval in cross section and often obscured by bowel gas. With deep inspiration the vein dilates, with deep expiration the venous return improves and the IVC decreases in diameter.

Adrenal Glands (Figs. 9.71 to 9.73)

The right adrenal gland is best evaluated intercostally at the midaxillary or anterior axillary line, with liver as the acoustic window. A subcostal oblique approach parallel to the rib cage at the midclavicular line can be also used. The left-adrenal gland is best evaluated intercostally at the posterior axillary or midaxillary line through the spleen or kidney. Both adrenal glands lie anteromedial to the upper poles of the kidneys. Both comprise of three parts; an anteromedial ridge from which the medial and lateral wings extend posteriorly. The right adrenal gland is triangular in shape, and is located posterior to the IVC. The medial wing is related to the right crux of diaphragm medially and the left wing has the posteromedial margin of liver on its lateral aspect. The left adrenal gland is crescentic in shape with shorter medial and lateral wings. The gland lies posterolateral to the aorta and the left crux of diaphragm. It is posterior to the lesser sac superiorly and posterior to pancreas inferiorly. The adrenal cortex is seen as a hypoechoic structure surrounded by echogenic perirenal fat and the medulla is seen as a thin echogenic central linear structure. Each gland measures 2.3 cm in width, 4–6 cm in length and 3.6 mm in thickness.

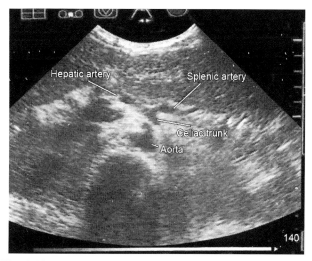

Fig. 9.66: Hepatic and splenic artery from the celiac trunk, the first branch of abdominal aorta seen in a transverse section.

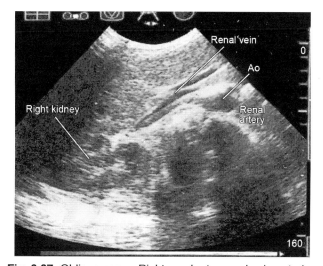

Fig. 9.67: Oblique scan—Right renal artery and vein entering the hilum of right kidney.

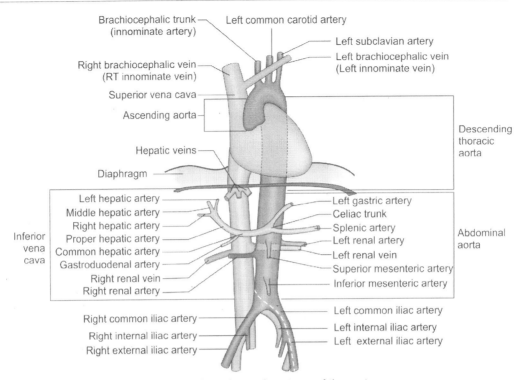

Fig. 9.69: Location and anatomy of the aorta.

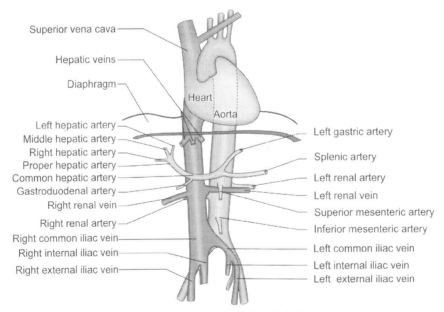

Fig. 9.70: Location and anatomy of the inferior vena cava.

Peritoneum

Multiple peritoneal ligaments and folds connect the viscera to each other, and to the abdominal and pelvic walls. The lesser omentum is the fold connecting the liver to the stomach and the duodenum. The greater omentum is the largest fold, and it extends inferiorly from the greater curvature of the stomach to cover the anterior aspect of the transverse colon and hangs down further like a curtain in front of the small bowel. The mesenteries refer to the peritoneal folds which suspend the small bowel, and colon from the posterior abdomen and pelvic wall. They include the mesenteries of the small bowel, the mesoappendix, transverse and sigmoid mesocolon. The peritoneal cavity is divided into the supramesocolic and inframesocolic compartment by the transverse mesocolon. The supramesocolic compartment is divided by the falciform ligament into the right and left supramesocolic spaces. The right supramesocolic space

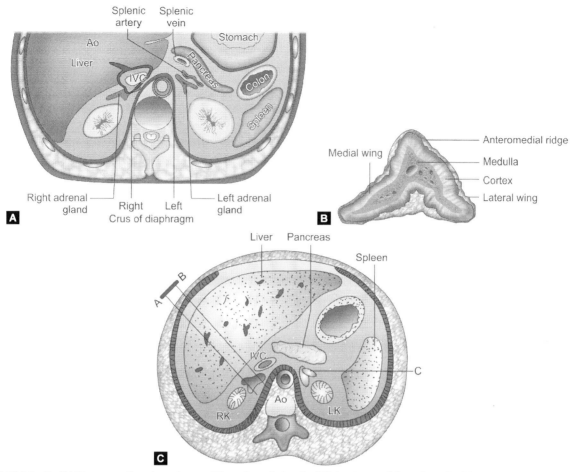

Figs. 9.71A to C: (A) Cross-sectional anatomy of the adrenal glands; (B) Anatomy of the adrenals. Diagrammatic representation of the general shape and make up of the adrenal gland; (C) Anatomy of the adrenals. Diagrammatic section to show the ideal scanning approach to the two sides. Scan lines A and B will show the wings and anteromedial ridge of the right gland respectively. Scan line C through the spleen will show the left adrenal gland.

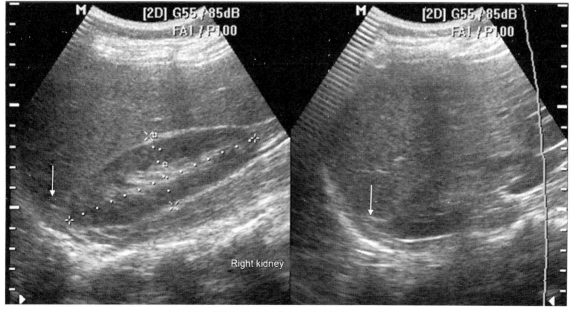

Fig. 9.72: Right adrenal (white arrows).

consists of the lesser sac and right perihepaticspaces. The right perihepatic space consists of the right subphrenic and right subhepatic spaces, the latter further comprise of an anterior compartment and a posterior compartment also called the hepatorenal recess or the Morrison's pouch.

The left supramesocolic spaces consist of four compartments anterior and posterior left perihepatic spaces and anterior and posteriorleft subphrenic spaces. The oblique root of the small bowel mesentery, extending from the duodenojejunal flexure to the ileocecal junction divides the inframesocolic compartment into a smaller right space and larger left space. When the peritoneal spaces fill with fluid or tumor or when their membranes thickened by disease they can be identified by sonography.

URINARY TRACT

A minimum fast of six hours is required, to limit bowel gas, before the examination. High resolution, real time sector scanners are used. The kidneys should be assessed in the transverse and coronal plane, with patient in supine, oblique, lateral decubitus and occasionally prone position. A nondilated ureter may be impossible to visualize because of overlying bowel gas. However, the proximal ureter may be visualized using a coronal oblique view, with the kidney as an acoustic window. A dilated ureter may be visualized by transverse and sagittal imaging and in women a dilated distal ureter may be visualized by TVS. Bladder is best evaluated when moderately filled. It should be scanned in the transverse and sagittal plane and occasionally in a decubitus position. TVS may be used in women to better visualize the bladder wall. The urethra in a woman can be scanned with transvaginal, transperineal or translabial sonography. The posterior urethra in men is best visualized with endorectal probes.

Normal Sonographic Anatomy (Figs. 9.74A and B)

The kidneys (**Figs. 9.75 to 9.87**) are retroperitoneal structures located on either side of the midline, at the level of D_{12}-L_3 vertebrae, in the supine position. The left kidney lies 1–2 cm higher than the right kidney. The upper poles are directed posteromedially. The normal adult kidney is bean shaped with a smooth convex contour anteriorly, posteriorly and laterally. Medially the surface is concave and is known as the renal hilum. The renal hilum is continuous with a central cavity called the renal sinus. The renal sinus contains blood vessels, pelvicalyceal system and fibrofatty tissue and appears as a central echogenic complex. The peripheral hypoechoic rim of tissues is the renal parenchyma, composed of outer cortex and inner, relatively hypoechoic renal medullary pyramids. Renal cortical echogenicity is either less or equal to that of the adjacent liver and spleen. Parenchymal junctional defect may be seen in normal kidney and should not be confused with renal scars and angiomyolipoma. It is seen as an echogenic line, located

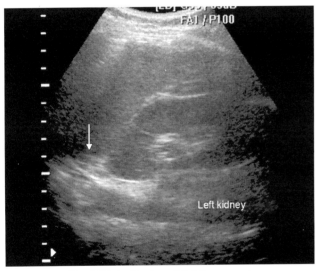

Fig. 9.73: Left adrenal (white arrows).

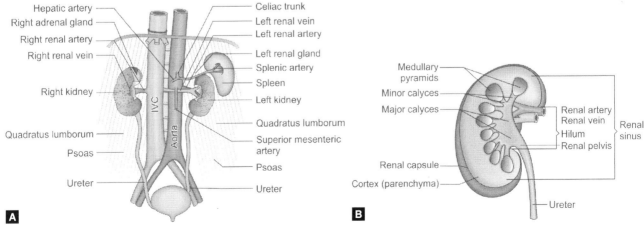

Figs. 9.74A and B: (A) Location of the urinary system; (B) Anatomy of the kidney.

CHAPTER 9: Basic Sonographic Anatomy

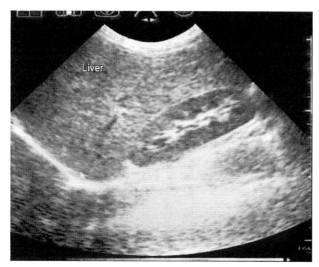

Fig. 9.75: Right kidney seen in posterior relation to the liver in the sagittal scan.

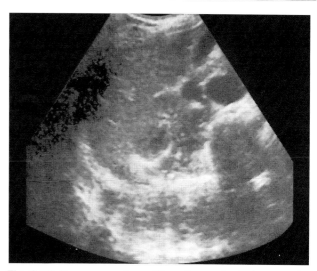

Fig. 9.78: Transverse view of liver. Appearing kidney can be confused with a lesion in the liver.

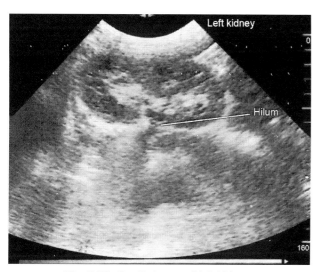

Fig. 9.76: Sagittal scan of left kidney.

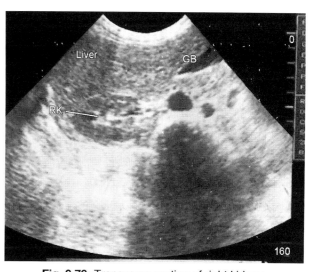

Fig. 9.79: Transverse section of right kidney.

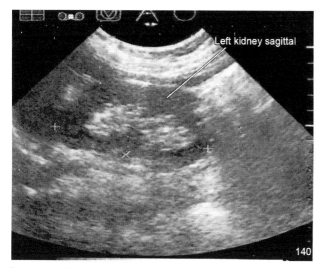

Fig. 9.77: Sagittal scan of left kidney showing length and AP dimension.

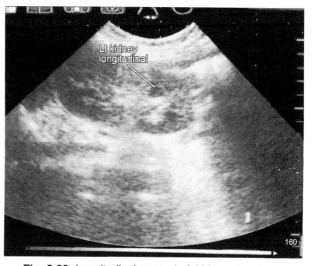

Fig. 9.80: Longitudinal scan—Left kidney showing a prominent pyramid.

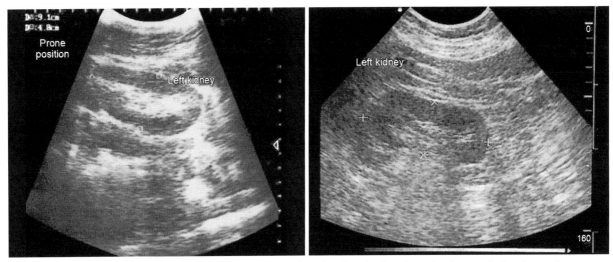

Fig. 9.81: Sagittal scan of left kidney in prone position showing the length and anteroposterior dimension.

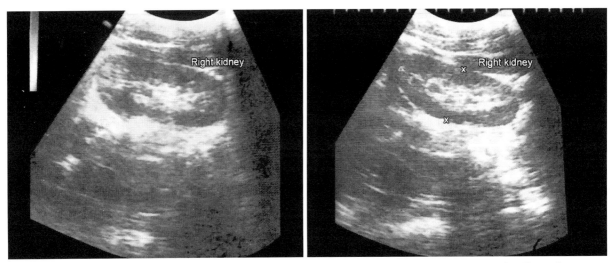

Fig. 9.82: Sagittal scan of right kidney in prone position showing the length and anteroposterior dimension.

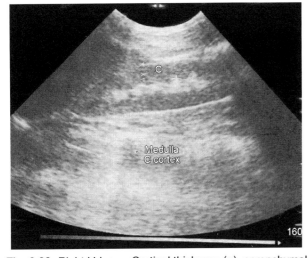

Fig. 9.83: Right kidney—Cortical thickness (×), parenchymal thickness (+).

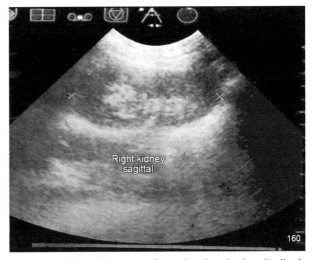

Fig. 9.84: Right kidney—caliper showing the longitudinal dimension.

anterosuperiorly extending from the perinepheric fat medially and inferiorly into the renal sinus. Hypertrophied column of Bertini (HCB) is a normal variant and represents unresorbed polar parenchyma from one or both of the two subkidneys that fuse to form the normal kidney. HCB is usually located at the junction of the upper and middle thirds of the kidney and indents the renal sinus laterally. It is bordered by a junctional parenchymal line and defect. It is continuous with the adjacent renal cortex, contains renal pyramids and is less than 3 cm in size. The kidney has a thin fibrous true capsule, perirenal fat surrounds this capsule. The fat is encased anteriorly by the fibrous fascia of Gerota and posteriorly by the fibrous fascia of Zuckerkandl. The renal capsule appears as a thin bright smooth echogenic line around the kidney.

Renal length correlates with body height and renal size decreases with advancing age because of parenchymal reduction. Normal renal measurements are: length—9–12 cm, width—4–6 cm, and thickness 3.5 cm. A difference of more than 2 cm in the lengths of the 2 kidneys is significant.

Ureter

It is a long 30–34 cm mucosal lined tube that delivers urine from the renal pelvis to the bladder. Its diameter varies between 2–8 mm.

Bladder (Figs. 9.88 to 9.90)

The bladder is situated in the pelvis, anteroinferior to the peritoneal cavity and posterior to the pubic bones. The shape, position and wall thickness of the bladder varies with degree of bladder distention. When distended it appears as a large anechoic area with smooth, uniformly thin walls, less than 4 mm. Following micturition, residual urine volume is normally less than 60 cc.

PROSTATE AND SEMINAL VESICLES (FIGS. 9.91 TO 9.93)

Transabdominal technique is used for estimation of size and radiotherapy planning and transrectal technique is used to evaluate for prostatic carcinoma. Transverse axial sections of the prostate provide anatomical detail of the gland symmetry, the seminal vesicles, and zonal anatomy. Sagittal sections are essential for imaging the urethra and its surrounding tissue and the configuration of the prostate at the bladder base. The normal prostate gland has a top like configuration with its base abutting against the bladder and apex directed downwards. The prostatic urethra runs through the centre of the gland in the midline. Volume of normal gland is up to 20 cc.

The normal prostate **(Figs. 9.94A to E)** measures 2.5 cm in its AP dimension 4 cm side to side and 3.5 cm from the bladder neck to its apex.

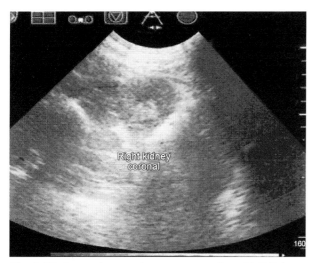

Fig. 9.85: Coronal scan—transverse section of left kidney.

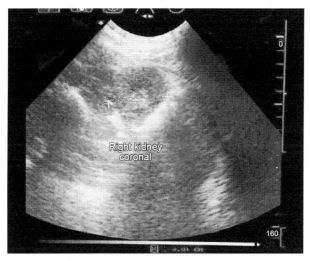

Fig. 9.86: Coronal scan—Transverse section of left kidney showing anteroposterior and mediolateral dimension.

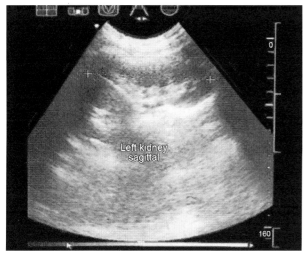

Fig. 9.87: Longitudinal scan showing normal left kidney.

Three glandular zones (peripheral, central and transitional) and one nonglandular zone the fibromuscular stroma can be identified on transrectal ultrasound (TRUS).

A fourth glandular zone, constituting 1% of the glandular volume consists of glands embedded in the longitudinal smooth muscles of the proximal urethra. The transitional zone located around the proximal urethra accounts for 5% of prostate volume. It is within this zone that hyperplasia and 10% of cancers develop. The central zone constitutes 25% of the normal glandular volume and is cone shaped, located near the prostatic base, and narrows at its apex near the veru montanum. The peripheral zone constitutes 70% of the normal glandular tissue. It envelops the other zones to form the posterolateral and apical parts of the prostate and is the site of origin of 70% of cancers. It is separated from the transition zone and central zone by the surgical capsule which is often hyperechoic as a result of corpora amylacea or calcification. The anterior portion of the prostate is the non-glandular fibromuscular stroma.

The transitional and central zones are both hypoechoic and heterogeneous. The peripheral zone is more reflective and homogeneous. The urethra and surrounding glands and smooth muscles are usually hypoechoic, but when corpora amylacea fill the periurethral glands urethra is collapsed, it appears as an echogenic line coursing through the prostate to its apex **(Figs. 9.95A and B)**.

The seminal vesicles are seen as paired, relatively hypoechoic multiseptate structures surrounding the rectum, cephalad to the base of the prostate gland. They usually measure less in width but may be very large and contain cysts occasionally **(Figs. 9.96A and B)**.

UTERUS AND ADNEXA

The standard transabdominal sonogram is performed with a distended urinary bladder, with 3.5 MHz transducer. The urinary bladder is considered ideally filled when it covers the entire fundus of the uterus. The distended bladder displaces the bowel out of the pelvis and displaces the pelvic organs

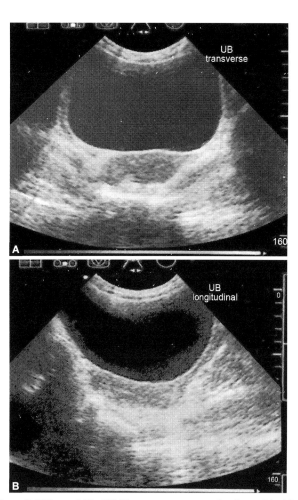

Figs. 9.88A and B: (A) Transverse scan of urinary bladder (UB) in a female pelvis. The uterus is seen posterior to it; (B) Longitudinal scan of urinary bladder in the same patient.

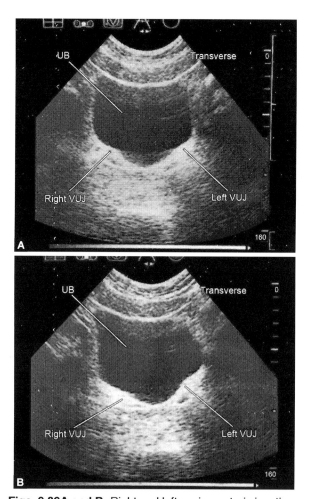

Figs. 9.89A and B: Right and left vesicoureteric junctions (VUJ) seen in transverse section of urinary bladder.

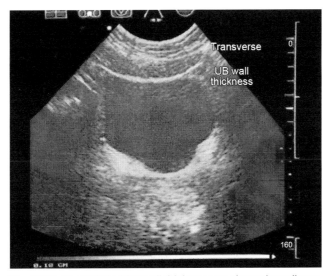

Fig. 9.90: Normal bladder wall thickness as shown by calipers.

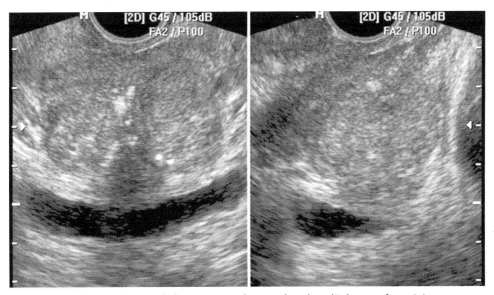

Fig. 9.91: High resolution transrectal coronal and sagittal scan of prostate.

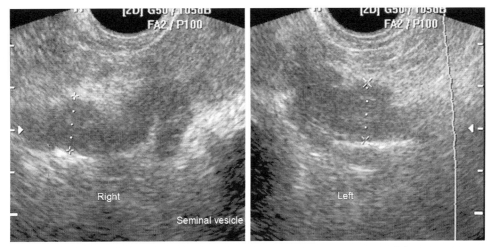

Fig. 9.92: High resolution transrectal scan showing seminal vesicles.

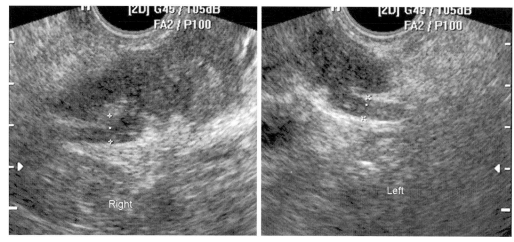

Fig. 9.93: High resolution transrectal scan of showing distal part of ductus deferens.

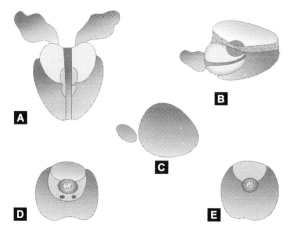

Figs. 9.94A to E: Diagram of prostate zonal anatomy. (A) Coronal section, mid-prostate; (B) Sagittal midline section; (C) Sagittal section, lateral prostate and seminal vesicle; (D) Axial section, prostatic base. Paired ejaculatory ducts are seen posterior to urethra and periurethral glandular area zone encompasses most of posterior and lateral aspect of gland; (E) Axial section, apex or gland showing mostly peripheral zone, and urethral and periurethral glandular area.

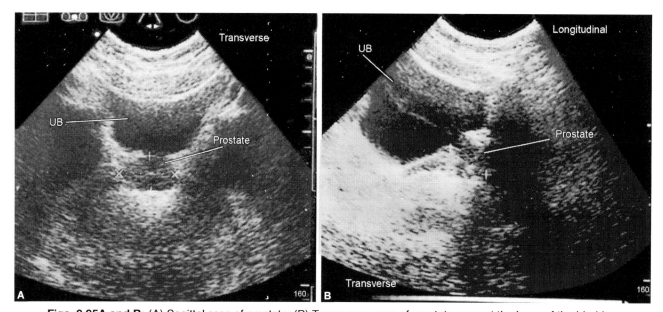

Figs. 9.95A and B: (A) Sagittal scan of prostate; (B) Transverse scan of prostate seen at the base of the bladder.

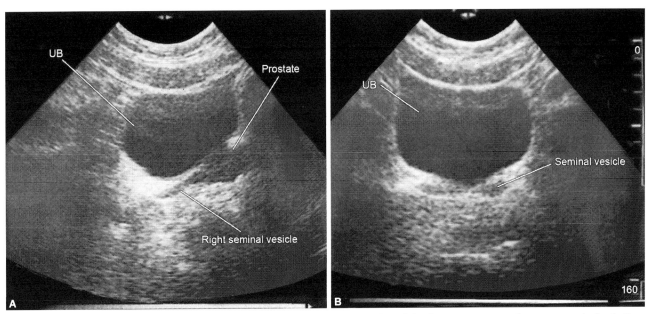

Figs. 9.96A and B: (A) Sagittal scan of right seminal vesicle, (B) Seminal vesicles in transverse section seen posterior to the urinary bladder.

5-10 cm from the anterior abdominal wall, besides providing an acoustic window to view them. Imaging of the uterus and adnexa is performed in both sagittal and transverse planes. The adnexa may be visualized scanning obliquely from the contralateral side or by scanning directly over it. For transvaginal sonography, the bladder must be empty to bring the pelvic organs into the focal zone of the transducer. A 5.0 MHz or 7.5 MHz transvaginal transducer is used. The transducer is prepared with ultrasound gel and then covered with a protective rubber sheath, usually a condom. Air bubbles should be eliminated to avoid artifacts. An external lubricant is then applied to the outside of the protective covering. The patient lies, supine, knees gently flexed and hips elevated slightly on a pillow. The transducer is inserted into the vagina and rotated and angulated such that both sagittal and coronal images are obtained **(Figs. 9.97A and B)**.

Transabdominal and transvaginal sonography are complementary technique. In most clinics transabdominal sonography is the initial pelvic examination, with transvaginal sonography reserved for a more detailed evaluation, if required. The transabdominal approach visualizes the entire pelvis and gives a global overview. Transvaginal sonography provides better anatomic detail and image quality as higher frequency transducers are used and is particularly useful in obese patients, those patients who are unable to fill their bladders and those with a retroverted uterus. Specific indications for transvaginal sonography:
- Uncertain transabdominal findings.
- Better characterization of a lesion.
- Strong family history of ovarian cancer.
- Suspected endometrial disorders.
- Assessment of a retroverted or retroflexed uterus.

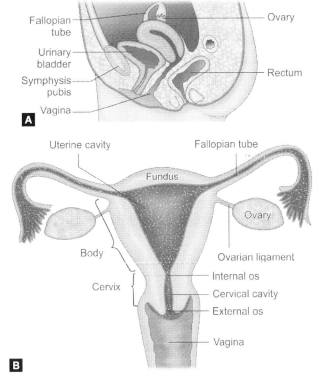

Figs. 9.97A and B: (A) Female pelvis; (B) Anatomy of uterus, fallopian tubes, ovaries, and vagina.

Uterus and adnexa: Normal sonographic anatomy **(Figs. 9.98 to 9.107)**.

The uterus lies in the true pelvis between the urinary bladder anteriorly and the rectosigmoid colon posteriorly. The body of uterus is very mobile and may lie in the midline (usually) or obliquely on either side of the midline.

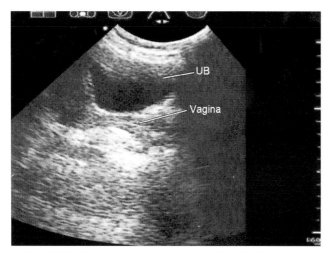

Fig. 9.98: Normal vagina as seen in a longitudinal scan.

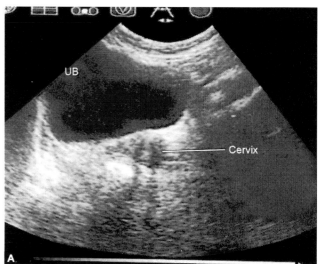

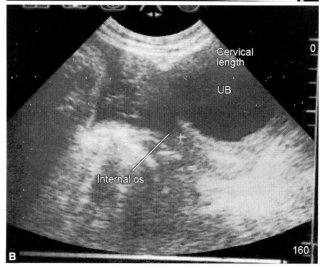

Figs. 9.99A and B: (A) Normal cervix as seen in a transverse scan; (B) Internal os and cervix are seen in sagittal scan with a partially full bladder cervix length is shown by calipers.

The cervix is fixed in the midline. The uterus is usually anteverted and anteflexed. Flexion refers to the axis of the uterine body relative to the cervix, whereas version refers to the axis of the cervix relative to the vagina. The uterus may be retroflexed when the body is tilted posteriorly relative to the cervix or retroverted when the entire uterus is tilted backwards relative to the vagina. Size and shape of uterus varies with age, parity and hormonal status. The infantile or pediatric uterus increases 2.0-3.5 cm in length, with body to cervical length ratio of 1:2 and AP diameter ranging from 0.5-1.0 cm. The prepubertal uterus has a tubular or inverse pear shape, with AP diameter of the cervix being greater than that of the body or fundus. In the immediate neonatal period because of residual maternal hormone stimulation the neonatal uterus is approximately 0.6-0.9 cm longer and 0.7-0.8 cm greater in AP diameter than the prepubertal uterus. Endometrium is echogenic and small amount of endometrial fluid may be present. After seven years of age, the uterus gradually increases in size until puberty and measures 6 cm in length by 13 years of age. At puberty there is rapid growth of the uterine body, such that ratio of body to cervical length becomes 2:1 and the uterus acquires a pear shape. The normal postpubertal nulliparous uterus measures 4.5-9.0 cm in length, 1.5-3 cm in AP and 4.5-5.5 cm in transverse diameters. Uterine dimensions increase by 1-1.2 cm with parity and the body becomes more rounded. After menopause the uterus atrophies rapidly, and in women over the age of 65 years its size ranges from 3.5-6.5 cm in length and 1.2-1.8 cm in AP diameter. The shape of postmenopausal uterus resembles that of premenopausal uterus. The normal myometrium comprises three layers. Of these the intermediate layer is the thickest and has a homogeneous texture of low to moderate echogenicity. The inner and outer layer is relatively hypoechoic to the intermediate layer. The normal endometrial cavity is seen as a thin echogenic line.

The sonographic appearance of the endometrium varies during the menstrual cycle. In the menstrual phase endometrium consists of thin broken echogenic line. During the proliferative phase the endometrium thickens, and the combined thickness of anterior and posterior layers of endometrium reaches 4.8 mm. It has a typical triple layer appearance central echogenic line, due to apposed endometrial surfaces surrounded by thicker hypoechoic functional layer, bounded by outer echogenic basal layer. Following ovulation the hypoechoic functional layer of endometrium becomes hyperechoic and the overall endometrial thickness increases to 7-14 mm. Following menopause the endometrium atrophies and is seen as a thin echogenic line not more than 8 mm thick.

Vagina

The vagina runs anteriorly and caudally from the cervix between the bladder and rectum. It is best seen sonographically on midline sagittal sections with a slight

CHAPTER 9: Basic Sonographic Anatomy

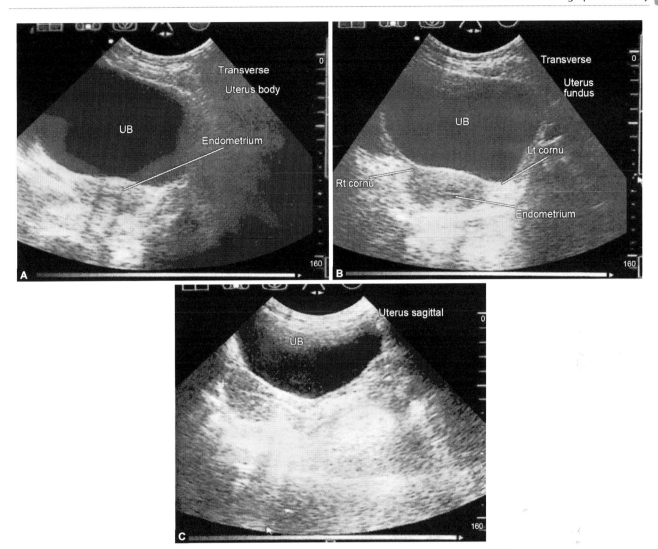

Figs. 9.100A to C: (A) Transverse scan of fundus of uterus showing both the cornu; (B) Transverse scan—Body of uterus showing the central echogenic endometrial cavity; (C) A normal retroverted uterus seen in a longitudinal view.

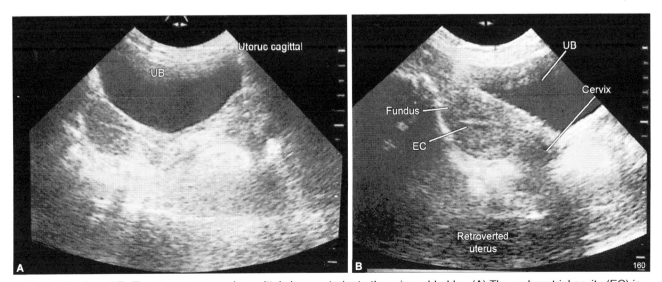

Figs. 9.101A and B: The uterus as seen in sagittal view posterior to the urinary bladder. (A) The endometrial cavity (EC) is seen as echogenic line; (B) Longitudinal scan of uterus showing its longitudinal and AP dimension.

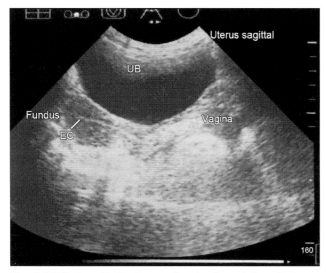

Fig. 9.101C: Longitudinal scan showing the relation of uterus, cervix and vagina to the urinary bladder.

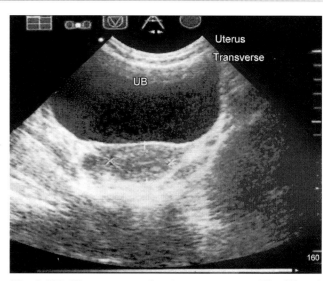

Fig. 9.103: Uterus as seen in a transverse scan. The AP and transverse dimension have been shown.

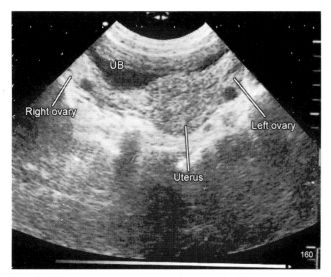

Fig. 9.102: Transverse section of the body of the uterus and bilateral ovaries are seen posterior to a partially full urinary bladder.

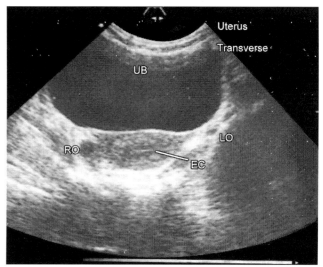

Fig. 9.104: Endometrium is seen as a dense echogenic line within the uterus. Both the ovaries are seen along side of uterus.

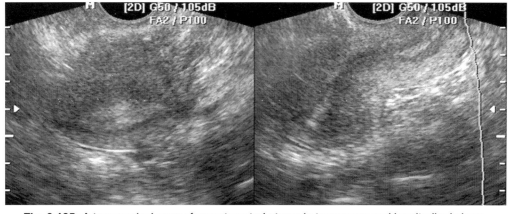

Fig. 9.105: A transvaginal scan of an anteverted uterus in transverse and longitudinal views.

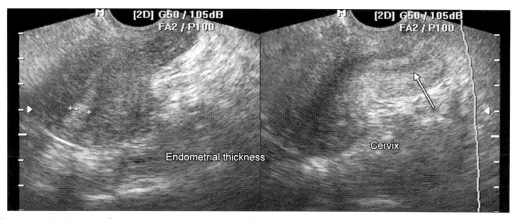

Fig. 9.106: A transvaginal scan of an anteverted uterus showing single layered echogenic endometrium (between the calipers) and cervix (white arrow).

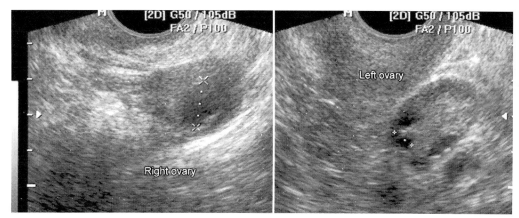

Fig. 9.107: A transvaginal scan through ovaries with multiple follicles.

caudal angulation of the transducer. It appears as a collapsed hypoechoic tubular structure with central, high amplitude, linear echo representing apposed mucosal surfaces.

Rectouterine recess/Posterior cul-de-sac/Pouch of Douglas is the most posterior and inferior reflection of the peritoneal cavity and is located between the rectum and vagina. Small amount of fluid may be seen in the cul-de-sac in asymptomatic women, during all phases of menstruation.

Ovary (Figs. 9.108 A and B)

Ovaries have a very variable position and may lie high in the pelvis, or in the cul-de-sac or be extremely laterally placed. Usually they lie lateral or posterolateral to the anteflexed midline uterus.

The ovaries are ellipsoidal in shape, with their craniocaudal axes paralleling the internal iliac vessels, which lie posteriorly. A normal ovary has a relatively homogenous echotexture with a central more echogenic medulla. Well defined, small anechoic or cystic follicles may be seen peripherally in the cortex. During the proliferative phase of the menstrual cycle many follicles are stimulated and they develop and increase in size until about the day eight or nine of the cycle. At that time one follicle becomes dominant and increases in size to up to 2–2.5 cm. The other follicles become atretic. Following ovulation the corpus luteum develops and may be identified as a small hypoechoic or isoechoic structure peripherally within the ovary. It involutes before menstruation.

Ovaries vary in shape, ovarian volume is thus the best indicator of ovarian size. The volume measurement is based on the formula for a prolate ellipse (0.52 × length × width × height).

Mean ovarian volume in the 1st year of life is a little more than 1 cc, 3.6 cc being the upper limit, in the first 3 months and 2.7 cc between 4–12 months. In the second year, the mean ovarian volume is slightly greater than 0.7 cc, the upper limit being 1.7 cc.

Ovarian volume remains relatively stable up to five years of age, and then gradually increases, when the mean volume is 4.2 ± 2.3 cc, with an upper limit of 8.0 cc. Small follicles are seen in the neonatal and premenarchal ovaries, usually <9 mm in size, but may be as large as 17 cc. After puberty, i.e. onset of menstruation, the mean ovarian volume = 9.8 ± 5.8 cc, 22 cc being regarded the normal upper limit following menopause, the ovaries atrophy and the follicles usually

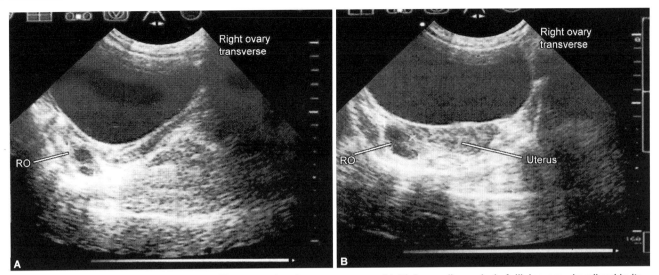

Figs. 9.108A and B: (A) Right ovary (RO) as seen in a transverse scan. Multiple small anechoic follicles are visualized in it; (B) Right ovary is seen along the uterus, the longitudinal and transverse dimensions of right ovary have been shown.

disappear. Mean ovarian volume ranges between 1.2–5.8 cc, with 8.0 cc being the upper limit of normal. Small anechoic cysts less than 3 cm in diameter may be seen sometimes in normal postmenopausal ovaries.

SCROTUM

The patient lies supine with thighs adducted and a towel placed underneath the scrotum. A high frequency 7.5 MHz or 10 MHz transducer is placed directly over the skin or over an interposed water bath.

The scrotum **(Figs. 9.109A to D)** is divided into two chambers by a midline scrotal septum. The scrotal wall comprises of the following layers from without inwards—(i) skin, (ii) dartos muscle, (iii) external spermatic fascia, (iv) cremasteric fascia and, (v) internal spermatic fascia, all which appear as an inseparable single echogenic stripe **(Figs. 9.110 to 9.112)**.

The adult testis is an ovoid organ measuring 3–5 cm in length 2–4 cm in width and 3 cm in AP diameter. The long axis of the testis is in a craniocaudal orientation. Each testis is surrounded by a dense fibrous capsule the tunica albuginea which may be visualized as a thin echogenic line on sonography. Multiple thin septations (septula) arise from the capsule and converge posteriorly to form the mediastinum testis. They divide the testis into lobules that contain the seminiferous tubules. These tubules join each other to form larger ducts known as tubuli recti, which enter the mediastinum testis, forming a network of channels within the testicular stroma, called the rete testis. The rete terminates in 10–15 efferent ductules at the superior portion of the mediastinum and carries seminal fluid from the testis to the epididymis.

The testis has a uniform echotexture composed of medium level echoes. The mediastinum testis is seen as a linear echogenic band extending craniocaudally within the testicular substance. The septula testis may be seen as linear echogenic or hypoechoic structures. The rete testis may be visualized as a hypoechoic or septated cystic area adjacent to the head of the epididymis.

The epididymis is a curved structure, 6.7 cm long, lying posterolateral to the testis. It is composed of a head, body and a tail. The head of the epididymis is known as the globus major and is located adjacent to the superior pole of the testis and is the largest portion of the epididymis. It is 10–12 mm in diameter and iso to hyperechoic to the testis.

The body or the corpus lies posterolateral to the testis, and is isoechoic or hypoechoic to the testis and measures usually 1–2 mm and up to 4 mm in diameters. The tail, appendix epididymis and appendix testis are identified as separate structures when a hydrocele is present. Occasionally a prominent vessel is seen traversing the substance of testis, as a tubular structure.

The normal spermatic cord lies just beneath the skin and is thus difficult to visualize sonographically.

The testis is covered on all sides by a double layer of tunica vaginalis, (which is the lower persistent portion of the processes vaginalis) except the posterior aspect. The inner or the visceral of tunica vaginalis covers the testis epididymis and the lower portion of the spermatic cord. The outer or parietal layer of the tunica vaginalis lines the walls of the scrotal pouch and is attached to fascial covering of the testis. A small amount of fluid is normally present between these layers.

PENIS

Patient lies supine and the penis is placed over the anterior abdominal wall. High frequency 7.5 MHz or 10.0 MHz linear array probes are used. The transducer is placed transversely on the ventral surface, starting at the level of the glans and moving down to the base of penis.

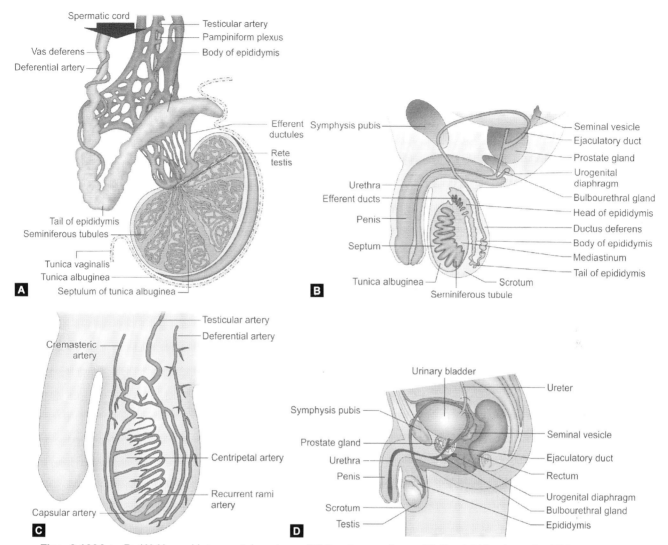

Figs. 9.109A to D: (A) Normal intrascrotal anatomy; (B) Scrotum anatomy; (C) Scrotal blood supply; (D) Male pelvis.

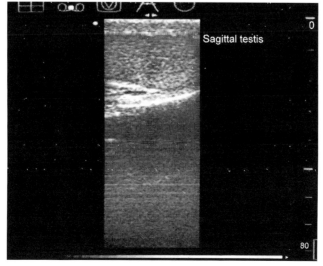

Fig. 9.110A: Sagittal scan of testis showing a homogeneous echotexture.

100 Principles and Practice of Ultrasonography

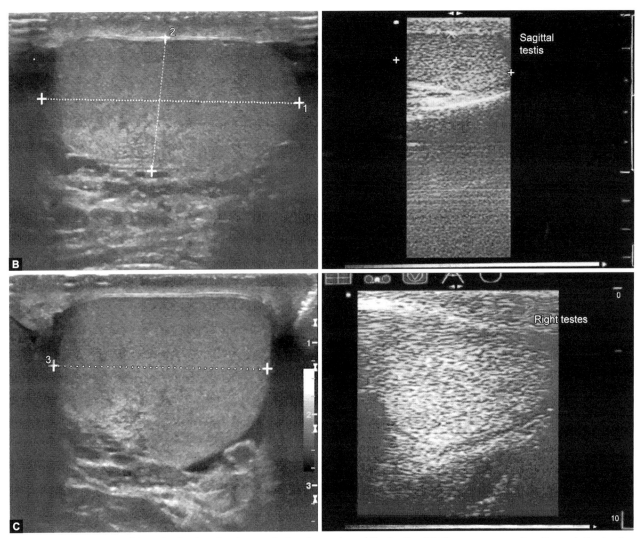

Figs. 9.110B and C: (B) Longitudinal and anteroposterior dimension of the testis; (C) Transverse section through the testis.

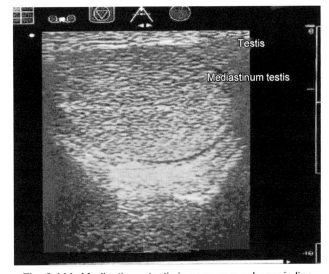

Fig. 9.111: Mediastinum testis is seen as a echogenic line through the testis.

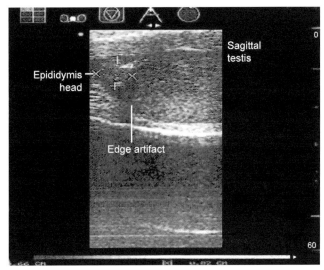

Fig. 9.112A: Head of epididymis of normal size.

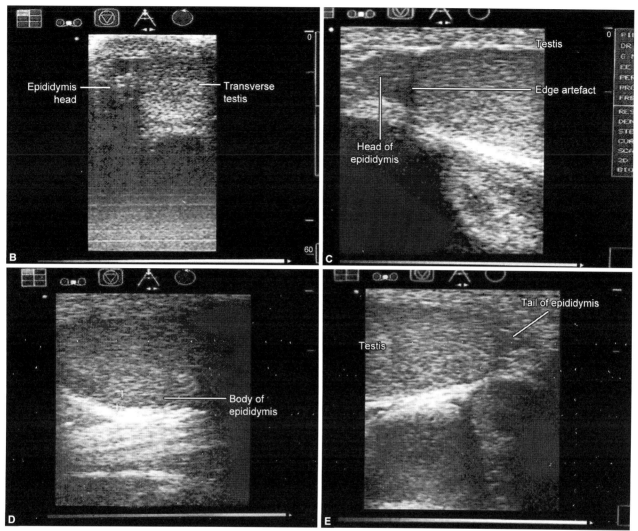

Figs. 9.112B to E: (B) Transverse scan showing the head of epididymis and superior pole of the testis; (C) Edge artifact from the head of epididymis; (D) Sagittal scan showing body of epididymis; (E) Tail of epididymis seen at the inferior pole of the testis in this sagittal scan.

Longitudinal evaluation is also done from the ventral surface. Copious amounts of the acoustic gel or an acoustic pad and gentle compression aid the visualization of the corpus spongiosum. Visualization of the penile urethra is optimally performed by distending it preferably by injecting a lidocaine gel in a retrograde fashion through the urethral meatus and then clamping the distal penis.

The penis **(Fig. 9.113)** is composed of three cylindrical structures of cavernous tissue, two dorsally lying corpora cavernosa and a single ventrally placed corpus spongiosum. These are enveloped in a thick fascial sheath, the tunica albuginea. The urethra travels through the centre of the corpus spongiosum. Distally the penis exhibits a conical extremity the glans penis, formed by an expansion of the corpus spongiosum, which fits over the blunt terminations of the corpora cavernosa. The paired dorsal arteries lie dorsally posterior to the tunica albuginea and supply blood to the skin and glans penis. The cavernosal arteries lie in the center of each corpus cavernosum. The deep dorsal vein travels on the dorsal aspect of the penis along the dorsal arteries and is sonographically visible.

On transverse scanning through the ventral surface, the two corpora cavernosa are easily identified as circular structures, adjacent to each other, separated by the septum penis. They have a uniform echotexture and are slightly echogenic compared to the corpus spongiosum. The fascial planes including the tunica albuginea are seen as their echogenic lines surrounding the corporal structures. The penis should be scanned to include the possibility of excessive amounts of fibrosis within the corporal bodies and/or in the fascial layers around the corporal bodies. Palpable abnormalities should be scanned and their exact location and sonographic features be noted. Cavernosal arteries are seen as tubular anechoic structures with echogenic walls in the center of corpora cavernosa. A central

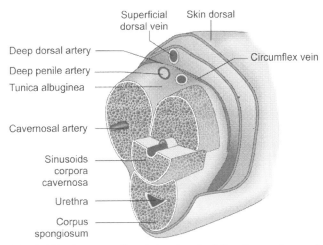

Fig. 9.113: Cross-sectional drawing depicting the anatomy of the penis.

echopoor lumen in the corpora spongiosum corresponds to the urethral lumen.

Thorax

Indications for chest sonography include:
- Differentiating pleural fluid from pleural masses.
- Identifying fluid in presence of pulmonary consolidation or collapse.
- To differentiate pleural from parenchymal lesion.
- To characterize the type of pleural fluid and to detect associated pleural abnormalities.
- To visualize the diaphragm and to differentiate subphrenic abscess from subpulmonic effusion.
- To aspirate/drain pleural collections under ultrasonic guidance that is small or difficult to localize clinically.

A direct intercostal approach using a 5 or 7.5 MHz linear transducer is used to visualize the pleural surface. The lower limit of the pleural space is effectively examined by using a 3.5 MHz sector transducer directed superiorly from the abdomen, i.e. by abdominal approach. Patient is examined in sitting and supine positions.

Direct intercostal approach with the linear probe oriented perpendicular to the intercostal spaces, the ribs are seen as rounded echogenic interfaces with prominent acoustic shadowing. Intercostal muscles are visualized between the rib shadows. The pleural space is located within 1 cm depth from the rib interface. The air filled lung covered by visceral pleura reflects the sound waves and produces a bright echogenic linear interface that moves with respiration also called "gliding sign". A thin hypoechoic line of pleural fluid is normally present separating the parietal and visceral pleura. The parietal pleura is seen as a less distinct weakly echogenic line often obscured by artifacts.

Abdominal approach: Through the abdomen the diaphragm which is about 5 mm thick, and appears as a bright curved echogenic line that moves with respiration. It is covered by the parietal pleura on its thoracic side and by peritoneum on its abdominal side. With an air filled lung the diaphragm-lung interface acts as a specular reflector and produces an artifactual mirror image of the liver or spleen above the diaphragm which is a definitive evidence of presence of air filled lung and absence of pleural fluid above the diaphragm.

NECK

Thyroid and Parathyroid Glands (Figs. 9.114 and 9.115)

Patient lies in the supine position. With a pad placed under the shoulders to extend neck. A preliminary scan of the entire thyroid region is done using a 5 MHz linear transducers and the size and relationship with adjacent structures of the gland are noted. A stand-off pad is used to reduce near field artifacts. A more detailed study is performed using high frequency transducers (7.5–15 MHz). The thyroid gland must be examined thoroughly in both transverse and longitudinal planes. Imaging of the lower poles can be enhanced by asking the patient to swallow, which momentarily raises a retrosternal thyroid gland in the neck. The examination should include the carotid artery, jugular vein and the jugular chain of lymph nodes laterally, submandibular lymph nodes superiorly and supraclavicular lymph nodes inferiorly **(Figs. 9.116 to 9.120)**.

The thyroid gland is located in anteroinferior part of the neck and consists of two lobes lying on either side of the trachea, connected across the midline by the isthmus, at the level of junction of middle and lower thirds of the gland. In many younger patients, a third pyramidal lobe is seen arising superiorly from the isthmus and lying in front of the thyroid cartilage.

In thin people, lateral lobes of normal glands may measure 7–8 cm in length and up to 1 cm in AP diameter,

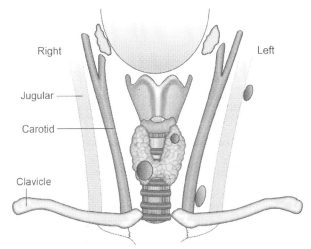

Fig. 9.114: Cervical "map" helps communicate relationships of pathology to clinicians and serves as a reference for follow-up examinations. (SMG, submandibular gland).

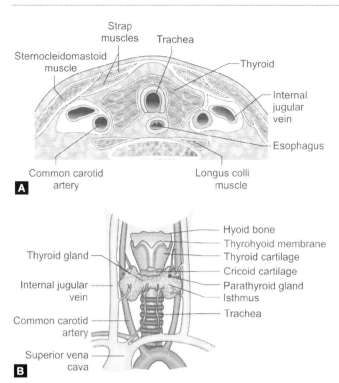

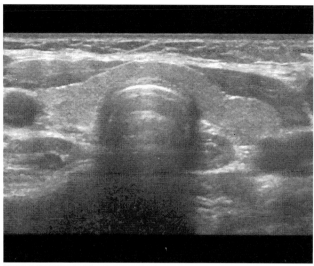

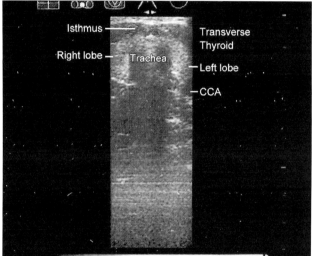

Figs. 9.115A and B: (A) Normal thyroid gland. Transverse diagrammatic representation; (B) Location and anatomy of thyroid gland.

Fig. 9.116: Thyroid gland in transverse section showing both the lobes and the isthmus.

but in obese people the length is usually less than 5 cm and the normal AP diameter may be up to 2 cm. The isthmus measures up to 4.6 mm in thickness. A thickness of >2 cm is suggestive of gland enlargement.

The normal thyroid gland is homogeneous in echotexture, and is hyperechoic compared to the adjacent strap muscles. It has a thin echogenic capsule and its texture may be interrupted by views, particularly at the poles. Small 2–3 mm echofree areas probably collard collections may be seen and in elderly people, nodular calcifications or linear bands of fibrous tissue may be seen.

The sternohyoid and omohyoid muscles are seen as thin hypoechoic bands anterior to the gland and sternocleidomastoid muscle is seen as a larger oval band lateral to the gland. The longus colli muscle is located posterior to each thyroid lobe. On longitudinal scan the recurrent laryngeal nerve and the inferior thyroid artery are seen a thin hypoechoic bands between the thyroid lobe and esophagus on the left and the thyroid lobe and longus colli muscle on the right side.

Parathyroid Glands

Most adults have four parathyroid glands two superior and two inferior each measuring 5 × 3 × 1 mm in size. A fifth supernumerary gland may be present in some people, usually in the anterior mediastinum associated with the thymus. The posterior thyroid glands lie adjacent to the posterior wall of the thyroid in the tracheoesophageal groove. The superior parathyroid gland usually lie at the junction of mid and upper third of the thyroid, just superior to the crossing of recurrent laryngeal nerve and inferior thyroid artery. The inferior parathyroids are very variable in position, but most lie close or at the inferior poles of thyroid lobes. The parathyroid glands are usually oval or bean shaped. They are isoechoic to the thyroid parenchyma and thus difficult to identify.

EYEBALL AND ORBIT

The eyeball is the dominant structure in the anterior orbit, embedded in fat, but separated from it by a membranous sac—Tenon's capsule. The eyeball is composed of two segments. The transparent anterior segment forms about 1/6th the size of eyeball and opaque posterior segment forms about five-sixth of the eyeball. The optic axis is an imaginary line joining the anterior pole—the central point of the anterior curvature of the eyeball to the posterior

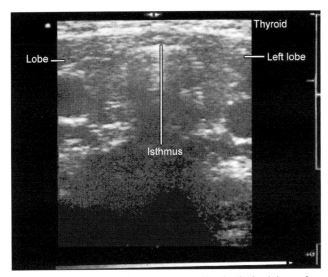

Fig. 9.117: Isthmus is seen connecting both the lobes of thyroid anterior to the trachea.

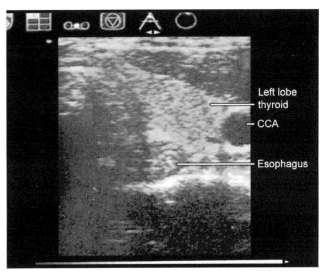

Fig. 9.118: Left lobe of thyroid in transverse section. Trachea is shown on the right side, esophagus is posterior and common carotid artery (CCA) is lateral to it.

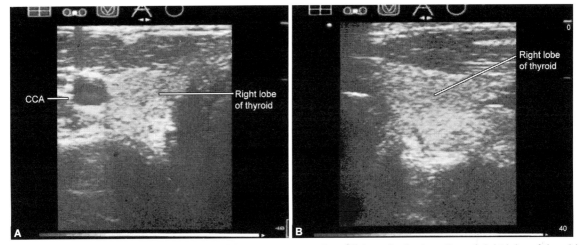

Figs. 9.119A and B: (A) Right lobe of thyroid in transverse section; (B) Longitudinal section of right lobe of thyroid.

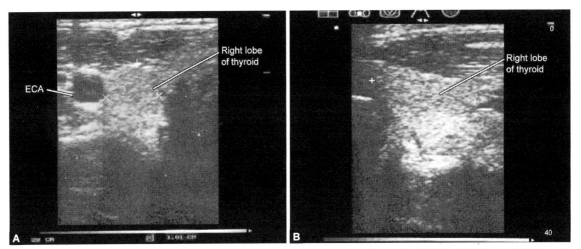

Figs. 9.120A and B: (A) Normal anteroposterior and mediolateral dimensions of the thyroid lobe; (B) Superoinferior dimension of the right lobe of thyroid.

pole—the central point of its posterior curvature. The normal axial length of the eye is 24 mm. The wall of the eyeball is made of three coats. The outer coat comprises the sclera and cornea. The sclera may be regarded as a up line expansion of the dural sheath of the optic nerve. It is thicker posteriorly (1 mm) than anteriorly (0.6 mm), or at the equator (0.5 mm). The optic nerve pierces the sclera, posteriorly 3 mm medial to the posterior pole and slightly above the horizontal meridian. The transparent cornea bulges forward from the sclera and measures 0.9 mm at its center and 1.2 mm at its periphery **(Figs. 9.121 to 9.125)**.

The intermediate coat comprises the choroid, the ciliary body and the iris. The choroid is up to 1 mm thick, and hypoechoic compared to the retina and sclera. It is separated from the sclera by the subchoroidal space. Anteriorly the choroid merges into the pars plana of the ciliary body at the ora serrata. The ciliary body is triangular in cross section being thicker anteriorly. It extends from the

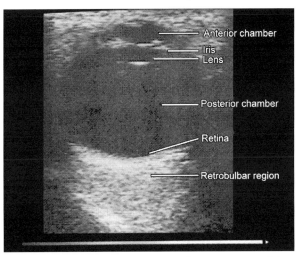

Fig. 9.123: Homogeneous echogenic appearance of the retrobulbar region is shown in this transverse section.

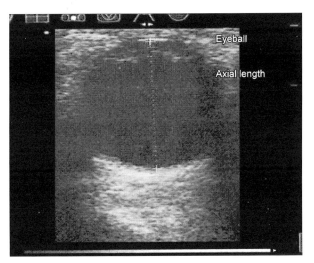

Fig. 9.121: Axial length of the eyeball as shown by calipers.

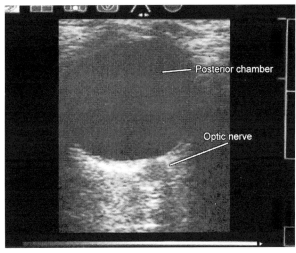

Fig. 9.124: Optic nerve is seen as a hypoechoic band in the retrobulbar region.

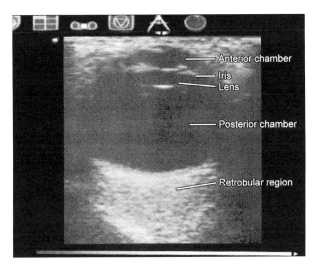

Fig. 9.122: Transverse section of the eyeball showing the anterior and the posterior chambers.

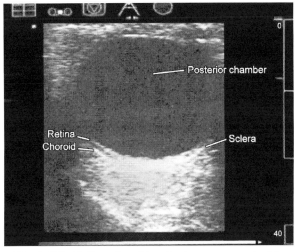

Fig. 9.125: Retina, choroid and sclera are seen in this transverse section.

corneoscleral junction backwards just over half way to the equator. The iris is a contractile diaphragm up to 1 mm in thickness, situated in front of the lens obscuring the anterior lens surface, the pupil is the circular aperture positioned slightly towards the nasal side of the center of the iris. The iris partially divides the space between the cornea and lens into aqueous filled anterior and posterior chambers of the eye. The retina is the innermost layer comprising of an anterior and posterior surface. It originates from the entrance of optic nerve and ends at the posterior edge of the ciliary body in a dentate line named the ora serrata. It is 0.4 mm thick near the optic nerve and decreases to 0.1 mm near the ora serrata. The retina is more firmly attached at the optic disc and ora serrata. The optic disc has a diameter of 1.5 mm and has slightly raised circumference. The macula is positioned 4 mm lateral to the optic disc and 1 mm inferior to it.

The refracting media of the eyeball comprise the cornea, aqueous humor, the lens and the vitreous body. The lens is a transparent biconvex body enclosed in a transparent elastic capsule. It is 10 mm in diameter and 3–4 mm thick. Its posterior surface indents the vitreous and is more convex than the anterior surface. A normal lens has an echofree interior, but echoes arise from the central part of the posterior lens cortex giving rise to a fine curved echogenic line on sonography.

The suspensory ligament is a series of fibrils attached to the ciliary processes and further back to the ora serrata. These fibrils pass centrally and attach themselves to the lens mostly anterior to the circumference and may be seen as fine linear echoes. The vitreous body is a transparent gel occupying the posterior four fifth of the eyeball. It is also attached to the optic disc, but more firmly at the pars plana, just in front of the ora serrata. Elsewhere, it lies in contact with the retina and is separated from it by the subretinal or retrohyaloid space. It is anechoic on sonography, but its posterior surface is sometimes seen undulating off the retina when scanning during eye movements.

Indications

- Opaque light conducting media, making direct vision by ophthalmoscopy difficult.
- Suspected intraocular tumor.
- To differentiate serous and solid retinal detachment.
- Examination of the vitreous.
- Localization of foreign bodies.
- Ocular measurements.
- Proptosis.
- Doppler investigation of orbital vascular disease and tumors.

Patient lies supine, and a 7.5 MHz or 10 MHz small part probe is placed directly over the closed eyelid direct contact method or a water bath may be used. Image of the globe is taken both when static and during rapid eye movements, and any after movements of pathological structures is noted.

The orbit is a pear shaped bony cavity whose stalk is the optic nerve, passing through the optic canal. Its medial and lateral walls are best demonstrated in a horizontal plane and the roof and floor in the vertical plane. The lacrimal gland is located in the lacrimal fossa, situated anterolaterally in the upper outer quadrant of the orbit, but is difficult to visualize sonographically unless enlarged. The orbit contains the eyeball, the nerves which innervate it including the optic nerve, the extrinsic muscles which move the eyeball and nerves and vessels which supply them. The optic nerve and ocular muscles pass anterolaterally from the apex of the orbit to their ocular attachments. The four recti arise from a tendinous ring at the apex and broaden out to form a cone of muscles around the eyeball. Within this cone lies the highly echogenic mass of fat which is traversed by the hypoechoic optic nerve, which is 25 mm in length in its intraorbital portion. The ocular muscles are seen as thin hypoechoic straps, their tendons are narrow anteriorly, and they have a fusiform muscle belly which tapers posteriorly into the orbital apex. The medial and lateral recti are readily seen in the horizontal plane. The superior and inferior muscles are seen in the vertical sections. The inferior oblique lies inferior and immediately behind the globe below the macula. The superior oblique is in the upper medial orbit.

BREAST (FIG. 9.126)

A high frequency probe 7–10 MHz with focal zones of up to 3 cm is used. An offset acoustic pad may be used to visualize the superficial structures. Sonography of the outer breast is performed with patient in supine oblique position. The side to be examined is elevated by placing a pillow behind that shoulder and torso, the ipsilateral arm is elevated and flexed at the elbow and hand rests under the neck. This position minimizes the thickness of the upper outer quadrant of breast tissue. Adequate sonographic penetration is assured of the underlying pectoral muscles and ribs are visualized. For imaging the other three quadrants of the breast the patient should lie supine both transverse and sagittal scans

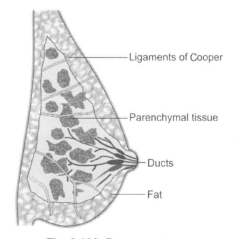

Fig. 9.126: Breast anatomy.

are obtained. The mammary ducts are visualized radially and in orthogonal antiradial direction. The nipple-areola complex is visualized using an offset pad or a fluid filled bag to improve the resolution of the near field structures. The tissue beneath the nipple is imaged by placing the transducer adjacent to the nipple and angling into the retroareolar area **(Figs. 9.127 to 9.133)**.

The anatomic components of the breast and surrounding structures have characteristic sonographic features. The skin complex is seen as two thin echogenic lines with a narrow hypoechoic band of dermis in between. The normal skin measures up to 2 mm in thickness. The mammary tissue is enclosed within a fascial envelope composed of superficial and deep layer which are usually not identified on sonography. The superficial layer is sometimes seen below the dermis and the deep layer lies over the retromammary fat and pectoralis muscle. The ribs appear as

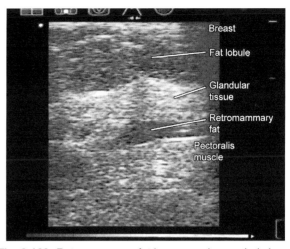

Fig. 9.129: Retromammary fat is seen as hypoechoic band under the echogenic glandular breast.

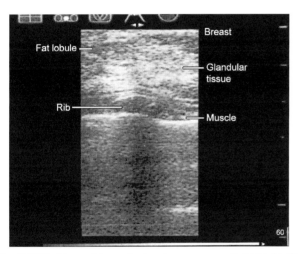

Fig. 9.127: Normal breast structures are well seen in this transverse scan. Glandular part of the breast appears echogenic while fat lobules are seen as oval hypoechoic structures.

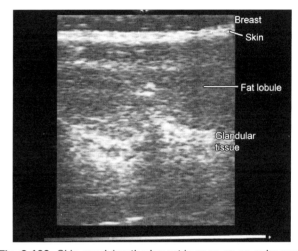

Fig. 9.130: Skin overlying the breast is seen as an echogenic thin band.

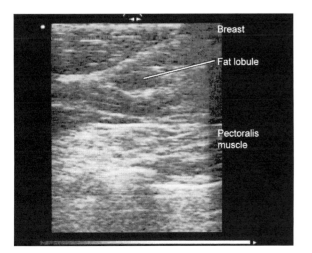

Fig. 9.128: Section taken from the upper lateral quadrant reveals fat lobules and the overlying muscle.

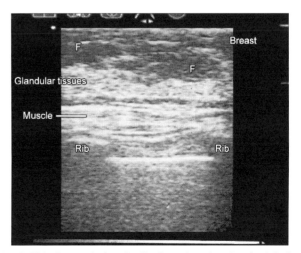

Fig. 9.131: Breast in longitudinal section showing fat lobules, echogenic glandular tissue, subareolar fatty layer and pectoralis muscle.

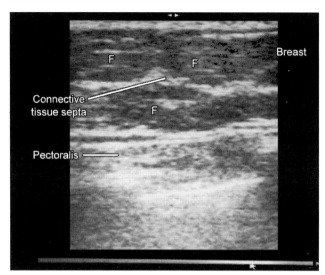

Fig. 9.132: Breast showing connective tissue septa as echogenic bands.

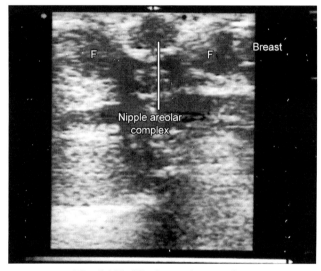

Fig. 9.133: Nipple areolar complex.

not identified. The mammary ducts are 7-20 in number and arranged radially around the nipple and become larger as they converge on the nipple. These are difficult to identify but are seen as tubular structures measuring 1-8 mm in diameter. These ducts become smaller and arborize in the peripheral portions of the breast. The nipple is of medium level echogenicity and attenuated sound, resulting in a posterior acoustic shadow. The normal nipple may sometimes appear as a well defined hypoechoic oval structure resembling a superficial adenoma if imaged from an oblique angle. Normal lymph nodes may be seen in the axilla and within breast parenchyma. They are reniform in shape and may have echogenic fatty hilum and hypoechoic parenchyma. The axillary vessels present as tubular pulsating structures.

Musculoskeletal System

Adult Hip

Bone obscures, the majority of the joint space in the mature hip **(Figs. 9.134 to 9.138)**. Fortunately the vertical recess of the joint capsule and the anterior extension of the joint space are readily seen on ultrasound images and so joint effusion or synovial thickening are easily diagnosed.

The iliofemoral ligament is applied closely to the anterior surface of the joint and provides a important landmark. The adjacent muscles are divided by distinct facial planes. The articular cartilage is thin 1-2 mm hypoechoic rim on the femora. In children the immature femoral head has a layer of unossified cartilage deep to the articular cartilage and both merge to form a thick hypoechoic band on ultrasound images.

Tendons (Fig. 9.139)

Tendons are made of densely packed parallel bundles of collagen fibers separated by ground substance and

oval hypoechoic periodic structures behind the pectoralis muscle and produce a posterior acoustic shadow. Intercostal muscles are identified between ribs.

The Cooper's ligaments provide connective tissue support for the breast and straddle the fascial envelope of the breast. They appear as thin echogenic arcs. Fat tubules are oval in one plane and elongate in the orthogonal plane. They are hypoechoic relative to the surrounding glandular tissue and may have a central echogenic focus of connective tissue. The glandular parenchyma appears homogeneously echogenic but may have hypoechoic zones caused by fatty tissue. The terminal duct lobular units (TDLU) are important anatomic units from which many benign (cysts, adenosis, and fibroadenomas) and malignant processes originate. They may enlarge or involute, reflecting age and physiologic differences. Hyperplastic TDLU are hypoechoic areas that can be visualized but a normal small TDLU is

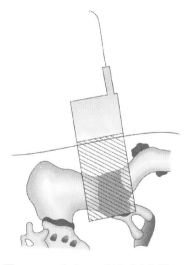

Fig. 9.134: The coronal plane of hip joint. Diagram to show the main anatomical structures.

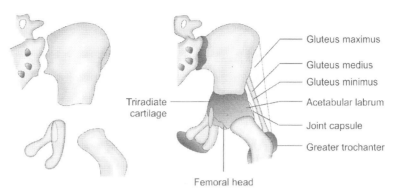

Fig. 9.135: Comparison of the X-ray and ultrasound anatomy. Anatomy as seen on a radiograph compared to the ultrasound coronal section of an infant's hip.

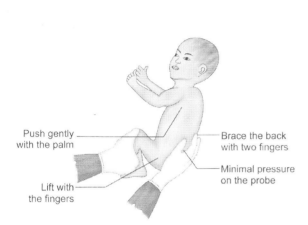

Fig. 9.136: Dynamic study of the infant hip. Direction of pressure exerted during the dynamic study of an infant's hip.

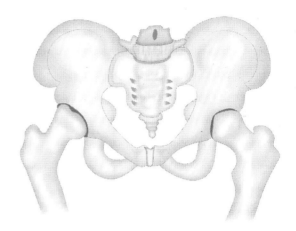

Fig. 9.137: Plane of the routine examination of irritable hip.

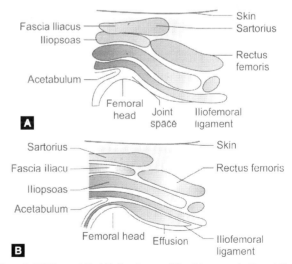

Figs. 9.138A and B: (A) Anatomy of the hip seen in the oblique sagittal plane; (B) Diagram of a hip containing an effusion.

fibroblasts. The peritoneum, a layer of loose connective tissue wraps around the tendon and sends intratendinous septae between the bundles of collagen fibers. In areas of mechanical constraint, tendons are associated with additional structures that provide mechanical support or protection. These include fibrous sheaths, sesamoid bones, synovial sheaths, and synovial bursae. High frequency 7.5–10 MHz linear array electronic probes are used to visualize the tendons at rest and during active and passive movements through flexion and extension maneuvers. A stand-off pad is used to visualize very superficial tendons and for evaluating tendons in regions with uneven surface. Care should be taken to always maintain the ultrasound beam perpendicular to surface of the tendon being examined, to avoid unnecessary artifacts like false hypoechogenicity. The contralateral extremity or region should always be examined for comparison.

On ultrasound examination, all tendons appear moderately echogenic and display a fibrillar texture on longitudinal scan and a finely punctate appearance on transverse scanning with high frequency transducers. Transverse scans are essential for measurement of maximum width thickness of tendons. Sesamoid bones are seen as echogenic structures with posterior acoustic shadowing. Synovial sheaths when seen with very high frequency (15 MHz) transducer, appear as hypoechoic area around the tendon. The large synovial bursae appear as flattened, fluid filled structures 2–3 mm thick.

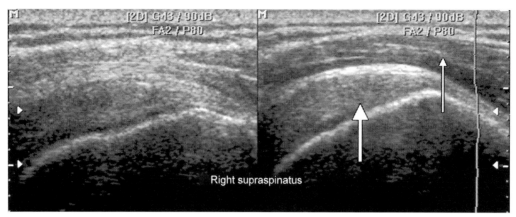

Fig. 9.139: Deltoid muscle belly (thin white arrow) and tendon of supraspinatus (thick white arrow).

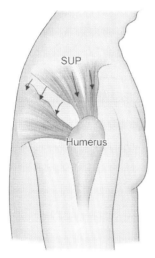

Fig. 9.140: General anatomic landmarks. Lateral photograph shows the bony structure, which limits the acoustic window for the examination of the cuff. SUP—Supraspinatus muscle and tendon; infraspinatus muscle and tendon (arrowheads), scapular spine (arrows), acromion.

Rotator Cuff (Figs. 9.140 to 9.145)

High resolution linear array transducer of 7.5 MHz frequency is used to visualize the rotator cuff tendon which is made of tendon of four muscles—the subscapularis, the supraspinatous, the infraspinatous, and the teres minor. The rotator cuff tendons are echogenic relative to the deltoid muscle belly and are surrounded by a thin hypoechoic synovial layer, less than 1.5 mm thick. The subacromial subdeltoid bursa shows as a hypoechoic stripe thinner than the thickness of the hypoechoic hyaline coartilage over the humeral head. The bursa is loaf-shaped in cross-section and extends from the coracoid anteriorly around the lateral shoulder and posterior part of the glenoid. The bursa is a potential space, and contains small amount of synovial fluid, not visualized on routine ultrasonography. The echogenic peribursal fat separates the bursa from the deltoid muscle.

The patient is scanned while sitting on a stool without armrests, and the examiner sits 5 cm above the patient, on another stool. To begin with the patient sits with his forearm on his thigh, hand palm pronated. Transverse images are taken through the proximal long biceps tendon, which appears as an echogenic oval structure in the bicipital groove. The bicipital groove is an important landmark over the anterior surface of the proximal humerus and is seen as a concave echogenic line. The long biceps tendon courses through the rotator cuff interval and divides the subscapularis from the supraspinatus tendon. As the transducer is moved superiorly above the bicipital groove the intracapsular portion of the tendon is seen obliquely in the shoulder capsule. Inferiorly the transverse scanning should be done up to the musculotendinous junction of the biceps to allow detection of the smallest fluid collection in the medial triangular recess at the distal end of the biceps tendon sheath. The transducer is rotated by 90° and aligned along the biceps groove to visualize the biceps tendon longitudinally. The transducer position is then returned to the transverse plane and moved proximally along the humerus to visualize subscapularis tendon which is viewed parallel to its axis and appears as a band of medium level echoes, deep to the subdeltoid fat and bursa. Scanning is also done during passive and external rotation to assess the integrity of the subscapularis tendon. Longitudinal scans of the tendon are obtained by rotating the transducer head by 90°. The normal subdeltoid bursa is recognized between the deltoid muscle on one side of the rotator cuff tendons and biceps tendon on the deep side. Next, the supraspinatous tendon is scanned, perpendicular to its axis, by moving the transducer posteriorly, over the humeral head, such that the probe head is directed downwards and slightly medially. The tendon is visualized as a band of medium level echoes deep to the subdeltoid bursa and superficial to the echogenic bony surface of the greater tuberosity.

The rest of the examination is done with the arm adducted and hyperextended and the should be in moderate internal rotation, as if the patient is reaching the opposite back pocket, longitudinal and transverse

CHAPTER 9: Basic Sonographic Anatomy

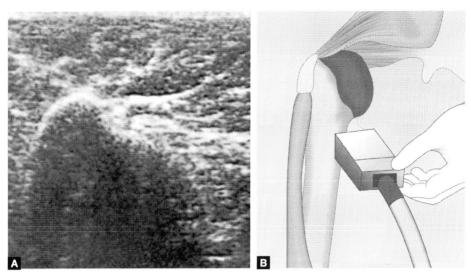

Figs. 9.141A and B: (A) Biceps tendon (transverse); (B) Transverse section of biceps tendon seen inside the bicipital groove.

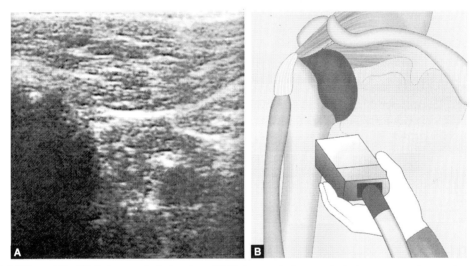

Figs. 9.142A and B: (A) Subscapularis tendon; (B) Subscapularis muscle in transverse plane subscapularis muscle in sagittal plane.

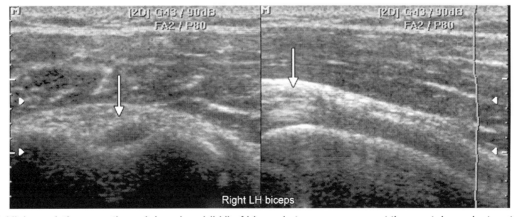

Fig. 9.143: High resolution scan through long head (LH) of biceps in transverse scan at the most dependant part of shoulder cavity and longitudinal scan in the upper part (white arrows).

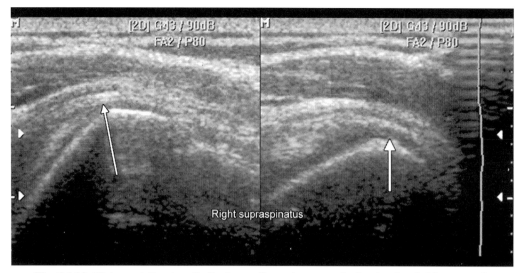

Fig. 9.144: High resolution longitudinal scan through supraspinatus tendon (white arrows).

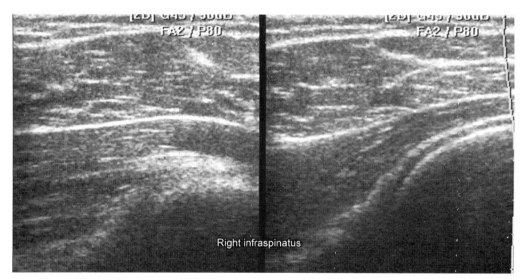

Fig. 9.145: High resolution longitudinal scan through infraspinatus tendon.

views of the supraspinatus tendon are obtained. During longitudinal scanning, the transducer overlays the acromion medially and lateral aspect of the greater tuberosity laterally. The transducer sweeps around the femoral head circumferentially starting anteriorly next to large biceps tendon and covering an area of 2.5 cm laterally. The infraspinatous tendon is scanned beyond this point. The musculotendinous junction shows as hypoechoic muscle surrounding the echogenic infraspinatous tendon. The transverse scanning of the supraspinatous tendon begins just lateral to the acromion and translates downward over the tendon and the greater tuberosity.

The transducer is then moved posteriorly, in the plane parallel to the scapular spine. The infraspinatous tendon appears as a beak shaped soft tissue structure as it attaches to the posterior surface of the greater tuberosity. The tendon is examined during internal and external rotation of the shoulder that relaxes and contracts the tendon respectively. At this level a portion of the posterior glenoid labrum is seen as an echogenic triangular structure surrounded by the hypoechoic fluid of the infraspinatous recess. The hypoechoic articular cartilage of the humeral head appears lateral to the labrum. Scanning is extended medially to visualize the suprascapular vessels and nerve in the spinoglenoid notch. The transversely oriented transducer is moved distally and trapezoid shaped teres minor is visualized. It is differentiated from the infraspinatious tendon by its broad and more muscular attachment. At the end of the examination, coronal images through the acromioclavicular joint are obtained. The superior glenoid labrum is shown with the transducer aligned posterior to the acromioclavicular joint and oriented perpendicular to the superior glenoid. Right and left sides are compared.

Elbow

With the elbow flexed at 90°, the tendons that are readily visualized include the lower tendon of triceps brachii and, the common tendon of flexor and extensor muscles of the forearm inserting into the medial and lateral epicondyle respectively. The lower tendon of the biceps brachii is rarely visualized inserting into the radial tuberosity.

Hand and Wrist (Fig. 9.146)

When the wrist is moderately flexed, the echogenic flexor tendons of the fingers are seen surrounded by the hypoechoic ulnar bursa, in the carpal tunnel. The median nerve which is slightly less echogenic than the tendons, courses anterior to the flexor tendons of the second finger outside the ulnar bursa. In the palm, the pairs of superficial and deep flexor tendons of the fingers are seen adjacent to the corresponding hypoechoic lumbrical muscles. At the fingers the flexor tendons lie in the concavity of the phalanges and this appear falsely echopoor along most of their course. Visualization of external tendon of the fingers requires the use of stand off pads.

Knee (Figs. 9.147 to 9.152)

As both the quadriceps and patellar tendons are slightly concave anteriorly when the knee is extended and at rest, scans should be obtained during active extension of the knee, or with the knee flexed, which straightens the tendons and eliminates the hypoechoic artefact. The quadriceps tendon lies under the subcutaneous fat and anterior to a fat pad and to the collapsed suprapatellar bursa. On transverse scans, the quadriceps tendon is oval, while the patellar

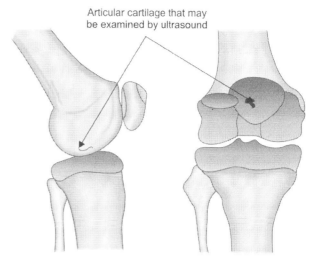

Fig. 9.147: Areas of the knee that may be examined by ultrasound.

tendon shows a convex anterior and flat posterior surface. The patellar tendon is a flat band extending from the patella to the tibial tuberosity over a length of 5–6 cm. It is 2–2.5 cm wide and 4–5 mm thick. The subcutaneous prepatellar and infrapatellar bursae are not visible. The deep infrapatellar bursa appears as a flattened anechoic structure 2–3 mm thick. Prepatellar fibers connect quadriceps tendon with the patellar tendon.

The collateral ligaments of the knee blend with the articular capsule and are poorly differentiated from the surrounding subcutaneous tissues. Because of their deep location and limited ultrasound window the cruciate ligaments cannot be reliably visualized with ultrasound.

Foot and Ankle

The Achilles tendon inserts into the posterior surface of the calcaneum. The echogenic, fatty Kager's triangle lies anterior to the distal half of the tendon. More anteriorly lies the hypoechoic flexor hallucis longus muscle and the echogenic posterior surface of the tibia. The flattened hypoechoic subtendinous calcaneal bursa is sometimes seen in the angle formed by the tendon and calcaneum. The tendon fibers have an oblique course forward and medially and in cross section the tendon appears elliptical, tapering medially. At 2–3 cm above its insertion, the tendon is 5–7 mm thick and 12–15 mm wide. The tendons of peroneus longus and brevis muscles are readily demonstrated posteriorly and that of tibialis posterior muscle medially. The tendons of the flexor digitorum longus and flexor hallucis longus muscles are also identified behind the medial malleolus, whereas the tendon of the tibialis anterior, extensor hallucis longus, and extensor digitorum longus are seen at the anterior aspect of the ankle, all enveloped in synovial sheaths. In the foot, the flexor and extensor tendons of the toes are evaluated similar to tendon of the fingers.

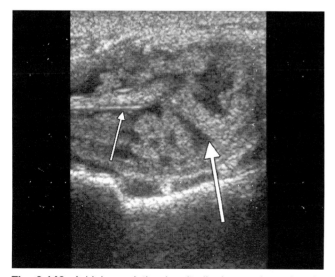

Fig. 9.146: A high resolution longitudinal scan through wrist showing tendon (thin white arrow) with proliferative synovial thickening surrounding it (thick white arrow) in a case of tenosynovitis.

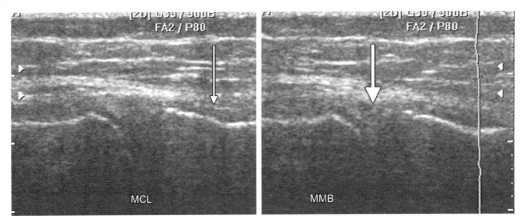

Fig. 9.148: High resolution longitudinal scan through medial side of knee joint showing medial collateral ligament (thin white arrow) and medial meniscus (thick white arrow).

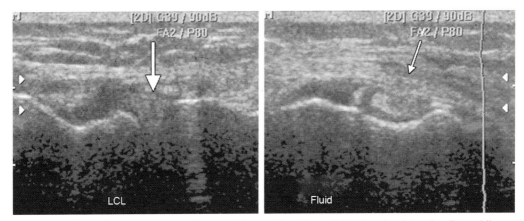

Fig. 9.149: High resolution longitudinal scan through lateral side of knee joint showing lateral collateral ligament (LCL) (thin white arrow) and lateral meniscus (thick white arrow) associated with some anechoic joint fluid.

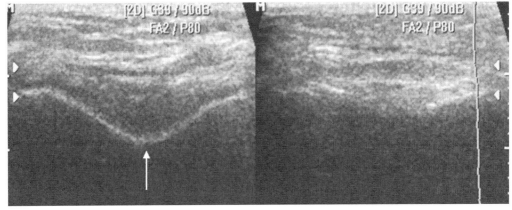

Fig. 9.150: High resolution scan through intercondylar region of femur showing no evidence of any joint collection (thin white arrow).

Skin and Subcutaneous Tissue (Fig. 9.153)

The normal layers of the skin from without inwards include the epidermis, dermis, and subcutaneous fat. The superficial fascia separates the skin from muscles. The epidermis appears as an echogenic band like structure measuring 1–3 mm in thickness. The dermis is homogeneously, relatively hypoechoic and measures 1–3.5 mm in thickness according to the site. The dermis is poorly separated from the subcutaneous fat, this layer is also relatively hypoechoic. It often contains thin echogenic strand due to connective to tissue fibers and measures 5 mm to 1 cm in thickness.

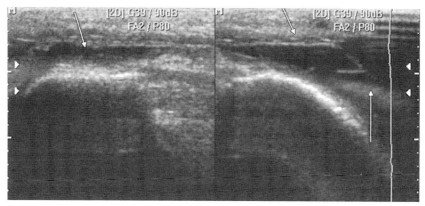

Fig. 9.151: High resolution transverse and longitudinal scans through prepatellar region showing anechoic septate collection (thin white arrows).

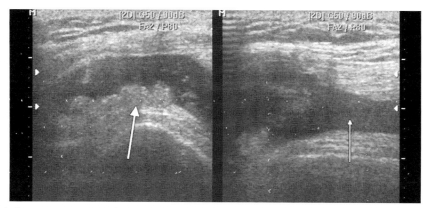

Fig. 9.152: High resolution transverse and longitudinal scans through suprapatellar bursa showing collection (thin white arrow) with thickened nodular synovium (thick white arrow).

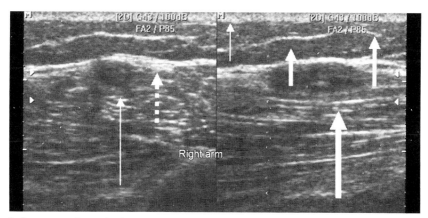

Fig. 9.153: High resolution scan through thigh revealing echogenic epidermis (thin white arrow), hypoechoic dermis and subcutaneous fat containing lipoma (thick white arrows), deep fascia (broken white arrow) and muscle (thick large arrow). Incidental note is made of healed cysticercus (thin long arrow).

The superficial fascia forms a linear echogenic, layer parallel to the skin surface sharply delineating the subcutaneous fat/muscle interface.

While scanning, the axis of the probe should be strictly perpendicular to the skin surface. A 7.5 MHz probe with a 2 cm stand-off pad should be used and plenty of gel helps to maintain a good contact especially while scanning lesions with irregular surface. Excessively hairy skin ought to be shaved prior to examination. Comparative scans of normal skin areas are very useful.

Muscles

Normal muscles have a striped pattern on longitudinal scans and the plane of striations varies with the orientation of the fibers. Sections at 90° to this alignment show speckled or uniformly mottled pattern. Adjacent muscles may demonstrate a confusing variation in reflectivity. Comparison with the opposite side of the body can avoid errors. Each muscle is surrounded by an echogenic capsule, sometimes adjacent to layers of reflective fat. Vessels may be seen within the muscles as echofree stripes. On contraction the striations become more prominent and the muscle widens and shortens with moderate increase in echogenicity. Small veins are temporarily obliterated.

PEDIATRIC SONOGRAPHY

Neonatal and Infant Brain Imaging

A 7.5 MHz transducer in premature infants to 5 MHz transducer in larger infants (up to 6 months) is placed over the anterior fontanelle and the brain is scanned in sagittal and coronal planes **(Figs. 9.154 to 9.160)**.

Coronal brain scans **(Figs. 9.161 to 9.169)**: The transducer head is placed transversely over the anterior fontanelle and the ultrasound beam is swept in an anterior and posterior direction, completely scanning the brain. Six standard sections are obtained.

- Most anterior section is just anterior to the frontal horns of the lateral ventricles. The anterior cranial fossa, frontal lobes and the orbits deep to the floor of skull base are visualized.
- Moving posterior, the frontal horns of lateral ventricles appears as symmetric, comma shaped areas with the hypoechoic caudate heads within the concave lateral border, outside the ventricles. Moving laterally the caudate nucleus is separated from the putamen by the internal capsule. Lateral to the putamen is the Sylvian fissure which appears echogenic because it contains the middle cerebral artery. Inferiorly the internal carotid arteries bifurcate to form the echogenic anterior and middle cerebral arteries.
- Further posteriorly the bodies of the lateral ventricle are visualized on either side of the cavum septi pellucidi. The thalami lie on either side of the third ventricle which is usually too thin to visualize in normal infants. Deep to the thalami the brainstem begins to be visualized.
- At a further posterior transducer angulation, the bodies of the lateral ventricle become more rounded, echogenic material seen in its floor is the choroid plexus. Choroid plexus is also seen in the roof of the third ventricle and the thalamic are more prominent on either side of the third ventricle. Deep to the thalami the tentorium covering the cerebellum is visualized. In the posterior fossa the echogenic midline vermis is surrounded by the more hypoechoic cerebellar hemispheres.
- Further posterior the trigone or atrium of the lateral ventricle is visualized and the choroid plexus nearly fills the ventricle in this area. In the midline the visualized portion of the corpus callosum deep to the cingulate sulcus is the splenium. Inferiorly the cerebellum is separated from the occipital cortex by the tentorium cerebelli.
- The most posterior section visualizes predominantly occipital lobe cortex and the occipital horns of the lateral ventricles. This section is angled posterior to the cerebellum.

Sagittal brain scans are obtained by placing the transducer longitudinally across the anterior fontanelle

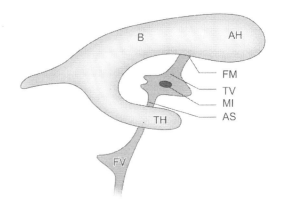

Fig. 9.155: Ventricular system. (AH: anterior horn; B: body; FM: foramen of Monro; MI: massa intermedia; TV: third ventricle; AS: aqueduct of Sylvius; TH: temporal horn; FV: fourth ventricle).

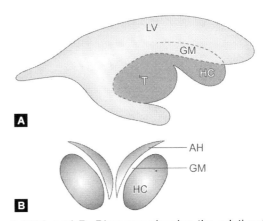

Figs. 9.156A and B: Diagrams showing the relationship of the caudate nucleus and germinal matrix (GM) to the lateral ventricle (LV). (A) sagittal, and (B) coronal. HC—head of caudate, T—thalamus, AH—anterior horn.

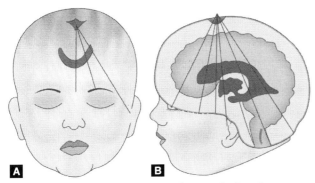

Figs. 9.154A and B: Technique for transfontanellar scan. (A) Sagittal; (B) Coronal.

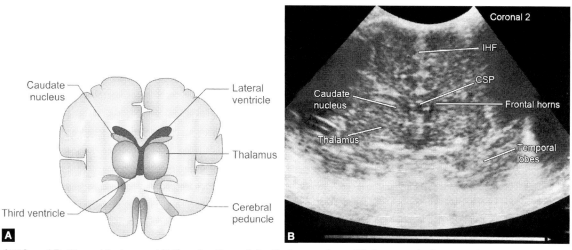

Figs. 9.157A and B: Normal thalamus. (A) Drawing through the thalamus plane; (B) Sonography in transaxial view showing thalamus.

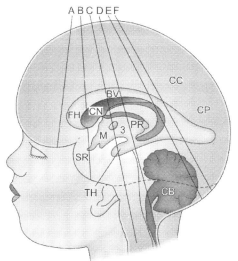

Fig. 9.158: Schematic representation of coronal planes used in brain scanning through anterior fontanelle (A to F correspond front to back). (CC: cerebral cortex; BV: body of lateral ventricle; FH: frontal horn; CN: caudate nucleus; M: massa intermedia; PR: pineal recess; 3: third ventricle; TH: temporal horn; SR: supraoptic recess; CP: choroid plexus; CB: cerebellum).

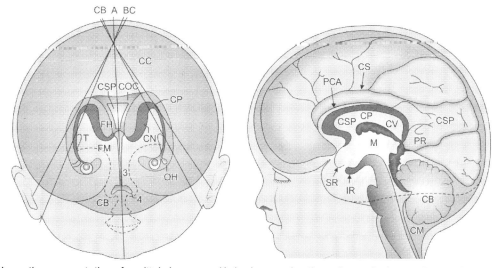

Fig. 9.159: Schematic representation of sagittal planes used in brain scanning through anterior fontanelle. A to C correspond to midline to lateral. (CB: cerebellum; CC: cerebral cortex; COC: corpus callosum; CN: caudate nucleus; CP: choroid plexus; CSP: cavum septi pellucidi; FH: frontal horn; FM: foramen of Monro; OH: occipital horn; T: temporal horn; 3: third ventricle; 4: fourth ventricle).

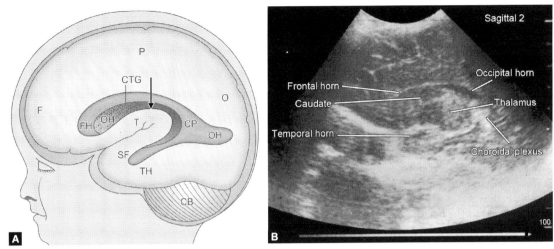

Figs. 9.160A and B: Normal paramedian sagittal anatomy. (A) Schematic drawing. F—frontal lobe; P—parietal lobe; O—occipital lobe; FH—frontal horn; CTG—caudothalamic groove (arrow)—body of lateral ventricle; OH—occipital horn; TH—temporal horn; SF—Sylvian fissure; T—thalamus; CB—cerebellum; CP—choroid plexus. (B) Sagittal sonogram, paramedian view. FL—frontal lobe; P—parietal lobe; T—thalamus; c—caudate nucleus; CP—choroid plexus.

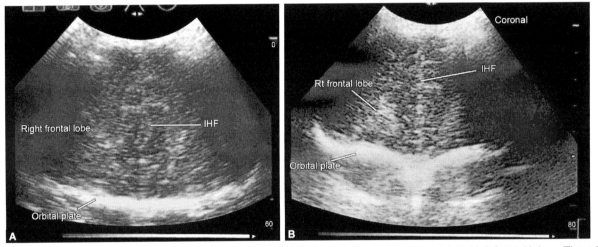

Figs. 9.161A and B: Coronal 1 scan—The midline echogenic IHF is seen separating the right and left frontal lobes. The orbital plate is also shown.

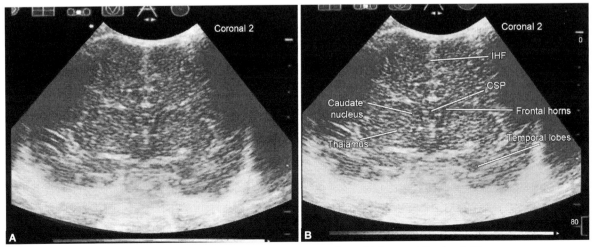

Figs. 9.162A and B: Coronal 2-scan showing the frontal lobes and the frontal horns.

CHAPTER 9: Basic Sonographic Anatomy

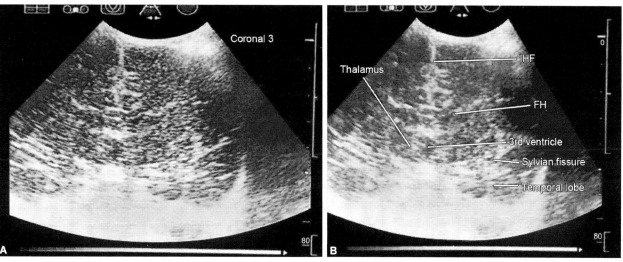

Figs. 9.163A and B: Coronal 3-scan—the frontal horns and the 3rd ventricle are seen.

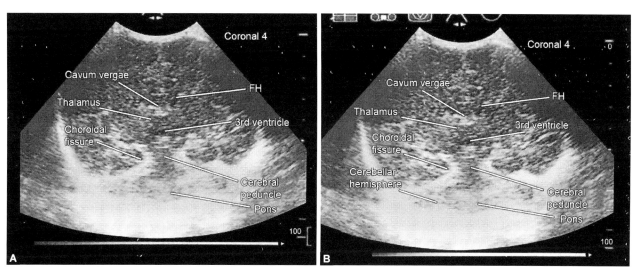

Figs. 9.164A and B: Coronal 4-scan—3rd ventricle is shown clearly.

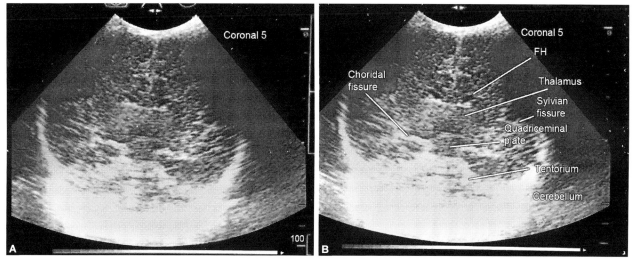

Figs. 9.165A and B: Coronal 5-scan showing frontal horn, thalami, Sylvian fissure, choroidal fissure.

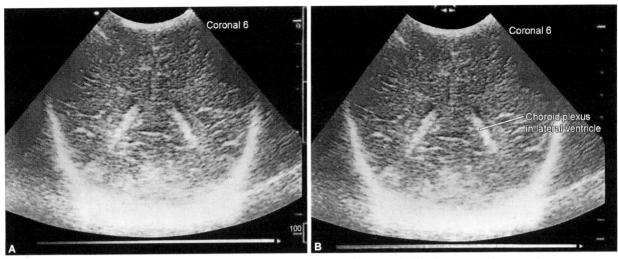

Figs. 9.166A and B: Coronal 6-scan—echogenic choroid is seen inside the body of the ventricle.

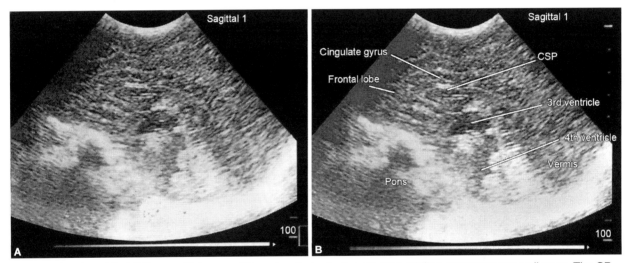

Figs. 9.167A and B: Midline sagittal scan—Through anterior fontanelle. The midline structures are well seen. The CP, 3rd ventricle, 4th ventricle appear anechoic, vermis is echogenic.

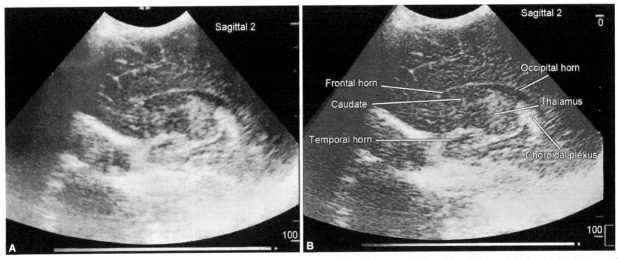

Figs. 9.168A and B: Sagittal scan through the anterior fontanelle with slight angulation. Frontal, occipital and the temporal horns are seen.

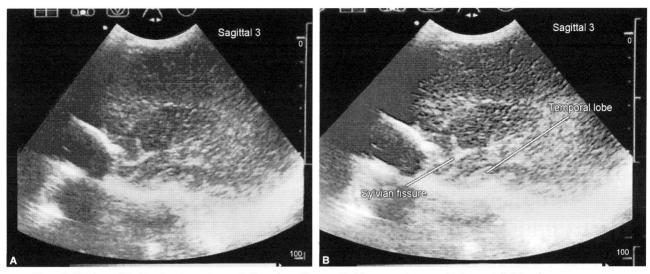

Figs. 9.169A and B: Further lateral angulation gives the sagittal 3-scan. Temporal lobe and Sylvian fissure are seen.

and angling it to each side. The midline is first identified through the interhemispheric fissure by recognition of the curving line of the corpus callosum, above the cystic cavum septi pellucidi, the third and fourth ventricles and the highly echogenic cerebellar vermis. A shallow angulation to each side by about 10° will show the entire lateral ventricles, provided the anterior ends of the probe is directed more medially than the posterior end, because the lateral ventricles oriented slightly obliquely in the parasagittal planes. Above the lateral ventricle is the cerebral cortex and below it is the cerebellar. The caudate nucleus and the thalamus are within the arms of the ventricle. More pronounced lateral angulation will demonstrate the peripheral aspect of the ventricles and more lateral cerebral hemisphere including the temporal lobes.

Infant Spine

The spinal canal and its contents are best visualized in the neonates because at birth the posterior portion of the neural arches and spinous processes are still cartilaginous and provide an acoustic window through which the content of spinal canal can be imaged in both sagittal (longitudinal) and axial (transverse) planes. By the end of the 1st year union of the laminae into a bony arch occurs in the lumbar region and ossification progresses cranially and is complete in the cervical region by the age of two years.

The most common indication for spinal sonography is to determine the level of conus medullaris and to look for tethering of the cord. Other indications include cases of obvious dysraphism like meningomyelocele and myeloschisis. Increasing age and severe spinal deformity are relative contraindication. Open neural tube defect is an absolute contraindication.

The patient is examined in the prone or lateral decubitus position with the spine slightly flexed, so that the spinous processes are separated and the acoustic window to the spinal canal is widened. Flexion is best achieved by placing the infant prone over a pillow, or in the lap of the attendant in case of smaller infants. In case there is a dorsal soft tissue mass the patient should be tilted foot down to shift the CSF into the lumbar and sacral theca. The highest frequency transducer that provides adequate tissue penetration (usually a 7.5 MHz linear transducer) and plenty of good quality thick coupling gel used to visualize the entire length of the spine from the craniocervical junction to the coccyx in both the sagittal and axial planes. Neonates and young infants are scanned over the midline between the spinous processes and as the posterior vertebral elements are unossified a broad longitudinal view of several spinal segments is obtained. In older infants and larger children the transducer is placed slightly lateral and parallel to the spinous processes and the transducer is aimed medially into the spinal canal from this parasagittal position. Since access is limited to the spaces between the vertebral laminae a segmental view of the spinal canal is obtained.

The spinal canal contents can be seen throughout the length of the spine from the medulla oblongata to the filum terminale. Longitudinal sector scanning over the posterior lip of the foramen magnum demonstrated a moderately echogenic vermis and very hypoechoic medulla. The cisterna magna is seen as a triangular an echoic space posterior to the medulla. Transverse scans show the cisterna magna bordered by cerebellar to with posterolateral to the medulla. Linear array scanning of the rest of the spinal canal reveals the spinal cord, which is relatively hypoechoic and is identified by its highly reflective anterior and posterior borders. The center of the cord contain 1 or 2 echogenic dots in the transverse plane and correspondingly 1 or 2 echogenic lines in the longitudinal plane in a dorsoventral relationship, which are referred to as the central echo complex. The size and shape of the spinal cord varies with the vertebral level. The cervical cord appears oval in transverse scanning, with the major axis in horizontal plane, it becomes more circular at the thoracic level and expands to a larger circle in the thoracolumbar and upper lumbar region. The conus medullaris appears as a diminishing circle in the transverse plane on sequential caudal scanning, surrounded by echogenic nerve roots. In the longitudinal view, the conus is tapered appearing like a horizontally oriented carrot. The tip of the conus medullaris usually lies at L_{2-3} IVD space level. The roots of the cauda equina appear as echogenic strands on longitudinal views and or dots on transverse views. Dorsal and ventral nerve roots can be separately identified on transverse views. The dentate ligaments can be noted in the thoracic cord extending horizontally from the cord at 9 O'clock and 3 O'clock positions. The anterior spinal artery and the epidural veins are apparent with color flow Doppler imaging, especially in the cervicothoracic and lower lumbar canal regions respectively.

The spinal cord and cauda equina oscillate in the dorsoventral and cephalocaudal directions synchronously with the heart beat.

Pediatric Head and Neck

The neck can be divided into three anatomic areas:

Face and Upper Neck

Salivary gland: These include the parotid glands, the submandibular glands and sublingual glands.

The parotid gland **(Figs. 9.170A to 9.171)** is the largest of all salivary gland and is located within a triangle bounded by the tip of the mastoid process, the mid-portion of the zygomatic arch and the angle of the mandible. The seventh cervical nerve and its five major branches that predominantly supply the facial muscles divide the gland into the deep and superficial lobes. The Stenson's duct drains the gland and its approximate location in adolescent can be obtained by placing the index finger on the inferior margin of the zygomatic arch. The duct will be located on the lower surface of the finger.

The gland is best evaluated in the axial and coronal planes using a high frequency linear, small parts transducer with or without a stand off pad. For the axial images, the transducer should be placed perpendicular to the ear, with its superior margin touching the ear lobule. In this position the mastoid is seen posteriorly as an echogenic line with posterior acoustic shadowing. As the transducer is moved inferiorly the sternocleidomastoid muscle can be seen originating from the mastoid. Anteriorly the mandible is identified as an echogenic line with posterior acoustic shadowing. The masseter muscle is seen superficial to the mandible. The muscle mass deep to the mastoid tip is the posterior belly of the diagnostic muscle and both these structures pass inferiorly and anteriorly towards the angle of mandible and are located deeper than the mandibular ramus. The parotid gland is seen as a homogenous mass located just below the skin surface. It extends anteriorly over the masseter muscle, medially behind the posterior aspect of mandible

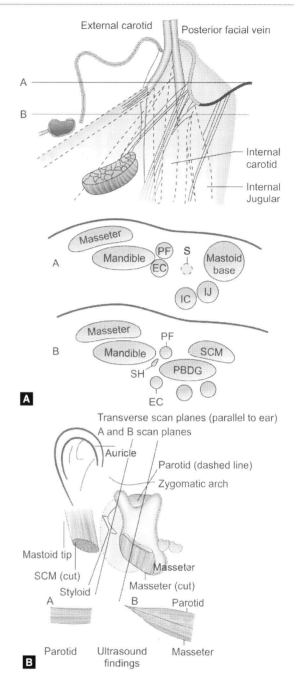

Figs. 9.170A and B: (A) Normal parotid gland diagram in axial or perpendicular scans. Normal landmarks such as the sternocleidomastoid muscle—SCM • Posterior belly of the digastric muscle—PBDG • Styloid process—S • Internal carotid artery—IC • External carotid artery—EC • Posterior facial vein—PF and stylohyoid muscle—SH can be seen. The parotid gland lies between the sternocleidomastoid muscle and mastoid tip posteriorly and the masseter muscle and mandible anteriorly; (B) Normal parotid gland.

and posteriorly to the mastoid tip and sternocleidomastoid. It is more echogenic and homogenous than the adjacent muscles and fat. The retromandibular or posterior facial vein is identified within the substance of the parotid gland just posterior to the mandible. The course of the facial nerve can be estimated by drawing a line from the upper aspect of the posterior belly of the digastric muscle to the posterior facial vein and then to the lateral aspects of the mandibular ramus.

The coronal images are obtained by placing the transducer just anterior and parallel to the ear. The transducer is then angled anteriorly and posteriorly. The parotid glands are seen as an elliptical, homogenous, echogenic area below the skin.

Submandibular gland **(Fig. 9.172)** lies in the submandibular space which is bounded laterally by the body of the mandible and superiorly and medially by the mylohyoid muscle. A small portion of this gland may pass posterior to the back of the mylohyoid muscle and lie within the sublingual space. It is drained by Wharton's duct, which passes between the lateral mylohyoid muscle and medial hyoglossus muscle. The gland is best evaluated by sonography from a submental position with the transducer angled in both the sagittal and coronal planes. The gland is located medial to the body of mandible and superficial to the anterior belly of digastric and mylohyoid muscles. The Wharton's duct runs in the plane between the mylohyoid and hyoglossus muscles and can be seen by having patients move their tongue.

Sublingual glands are multiple in numbers and lie in the floor of the mouth, deep to the mylohyoid muscle and superficial to the hyoglossus and the intrinsic muscles of the tongue and are difficult to visualize sonographically.

Lateral neck: The neck is divided anatomically into anterior and posterior triangle by the sternocleidomastoid muscle which extends from the mastoid tip anteroinferiorly. Inferiorly this muscle has a medially located sternal head and a lateral clavicular head. The posterior aspect of the posterior triangle is bounded by the trapezius muscle and the anterior aspect of the anterior triangle in the midline. The common carotid artery and the internal jugular vein lie just deep to the sternocleidomastoid muscle, with the vein lying posterolateral to the artery in the upper neck and anterolateral to the artery in the lower neck. The cervical lymph node chains are divided into four or five major groups, of which the two major groups. Located in the anterior and posterior triangle are sonologically important. As a general rule the posterior triangle lymphadenopathy tends to be benign. Normal cervical nodes are oval and hypoechoic with an echogenic linear hilum. Power mode Doppler imaging will often identify a central vessel in the hilum of the normal node.

Thyroid and Parathyroid Glands

During development the thyroid diverticulum migrate inferiorly to below the larynx where it develops into the thyroid gland. The remnant of this thyroid diverticulum is known as the thyroglossal duct. The right and left lobes of the thyroid gland are homogeneous echogenic structures

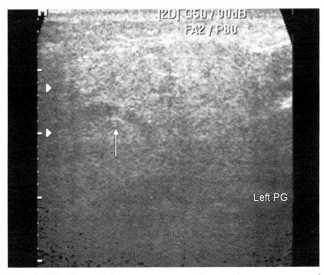

Fig. 9.171: Normal homogeneous echogenic appearance of parotid gland (PG) with mildly dilated Stenson's duct (white arrow).

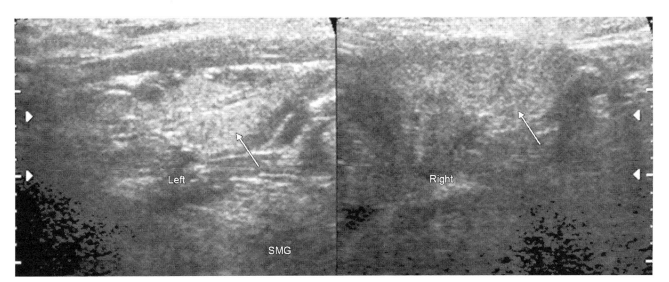

Fig. 9.172: Normal homogeneous echogenic appearance of submandibular gland (SMG) (white arrows).

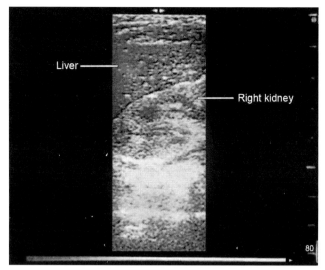

Fig. 9.173: Right kidney in relation to liver, cortical echotexture is more than that of liver in a normal neonate.

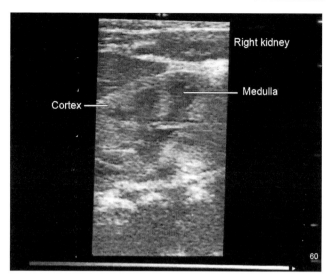

Fig. 9.175: In this oblique scan of a neonate the cortex and medulla of the kidney are obliquely visualized.

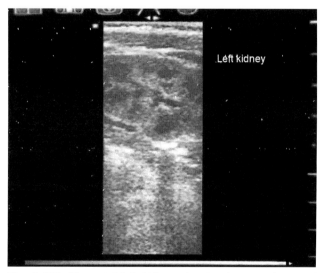

Fig. 9.174: Neonatal left kidney showing increased central echotexture and accentuated corticomedullary appearance—A normal appearance.

located on either the larynx or trachea, which are seen as markedly echogenic areas with shadowing in the midline in the lower neck. The great vessels are seen on the posterolateral aspects of both lobes. The parathyroid glands are usually not identified, but can be seen as hypoechoic masses along the posteromedial aspects of the thyroid lobes.

Pediatric Renal Anatomy (Figs. 9.173 to 9.175)

Neonatal kidneys appear markedly different from the adult kidneys on ultrasound scanning. The cortex is thinner and more echogenic then the liver. The renal pyramids are larger and more prominent. They are recognized by their relative hypoechoic echotexture, triangular shape, with the base on the cortex and arrangement around the central echocomplex. The corticomedullary differentiation is greater in the infant kidney, and the arcuate vessels are usually recognized as highly reflective foci on the base of the triangular pyramids as they pass between the cortex and medullae.

The renal capsule is less well defined and the central echo complex is also much less prominent as compared to the renal parenchyma because there is less peripelvic fat in the infant than in the adult. Mild degree of separation of sinus echoes can be seen in normal infants who are well hydrated and have a full bladder. Separation of the central sinus echoes by more than 10 mm is suggestive of obstruction.

The age of transition from the neonatal appearance to the adult pattern usually occurs at 2–3 months after birth, but may persist up to six months of age. The neonatal kidney is 4.5–5 cm long and 2 cm wide. A difference of more than 15% between the renal lengths is suggestive of scarring.

Pediatric Urinary Bladder

The normal fluid filled bladder has an elliptical shape with a smooth muscular wall, 3 mm thick when the bladder is full and 5 mm when empty (independent of age). A postmicturition bladder volume of 30 mL is abnormal. The bladder neck and urethra can be demonstrated in both males and females by angling the transducer inferiorly.

Adrenal Gland (Figs. 9.176 and 9.177)

In the neonatal period, the normal adrenal gland is readily visualized in the suprarenal location and has a V, Y or Z shaped configuration. The gland has a thin echogenic core representing the medulla, which is surrounded by a hypoechoic rim of cortex. The thick fetal zone that comprises 80% of the cortex of the gland undergoes involution after birth and is replaced by connective tissue by one year of age. The adrenal length varies between 0.9–3.6 cm and the width

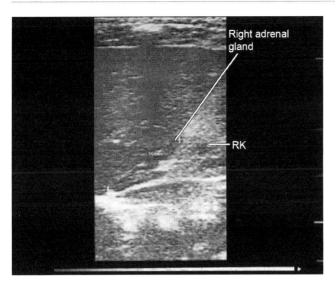

Fig. 9.176: Right adrenal gland is seen superior to the right kidney in this neonate.

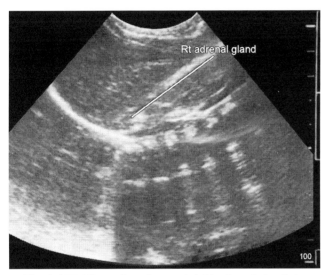

Fig. 9.177: Dimension of normal right adrenal gland are shown in this neonatal scan.

ranges from 0.2–0.5 cm in infants. In case of renal agenesis the neonatal adrenal appears as a long linear structure, still recognizable by normal cortex and medulla. The adrenal gland in the older child becomes relatively smaller and obscured by perirenal fat and thus difficult to visualize.

GASTROINTESTINAL TRACT

Pediatric stomach: The stomach should be examined in the distended state, filled with clear glucose water. Most abnormalities in infants and children involve the distal third of the stomach, which can be examined, using liver as the acoustic window. The normal gastric mucosae including the muscularis mucosae and submucosal layers measure 2–3 mm whereas the outer circular muscle layer measures 1–2 mm in thickness.

Pediatric Pelvis

The uterus: In the newborn female, the uterus is spade shaped and measures 3.5 cm in length with a fundus to cervix ratio of 1:2. The endometrium is thick and brightly echogenic due to hormonal stimulation in utero. At 2–3 months of age the uterus regresses to a prepubertal size and tubular configuration, with the length measuring 2.5–3 cm and fundus to cervix ratio becomes 3:1.

Ovary

The neonatal ovaries may be found anywhere between the lower pole of the kidneys and the true pelvis, because of their long pedicles and a small pelvis. They have a heterogeneous appearance secondary to small cysts and these cysts may be more than 9 mm in diameter. After the age of eight years and before puberty the ovaries have a multicystic appearance and each ovary may have six or more follicles more than 4 mm in diameter. The mean ovarian volume in neonates and girls less than six years of age is 1 cm^3. Ovarian volume gradually increases at about six years and in girls between 6–11 years the mean ovarian volume ranges between 1.2 cm^3–2.5 cm^3. There is marked enlargement in ovarian size, post-puberty and the ovarian volume may range between 2.5 cm^3 and 21.9 cm^3 with a mean volume of 9.8 cm^3.

Prostate

The prostate is ellipsoid in boys compared with the conical shape seen in adults. It is more homogeneous and hypoechoic than the adult prostate. Between the ages of 7 months to 13.5 years the prostate volume ranges between 0.4–5.2 ml. The seminal vesicles are best identified in the transverse plane as small hypoechoic structures giving an appearance similar to a Seagull's wings.

The scrotum: The normal newborns testes have homogeneous low to medium level echoes and are spherical or oval in shape, with a diameter of 7–10 mm. The epididymis and mediastinum are usually not seen in the neonate. It may also not be possible to detect color flow in normal, small prepubertal testes and epididymis. By puberty the testes contain homogeneous medium level echoes, mediastinum testes and epididymis are seen and of the testis measure 3–5 cm in length and 2–3 cm in depth and widen.

Pediatric Chest (Fig. 9.178)

Indications for chest sonography include:
- Pleural effusions
- Diaphragmatic paralysis
- Cystic versus solid masses
- Diaphragmatic hernia
- Diaphragmatic defect
- Subpulmonic versus subphrenic fluid
- Pericardial effusion
- Vascular thrombi, e.g. cardiac, SVC, IV
- Tumor versus large or persistent pleural effusion
- Chest wall mass versus plural fluid

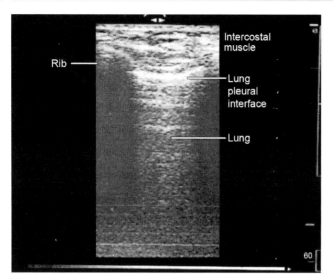

Fig. 9.178: Normal lung as seen in transverse section. Ribs with distal shadowing are shown with intercostal muscles. The lung pleural interface is seen as an echogenic line.

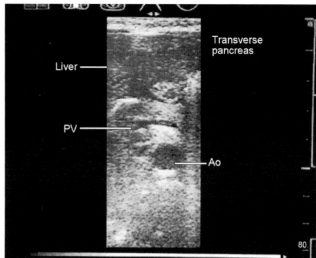

Fig. 9.179: Pancreas in transverse section, portal vein and splenic vein are also seen.

- Mediastinal masses
- Relationship of thymus to masses
- Extension of neck masses into the chest
- Catheter position in vessels
- Endotracheal tube placement
- Needle biopsy of masses.

In children the normal thymus is an excellent acoustic window to view normal mediastinal structures and mediastinal masses. The thymus is located anterior to the great vessels and extends down to the upper portion of the heart. The echogenicity of thymus is usually less than that of liver, spleen and thyroid. The great vessels, the SVC, the aorta and the pulmonary artery are well image through the thymus.

Pediatric Pancreas (Fig. 9.179)

The pancreas in a child, compared to the adults is poorly reflective and relatively bulky with a prominent tail. At any age the diagnosis of pancreatic enlargement is made if the width of the body of the pancreas is more than 1.5 cm. Normal dimensions of the pancreas at different ages are:

Age	Head	Body	Tail
< 1 month	1.0–1.4	0.6–0.8	1.0–1.4
1 month–1 year	1.5–2.0	0.8–1.1	1.2–1.6
1–10 years	1.7–2.0	1.0–1.3	1.8–2.2
10–19 years	2.0–2.5	1.1–1.4	2.0–2.4

Normal pancreas in neonates can be marked hypoechoic.

Pediatric Hepatobiliary System and Spleen (Figs. 9.180 and 9.181)

The ultrasound appearances of the normal liver in a child do not differ greatly from those of the adult liver. The normal common bile duct should not measure more than 1 mm in thickness in neonates and 6 mm in adolescents. The size of the gallbladder varies with patients' age and degree of fasting. The normal gallbladder should be approximately triangular in cross section whereas an abnormally distended gallbladder is more circular in this view. The echotexture of the normal spleen in children is homogeneous and with a reflectively between that of the kidney and liver.

Size of Spleen

Age	Maximum length in cm
0–3 months	6.0
3–6 months	6.5
6–12 month	7.0
1–2 years	8.0
2–4 years	9.0
4–8 years	10.0
8–12 years	11.5
12–15 years	12.8

Joints

Neonatal Hips

A 7.5 MHz linear transducer and a 5 MHz linear transducer is used for an infant up to three months and between 3–7 months respectively. All scanning is performed from the lateral or posterolateral aspect of the hip from the neutral position at rest to one in which the hip is flexed, and four standard views are obtained. Dynamic hip assessment is done to determine the position and stability of the femoral head and to assess the development of the acetabulum. With the hip flexed at 90°, the femur is moved through a range of abduction and adduction with stress views performed in the flexed position. The stress maneuvers are the imaging counterparts of the clinical Barlow and Ortolani

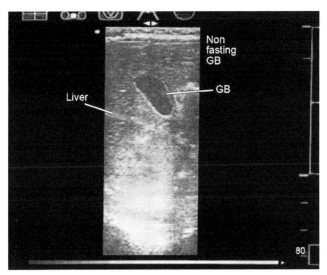

Fig. 9.180: Normal non-fasting gallbladder.

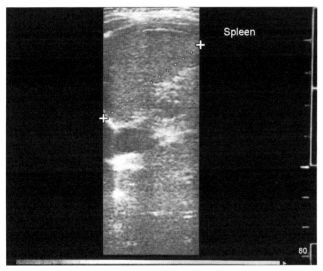

Fig. 9.181: Spleen in longitudinal section.

maneuvers and which are used clinically to determine hip abnormality. The Barlow test determines whether the hip can be dislocated. The hip is flexed, thigh adducted and a gentle push applied posteriorly. An unstable femoral head moves out of the acetabulum. The Ortolani test determines if the dislocated hip can be reduced. As the flexed, dislocated hip is abducted the examiner feels a vibration of click that results when the femoral head returns to the acetabulum at rest, with abduction and adduction motions when the hip is flexed and during the application of stress.

At birth the proximal femur and much of the acetabulum are composed of cartilage, which is hypoechoic compared with soft tissue and easy to distinguish. The cartilaginous femoral head has low ultrasound attenuation and provides a window into the acetabulum, allowing a detailed examination of the joint. Ossification begins between six weeks and eight months in the femoral head which blocks further transmission of sound and makes hip sonography practical only up to one year of age.

The acetabulum is composed of both bone and cartilage. At birth the bony ossification centers in the ilium, ischium and pubis are separated by a Y-shaped triradiate cartilage. The acetabular labrum is a rim of hyaline cartilage extending outwards from the acetabular margin and it form the cup that normally contains the femoral head. The labrum is poorly reflective and has echogenic fibrocartilage at its lateral margin. The joint space may be identified as a line between the femoral and acetabular cartilage. The echogenic hip capsule, composed of fibrous tissue is seen lateral to the femoral head.

- Coronal/neutral view with the patient supine the linear transducer is placed vertically on the lateral aspect of the hip and the hip is scanned until a standard plane of section is obtained. This plane demonstrates the mid portion of the acetabulum, with the straight iliac line superiorly and the inferior tip of the os ilium seen medially within the acetabulum. The echogenic tip of the labrum is also visualized. In the normal hip, the acetabular roof has a concave configuration and covers at least half of the femoral head. The acetabulum can be assessed visually or with alpha and beta angles, noting the depth and angulation of the acetabular roof as well as the appearance of the labrum. The alpha angle measures the inclination of superior osseous acetabular rim with respect to the lateral margin of the iliac bone. The beta angle is formed by the baseline iliac bone and the inclination of the cartilaginous acetabular roof for which the tip of the labrum is the key landmark.

- *Coronal/flexon view:* With the same transducer position as in coronal neutral view, the hip is flexed at 90° and the transducer moved in an anteroposterior direction to visualize the entire hip. The curvilinear margin of the bony femoral shaft is identified anteriorly to the femoral head. In the mid portion of the acetabulum, the normally positioned femoral head is surrounded by echoes from the long acetabular components. The transducer position should be so adjusted that superiorly the lateral margin of the iliac bone is seen as a straight horizontal line. This plane ensures that the mid-acetabulum is accurately visualized and the maximum acetabular depth obtained. A normal hip gives the appearance of 'a ball on a spoon' in the mid acetabulum. The femoral head represents the ball, the acetabulum forms the bowl of the spoon and the iliac line form the handle. When the transducer is moved posteriorly the posterior lip of the triradiate cartilage is visualized. The bone above and below the cartilage notch is flat and the normal femoral head is never seen over the posterior lip of the acetabulum, while the push and pin maneuvers are used during dynamic scanning. Also, with the plane of scan comprising the mid acetabulum, a Barlow type maneuver is performed with adduction and gentle pushing against the knee, a normal hip remains in place against the acetabulum.

- *Transverse/flexion view:* The transducer is rotated through 90° and moved posteriorly, so that it is posterolateral to the joint. The bony shaft and metaphysis of the femur produce a bright echogenic line anteriorly adjacent to the sonolucent femoral head. The echoes from the bony acetabulum are posterior to the femoral head and produce a U shape configuration in the normal hip. The flexed hip is moved from maximum adduction to wide abduction and the deep U configuration of the acetabulum seen in maximum abduction, changes to a shallower V appearance in adduction. In adduction the hip is stressed with a gentle push (a Barlow test), in the normal hip the femoral head remains deeply in the acetabulum, in contact with the ischium.

- *Transverse/neutral view:* The leg is brought down and transducer directed horizontally into the acetabulum from the lateral aspect of hip. The plane of interest passes through the femoral head into the acetabulum at the center of the triradiate cartilage. In the normal hip the sonolucent femoral head is positioned against the bony acetabulum over the triradiate cartilage. The elements of the sonogram resemble the components of a flower. The femoral head represent the flower, echoes from the ischium posteriorly and pubis anteriorly forms the leaves at its base. The stem is formed by echoes that pass through the triradiate cartilage into the area of acoustic shadowing created by osseous structures. The presence and size of the ossific nucleus are evaluated in this view.

VASCULAR SYSTEM

Blood Vessels Veins and Arteries

Carotid Artery Anatomy (Fig. 9.182)

The innominate or the brachiocephalic artery is the first major branch of the aortic arch and it divides into the right common carotid and right subclavian arteries. The left common carotid is the second and the left subclavian artery the third major branches of the arch of aorta. The common carotid arteries ascend into the neck, posterolateral to the thyroid gland, and lie deep to the jugular vein sternocleidomastoid muscle. At the carotid bifurcation they divide into the external carotid artery and the internal carotid artery. The ICA has no branches in the neck and may demonstrate an ampullary region of mild dilatation just beyond its origin. The ECA has multiple branches in the neck that supply the fascial musculature.

Vertebral Artery Anatomy

Vertebral artery is the first branch of the subclavian artery. In 6–8% of cases the left vertebral artery arises directly from the aortic arch, proximal to the origin of left subclavian artery. In 90% of people the proximal vertebral artery ascends superomedially passing anterior to the C7 transverse process and enters the transverse foramen of C6 vertebrae. 10% of vertebral arteries enter into the transverse foramens above or below C6 level. Size of the vertebral arteries is variable and with left larger than the right in most cases. One vertebral artery may even be congenitally absent.

Peripheral Arteries

Lower extremity—anatomy—the deep arteries of the leg travel with an accompanying vein. The common femoral artery starts at the level of inguinal ligament and continues for 4–6 cm until it branches into the superficial femoral and deep femoral arteries. The deep femoral artery quickly branches to supply the region of the femoral head and the deep muscles of the thigh. With peripheral artery disease, collateral pathways often form between this deep femoral artery and the lower portions of the superficial femoral or the popliteal arteries. The superficial femoral artery continues along the medial aspect of the thigh at a depth of 4.8 cm until it reaches the adductor canal through the adductor hiatus and continues as the popliteal artery. The popliteal artery crosses posterior to the knee and gives off small geniculate branches and terminates as two major branches the anterior tibial artery and the tibioperoneal trunk. The anterior tibial artery courses in the anterior compartment of the lower leg after crossing through the interosseous membrane. It finally crosses the ankle joint as the dorsalis pedis artery. The tibioperoneal trunk gives off the posterior tibial and the peroneal arteries, which supply the calf muscles. The posterior tibial artery is more superficial than the peroneal artery and can be followed behind the medial malleolus.

Upper extremity: The arteries of the upper extremity are accompanied by solitary veins at the subclavian and axillary level and duplicated veins at the brachial levels and distally. The axillary artery is the continuation of the subclavian artery at the outer border of 1st ribs. The axillary artery courses medially over the proximal humerus and becomes the brachial artery, which in most people can be visualized up to the antecubital fossa, where it trifurcates into the radial, ulnar, and interosseous branches. The radial and ulnar arteries can normally be imaged to the level of the wrist.

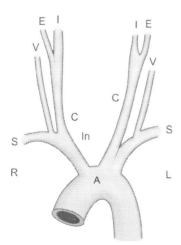

Fig. 9.182: Branches of the aortic arch and extracranial cerebral arteries. (A: Aortic arch; In, innominate artery; C: common carotid artery; V: vertebral artery; S: subclavian artery; I: internal carotid artery; E: external carotid artery; R: right side; L: left side).

CHAPTER 9: Basic Sonographic Anatomy | 129

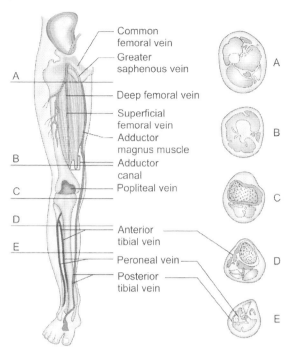

Fig. 9.183: Anatomy of lower extremity veins.

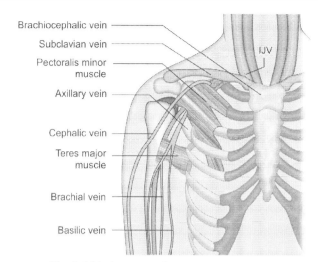

Fig. 9.184: Anatomy of upper extremity veins. (IJV: internal jugular vein).

Peripheral Veins (Fig. 9.183)

The lower limb veins: The venous system of the lower extremity consists of a superficial, and a deep system connected by a third system of perforating veins. The superficial system consists of the greater and lesser saphenous veins and their tributaries. The greater saphenous vein is formed on the medial aspect of the dorsum of the foot, from here it passes upwards in front of the medial malleolus, crosses obliquely the lower 1/3rd of the medial surface of tibia and then ascends in the subcutaneous tissues of the medial aspect of the leg and thigh, to drain into the common femoral vein in the proximal thigh, inferior to the inguinal ligament and proximal to the bifurcation of the common femoral vein. The greater saphenous vein measures 1-3 mm in diameter at the ankle and 3-5 mm in diameter at the saphenofemoral junction. The lesser saphenous vein arises on the lateral aspect of the dorsum of the foot and then passes upwards behind the lateral malleolus and ascends along the posterior aspect of the calf in the subcutaneous tissues and drains into the popliteal vein. It measures 1-2 mm distally and 2-4 mm at its junction into popliteal vein.

The deep system: The anterior tibial vein is formed on the dorsum of the foot, and ascends anterior to the interosseous membrane, along the corresponding artery in the anterior compartment of the leg and drains into the popliteal vein. The paired peroneal veins lie along peroneal artery, medial to the posterior aspect of fibula. The paired posterior tibial veins lie posterior to the medial malleolus and ascend along the posterior tibial artery deep in the calf musculature. The popliteal vein is formed by the veins accompanying the anterior tibial and posterior tibial arteries. It is medial to the popliteal artery in lower part of the popliteal fossa, posterior to it in the middle and posterolateral to it in the upper 3rd. It continues as the superficial femoral vein at inferior end of the adductor canal. The superficial femoral vein lies medial to the superficial femoral artery as it ascends in the fascial space deep to the sartorius muscle. It unites with the deep femoral vein, 6-8 cm distal to the inguinal ligament, in the proximal thigh to form the common femoral vein. The deep femoral vein lies medial to the deep femoral (profunda) artery, branches extensively and drains the muscles of the thigh. The common femoral vein lies deep and medial to the common femoral artery and continues as the external iliac vein at the level of the inguinal ligament.

Upper Extremity Veins (Fig. 9.184)

Venous return from the arm is primarily through the superficial cephalic and deeper basilic veins. The cephalic vein travels in the subcutaneous fat of the lateral aspect of the arm and joins with the deep venous system at the superior aspect of the axillary or distal subclavian vein. The basilic vein is located superficially on the medial aspect of the arm and is joined by the paired deeper and smaller brachial veins at the level of the teres major muscle, thus forming the axillary vein. The axillary vein is superficial to the axillary artery and becomes the subclavian vein at the level of the outer border of 1st rib. The subclavian vein is inferior and superficial to the adjacent artery as they pass medially deep to the clavicle. In the base of the neck the smaller external jugular vein and the larger, internal jugular veins join the subclavian to form the brachiocephalic vein. The internal jugular vein extends from the jugular foramen in the base of skull and travels inferiorly in the carotid sheath, superficial and lateral to the common carotid artery in the anterior neck. The right brachiocephalic vein travels along the superficial aspect of the superior right mediastinum. The left brachiocephalic is longer and passes from the left superior mediastinum to the right just deep to the sternum. The right and left brachiocephalic veins join to form the superior vena cava.

10

CHAPTER

Abdomen: Hepatobiliary System and Spleen

BENIGN FOCAL LIVER LESIONS

Simple Cyst (Fig. 10.1)

Simple cysts are posteriorly enhancing anechoic, well defined lesions with thin regular walls without internal echoes. Sometimes septations are seen inside the cyst. Simple liver cysts are primary or secondary. Primary liver cysts are developmental defects in the formation of bile ducts. It is an incidental finding or occasionally present with pain. These are more common in the right lobe and the average size is 3 cm. Secondary liver cysts are acquired cysts usually secondary to trauma, inflammation or parasitic infection.

US-guided percutaneous aspiration may be performed with cytological analysis to confirm the diagnosis.

Polycystic Liver Disease (Fig. 10.2)

Multiple cysts in the liver occasionally occur as an isolated phenomenon; however, they are most commonly seen in patients with underlying polycystic disease. Approximately one-third of patients with autosomal dominant polycystic kidney disease have liver cysts. Liver function tests are usually normal in these patients presenting most commonly with hepatomegaly. Indeed if LFT is abnormal complications like tumor, cyst infection and biliary obstruction should be excluded. The main differential diagnoses include marked intrahepatic biliary duct dilatation and Caroli's disease.

Peribiliary Cysts

These are usually a consequence of severe hepatic disease and are believed to arise from the dilated and obstructed periductal glands of biliary ducts. Presence of solitary or multiple small cysts or clusters of tortuous tubular anechoic channels along biliary ducts and portal vein radicles at the porta hepatis or junction of left and right hepatic ducts is characteristic on US. They are mostly detected incidentally and rarely may be the cause of obstruction.

Von Meyenburg Complexes (also known as Biliary Hamartomas)

It is rare benign developmental hepatic malformation detected incidentally in a small percentage of population.

Histologically, presence of multiple dilated intrahepatic ducts packed densely in collagenous stroma, often with

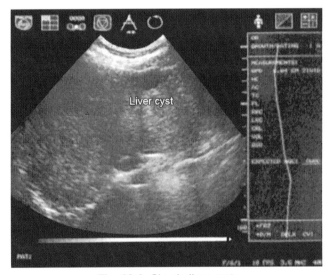

Fig. 10.1: Simple liver cyst.

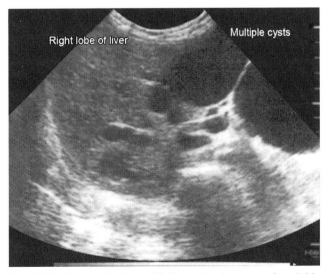

Fig. 10.2: Polycystic liver—Multiple simple cysts of variable sizes are seen in transverse scan of adult liver in a case of polycystic kidney disease.

presence of cholesterol crystals is characteristic. It is associated with congenital hepatic fibrosis, polycystic disease, recurrent attacks of cholangitis and cholangiocarcinomas.

It is characterized sonographically by the presence of multiple, solid, hypoechoic, subcentimeter nodules. Presence of cholesterol crystals within the lesion give rise to echogenic foci with ring down or reverberation artefact. The important differential diagnosis is metastases and intraductal calculi.

Hydatid Disease (Figs. 10.3A to G)

Liver is the organ most frequently involved by hydatid disease. The parasite is endemic in areas where sheep and cattle grazing is common. The eggs of *Echinococcus granulosus* are excreted in the feces of infested dogs. Human beings serve as intermediate hosts. The embryos are released in the duodenum and pass through the mucosa to reach the liver through the portal venous system. In the liver the surviving embryos form slow-growing cysts. The cyst wall has an outer ectocyst and an inner germinal layer called endocyst. The endocyst gives rise to brood capsules and the ectocyst may calcify. The host inflammatory reaction forms a dense capsule around the cyst the pericyst.

A variety of US findings may be found.

- Solitary cyst occurs as a single cyst may vary widely in size and are indistinguishable from simple liver cysts. The following features may suggest the diagnosis of hydatid cyst:

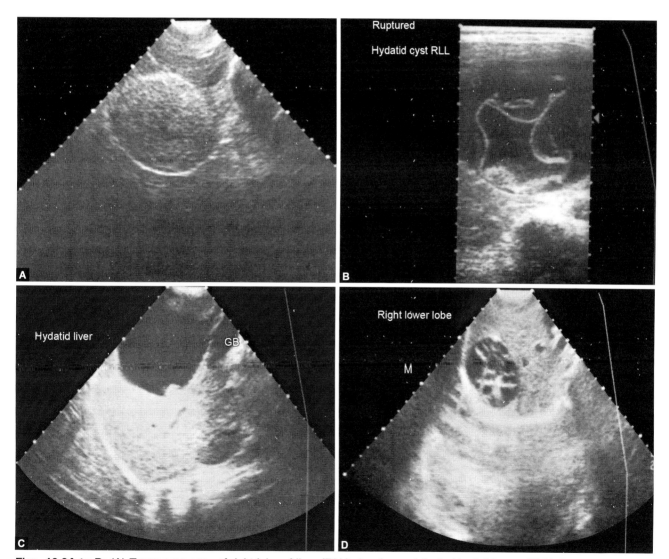

Figs. 10.3A to D: (A) Transverse scan of right lobe of liver (RLL) showing an infected hydatid cyst; (B) Hydatid cyst in a liver showing complete detachment of membranes giving the pathognomonic appearance of ultrasound Waterlily sign. Hydatid sand is also seen at the bottom of the cyst; (C) subcostal scan of liver shows a large cyst with a small mural nodule. Complement fixation test revealed hydatid cyst; (D) Classical hydatid cyst: Pathognomonic appearance of hydatid cyst with multiple daughter cysts producing the characteristic cart wheel or honeycomb appearance.

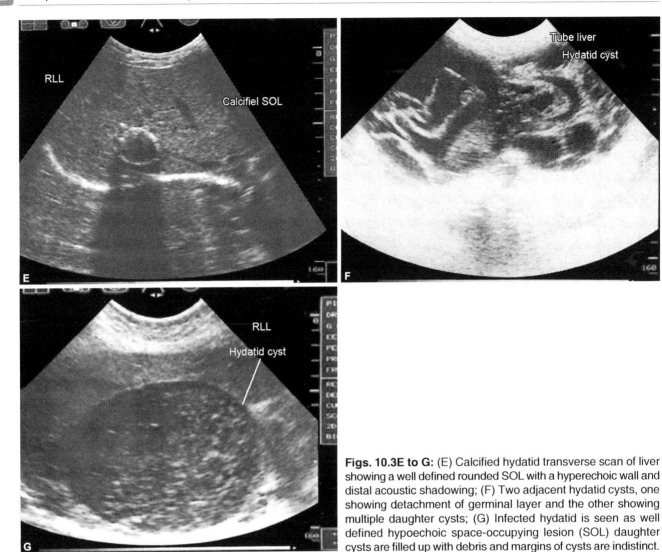

Figs. 10.3E to G: (E) Calcified hydatid transverse scan of liver showing a well defined rounded SOL with a hyperechoic wall and distal acoustic shadowing; (F) Two adjacent hydatid cysts, one showing detachment of germinal layer and the other showing multiple daughter cysts; (G) Infected hydatid is seen as well defined hypoechoic space-occupying lesion (SOL) daughter cysts are filled up with debris and margins of cysts are indistinct.

- Wall calcification
- Debris (sand or scolices)
- Two layers of the wall
- Lobulated wall.

- Separation of membrane produces a pathognomonic appearance for hydatid disease. Detatchment and collapse of the inner germinal layer from the ectocyst produces on US a "Waterlily sign".
- Daughter cysts give rise to a characteristic appearance; "cysts within a cyst", "cartwheel appearance" or "honeycomb cyst".
- Multiple cysts with heavy or continued infestation multiple primary parent cyst may develop within the liver. This produces hepatomegaly. Membrane separation or daughter cyst formation may give a clue to the diagnosis.
- Cyst with echoes may be seen in secondarily infected hydatid cysts; sometimes producing an almost solid appearance of the lesion.

ABSCESS

Pyogenic Abscess (Figs. 10.4A to C)

Intrahepatic abscesses most frequently arise as a complication of an intra-abdominal infection with direct portal venous spread to the liver. Presentation is with fever, pain, pleurisy, nausea, and vomiting. US shows a spherical, oval or slightly irregular echopoor lesion with distal enhancement in 3/4th cases. Internal fluid ranges from echo-free to highly echogenic. Presence of gas gives rise to echogenic foci with posterior reverberation artifact, fluid-filled interfaces, internal septations and debris can also be observed. The abscess wall can vary from well defined to irregular and thick. Sometimes, multiple small sized lesions may coalesce or arise adjacent to each other producing a "cluster sign". The latter is more common in hepatic abscess of biliary origin. The presence of multiple, small to moderate sized, hypoechoic lesions involving multiple lobes of liver surrounded by altered echotexture

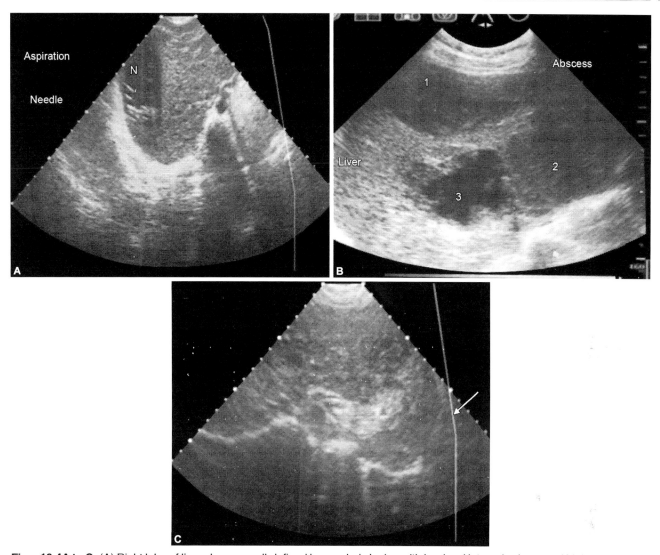

Figs. 10.4A to C: (A) Right lobe of liver shows a well-defined hypoechoic lesion with low level internal echoes and highly echogenic foci suggestive of air inside it. Needle tip is seen inside the abscess; (B) Multiple liver abscess seen as large hypoechoic lesions showing internal echoes and posterior acoustic enhancement, (C) Liver abscess in formation seen as an ill defined hypoechoic lesion in the left lobe of liver (arrow).

in the adjacent hepatic parenchyma (secondary to edema) is characteristic of pyogenic abscess.

Main differential diagnoses are amebic abscess or hydatid disease, simple cyst with hemorrhage or infection, hematoma and necrotic or cystic neoplasm.

Amebic Abscess (Figs. 10.5A to C)

Entamoeba histolytica primarily infest the colon and in 25% of these patients hepatic abscess formation occurs. US characteristics are—oval or round lesion of lower reflectivity than liver with a homogeneous pattern of internal echoes and presence of distal acoustic enhancement. Lack of a significant wall echo gives it a punched-out appearance. The lesion is usually subcapsular in location involving mainly the posterior and superior aspect of the right lobe of liver.

Serial follow-up after therapy shows a decrease in the size of the lesion and a decrease in reflectivity.

Fungal Abscesses/Candidiasis

Hepatic candidiasis is an uncommon condition and occurs in immunologically compromised patients by blood spread from other organs, most commonly lungs. US features are:
- Wheel within a wheel—peripheral hypoechoic zone with an inner echogenic wheel and central hypoechoic nidus.
- Bulls eye—1–4 cm lesion having a hyperechoic center and a hypoechoic rim.
- Uniformly hypoechoic—This is the most common US presentation. The important differential diagnoses are lymphoma and leukemia.

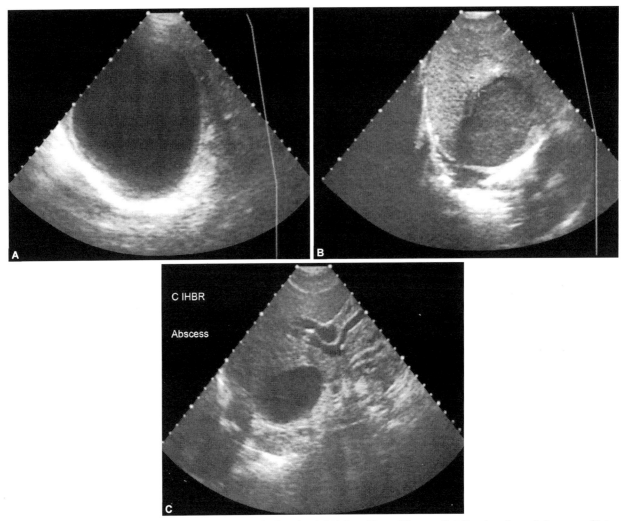

Figs. 10.5A to C: (A) A large amebic abscess seen replacing the right lobe of liver. It has well-defined walls and absence of internal echoes, distal acoustic enhancement is present; (B) Amebic liver abscess—A hypoechoic SOL is seen in the posterosuperior aspect of liver with evidence of posterior enhancement. It is extending into subdiaphragmatic space; (C) An oval well defined anechoic cystic lesion in posterior aspect of right lobe suggestive of amebic liver abscess.

- Echogenic—due to variable amount of calcification multiple lesions are characteristic.

Cavernous Hemangioma (Fig. 10.6)

This is the most common benign tumor of the liver. The majority is asymptomatic and discovered incidentally not requiring any form of treatment. Lesions may be single or multiple but usually less than 2 cm in diameter and located in a peripheral location more commonly in the right lobe. On US it appears as a sharply defined, highly echogenic round tumor with a homogeneous echo pattern. Tumor larger than 2.5 cm can show posterior acoustic enhancement and may develop a lobular margin. On undergoing degeneration the reflectivity of the lesion becomes more heterogeneous.

With the typical US features and no known history of malignancy the lesion is safely considered to be a hemangioma and a 3–6 months follow-up is all that is required. In a patient with a known malignancy, abnormal results of liver function test (LFT), clinical liver symptoms or an atypical US pattern, further workup is mandatory to rule out echogenic metastases.

Focal Fatty Change (Fig. 10.7)

Fatty infiltration of the liver arises from a variety of nutritional disturbances or toxic insults to the liver. Characteristically, the involvement is uniform or geographic in distribution, but occasionally it may be nodular or multifocal. US features suggesting the diagnosis are typical high reflectivity of lesions with sharp angular boundaries and no evidence of displacement or effacement of vascular structures.

Those occurring centrally usually lie close to the main hepatic veins.

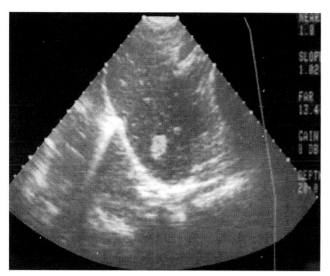

Fig. 10.6: Right lobe of liver shows a tiny highly reflective cavernous hemangioma.

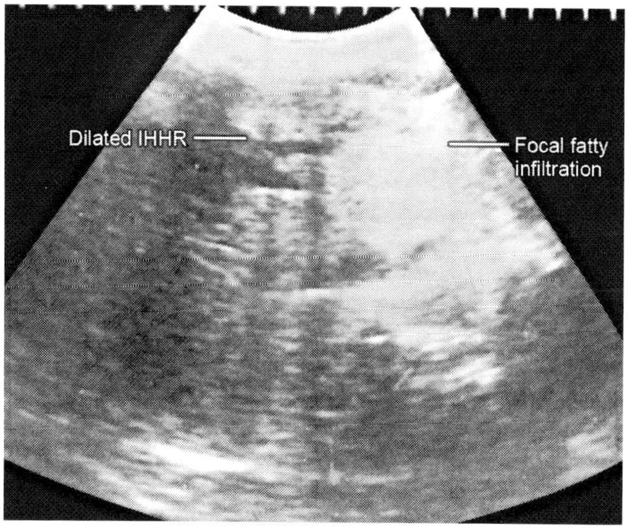

Fig. 10.7: Focal fatty infiltration in transverse scan of liver showing focal fatty change as hyperechoic well defined lesion with no distortion of normal vascular architecture.

Hematoma (Fig. 10.8)

Hematoma in the liver may be caused by blunt abdominal trauma or rupture of a neoplasm such as hepatic adenoma or cavernous hemangioma. In the acute situation, a central hematoma is highly echogenic. With time the clot undergoes liquefaction which corresponds with decreasing reflectivity and an apparent increase in the size of the lesion. Over a period of months the hematoma may become cystic and develop internal stranding.

Calcification

Liver calcification is seen as an end result of conditions including tuberculosis, syphilis, parasitic disease, chronic liver abscesses and hematoma. US features are a focus of very high reflectivity and clear cut distal acoustic shadowing.

Focal Nodular Hyperplasia (Fig. 10.9)

It is an incidentally detected developmental malformation of the liver, usually in females of reproductive age group representing the second most common benign tumor of liver. On US, the characteristic feature of focal nodular hyperplasia (FNH) is that of a solitary, well circumscribed, slightly hypoechoic to isoechoic, solid mass, usually lesion less than 5 cm in diameter, detected incidentally by contour abnormality of liver or mass effect on the adjacent vascular structure. It may reveal a central linear or stellate hypoechoic scar. These lesions are highly vascular and hence Doppler scanning is useful.

Hepatic Adenoma

It is a rare benign hepatic tumor that is detected incidentally or becomes symptomatic secondary to internal hemorrhage

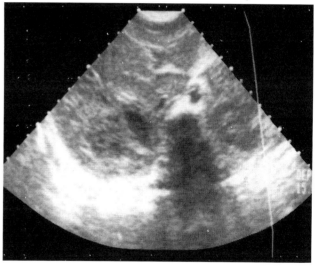

Fig. 10.8: An ill-defined lesion is seen in right lobe with multiple areas of hypo and hyperechogenicity suggestive of resolving hematoma in a patient of blunt abdominal trauma.

or infarction. It may present as an abdominal catastrophe with severe pain abdomen, severe hemorrhage, and ascites. It is commonly associated with oral contraceptive use and glycogen storage disease especially von Gaucher's disease. Surgical resection of the tumor is recommended due to the propensity of tumor to undergo hemorrhage and malignant degeneration.

It is difficult to differentiate the lesion from FNH by US and Doppler studies and many a times with CT and MRI as well.

Hepatic Lipoma

This is a very rare tumor of liver seen as highly echogenic mass with posterior acoustic enhancement that is usually

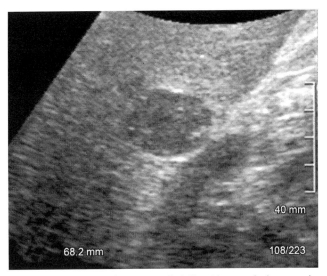

Fig. 10.9: US scan shows a well-defined hypoechoic mass in liver in a case of FNH.

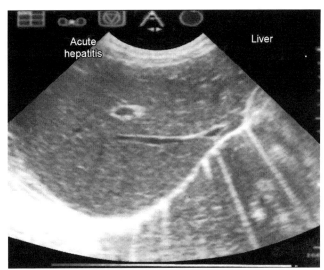

Fig. 10.11: Acute hepatitis.

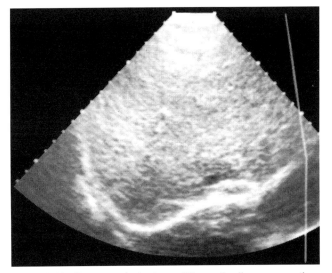

Fig. 10.10: Coarse echotexture of the entire liver suggestive of diffuse infiltrative pathology.

indistinguishable from cavernous hemangioma, focal fatty infiltration and echogenic metastasis. The classical appearance is that of an echogenic mass located in hepatic segments adjacent to the dome of diaphragm which is seen as interrupted echogenic curvilinear line due to differential sound through transmission.

BENIGN DIFFUSE LIVER DISEASE

Conditions affecting the liver diffusely.

Fatty Infiltration (Fig. 10.10)

This reversible disorder occurs due to accumulation of fatty droplets within the liver cells. The causes are obesity, alcohol, diabetes, pregnancy, drugs (especially corticosteroids), toxic substances, malnutrition due to dietary deficiency or wasting diseases and inborn errors of metabolism. US appearance is of a bright liver with increased attenuation of the US beam. Depending upon the amount of fat deposited, it is:

- Mild or Grade I—minimal increase in hepatic echogenicity with normal visualization of diaphragm and intrahepatic vessel borders
- Moderate or Grade II—increase in hepatic echogenicity with impaired visualization of intrahepatic vessels and diaphragm
- Severe or Grade III—marked increase in echogenicity with poor or nonvisualization of the hepatic vessels and diaphragm.

Focal fatty infiltration: Fatty infiltration may be patchy with angulated boundaries with no features of mass effect and normal vessels can be seen to pass through the affected portions of the liver without displacement. Single or multiple focal fatty deposit need to be differentiated from an echogenic metastasis.

Hepatitis

Acute Viral Hepatitis (Fig. 10.11)

Presentation is with fever, nausea, vomiting, pain in the right hypochondrium, jaundice, and deranged liver function tests. Main role of ultrasound (US) is in excluding an obstructive (surgical) cause of jaundice by demonstrating nondilatation of bile ducts. US examination reveals 'dark liver', i.e. a less reflective liver parenchyma with high echo amplitude of the portal vein walls. This appearance is often referred to as a "starry sky appearance". Another striking feature is contracted gallbladder with thickened wall. Liver could be enlarged **(Figs. 10.12A to C)**. US findings of a dark liver should be interpreted with caution as it is present in other conditions as well like congestive cardiac failure

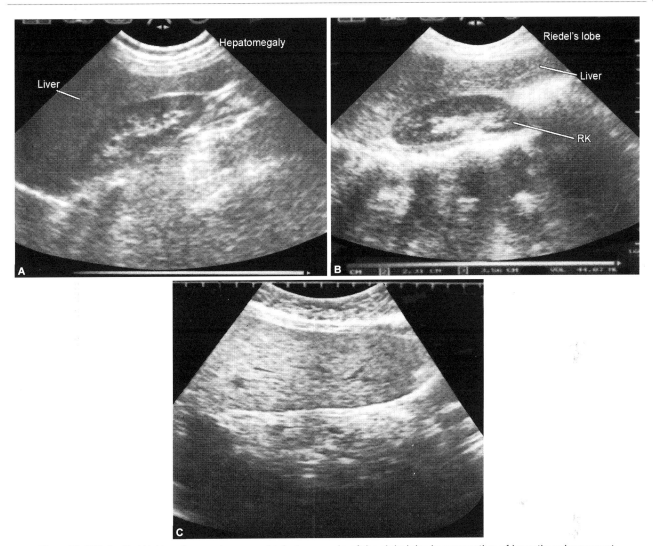

Figs. 10.12A to C: (A) Hepatomegaly—round inferior margin of the right lobe is suggestive of hepatic enlargement; (B) Riedel's lobe—It is an extension (inferior) of the right lobe which often overlies the kidney; (C) Hepatomegaly.

(CCF), AIDS, radiation injury, leukemic infiltration, and even in normal individuals.

Acute Alcoholic Hepatitis

This causes an enlarged 'bright' liver with increased attenuation of US due to fatty infiltration.

Chronic Hepatitis

Abnormal US findings are due to diffuse inflammation with varying degrees and distribution of necrosis, fatty change and fibrosis. There is increased parenchymal reflectivity and altered echo pattern. Increased attenuation sometimes occurs depending upon the amount of fatty infiltration.

Granulomatous Hepatitis (Figs. 10.13A and B)

Most common cause is tuberculosis. This produces a 'bright liver' with multiple small, moderately reflective lesions measuring 3–5 mm in diameter surrounded by an echo poor halo are present. Occasionally echo poor nodules occur in tubercular hepatitis which has to be distinguished from metastatic disease. Presence of portal adenopathy especially necrotic in nature is highly suggestive of tubercular etiology.

Cirrhosis (Figs. 10.14A and B)

Cirrhosis is a diffuse process of architectural distortion of liver due to parenchymal destruction accompanied by nodular regeneration and fibrosis.

The classic clinical presentation is hepatomegaly, jaundice and ascites, however, only 60% patients with cirrhosis have signs and symptoms of liver disease.

The most common causes of cirrhosis are alcohol consumption and chronic viral hepatitis. Other causes are biliary cirrhosis (primary and secondary), Wilson's disease, hemochromatosis, etc. US detects cirrhosis in only 2/3rd cases. Sonographic findings are:

- Liver size in early stages—the liver is enlarged, whereas in advanced stages liver is smaller than normal. Relative enlargement of the caudate lobe may be present. A caudate lobe (CL) to right lobe (RL) width ratio of 0.65 or greater is an indicator of cirrhosis
- Coarse echotexture—with concomitant loss of definition of portal vein walls. There is no significant increase in attenuation of US beam
- Nodular surface—due to regenerating nodules and fibrosis an irregular liver surface is appreciated especially in the presence of ascites
- Regenerating nodules are only detected when they appear hypoechoic with a thin echogenic border. Isoechoic lesions are missed, larger nodules (> 1 cm) are considered premalignant. Doppler settles confusion between the two as hepatomas are vascular while regenerating nodules are not. Cirrhosis is a risk factor for hepatoma and US is also used to screen for this complication.

Budd-Chiari Syndrome

This syndrome is caused by partial or complete obstruction of hepatic venous outflow (major hepatic veins or IVC). The obstruction is frequently a result of thrombus formed due to a hypercoagulable state. Patients with complete obstruction of rapid onset die of acute liver failure even before presenting for imaging investigations. US features in acute phase of incomplete, slow onset obstruction of hepatic veins are hepatomegaly, ascites with normal spleen size. Throm-

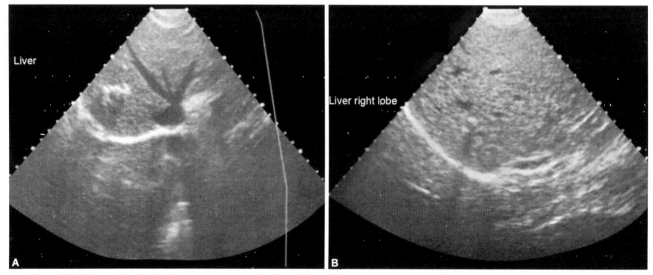

Figs. 10.13A and B: Healed granuloma seen in right lobe of liver as hyperechoic focus with distal acoustic shadowing.

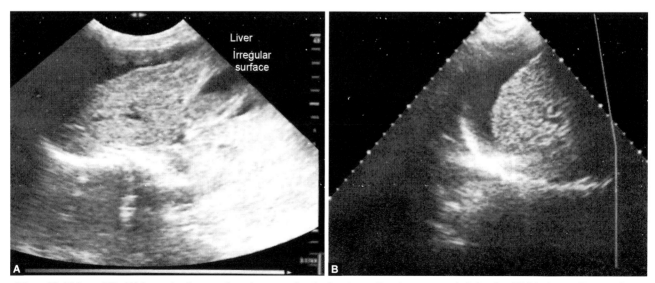

Figs. 10.14A and B: (A) Irregular liver surface is seen clearly due to ascites in a case of cirrhosis; (B) Moderate liver surface irregularity is seen well due to ascites.

bus may be seen within the major hepatic veins or IVC. As the disease progresses, compensatory hypertrophy of the caudate lobe occurs with dilated serpiginous veins and progressive splenomegaly. In chronic patients, liver texture is abnormal with small focal areas of high attenuation giving rise to acoustic shadow due to presence of calcification.

PORTAL HYPERTENSION (FIGS. 10.15A TO D)

Cirrhosis is the most common cause of intrahepatic portal hypertension. Thrombotic diseases of IVC and hepatic veins over time will also result in cirrhosis and finally portal hypertension (PHT). Presinusoidal PHT can be divided into extrahepatic and intrahepatic forms. Extrahepatic presinusoidal PHT is caused by portal vein or splenic vein thrombosis and is suspected in patients with clinical signs of PHT-ascites, splenomegaly, and varices with a normal liver biopsy. Thrombosis of portal venous system occurs due to neonatal sepsis, umbilical vein catheterization, trauma, hepatocellular carcinoma, pancreatic carcinoma, pancreatitis, splenectomy, and hypercoagulable state. Intrahepatic presinusoidal PHT is due to schistosomiasis, primary biliary cirrhosis and toxic insults.

Sonographic findings of PHT are:

Portal vein diameter more than 13 mm (measured at the head of pancreas), and dilated splenic vein, and superior mesenteric vein (more than 10–12 mm). Diameter of superior mesenteric vein more than 13 mm is a specific sign for PHT. Diameter of splenic vein more than 20 mm is also considered as being specific for PHT. Diameter of portal vein more than 17 mm is indicative of large portosystemic collaterals. Lack of more than 20% increase in the diameter of portal and superior mesenteric vein with

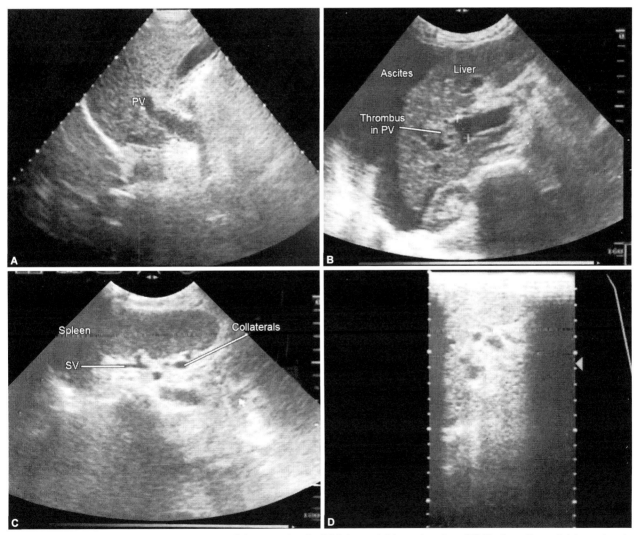

Figs. 10.15A to D: (A) Increased diameter of the portal vein (PV) in portal hypertension; (B) Prehepatic portal hypertension caused by portal vein thrombosis. Thrombus appears as an immobile echogenic material inside the lumen of dilated portal vein. Ascites is also seen; (C) Multiple small anechoic channels suggestive of collaterals are seen at the splenic hilum in a case of portal hypertension; (D) Collaterals at the porta.

deep inspiration is a specific sign for early PHT secondary to cirrhosis. Secondary signs are gross splenomegaly, ascites and portosystemic venous collaterals. Major sites of portosystemic venous collaterals, visualized by US are:
- Gastroesophageal junction—dilatation of coronary vein (> 7 mm suggests severe PHT)
- Paraumbilical vein—runs in the falciform ligament
- Splenorenal and gastrorenal
- Intestinal—seen in regions where the GI tract is retroperitoneal
- Hemorrhoidal—perianal region.

Portal Vein Thrombosis (Figs. 10.16A and B)

Portal vein thrombosis has been associated with malignancy (hepatocellular carcinoma, pancreatic carcinoma), chronic pancreatitis, hepatitis, septicemia, trauma, splenectomy, portocaval shunts, hypercoagulable states (pregnancy), etc. In neonates, acute dehydration, umbilical vein catheterization, and omphalitis are the main causes of portal vein thrombosis.

US findings are echogenic thrombus within the lumen of portal vein, portal vein collaterals, expansion of the caliber of portal vein and cavernous transformation of portal vein (periportal collaterals). Acute thrombus is anechoic and can be easily detected on Doppler. On gray scale US, the acute thrombus can be suspected by the lack of respiratory variation in caliber of the portal vein.

MALIGNANT LIVER DISEASE

Malignant lesions of the liver are primary hepatocellular carcinoma, and secondary (metastatic) tumor.

Hepatocellular Carcinoma (HCC) (Figs. 10.17A to D)

It occurs more commonly in men. Predisposing factors are cirrhosis (alcoholic and postchronic hepatitis), alfatoxins. Patient presents with right upper quadrant pain, weight loss and abdominal swelling due to ascites. Jaundice appears late due to destruction of liver parenchyma or invasion and obstruction of the bile ducts. US appearance of hepatocellular tumor depends upon the form (a) nodular form (nodules < 5 cm) appear as solitary or multifocal nodules (b) massive nodular form (nodules > 5 cm) may present as diffuse parenchymal infiltration. Hepatocellular carcinoma is of variable echogenicity. The highly reflective pattern is the most frequent finding (found in > 50% cases). However, small (< 3 cm) nodules tend to be poorly reflective. Small echogenic nodules also display an echopoor rim around them. An echopoor nodule may be found inside a large mass (tumor in tumor phenomenon) with surface lobulations and central scar that are suggestive of fibrolamellar variety of hepatocellular carcinoma. In diffuse involvement the mass is indistinct and large portion of liver is involved appearing as heterogeneous echotexture with hepatomegaly. Hepatocellular carcinoma (especially infiltrative type) has a strong tendency to invade the portal venous system.

Important differential diagnosis of hepatocellular carcinoma are regenerating nodule in cirrhotic liver, hemangiomas, focal fatty change and metastatic deposit.

Metastatic Tumors (Figs. 10.18A to G)

Terminal metastatic involvement of the liver is the rule in all but CNS, head and neck malignancies. However, the liver

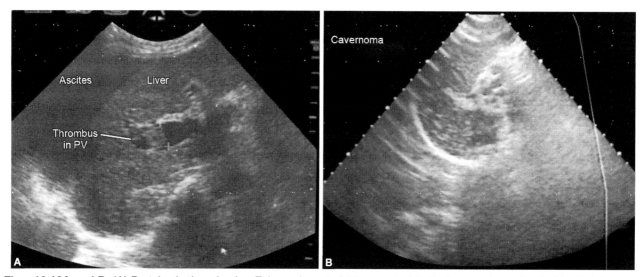

Figs. 10.16A and B: (A) Portal vein thrombosis—Echogenic material is seen inside the lumen of portal vein. The PV diameter is increased (17 mm). Free fluid surrounding the liver is also seen; (B) Portal cavernoma—multiple anechoic channels seen to replace the portal vein at porta hepatis.

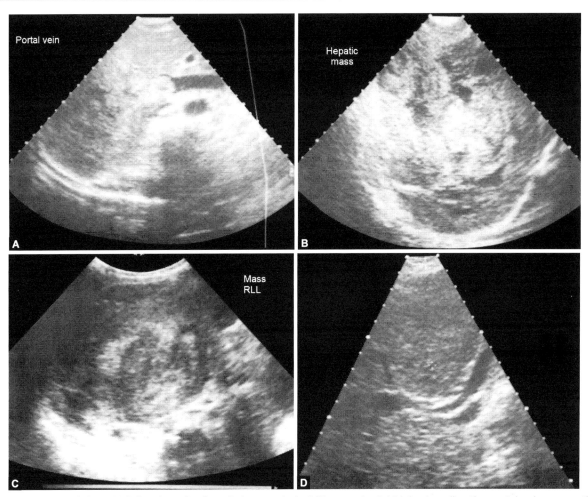

Figs. 10.17A to D: (A) An ill-defined predominantly hyperechoic SOL seen in right lobe invading the portal vein suggestive of hepatocellular carcinoma (HCC) with tumor thrombus in portal vein; (B) A large SOL of heterogeneous echotexture is seen occupying almost whole of the right lobe of liver. A rim of normal liver tissue is seen on the posteromedial aspect of the mass; (C) One year old child showing an ill defined large SOL in the liver. The lesion has a heterogeneous echotexture and few small areas of calcification. On histopathology it proved to be a hepatoblastoma; (D) Hepatocellular carcinoma: An isoechoic liver mass indenting the portal vein. The margins of the lesion are not apparent.

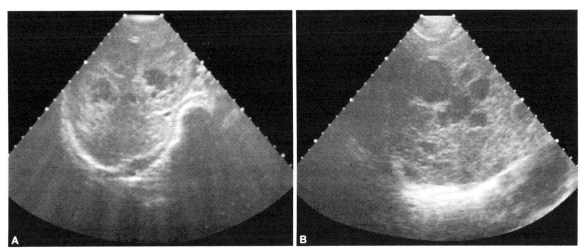

Figs. 10.18A and B: (A) Two large metastatic lesions are seen with central hypoechoic areas with irregular margins suggestive of necrosis. The patient was a case of carcinoma esophagus; (B) Multiple hypoechoic metastases are seen. Patient was a case of breast carcinoma.

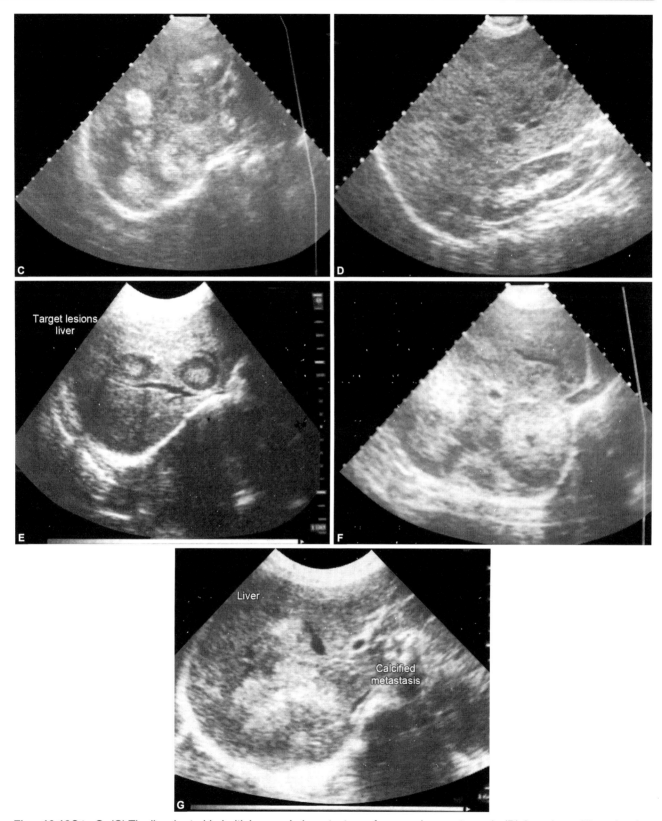

Figs. 10.18C to G: (C) The liver is studded with hyperechoic metastases from carcinoma stomach; (D) An enlarged liver showing multiple hypoechoic deposits; (E) Right lobe of liver shows the concentric ring pattern of the "target" or "bull's eye" lesion. This pattern is more often seen with larger lesions; (F) Right lobe of liver shows large hyperechoic metastatic lesions. Few are showing central necrosis; (G) Calcified metastases—multiple well-defined hyperechoic lesion with evidence of calcification within it. Patient was a case of adenocarcinoma stomach.

is involved early in the tumor arising in the splanchnic bed whose venous drainage passes directly to the liver. Liver metastases are characteristically multiple and show a range of sizes with a uniform distribution.

US appearances are variable. Focal hypoechoic lesions are the most common presentation. Bull's eye or target pattern is pathognomonic of metastasis. It appears as a highly reflective lesion with echopoor halo. Presence of multifocal solid lesions with hypoechoic halo is highly suggestive of metastatic lesions. Various US patterns are:
- Poorly reflective—typical of breast, bronchus, lymphoma
- Highly reflective—metastases from GI tract, urogenital tract especially bladder, carcinoid
- Cystic—mucin secreting, e.g. mucinous adenocarcinoma of ovary, colon and pancreas.
- Calcified—colorectal carcinoma, gastric carcinoma, melanoma, osteosarcoma, chondrosarcoma, neuroblastoma, mesothelioma, melanoma
- Confluent—any extensive secondary tumor

Diffuse involvement is a feature of lymphoma and leukemia along with liver enlargement.

SPLEEN

Diffuse Diseases of Spleen

Diseases affecting the spleen diffusely cause splenic enlargement **(Figs. 10.19 and 10.20)** with relative preservation of the shape and contour of the spleen and dilatation of splenic vessels at the splenic hilum **(Figs. 10.21 and 10.22)**. Splenic enlargement occurs in acute or chronic infections (malaria, TB) **(Fig. 10.23)**, blood dyscrasias, lymphoma, leukemia, Gauchers' disease, portal hypertension, amyloidosis, etc **(Fig. 10.24)**.

Tuberculosis of the spleen is usually miliary and causes enlargement with a heterogeneous echotexture and innumerable tiny hypoechoic lesions especially on high

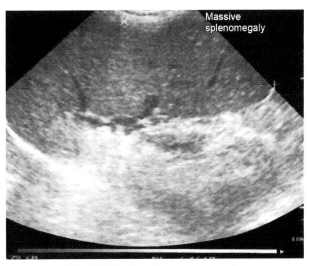

Fig. 10.20: Massive splenomegaly.

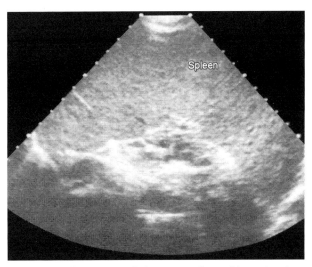

Fig. 10.21: Splenomegaly in a case of portal hypertension collaterals are seen at the splenic hilum.

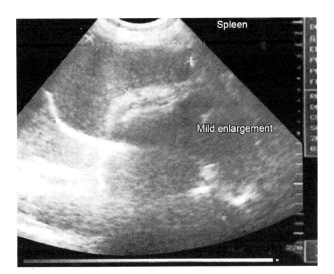

Fig. 10.19: Mild splenomegaly.

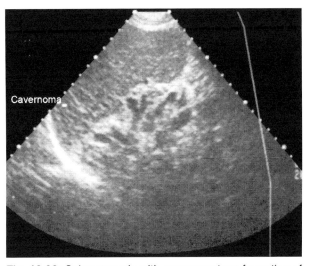

Fig. 10.22: Splenomegaly with cavernous transformation of splenic vein.

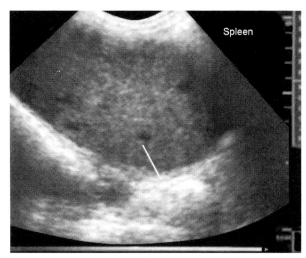

Fig. 10.23: Multiple hypoechoic lesions are seen in an enlarged spleen in this case of disseminated tuberculosis.

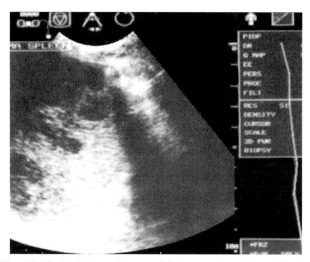

Fig. 10.25: Multiple echopoor SOLs seen in spleen. Similar lesions were seen in the liver and there was generalized lymphadenopathy.

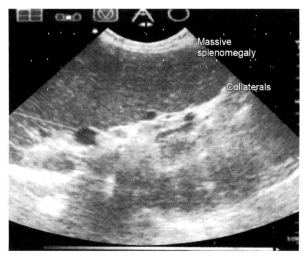

Fig. 10.24: Massive splenomegaly with collaterals in the splenorenal ligament.

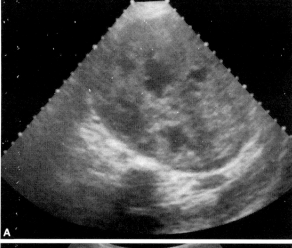

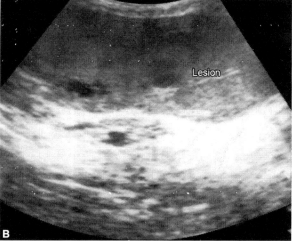

Figs. 10.26A and B: (A) A case of splenic abscess—A large SOL of heterogeneous echotexture with anechoic areas and slight posterior acoustic enhancement; (B) Fungal abscess—Multiple round echopoor SOLs seen in the splenic parenchyma. The walls are irregular and few of them show central echogenic focus.

resolution US in active stage. In healing or healed stage, innumerable tiny calcified lesions with high reflectivity may be seen.

FOCAL DISEASES OF SPLEEN

Lymphoma (Fig. 10.25)

Lymphomatous deposits in spleen can be diffuse, focal or multifocal. Focal involvement does not cause splenic enlargement. Focal lesion is seen as echopoor area with ill-defined margins. Larger lesions appear heterogeneous.

Abscess (Figs. 10.26A and B)

These are uncommon. Abscesses are usually caused by hematogenous spread of infection or may develop after trauma or infarction. US features are focal echo free defects or as complex lesions with cystic and solid components. The wall is often thick and irregular and they may contain echoes, septations or gas. In fungal abscesses various US pattern seen are 'wheel with in a wheel', 'bull's eye', uniformly echo-poor lesions or reflective foci with variable degrees of acoustic shadowing. Abscesses may be focal or multifocal. Inflammatory pseudotumors are solitary benign masses seen as well-defined reflective mass which are partially calcified. These are to be differcntiated from granulomas, hamartoma, venous congestion, splenic cysts and hemangioma.

Metastases (Fig. 10.27)

Splenic metastases are uncommon except from lymphoma.

Trauma (Figs. 10.28A and B)

Blunt abdominal trauma often involves the spleen in various manners:

Adrenergic stimulation causes splenic enlargement. Subcapsular hematoma is seen as echofree collection indenting the splenic parenchyma from outside.

Spleen hematoma in acute stage appears as highly reflective crescentic lesion either well or poorly defined. Later, it becomes echopoor following degradation of blood. Splenic rupture produces an irregular linear area of reduced reflectivity due to hemorrhage.

Cysts and Tumors (Figs. 10.29 and 10.30)

- Cystic lesions of the spleen are primary or epithelial cysts and secondary cysts. Primary splenic cysts are well-defined echo free lesions with posterior enhancement. Calcification may be present. Secondary cysts are post-traumatic cysts and parasitic hydatid cysts. The most common US finding of hydatid cysts is an echo free cyst with thick echogenic wall. Complicated cysts give an echogenic appearance. Post-traumatic cysts are indistinguishable from primary splenic cysts.
- Hemangiomas rarely involve the spleen. US appearances vary from well defined echo-poor lesions with posterior enhancement to homogeneous reflective lesions or mixed lesions.
- Lymphangiomas are benign congenital malformation of lymphatic system seen sonographically as multiple echopoor lesions.

GALLBLADDER

Congenital Variations

Gallbladder septations, bilobed GB and duplication anomalies can be detected on US. In cases of an elongated

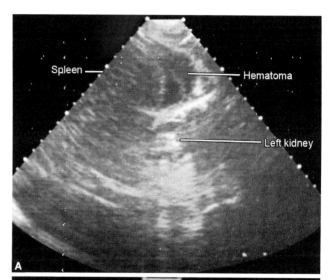

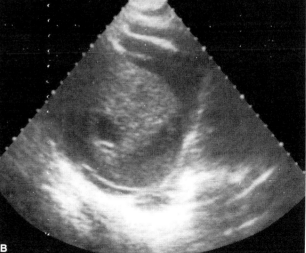

Figs. 10.28A and B: (A) Splenic trauma—Splenic laceration with hematoma; (B) An anechoic collection around the spleen—Perisplenic hematoma. There is also a parenchymal laceration with hematoma of the spleen.

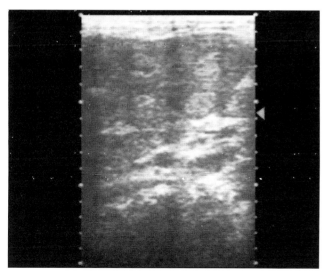

Fig. 10.27: Metastases—multiple echogenic areas seen in the spleen—Case of adenocarcinoma colon.

cystic duct or a long gallbladder (GB), mesentery of the GB is anomalous in location and is susceptible for torsion. Phrygian cap deformity is seen as the GB fundus folded on the body. Intrahepatic GB can be confused with a simple cyst.

Gallbladder Stones/Cholelithiasis (Figs. 10.31A to C)

Cholelithiasis has a high prevalence and two-third of gallstone carriers are asymptomatic.

Classical US appearances are a highly reflective intraluminal structure which is gravity dependent and casts a sharp and clean acoustic shadow. Shadowing beyond a stone is not affected by the chemical composition of the stone or the shape and size of the stone. Stones as small as 1 mm are picked up by US with optimal scanning techniques.

Contracted Gallbladder

In situations when the gallbladder lumen is completely filled by stones, or where the wall has been chronically inflamed and becomes fibrotic, or where the cystic duct is obstructed, there may be no fluid bile within the lumen. These contracted gallbladder initially recognized on US as 'nonvisualized' gallbladder are infact diseased. This diagnosis becomes more accurate if distal acoustic shadowing is present from the gallbladder fossa. This has to be differentiated from bowel gas in the duodenum. In the presence of wall-echo-shadow (WES) **(Fig. 10.32)** triad the diagnosis of gallstones is certain. This complex consists of reflective anterior wall of the gallbladder separated by a thin echopoor rim (residual bile or thickened gallbladder wall) from the reflective anterior surface of the stone which casts a complete acoustic shadow. Moving the patient during US examination (left decubitus position) helps to demonstrate the gravity dependence of stones and differentiates them from polyps. Movement also helps to demonstrate multiple small stones by clustering them in a group from where shadowing in readily visible. Sometimes floating stones are also encountered and easily demonstrated by movement of the patient. Layering of echoes on erect scans with evidence of shadowing from them is suggestive of milk of calcium bile.

Echogenic Bile/Biliary Sludge (Figs. 10.33A to C)

Nonshadowing, gravity dependent echoes in the gallbladder are referred to as biliary sludge. This may be due to pus or blood in the bile as a result of infection or trauma or it may be seen in association with gallstones. Sometimes echo-

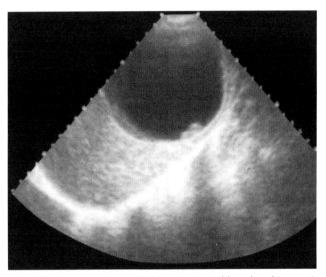

Fig. 10.29: Splenic hydatid—Large cyst with a daughter cyst and hydatid sand.

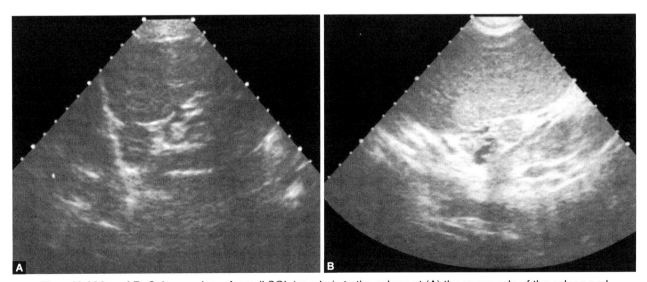

Figs. 10.30A and B: Splenunculus—A small SOL isoechoic to the spleen at (A) the upper pole of the spleen and (B) the splenic hilum.

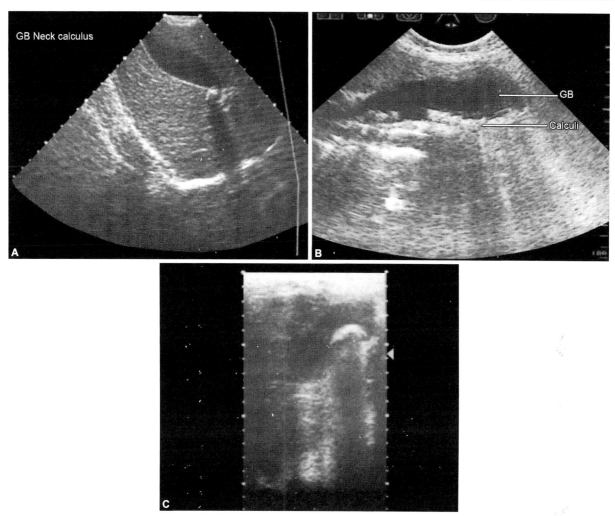

Figs. 10.31A to C: (A) GB calculus—A calculus is seen at the neck of gallbladder; (B) Cholelithiasis—GB lumen shows multiple small echogenic foci with distal acoustic shadowing in the dependent part; (C) A solitary echogenic focus with posterior acoustic shadowing is seen inside the lumen of the gallbladder.

genic bile is also seen in conditions leading to bile stasis, as pathological biliary obstruction or physiological reasons like prolonged fasting, patients on parenteral nutrition, after GI surgery. Rescanning after a normal diet causes disappearance of the echoes.

Occasionally nonshadowing echoes are clumped together within the gallbladder lumen and are called 'sludge balls' or tumefactive sludge. This causes confusion with growth in the gallbladder lumen. Movement of the echoes with gravity differentiates the two conditions. A repeat scan with normal diet also solves the diagnostic dilemma.

Gallbladder Wall Thickening (Figs. 10.34 to 10.37)

In the fasting state, the normal gallbladder is distended and has a wall thickness of less than 3 mm. Measurement of the anterior wall thickness is taken on a transverse scan at the level of the body. Various causes of gallbladder wall thickening are known:

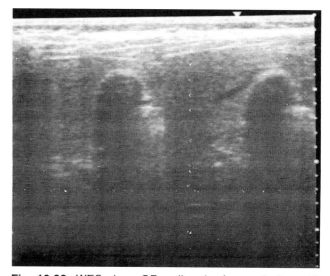

Fig. 10.32: WES sign—GB wall, echo from calculus with posterior acoustic shadowing are seen in the GB fossa suggestive of cholelithiasis with chronic cholecystitis.

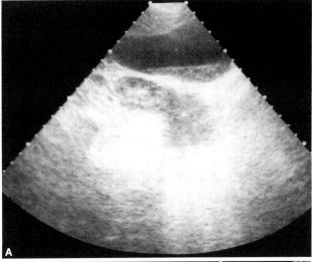
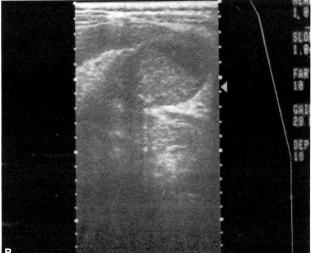
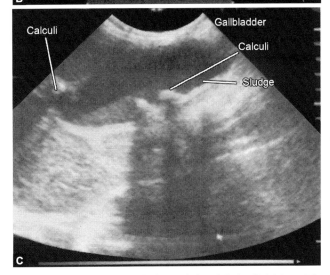

Figs. 10.33A to C: (A) A straight debris fluid level in the dependent portion of GB is diagnostic of sludge; (B) Sludge in gallbladder; (C) Cholelithiasis: Longitudinal and transverse scan of GB showing three calculi in it's lumen (1 at neck). Sludge is seen as echogenic material with a straight level in the dependent portion of GB.

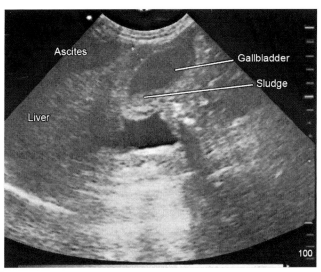

Fig. 10.34: Gallbladder wall thickening due to ascites. Sludge is seen inside gallbladder lumen. Shadowing is seen from the adjacent bowel loop.

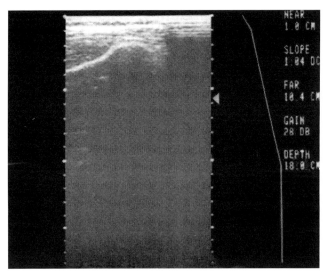

Fig. 10.35: Dense shadowing seen from the calcified anterior gallbladder wall in porcelain GB.

Physiological: Postprandial

Inflammatory diseases of gallbladder: Acute cholecystitis **(Figs. 10.38 A and B)**.

Chronic Cholecystitis (Fig. 10.39)

Noninflammatory diseases of gallbladder: Adenomyomatosis, carcinoma, and leukemia.
- Edema of gallbladder wall—ascites
  - Hypoalbuminemia
  - Portal hypertension
  - Malignant lymphatic obstruction
- Nearby inflammatory disease: Hepatitis
  - Acute pancreatitis

CHAPTER 10: Abdomen: Hepatobiliary System and Spleen

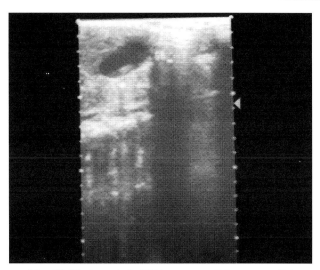

Fig. 10.36: Ascaris in GB is seen as 2 linear parallel echogenic lines.

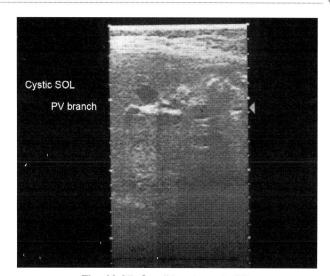

Fig. 10.37: Small intrahepatic GB.

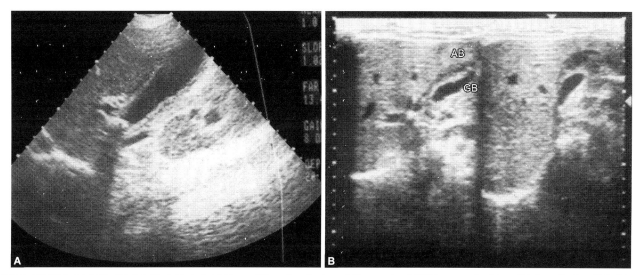

Figs. 10.38A and B: (A) Acute calculus cholecystitis—A calculus at the neck of GB is seen inside a thick walled gallbladder; (B) Thickened gallbladder wall, pericholecystic fluid and a hypoechoic collection at the fundus is evident in this case of acute acalculous cholecystitis.

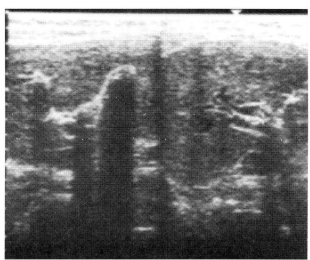

Fig. 10.39: Chronic cholecystitis with cholelithiasis—Dense acoustic shadowing is seen from the GB fossa. WES sign is positive. Adjacent scan shows a dilated CBD with an echogenic focus inside it's lumen.

Acute Cholecystitis

Acute cholecystitis occurs in approximately one-third of patients with gallstones and is caused by persistent calculous obstruction of the gallbladder neck or cystic duct and resultant inflammation of gallbladder wall. Patients present with pain in the right upper quadrant with nausea or vomiting and/or fever. US helps to establish the diagnosis more accurately in calculous cholecystitis rather than 5–10% of patients in whom acalculous cholecystitis occurs. US signs of acute cholecystitis are given here in the tabulated form.

Major	Minor
• Stones in GB	• Pericholecystic fluid (if gangrenous GB)
• Edema of GB wall	• Thickening of GB wall
• Nonvisualization of GB	• GB tenderness
• Gas in GB wall	• Intraluminal changes
	• GB enlargement
	• Round GB shape

Presence of one major sign and one minor sign has a sensitivity rate of 90–98% in diagnosing acute cholecystitis. Stones in gallbladder with a positive US Murphy's sign are highly specific for acute cholecystitis (92%).

Empyema of the Gallbladder

Empyema of the gallbladder is difficult to recognize on ultrasound as the typical finding of sludge (non-shadowing gravity dependent echoes) may be caused by many processes including debris or pus.

Emphysematous Cholecystitis

Emphysematous cholecystitis may occur in the absence of gallstones usually in diabetics. Its hallmark is the presence of gas in GB wall. It is seen as highly reflective areas within a thickened and edematous GB wall with shadowing and reverberations distally.

Acute Acalculous Cholecystitis

Acute cholecystitis is acalculous in approximately 5–10% of all patients. It occurs as a complication of prolonged or severe illness, major surgery, burns, sepsis and diabetes. Gangrene and perforation are more common in the acalculous variety. US features of distention of GB, wall thickening, presence of sludge and lack of response of the gallbladder to cholecystokinin are helpful diagnostic signs. US guided aspiration of GB bile for culture can also be performed.

Chronic Cholecystitis

Patients presenting with recurrent right upper quadrant pain, with nausea, dyspepsia, and intolerance to fatty diet are patients of this disease entity. It is almost always associated with gallstones. US features are a small contracted GB with gallstones with or without thickening of the gallbladder wall. Nonvisualization of the gallbladder at US is highly predictive of gallbladder disease.

Gallbladder Polyps (Figs. 10.40A and B)

Included in this group are pseudotumors like inflammatory polyps, cholesterol polyp, adenomyomas and localized adenomyomatosis. Adenomatous polyps occur in Peutz-Jeghers syndrome of which 10% are multiple and 10% show complains of carcinoma in situ. Polyps appear as small intraluminal reflective structures which are fixed to the gallbladder wall and do not cast an acoustic shadow.

Other benign neoplasms of gallbladder like fibroma, myoma, carcinoid, hemangioma are extremely rare.

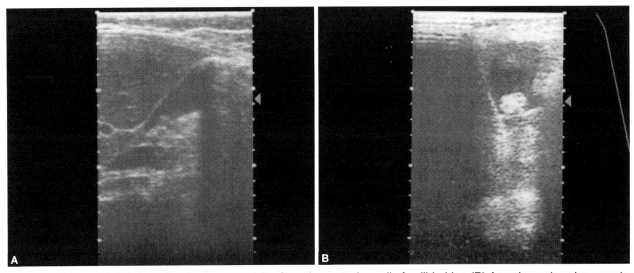

Figs. 10.40A and B: (A) A small polyp is seen arising from the posterior wall of gallbladder; (B) An echogenic polyp seen in the transverse scan of gallbladder.

Cholesterolosis and Adenomyomatosis of Gallbladder (Figs. 10.41 and 10.42)

The strawberry gallbladder or cholesterolosis is a noninflammatory, benign condition often detected incidentally arising secondary to accumulation of lipids (cholesterol) in the mucosa of the gallbladder wall. The resulting surface nodules are recognized by US, when they are 2 mm or greater in diameter. They are seen as single or multiple, echogenic, polypoidal excrescences attached to the wall with characteristic lack of distal acoustic shadow and mobility with patient posture. V-shaped comet tail artefact may be demonstrable in these lesions.

The hyperplastic changes in the gallbladder wall occurring in the absence of gallstones or inflammatory infiltrates is known as adenomyomatosis or cholecystitis glandularis proliferans. Excessive intraluminal pressure has been suggested as the possible etiology. The US features are characteristic and include diffuse or segmental thickening of the gallbladder wall, with intraluminal diverticula (Rokitansky-Aschoff sinuses or RAS) and echogenic foci with posterior reverberation artefacts within the thickened gallbladder wall. Segmental and eccentric wall thickening may produce midcavity strictures, and the highly echogenic periluminal foci due to aggregates of solid bile elements in the RAS give rise to a typical diamond ring appearance on axial scans of gallbladder.

Gallbladder Carcinoma (Figs. 10.43A to C)

GB carcinoma is the fifth most common malignancy of GI tract. It is a highly malignant tumor with a mean survival of less than five months from the time of diagnosis. Females are affected four times more commonly as males and has a high correlation exists with gallstones (80–90%) and chronic cholecystitis. Clinically the condition is not suspected until local spread or distant metastases have occurred. Therefore, US is a very useful investigation in detecting early resectable growths. Various ultrasonic appearances of gallbladder carcinoma have been described. The most common finding is of a large solid mass filling the gallbladder bed, lack of visualization of a separate gallbladder lumen or presence of stones within the mass. Gallbladder mass may also present as focal thickening or diffuse, irregular, asymmetric nodular thickening of the wall. Twenty five percent of patients with porcelain gallbladder will have associated carcinoma. On US it appears as a biconvex curvilinear reflective structure with shadowing. Carcinoma can be detected in this condition if there is focal or diffuse thickening of the gallbladder wall external to the calcified portion, or if there is an eccentric mass arising from the gallbladder wall,

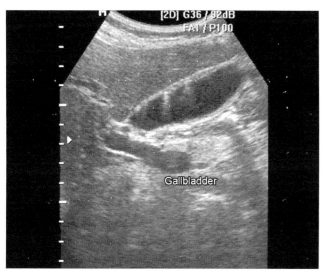

Fig. 10.41: Cholesterolosis of gallbladder with V-shaped comet tail artefact.

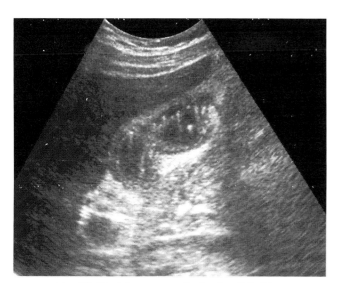

Fig. 10.42: Adenomyomatosis of gallbladder.

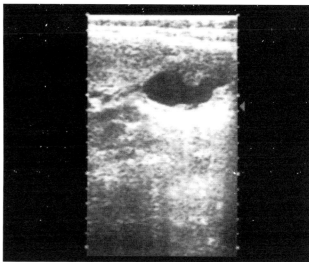

Fig. 10.43A: Small exophytic mass seen to arise from anterior wall of gallbladder.

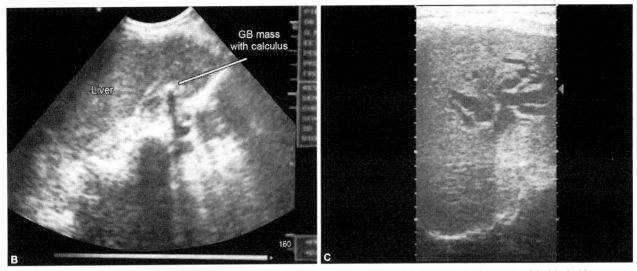

Figs. 10.43B and C: (B) The whole GB is occupied by an isoechoic mass which has a calculus embedded in it. However, gallbladder wall is intact; (C) Dilated intrahepatic bile ducts—Stellate branching pattern seen in transverse scan.

porta hepatis or peripancreatic lymphadenopathy or liver metastases are seen.

Hydrops (Fig. 10.44)

If the dimension of gallbladder exceeds 10 × 5 cm or becomes spherical in shape, it is an abnormally distended gallbladder. Many conditions cause gallbladder enlargement, e.g. diabetes, pregnancy, typhoid in children. 'Hydrops' is reserved for gallbladders which are distended due to blockage of cystic duct.

BILE DUCT PATHOLOGY/DILATATION

Intrahepatic bile duct dilatation is present when the ratio of duct to portal vein diameter ratio exceeds 1:4. Right and left bile ducts are termed dilated when they exceed 2 mm in diameter while CBD should be normally less than 5 mm at porta hepatis and less than 6 mm at the distal end within the head of the pancreas. Dilatation of the intrahepatic bile ducts will result in one or more of the following ultrasound findings **(Figs. 10.45 A to C)**:
- Parallel channel sign
- Double-barrel shot gun sign
- Too many tubes in the liver
- Stellate pattern near porta.

BILE DUCT STONES/ CHOLEDOCHOLITHIASIS (FIGS. 10.46A TO D)

Choledocholithiasis occurs in approximately 15% of the patients with stones in the gallbladder and in 4% of postcholecystectomy cases. The classical clinical presentation is biliary colic, jaundice and fever—Charcot's

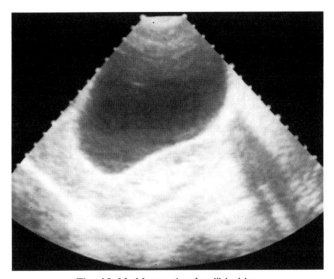

Fig. 10.44: Mucocele of gallbladder.

triad. US has a low sensitivity in detecting stones in the CBD. This is due to a confusion occurring due to the presence of gas in the duodenum; intermittently obstructing stones do not cause dilated bile ducts; 10% stones lack shadowing; or gas and sludge in the bile ducts may be confused with stones. To overcome this problem patients are scanned with water in their stomach and duodenum in both the right oblique and left oblique and semi-erect positions. Disproportionate dilatation of the extrahepatic biliary tree in comparison to the intrahepatic ducts gives a clue to the stone etiology. Stones appear as echogenic focus with acoustic shadowing if lying in a pool of bile inside the CBD.

Careful screening of CBD is to be done to find out associated cyst (choledochal cyst) **(Figs. 10.47A to C)**; gas in bile duct **(Figs. 10.49A and B)**; any other shadows **(Fig. 10.50)**.

CHAPTER 10: Abdomen: Hepatobiliary System and Spleen

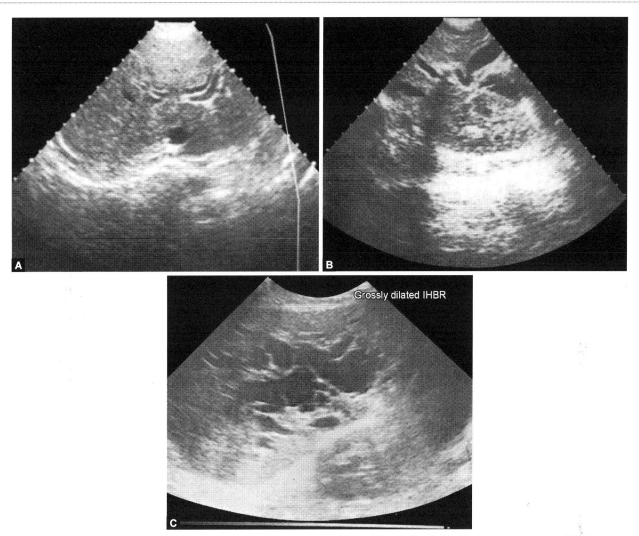

Figs. 10.45A to C: (A) Mildly dilated left hepatic duct is seen anterior to the portal vein in this transverse scan; (B) Cystic duct calculus—A small echogenic focus with acoustic shadow is seen in the cystic duct. Gallbladder appears normal; (C) Grossly dilated IHBR are seen as multiple tubular structures.

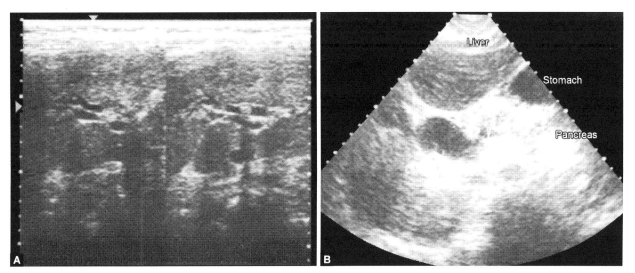

Figs. 10.46A and B: (A) Scan at porta shows a dilated CBD. Adjacent scan shows a calculus inside the lumen of CBD; (B) Choledocholithiasis—an echogenic focus with acoustic shadow seen inside a dilated CBD.

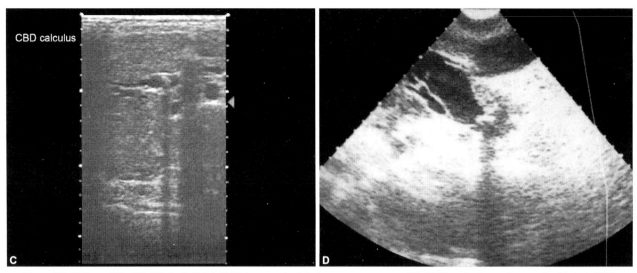

Figs. 10.46C and D: (C) Dilated distal CBD is seen in this transverse scan; (D) CBD calculus—A grossly dilated CBD (measuring 23 mm) is seen with a echogenic focus with shadowing at it's distal end.

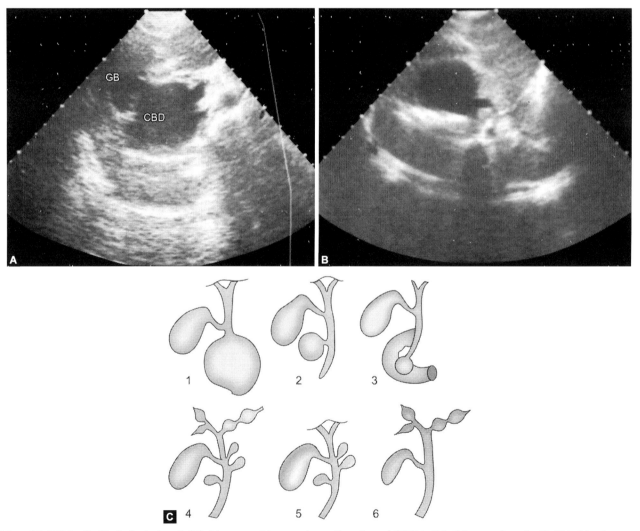

Figs. 10.47A to C: Choledochal cyst. (A) A large cyst is seen in continuation of CBD in this 24 years female. Gallbladder is seen adjacent to the cyst; (B) A large cyst is seen in continuation with CBD in this 4 years old female; (C) (1-6) Choledochal cyst.

CHOLEDOCHAL CYSTS (FIGS. 10.47 AND 10.48)

These are an uncommon congenital cause of biliary tract dilatation usually manifesting in childhood with a classic triad of icterus, right hypochondrium pain and palpable mass in subcostal region. It classified into five categories as follows:

Todani's classification of choledochal cysts:

Type I: Cystic fusiform dilatation of extrahepatic CBD (commonest)
Type II: Diverticulum arising from CBD
Type III: Choledochocele or cystic dilatation of intramural portion of distal CBD within the duodenal wall
Type IVA: Multiple intrahepatic and extrahepatic cysts arising from the biliary tract
Type IVB: Multiple extrahepatic cysts arising from the biliary tract.
Type V: Multiple intrahepatic cysts arising from the biliary tract (also known as Caroli's disease).

The important differential diagnoses include hepatic cysts, pancreatic pseudocyst and duplication cysts. The important clue to the diagnosis of choledochal cysts is demonstration of communication with biliary ducts. Hepatobiliary scans demonstrating excretion of the radiotracer in to the cysts are diagnostic.

Complications associated with choledochal cysts include cholangitis, obstructive jaundice, choledocholithiasis, and cholangiocarcinoma.

Pneumobilia (Figs. 10.49A and B)

Sonographically, it is characterized by a linear echogenic appearance with minimal or acoustic shadowing but presence of comet-tail artefact. It can be easily recognized by its movement with change in posture.

The most important causes include incompetence of sphincter of Oddi, enterobiliary fistula or biliary-enteric anastomosis

Biliary Ascariasis (Fig. 10.50)

It is the commonest parasitic biliary infestation in endemic areas. Ascaris is recognized on US as tubular, nonshadowing filling defect in the extrahepatic duct that may be straight or coiled. There is characteristic tram-track appearance with two echogenic lines separated by a sonolucent center. When live, its movement can be demonstrated by US. Macerated worm may be mistaken for a mass lesion especially in cases of obstructive jaundice.

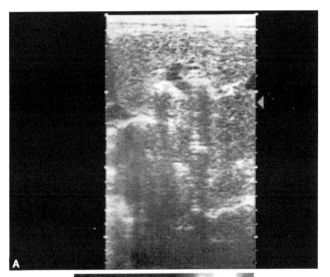

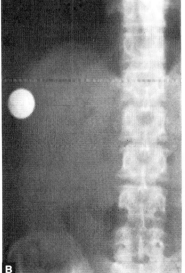

Figs. 10.49A and B: (A) Pneumobilia echogenic foci with dirty shadowing is suggestive of gas in the lumen of biliary tree; (B) Plain X-ray confirms pneumobilia seen as branching pattern of air in the biliary tree.

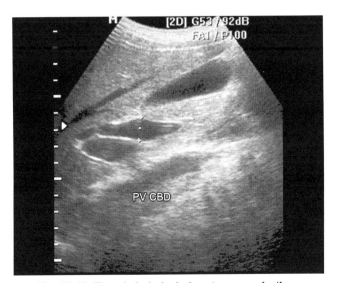

Fig. 10.48: Type I choledochal cyst seen as fusiform dilatation of extrahepatic portion of CBD.

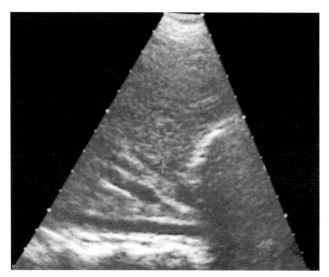

Fig. 10.50: Ascaris is seen as a linear echogenic shadow occupying the dilated CBD.

MIRIZZI SYNDROME

It is an uncommon condition characterized by extrahepatic biliary obstruction secondary to impaction of the calculus in the cystic duct or gallbladder neck with subsequent compression of the common hepatic duct. The condition usually arises when the cystic duct runs parallel to the common hepatic duct for considerable distance before finally joining it.

Occasionally the calculus may erode the cystic duct or GB wall to enter in to the common hepatic duct or adjacent bowel especially the duodenum resulting in cholecystobiliary or cholecystoenteric or cholecystoduodenal fistula.

BILE DUCT NEOPLASM (FIGS. 10.51A TO C)

Benign lesions of the bile duct are rare and include papillomas, adenomas, cystadenomas, etc. Cystadenomas

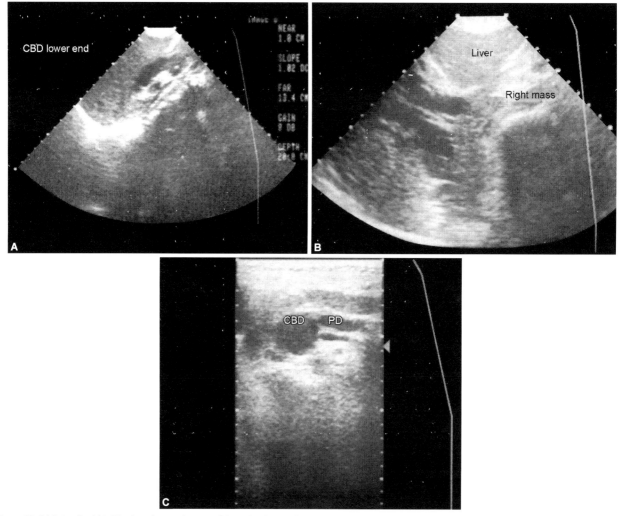

Figs. 10.51A to C: (A) Cholangiocarcinoma: Mass lesion at lower end of dilated common duct, and (B) mass lesion is seen to obstruct the distal CBD causing proximal dilation of the CBD, (C) Transverse scan showing a grossly dilated distal CBD at the head of pancreas. The pancreatic duct (PD) is also dilated. Double duct sign is suggestive of periampullary carcinoma.

are multilobulated cystic masses usually occurring in young females.

Primary malignant tumors of the bile ducts are cholangiocarcinomas. These patients present with features of obstructive jaundice. These may develop at any level within the biliary tree and when they involve the confluence of the left and right hepatic ducts at the porta hepatis they are referred to as Klatskin tumors. US features of cholangiocarcinomas are dilatation of the biliary tree up to the level of obstruction where a solid poorly reflective mass or a heterogeneous mass with ill-defined margins is present. Sometimes thickening of the walls of the bile duct may be the only evidence of tumor.

Abrupt tapering of the CBD with proximal dilatation may sometimes be the only clue to the presence of malignant lesion. Lymph node enlargement, hepatic metastases or direct invasion of portal vein is also looked as supportive evidence of bile duct malignancy for on US.

OTHER TUMORS OBSTRUCTING BILE DUCTS

The bile ducts may be obstructed by intrahepatic tumors, enlarged lymph nodes at porta hepatis, carcinoma of the head of the pancreas and ampullary tumors.

11

CHAPTER

Abdomen: Pancreas

CONGENITAL ANOMALIES

- Agenesis of dorsal anlage or hypoplasia of pancreas—is usually characterized by absence of the body and tail of the pancreas with compensatory hypertrophy of the head region.
- Congenital cysts—anomalous development of the pancreatic ducts results in cysts of the pancreas. These are found in association with cystic disease of liver, spleen and kidneys and VHL syndrome.
- Cystic fibrosis causes dysfunction of multiple glands including the exocrine portion of pancreas. Most common sonographic finding is increased echogenicity due to fibrosis and fatty change. The pancreas may be small; an enlarged pancreas indicates complication like pancreatitis especially if the echogenicity is reduced. Sometimes cysts are also seen in the pancreas.

Inflammatory Diseases

Acute Pancreatitis (Figs. 11.1A and B)

Diagnosis of acute pancreatitis is based on clinical and laboratory findings. Patients present with severe abdominal pain and markedly raised serum amylase levels. US has limited usefulness in diagnosing acute pancreatitis in the early stages. US is mainly used to detect the cause of pancreatitis as gallstones and CBD stones, extent of pancreatic necrosis, follow-up of complications and guidance of interventional procedures.

Sonographic finding of acute pancreatitis is often appreciated after 48 hours of acute episode as the ileus resolves and thus permits visualization of the pancreas. With the advent of present day scanners, it does not hold true. Moreover, US scanning in lateral decubitus position to allow the air movement resulting in visualization of pancreas even in severe pancreatitis.

Focal pancreatitis is seen as focal isoechoic or hypoechoic enlargement of the pancreatic head. These patients are usually alcoholics and acute disease occurs on a background of chronic pancreatitis. Presence of calcification in the lesion and abnormal ductal changes outside it suggests focal pancreatitis rather than a tumor mass.

Diffuse pancreatitis **(Figs. 11.2A and B)**: The size of pancreas is increased with decrease in its echogenicity

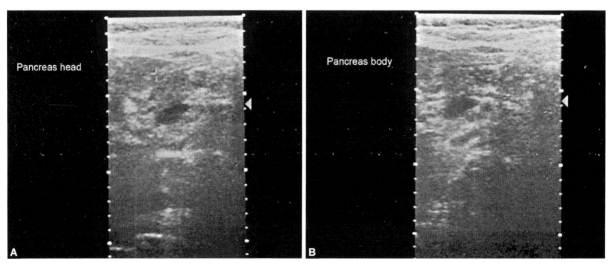

Figs. 11.1A and B: Acute pancreatitis—pancreas is bulky and hypoechoic.

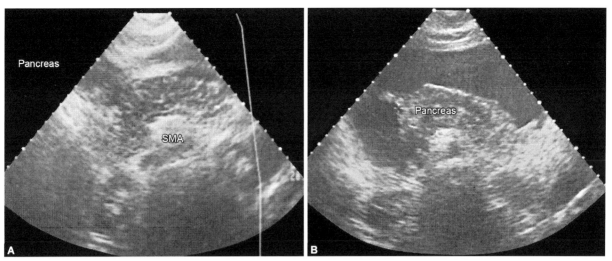

Figs. 11.2A and B: Acute pancreatitis. Pancreas is diffusely increased in size and appears hypoechoic and heterogeneous in echopattern. The borders are not well-demarcated. A small fluid collection is seen in the lesser sac anterior to the body of pancreas. Duodenum appears dilated; (B) Acute pancreatitis. Pancreas is bulky and heterogeneous in echotexture. There is evidence of a large collection anterior to pancreas. (SMA: superior mesenteric artery).

due to inflammation. In mild cases US findings may be that of a normal pancreas. With the increase in severity the US findings are more pronounced. The pancreas may also appear inhomogeneous with focal hemorrhagic areas seen as echogenic masses. Areas of fluid collections may be seen within the pancreas suggestive of pancreatic necrosis. The duct may be compressed and its walls may appear more reflective. US examination should also concentrate on the biliary tree to detect choledocholithiasis and gallstones. Extrapancreatic manifestations are important in patients with acute pancreatitis **(Fig. 11.3)**. These include fluid collections and edema along the lesser sac, anterior pararenal spaces and perirenal spaces etc. Others are ascites, thickening of the adjacent GI tract and thickened gallbladder wall.

Complications of Pancreatitis (Figs. 11.4A to C)

- Pseudopancreatic cyst—10–20% of patients with acute pancreatitis develop this complication after 4–6 weeks. Pseudocysts are spherical fluid collections with a well defined smooth wall of variable thickness without echoes and with posterior enhancement. Debris within it suggests hemorrhage or infection. A pseudocyst may be multiloculated or even show calcification in its wall. Clinically persistent pain and elevated serum amylase levels suggest the diagnosis.
- Obstruction of gastrointestinal tract (GIT) or bile ducts—this complication is found in 30–50% of patients with pseudocysts. Obstruction of bile ducts may cause obstructive jaundice which could later progress to obstructive cholangitis.
- GI hemorrhage may occur as pseudocyst sometimes erodes into the stomach wall or from variceal bleeding caused by local portal HT due to portosplenic compression or thrombosis.

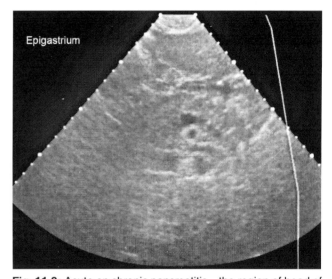

Fig. 11.3: Acute on chronic pancreatitis—the region of head of pancreas is swollen, hypoechoic and not well-demarcated. Body and tail of pancreas shows small echogenic specks suggestive of calcification.

- Rupture of the pseudocyst may cause acute peritonitis.
- Pancreatic abscess—occurs in postoperative patients and has to be distinguished from pseudocysts as they carry high mortality. Sonographically, it is seen as thick walled anechoic mass containing debris with bright echoes from gas bubbles or as a complex mass lesion. US-guided aspiration and culture settles the diagnosis.
- Pseudoaneurysms—are seen as complication of pancreatitis or pseudocyst. Presence of an echogenic crescent representing the thrombus at the periphery of a cystic mass lesion adjacent to the head of the pancreas is highly suggestive of an aneurysm. Doppler sonography is diagnostic in these cases.

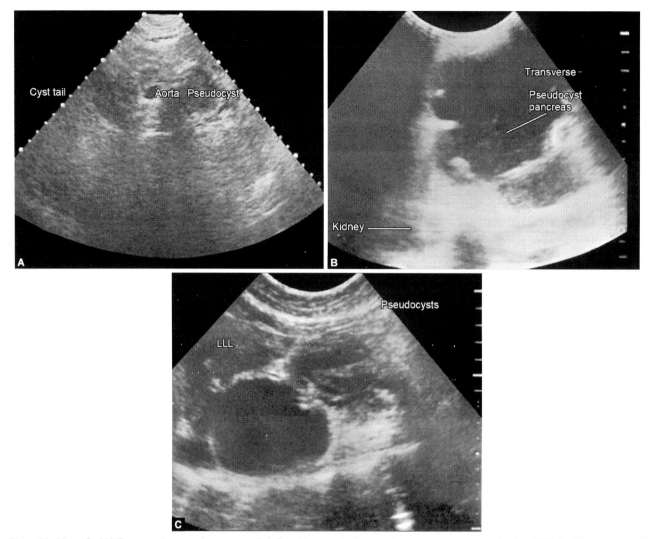

Figs. 11.4A to C: (A) Pancreatic pseudocyst—well defined hypoechoic rounded space-occupying lesion (SOL) with evidence of posterior enhancement seen in the region of tail of pancreas in a follow-up case of acute pancreatitis; (B) Pseudocyst pancreas—a large multiloculated collection seen in lesser sac with evidence of debris in it; (C) A large pseudocyst seen in lesser sac posterior to left lobe of liver (LLL). Another pseudocyst is seen adjacent to it with evidence of internal septae.

- Pancreatic ascites and pleural effusion—especially left sided pleural effusion is seen. Pancreatic ascites may be asymptomatic causing an enlarging abdomen.

Chronic Pancreatitis (Figs. 11.5 to 11.7)

Chronic alcohol intake or biliary tract disease cause repeated bouts of mild or subclinical pancreatitis to cause a progressive and irreversible destruction of the pancreas.

Sonographic findings are:

Size of pancreas varies from small and atrophic to enlarged in size with an irregular surface. Echotexture is usually heterogeneous; echogenic areas may be seen due to fibrosis and calcification while hypoechoic areas are seen due to associated inflammation. In 40% patients a focal mass may be seen. Calcification in the lesion differentiates it from a tumor mass.

Irregular dilatation of the pancreatic duct is also present. Pancreatic calcification is usually due to calcified protein plugs in the ductal system and is seen as echogenic foci with distal shadowing. Pseudocysts—intra or peripancreatic lesions are present which is better marked off than in acute pancreatitis. An inflammatory stricture at the lower CBD can cause dilated bile ducts. Portosplenic vein thrombosis with cavernous transformation occurs in 5% cases.

Neoplasms

Adenocarcinoma (Figs. 11.8 to 11.10)

Arises from the ductal system most commonly in the head of the pancreas and presents with obstructive jaundice (with a palpable nontender gallbladder), weight loss and pain. Tumors of the body and tail present later with less specific symptoms. Diagnosis on US depends upon:

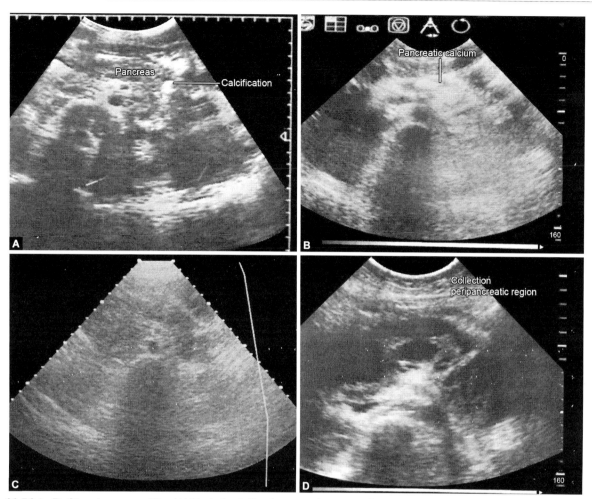

Figs. 11.5A to D: Chronic pancreatitis: (A) Foci of calcification seen in region of pancreatic tail; (B) A dense echogenic focus with distal acoustic shadowing is seen in region of pancreas representing calcification; (C) Transverse scan of pancreas showing a bulky pancreas with heterogeneous echotexture. Fascial planes are not well demarcated, echogenic areas in the region of head suggest hemorrhage in a case of necrotizing pancreatitis; (D) Acute necrotizing pancreatitis: anechoic collection seen surrounding the pancreas with necrotic pancreatic debris seen in it.

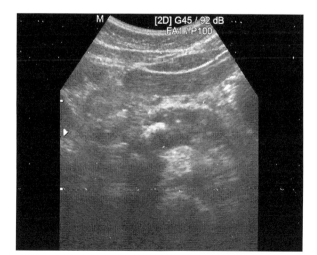

Fig. 11.6: US image through the neck and body region of pancreas shows a large calculus in the main pancreatic duct in the region of neck with distal dilatation in a case of chronic calcific pancreatitis.

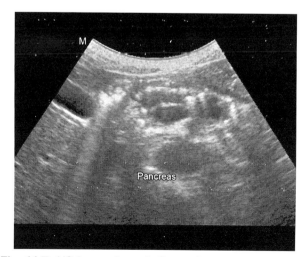

Fig. 11.7: US image through the neck and body region of pancreas shows a dilatation of main pancreatic duct with multiple tiny ductal calculi in a case of chronic calcific pancreatitis.

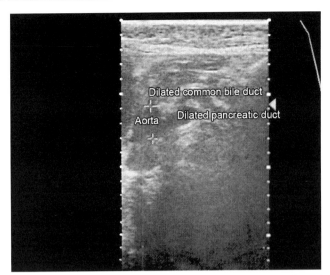

Fig. 11.8: Transverse scan of pancreas shows dilated pancreatic duct and terminal end of dilated common bile duct (CBD). This was a case of periampullary carcinoma.

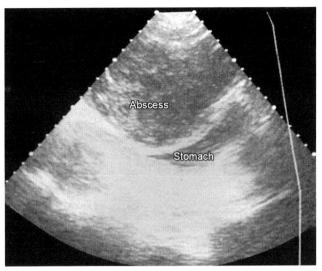

Fig. 11.10: Transverse and longitudinal scans of epigastrium show a large, well-defined rounded SOL with internal contents and posterior enhancement in the lesser sac region. The differential diagnosis was abscess and nonfunctioning pancreatic tumor. FNAC confirmed the latter.

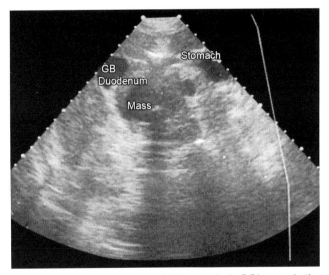

Fig. 11.9: A well defined rounded hypoechoic SOL seen in the region of head of pancreas. Fine needle aspiration cytology (FNAC) revealed it to be a well-differentiated adenocarcinoma.

Direct signs	Indirect signs
1. Mass lesion	1. Dilated pancreatic duct
	2. Bile duct dilatation
	3. Pancreatitis
	4. Atrophy

A poorly defined, homogeneous or inhomogeneous, solid hypoechoic mass is seen inside the pancreas. This may be associated with expansion of the pancreas. Rarely necrosis is seen as a cystic area with in the mass. The mass usually measures 2 cm at the time of diagnosis and has lobulated contours. Pancreatic duct dilatation appears as tortuous hypoechoic channel with nonparallel walls and ending abruptly. The lesions of the head of pancreas also obstruct the distal CBD causing bile duct dilatation up to the site of obstruction which is seen as an abrupt termination of the dilated system. This double-duct sign (dilated pancreatic and bile duct) usually indicates the presence of pancreatic adenocarcinoma. Features of pancreatitis or atrophy may be present proximal to the mass. In atrophy disproportionate size of the head with respect to body and tail gives a clue to the presence of a mass. US also helps in assessing the tumor resectability to avoid unnecessary surgery. Extension of the carcinoma beyond the pancreatic parenchyma-involvement of retroperitoneal fat, adjacent organs, lymphadenopathy, liver metastasis and venous invasion precludes the feasibility of surgery.

Main differential diagnoses of adenocarcinoma are focal pancreatitis, peripancreatic lymphadenopathy and ampullary adenocarcinoma. Echogenic septa are recognized between the lymph nodes and absence of jaundice with a large pancreatic head mass close to distal CBD favors lymphadenopathy. Periampullary adenocarcinomas are differentiated from carcinoma head of pancreas more accurately by endoscopic ultrasound.

Cystic Neoplasms

These represent 10–15% of all pancreatic cysts. These present in middle and old age with vague abdominal symptoms, weight loss, abdominal mass or jaundice. Microcystic adenomas are relatively well-defined on sonography with external lobulations. The mass is echogenic solid appearing, or solid with cystic areas or a multicystic. A central stellate shaped echogenic area with or without calcification is present and represents the scar within the lesion.

Macrocystic neoplasms—on US appear as well-circumscribed smooth surfaced thin-or thick-walled, unilocular or multilocular cystic lesions of variable sizes, usually more than 2 cm in diameter and less than six in number. These also vary from clear cysts to solid-looking cysts.

Islet Cell Tumors

Islet cell neoplasms are equally distributed throughout the gland and are of two types: functioning and nonfunctioning or silent tumors.

Functioning Tumors

Due to the small size of functioning tumors at the time of presentation, they are difficult to detect on ultrasound, except endoscopic ultrasound, where they appear as well-defined hypoechoic lesions without central necrosis or calcification.

Beta-cell tumor/Insulinomas are functioning tumors, usually benign more commonly found in the body and tail and present with hypoglycemic symptoms.

G-cell tumors (gastrinomas) are potentially malignant tumors presenting around 50 years of age with diarrhea and peptic ulcer disease.

Other rare functioning tumors are glucagonomas, VIPoma, somatostatinoma and carcinoid.

Nonfunctioning Islet-cell Tumors

These are large tumors arising in the head region of pancreas with a high incidence of malignancy. Nonfunctioning tumors are usually detected as large, echogenic masses with multifocal calcification or necrosis.

12
CHAPTER

Abdomen: Gastrointestinal Tract

Normal gut has a reproducible pattern or "gut signature", and a variety of gut pathologies create recognizable sonographic abnormalities. On sonography the gut signature varies from a bull's eye appearance in cross-section (an echogenic center with a hypoechoic rim) to full depiction of five sonographic layers. With 5.0 MHz probes the sonographic layers are alternately echogenic and hypoechoic; the first, third and fifth are echogenic and the second and fourth are hypoechoic **(Figs. 12.1 to 12.5)**.

Gut Wall Pathology

Gut wall pathologies creates a characteristic sonographic pattern **(Figs. 12.6A and B)**. The most familiar is a "target" pattern, symmetric if the echogenic mucosa is centrally placed or asymmetric if present on one side of the hypoechoic gut wall. The "pseudokidney" **(Fig. 12.7)** pattern is also specific for gut wall pathologies. The thickened gut wall corresponds to the hypoechoic external rim while the residual gut lumen or mucosal ulceration appears as the echogenic center. Gut wall masses are distinct from the thickened gut wall, and may be intraluminal, mural or exophytic. Intraluminal masses are frequently obscured by gut gas or luminal contents. The exophytic masses are more

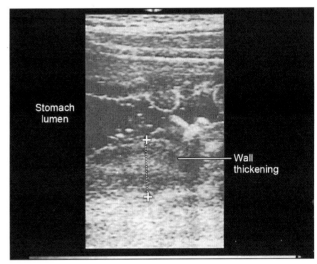

Fig. 12.2: Anterior and posterior wall of stomach irregularly thickened in a case of linitis plastica.

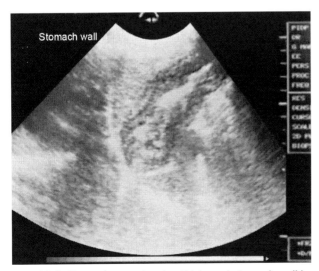

Fig. 12.1: Coronal scan showing thickened stomach wall in the region of the fundus in a case of carcinoma stomach.

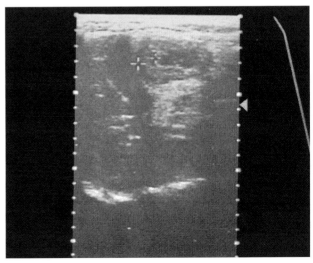

Fig. 12.3: Duodenal wall appears thickened.

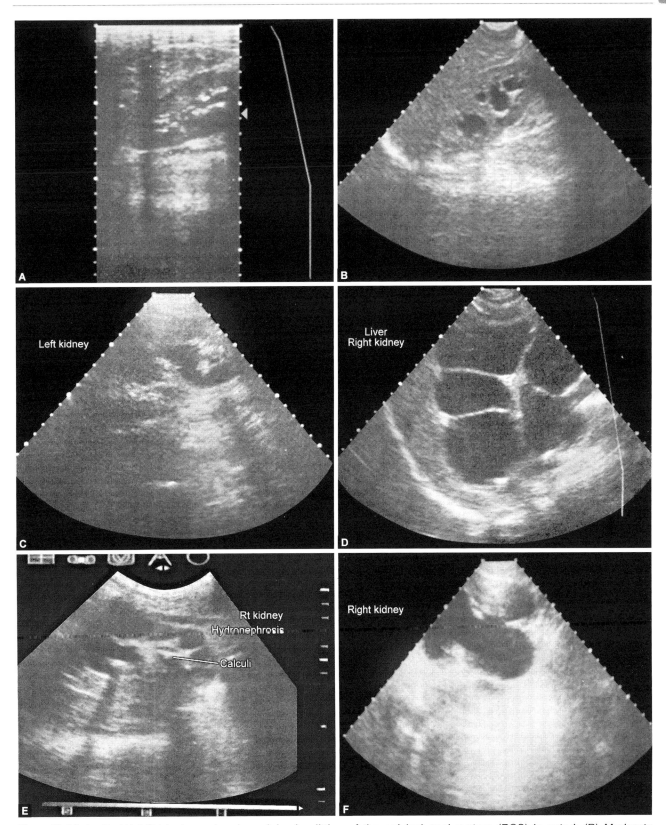

Figs. 13.6A to F: (A) Mild hydronephrosis—minimal splitting of the pelvicalyceal system (PCS) is noted; (B) Moderate hydronephrosis; (C) Moderate hydronephrosis—left kidney with dilated upper ureter; (D) Grossly enlarged hydronephrotic kidney with no perceptible parenchyma; (E) Longitudinal scan of right kidney showing gross dilatation of PCS with thinned out parenchymal tissue. Two echogenic foci with acoustic shadowing are seen in the dilated upper calyx and pelvis; (F) micky mouse appearance of pelvicalyceal system in a case of severe hydronephrosis.

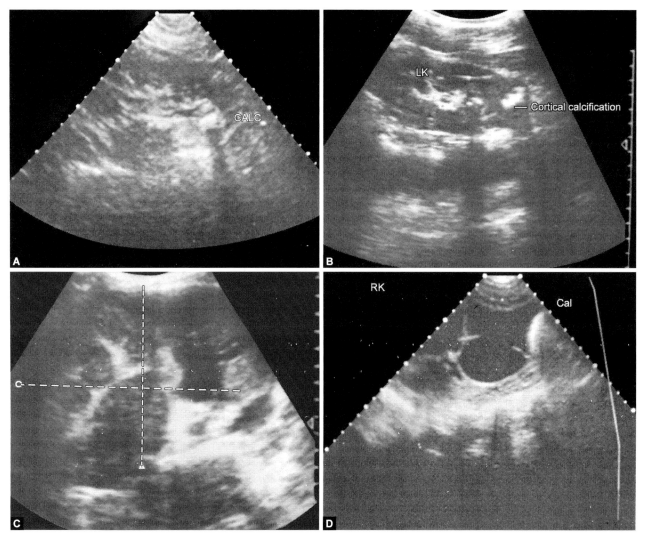

Figs. 13.7A to D: (A) Renal calculus—an echogenic foci with distal acoustic shadowing in lower calyx; (B) Dense echogenic focus with distal acoustic shadowing is seen in the renal cortex suggestive of old tubercular involvement. A calculus is also seen in lower pole; (C) A large SOL in lower pole of kidney showing heterogeneous echogenicity. Pelvicalyceal system appears hydronephrotic; (D) A grossly hydronephrotic kidney with large echogenic focus with acoustic shadow lying in pelvis.

junction are associated with mucosal edema at the trigone. US evaluation of ureteral orifices for jets is helpful to assess for obstruction.

Complication of calculus disease—infection (pyonephrosis, perinephric abscess) and rupture of a calyx or pelvis to produce a urinoma.

Urinoma **(Fig. 13.8)**: In an acutely obstructed urinary tract the high pressure generated proximal to the block leads to rupture of the most vulnerable part of the drainage system with subsequent extravasation of urine into the surrounding fat planes. This appears on US as anechoic collection usually.

- *Nephrocalcinosis (Fig. 13.9)*: Renal parenchymal calcification or nephrocalcinosis can occur in diseased or normal kidney. Calcification can occur in tumors, abscesses or hematomas and is called dystrophic calcification. Metastatic calcification occurs in hypercalcemic states like hyperparathyroidism, RTA and renal failure. Calcium deposition may be present in the cortex or the medulla. Cortical involvement occurs in acute cortical necrosis, chronic glomerulonephritis, and rejected transplants. Medullary nephrocalcinosis occurs in hyperparathyroidism, renal tubular acidosis, medullary sponge kidney, chronic pyelonephritis, papillary necrosis, and vitamin D excess, etc. On US cortical nephrocalcinosis is seen as increased cortical echogenicity which may produce acoustic shadowing. Medullary nephrocalcinosis appears as increased echogenicity (more than cortex) with or without shadowing.
- *Infections*
  - *Pyelonephritis (Fig. 13.10)*: Most cases (85%) of acute pyelonephritis are due to ascending

infection. Women are most commonly affected and present with flank pain, fever with evidence of bacteriuria or pyuria and raised total leukocyte count. On sonography, majority of the affected kidney appear normal. The following findings may be present—renal enlargement, compressed renal sinus, hypoechoic parenchyma with loss of corticomedullary differentiation; poorly marginated masses in the parenchyma or gas within the renal parenchyma.

- *Renal and perinephric abscess (Figs. 13.11A to H):* Untreated or inadequately treated acute pyelonephritis may progress to renal abscess which may decompress into the collecting system or perinephric space. Perinephric abscess may also occur from ruptured pyonephrosis, direct extension from peritoneal or retroperitoneal infections or following percutaneous procedures. On US, renal abscess appears as a solitary round, thick-walled hypoechoic complex mass often with evidence of posterior enhancement and internal mobile debris. Septations may be present. Air seen as echogenic specks with distal dirty shadowing may be present within the lesion. Perinephric abscess has a similar appearance but lie outside the renal capsule.

- *Pyonephrosis (Fig. 13.12):* An infected hydronephrotic pelvicalyceal system is termed pyonephrosis. On US, hydronephrosis with or without dilated

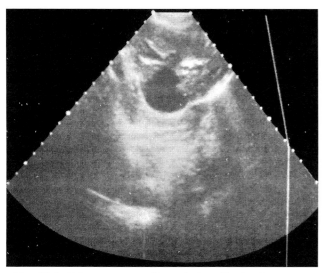

Fig. 13.8: Urinoma—a small anechoic collection is seen to communicate with pelvicalyceal system of right kidney.

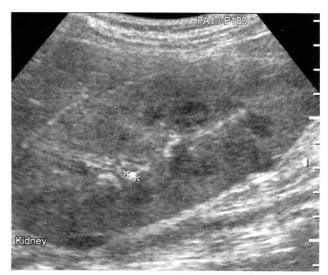

Fig. 13.10: Shows enlarged kidney with altered corticomedullary differentiation (CMD) and compressed renal sinus echoes suggestive of acute pyelonephritis.

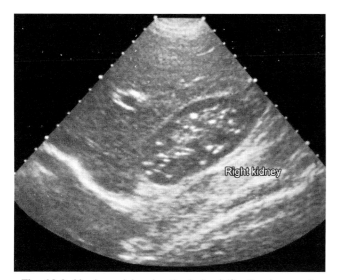

Fig. 13.9: Nephrocalcinosis-stippled calcification is seen in the region of the renal pyramid.

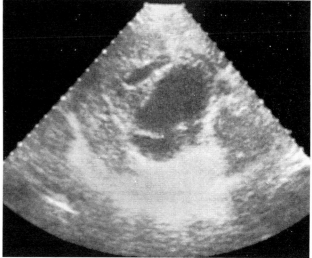

Fig. 13.11A: An anechoic collection with septae in it seen at the posterolateral aspect of right kidney. USG guided aspiration revealed it to be Abscess.

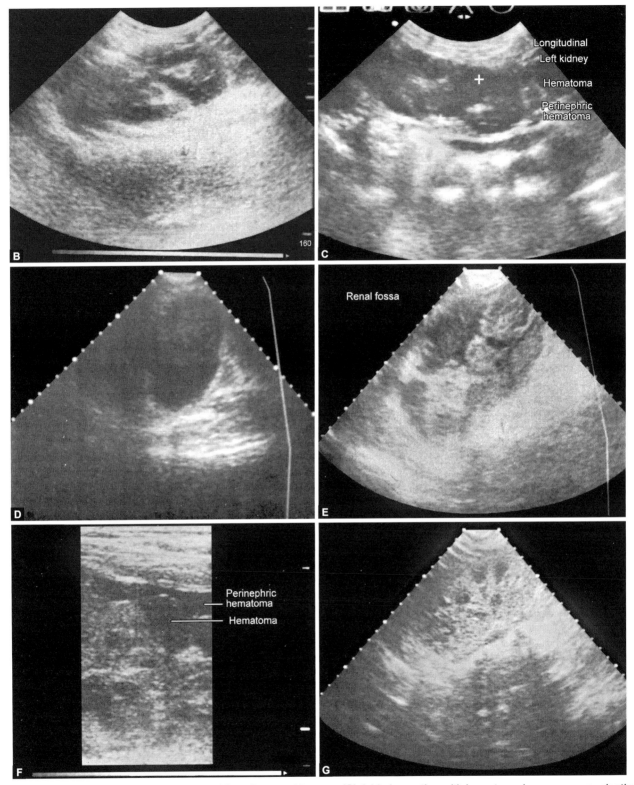

Figs. 13.11B to G: (B) Laceration in the middle pole—renal trauma; (C) A big laceration with hematoma is seen communicating with PCS at the junction of upper 2/3rd and lower 3rd of the left kidney. A small perinephric hematoma is also seen at its' lower pole; (D) Anechoic collection is seen in the perinephric region in the case of renal trauma; (E) An echogenic perinephric collection is seen surrounding the right kidney. There are areas of hyperechogenicity suggestive of organizing hematoma; (F) Hematoma is seen as a well-defined hypoechoic areas is seen in cortex. Perinephric hematoma is also present; (G) Abscess—a round hypoechoic SOL is seen in the region of upper pole of left kidney. The kidney also shows increased cortical echotexture with accentuated corticomedullary differentiation.

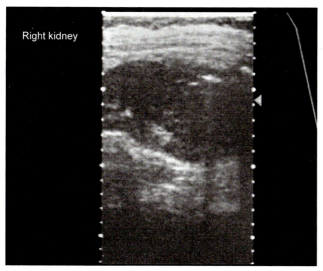

Fig. 13.11H: Renal abscess—a well-defined fluid filled mass containing low intensity echoes seen in right kidney. An echogenic focus with reverberating artifact is seen suggestive of gas.

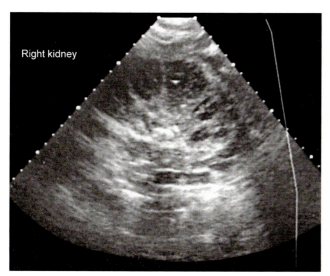

Fig. 13.12: Pyonephrosis—stone is seen in renal pelvis with polvicalyceal hydronephrosis with evidence of debris and air inside it.

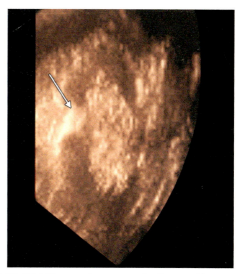

Fig. 13.13: 3D US scan shows a cortical scar with parenchymal atrophy (white arrow), a feature of chronic pyelonephritis.

ureter may be seen. Mobile collecting system debris, with or without a fluid debris level, collecting system gas and stones may be seen.

- *Emphysematous pyelonephritis:* An uncommon but life-threatening infection of renal parenchyma by gas forming organism usually affects diabetic women. At presentation most patients are extremely ill with fever, flank pain, hyperglycemia, acidosis, and electrolyte imbalance. On US presence of gas in the parenchyma, collecting system or perinephric renal collections appears as echogenic foci with distal dirty acoustic shadowing.
- *Chronic—Pyelonephritis* **(Fig. 13.13)***:* Chronic or recurrent episodes of vesicoureteric reflux occurring more commonly in childhood and in women leads to a nephropathy. Renal changes are unilateral or bilateral but asymmetric. The upper polar region is most commonly affected. On sonography, a dilated blunt calyx is seen associated with an overlying cortical scar or cortical atrophy. If the disease is unilateral, there may be compensatory hypertrophy of the contralateral kidney. If the disease is multicentric, hypertrophy of normal intervening parenchyma may create island of normal tissue simulating a tumor.
- *Xanthogranulomatous:* Pyelonephritis this is an inflammatory pathology of the kidney, usually seen in diabetics, where in, there is calculus disease associated with superadded bacterial infection usually due to *E. coli*. There is destruction of the parenchyma and replacement of it with lipid-laden macrophages. Patient presents with pain, mass, weight loss, and UTI. On US, diffuse variety shows an enlarged, normal shaped kidney with loss of corticomedullary differentiation. A dilated pelvicalyceal system is present with large echogenic focus with distal acoustic shadowing suggestive of a staghorn calculus. Multiple hypoechoic areas may be present in the parenchyma. Focal involvement is difficult to differentiate from tumor or abscess.
- *Papillary necrosis:* Many causes lead to ischemia and thus development of papillary necrosis and these are analgesic abuse, diabetes, urinary tract infection, obstructive uropathy, prolonged hypotension, sickle cell anemia, etc; US appearances vary with the stage of the disease. Swollen papillae appear as enlarged pyramids. With papillary cavitation, cystic collections within the medullary pyramids are seen. On sloughing of the papilla a clubbed calyx is present. The sloughed papilla can be seen in the

collecting system as an echogenic nonshadowing structure. On calcification it imparts a shadowing as well and then simulates a calculus. On passing into a ureter obstruction may be caused with resultant hydronephrosis.

- *Tuberculosis* **(Figs. 13.14A and B)**: Urinary tract tuberculosis occurs with hematogenous seeding of the kidney by *Mycobacterium tuberculosis* from as extraurinary source. Patients present with lower urinary tract signs and symptoms like frequency, dysuria, urgency, and hematuria (gross or microscopic). Though both kidney are infected. Clinical manifestations are usually unilateral. On US, early findings are small focal lesions which are echogenic or hypoechoic with an echogenic rim. Larger lesions are of mixed echogenicity with poorly defined borders. Later, the tubercles may emerge with evidence of cavitation and communication with the collecting system. It is now that US findings resemble those of papillary necrosis. Spread of infection to the ureters may cause spasm and edema in the VUJ giving rise to hydronephrosis and hydro-ureter. Chronic changes of tuberculosis include fibrosis and calcification. On US, focal caliectasis with evidence of an echogenic focus with distal acoustic shadowing is present. Cavitation, collecting system dilatation with parenchymal atrophy or perinephric abscess may also be seen. In cases of autonephrectomy a small calcified kidney is present.
- *Fungal infection—Candida albicans:* Patients with chronic debilitating illnesses or immunosuppression are at increased risk of developing fungal infections most commonly *Candida albicans*. On US parenchymal involvement appears as small hypoechoic parenchymal masses while fungal balls appear as nonshadowing mobile echogenic soft tissue mass without evidence of shadowing. These fungal balls may cause obstruction and thus hydronephrosis.
- *Parasitic:* Hydatid disease **(Figs. 13.15A and B)** 2–5% of patients with hydatid disease have renal involvement. Renal hydatid disease is solitary involving renal poles and cause symptoms only when large enough to cause pressure symptoms or get ruptured. On US, an anechoic cyst is present which may have a perceptible wall. Mural nodularity, multiloculated appearance suggests scolices and daughter cysts respectively. The membrane from the endocyst may detach and form hydatid sand. Calcification of the wall may be present in chronic cases.

RENAL TUMORS

Benign Tumors

Angiomyolipoma (AML)

Angiomyolipomas (AML) are benign renal tumors consisting of blood vessels, muscle tissue, and fat. These are usually unilateral and are found in middle-aged females or occur sporadically in patients of tuberous sclerosis. Classically, AML is hyperechoic due to predominance of fat. Other components impart a hypoechoic or isoechoic appearance. The tumor may be within the parenchyma or exophytic. Sometimes these tumors may bleed into soft tissues resulting in formation of extrarenal hematomas.

Multilocular Cystic Nephroma (Fig. 13.16)

This tumor is found in children below four years or later more commonly in females. On sonography, it appears as a localized, rounded multiloculated mass with anechoic appearance and thick septa.

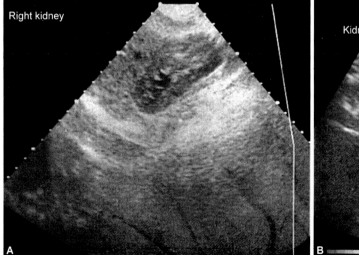
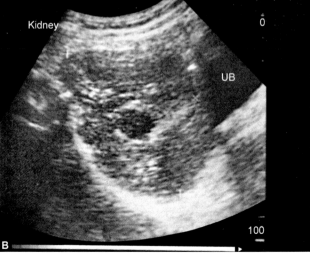

Figs. 13.14A and B: (A) Focal caliectasis seen in upper pole of right kidney, old case of TB kidney; (B) Pancake kidney—both the kidneys are completely fused and lie in the pelvis posterior to the urinary bladder.

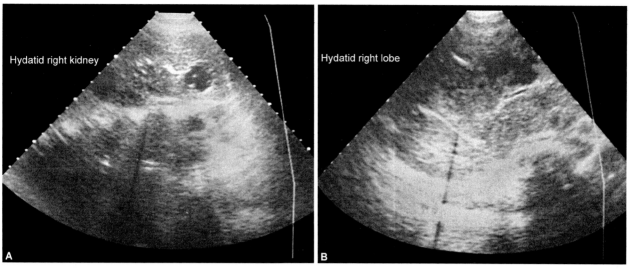

Figs. 13.15A and B: (A) Right kidney shows the presence of hydatid cyst with 3 daughter cysts inside it; (B) Hydatid cyst was also present in the right lobe of liver.

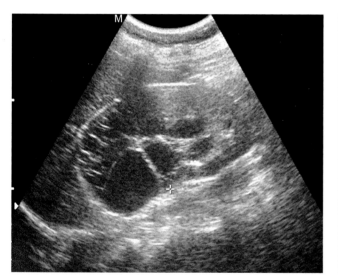

Fig. 13.16: A multilocular nephroma involving the superior and midpolar region of kidney.

Fig. 13.17: A large anechoic cyst is seen occupying the lower and middle pole of right kidney with a mural nodule inside it—renal cell carcinoma.

Oncocytomas

These occur most commonly in men with a peak incidence in sixth and seventh decades. These are solid tumors with a central stellate scar. On sonography, oncocytomas are variable in appearance and may be isoechoic, hypoechoic or hyperechoic, with a homogeneous or heterogeneous echotexture and a well or poorly defined wall. A central scar, central necrosis or calcification may be seen. These tumors can be confused with renal cell carcinoma.

Malignant Renal Tumors

Renal Cell Carcinoma (RCC) (Figs. 13.17 and 13.18)

Renal cell carcinoma (RCC) accounts for 85% of primary malignant renal parenchymal tumors. It occurs more commonly in males between 50–70 years. Presentation is with flank pain, gross hematuria, weight loss and palpable renal mass. Manifestation, secondary to hormone production may also occur like raised RBC count, hypercalcemia, galactorrhea, hypertension or gynecomastia. On sonography, most tumors are solid benign isoechoic (85%), hypoechoic (10%) or echogenic (5%). Tumors which are less than 3 cm appear echogenic than renal parenchyma, but the presence of cystic areas and hypoechoic rim differentiates them from angiomyolipomas. Calcification when present is seen as a hyperechoic focus with distal acoustic shadowing. Less common variety of cystic carcinomas appear as multiloculated cystic mass with internal septations more than 2 mm thick, unilocular debris-filled cystic mass with thick, irregular walls which may be calcified, or as a simple cyst with a mural nodule. On sonography involvement of the perirenal tissue, regional lymph nodes, liver metastasis and renal vein involvement is also looked for.

Transitional Cell Carcinoma (TCC) (Figs. 13.19A and B)

Transitional cell carcinoma (TCC) of the renal pelvis accounts for 7% of all primary renal tumors. They are four times more common in men and the mean age at diagnosis is 65 years. The most common presentation is with hematuria (gross or microscopic), only a few present with pain in the flank. The sonographic appearance may be of a hypoechoic lesion placed centrally in the renal sinus causing loss of the normal central sinus echogenicity. Proximal pelvicaliectasis may be associated. TCC should be differentiated from blood clots which may have a similar appearance but, however, are likely to shift with change in position with movement. The tumor may grow in a diffusely infiltrative pattern causing distortion of the renal architecture with enlargement but maintenance of the reniform shape. Flat tumors are not seen on sonography, although the associated pelvicaliectasis may be visualized. Transitional cell carcinoma may demonstrate calcification creating difficulty in differentiation of tumor from stones or sloughed calcified papilla.

Squamous Cell Carcinoma (SCC)

Squamous cell carcinoma (SCC) represents 6–15% of renal pelvic tumors. Distant metastases are usually present at the time of diagnosis. On sonography renal SCC is seen as a diffusely enlarged kidney with maintenance of its reniform shape. The normal renal echotexture is destroyed and often a stone is present. It is not possible to differentiate it from xanthogranulomatous pyelonephritis.

Adenocarcinoma (Fig. 13.20)

Almost all the patients with adenocarcinoma kidney have urinary tract infection and two-third will have a stone usually a staghorn. Presentation is with hematuria. On sonography, renal pelvic mass is present occasionally with evidence of calcification. Associated stone and hydronephrosis is evident.

Secondary Renal Tumors (Figs. 13.21A and B)

The kidneys may be unilaterally or bilaterally involved by hematogenous spread or by direct extension from contiguous retroperitoneal nodes. On sonography, the

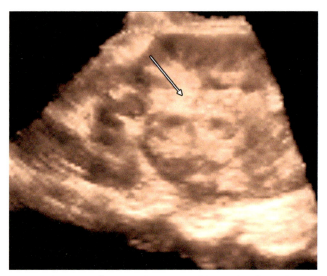

Fig. 13.18: 3D US scan shows a solid renal cell carcinoma (white arrow) arising from the inferior and midpolar region of kidney.

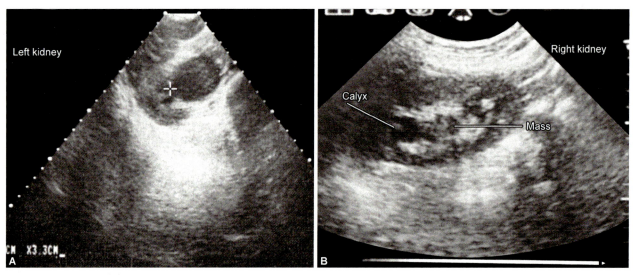

Figs. 13.19A and B: (A) Transitional cell carcinoma—a hypoechoic lesion is seen to occupy the whole of pelvis of right kidney; (B) Transitional cell carcinoma—a hypoechoic mass is seen splitting the central sinus echo-complex and causing focal caliectasis of the upper pole of right kidney.

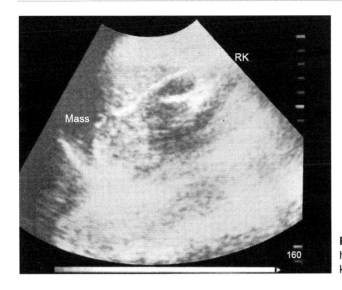

Fig. 13.20: Adenocarcinoma—a SOL of predominantly hyperechoic echotexture is seen to arise from upper pole of right kidney and bulging the cortex.

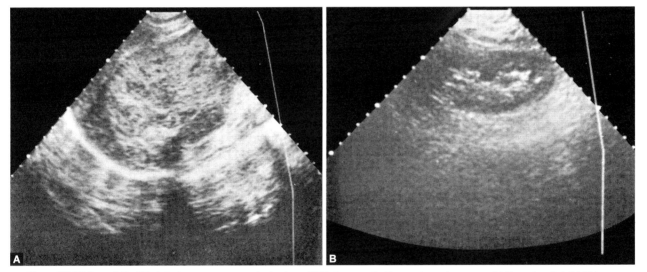

Figs. 13.21A and B: (A) A heterogeneous echotexture SOL is seen in the region of upper middle pole of right kidney; (B) Pseudotumor—the pelvicalyceal system is indented by a mass isoechoic to the cortex-hypertrophied column of Bertin.

involved kidney may appear large with a thickened, hypoechoic parenchyma. Occasionally there may be single or multiple discrete focal hypoechoic lesions. Direct invasion of the kidney by large retroperitoneal lymph node masses may occur with associated vascular and ureteral encasement. Large retroperitoneal hypoechoic lymph node masses will be seen extending into the kidney causing hydronephrosis. Rarely, perirenal involvement is seen as a surrounding hypoechoic perirenal mass.

Leukemia and Lymphoma (Fig. 13.22)

The kidneys are involved bilaterally. Sonographically, the diffuse variety caused massive increase in size with loss of corticomedullary distinction and distortion of the sinus echoes. The echogenicity of the cortex may be coarsened or decreased. Occasionally focal or multifocal renal masses with low level echoes may also be seen. Renal, subcapsular or perinephric hemorrhage may be present.

Secondary Deposits

These may be single or multiple and indistinguishable from a primary renal tumor. Diffuse, focal or multifocal involvement may be seen.

RENAL CYSTIC DISEASE

Cortical Cysts

Simple Cortical Cysts (Fig. 13.23)

This acquired benign lesion is found in 50% of people over the age of 50 years. Most are asymptomatic however, if large or infected, hematuria may occur. On sonography, a

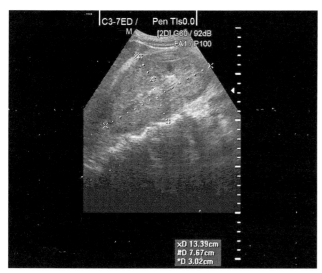

Fig. 13.22: Enlarged, echogenic kidney with loss of corticomedullary differentiation (CMD) and compressed renal sinus echoes in a case diffuse renal involvement by leukemia.

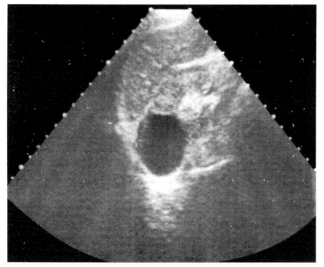

Fig. 13.23: Simple cortical cyst—a well defined anechoic SOL with posterior acoustic enhancement seen in upper pole of right kidney.

sharply defined, anechoic, rounded lesion with evidence of posterior acoustic enhancement is seen in the cortex of one or both kidneys. These have an imperceptible wall and are seen to bulge the renal outline if big enough to do so.

Complex Cortical Cysts (Fig. 13.24)

Cysts which do not meet the criteria of simple cyst are called complex cysts. On sonography these include cysts containing internal echoes, septations, calcification, perceptible defined thick wall and mural nodularity. These cysts require further evaluation by CT, US guided-aspiration and cytological analysis.

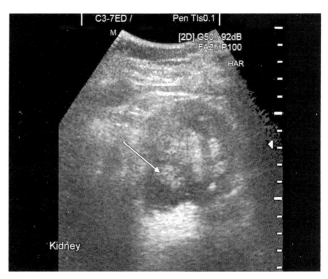

Fig. 13.24: A cortical renal cyst with internal clot (white arrow).

Parapelvic Cysts

These are lymphatic in origin and do not communicate with the collecting system. These are usually asymptomatic until they get infected or cause obstruction to the outflow tract. On sonography, these appear as well-defined anechoic renal sinus masses and can be confused with hydronephrosis.

Medullary Cysts

Medullary Sponge Kidney

This characterizes dilated, ectatic collecting tubules and there may be focal or diffuse involvement of the kidney. It usually occurs in third and fourth decades and is found in 12% of patients with renal stones. Uncomplicated disease is asymptomatic, however, with stone formation renal colic, hematuria and flank pain may occur. On sonography the condition is detected if nephrocalcinosis is present. Multiple, echogenic shadowing foci localized to the medullary pyramids are evident.

Medullary Cystic Disease

The adult form is an autosomal dominant form. Sonography demonstrates small echogenic kidneys with medullary cysts.

Polycystic Kidney Disease (Fig. 13.25)

Autosomal Dominant Form (ADPCK)

In this disorder there are multiple variable sized cortical and medullary cysts in both the kidneys. Patients become symptomatic in their fourth decade with palpable mass, pain, hypertension, hematuria or urinary tract infection. Renal failure develops in 50% of patients and is usually present by 60 years of age. Complications like infection, hemorrhage, stone formation and rupture and obstruction

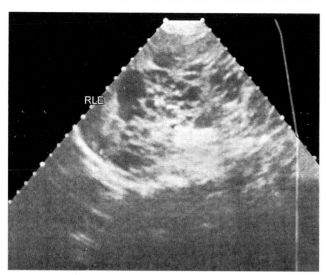

Fig. 13.25: Adult polycystic kidney disease (APKD)—a classical case of APKD showing innumerable cyst with complete architectural distortion of the right kidney. The kidney is also enlarged.

may occur. Associated anomalies include liver cysts, pancreatic and splenic cysts, cerebral artery or aortic aneurysms, cardiac disease and colonic diverticula. On sonography, the kidneys are enlarged with multiple bilateral asymmetric cysts of variable sizes. These do not communicate with each other. Complicated infected or hemorrhagic cysts show thick wall, internal echoes or septa or fluid-debris level. Echogenic foci with distal shadowing may be due to stones or calcification in the wall.

Multicystic Dysplastic Kidney

This developmental anomaly occurs due to urinary tract obstruction during embryogenesis. There is no function or very little renal function left. The disease is usually unilateral and occasionally may be bilateral or focal. Ultrasound findings range from a large multicystic mass present at birth to a kidney with smaller cysts not discovered until adulthood, depending upon the severity of malformation. In adults the cystic renal fossa mass is not large and cyst wall calcification is present. Multiple noncommunicating cysts with absence of normal renal parenchyma and renal sinus is seen.

Acquired Renal Cystic Disease

Renal cysts form in the kidneys of patients with renal failure undergoing dialysis. Ultrasound shows multiple small cysts (0.5 cm–3 cm) involving both cortex and the medulla. Three to five cysts in each kidney in a patient with chronic renal failure are diagnostic. Kidneys also appear small and quite echogenic.

von Hippel-Lindau Disease

This autosomal dominant disease is characterized by retinal angiomatosis, CNS hemangioblastomas, pheochromocytomas and renal cell carcinoma. In addition to this 76% patients show evidence of renal cysts which are mostly cortical in location.

Vascular

Renal Arterial Occlusion and Infarction

Renal artery occlusion may occur due to embolus or thrombosis. Whole kidney is affected if the main renal artery is occluded, whereas segmental and focal infarction may occur with peripherally located vascular occlusions. On sonography, acute complete renal arterial occlusion may demonstrate a normal kidney. Segmental or focal infarction appears as a hypoechoic, wedge shaped mass indistinguishable from acute pyelonephritis. Chronic occlusions causes an end-stage, small, and scarred kidney.

Renal Artery Stenosis

Renal artery stenosis commonly due to atherosclerosis or occasionally due to fibromuscular dysplasia is a cause of secondary hypertension. This disorder may affect one or both kidneys. On sonography the involved kidney is small in size with a smooth outline. Cortical thickness is uniformly reduced and the pelvicalyceal system is not dilated. The evaluation of site and extent of stenosis in the renal artery needs Doppler ultrasound.

Renal Vein Occlusion

Renal vein occlusion occurs due to invasion of the renal vein by tumors (Wilm's or renal cell carcinoma), dehydration, hypercoagulable status, pancreatitis or trauma, etc. Symptoms are present with acute onset disease-flank pain and hematuria. On ultrasound, in early stages the kidney is large with a thick hypoechoic cortex with lost corticomedullary differentiation. The pelvicalyceal system is normal and the vein appears to be distended with presence of internal echoes. In the later stages, recanalisation and collateral formation may revert the sonographic appearance to normal.

RENAL MEDICAL DISORDERS

On sonography these disorders cause a diffuse increase in cortical echogenicity with or without loss of normal corticomedullary distinction. In type 1 disease the corticomedullary distinction is preserved while it is lost in type 2 disease.

Acute Tubular Necrosis

This is the most common cause of acute reversible renal failure and occurs due to presence of cellular debris within the renal collecting tubules. Factors such as hypotension, dehydration, drugs, heavy metal, etc. may cause ischemic or toxic insult to the tubular epithelium. On sonography bilaterally enlarged, echogenic kidneys are seen except in cases of hypotension where normal renal scan is the usual finding.

Acute Cortical Necrosis

Ischemic necrosis of the cortex results in irreversible renal failure. This occurs in association with sepsis, burns, severe dehydration, snake bite and pregnancy complicated by placental abruption. On sonography the renal cortex appears hypoechoic initially which later demonstrates calcification.

Glomerulonephritis

- Acute glomerulonephritis affects the glomerulus with proliferative and necrotizing abnormalities. Patients present with hematuria, hypertension and azotemia. On sonography, bilateral involvement is present. Kidney size ranges from normal to large. The cortex is normal, hypoechoic or hyperechoic in appearance with a normal medullary pattern.
- Chronic glomerulonephritis appears as bilateral small, kidneys with global loss of parenchyma, smooth outline and normal pelvicalyceal system. The kidneys appear echogenic.

Diabetes Mellitus

This is the most common cause of chronic renal failure. On sonography findings vary according to the stage of the nephropathy. In the early stages kidneys are enlarged and, with time reduction in size and increase in cortical echogenicity with preserved corticomedullary differentiation are noted. With end stage disease, the kidneys are smaller and more echogenic with lost corticomedullary distinction.

Amyloidosis

Amyloidosis may be primary or secondary and is usually a systemic disease. Patients present with renal failure. Primary amyloidosis occurs in men, around 60 years of age. While secondary amyloidosis is present in cases of multiple myeloma, rheumatoid arthritis, tuberculosis, Hodgkin's disease, etc. On sonography, in acute stage the kidneys may be symmetrically enlarged. With disease progression, the kidneys shrink in size and demonstrate cortical atrophy with increased cortical echogenicity. Focal renal masses, a central pelvic mass or amorphous calcification may be present.

Sonography of the Ureters (Figs. 13.26 to 13.30)

The ureters are usually not well seen in the normal state. When dilated they are visualized over a variable length as an anechoic tube with echogenic walls arising from the pelvis of the kidney. They are, however, difficult to be seen in their middle third due to bowel gas shadows. Dilatation of the ureters should lead to a search for a cause. The most common cause of hydroureter is a ureteric calculus seen as an echogenic focus with distal acoustic shadowing at the lower end of a dilated ureter. Other causes are clots,

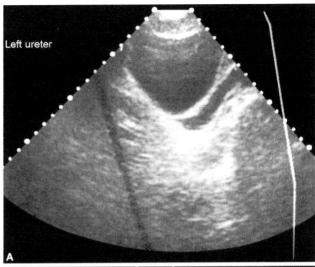
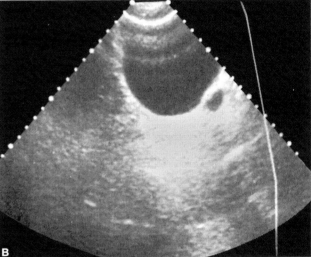

Figs. 13.26A and B: Transverse and longitudinal scans of a grossly dilated lower ureter.

tumor, and fungal balls seen as nonshadowing echoes in the dilated ureter. The tumors are nonmobile while clots and fungus balls may demonstrate mobility. Other causes like nodes, pregnancy, retroperitoneal fibrosis or bladder causes (mass lesions), spread of pelvic malignancy, etc. may be found. Bilateral dilated ureters are present in cases of bilateral reflux, or obstructive bladder or urethral lesions. Congenital abnormalities like double, retrocaval ureters are difficult to see. Obstruction of the upper moiety of a duplex collecting system due to a ureterocele appears as rounded, cyst-like mass in the bladder with a dilated ureter and dilated pelvicalyceal system of the upper moiety.

Urinary Bladder

Congenital Anomalies

Among the various congenital anomalies, urachal anomaly and bladder diverticulum are most likely to be diagnosed by ultrasound.

CHAPTER 13: Abdomen: The Urinary Tract

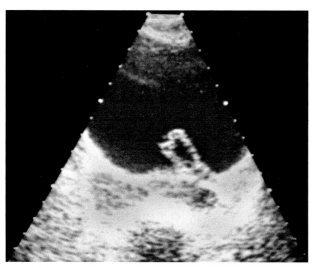

Fig. 13.27: Ureterocele—transverse scan of urinary bladder shows a cystic structure at the left UV junction.

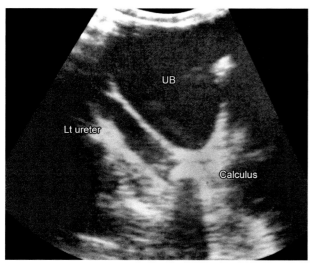

Fig. 13.28: An echogenic structure with distal acoustic shadowing seen in left lower ureter.

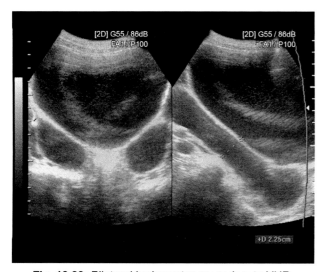

Fig. 13.29: Bilateral hydroureter secondary to VUR.

- Urachal Anomalies—the urachal anomaly could be a diverticulum or a cyst. A diverticulum is a tubular structure which is seen in the midline extending from the anterosuperior aspect of the bladder, towards the umbilicus. Its wall has the same appearance and thickness as those of the bladder. The lumen may appear anechoic if fluid filled.

  A urachal cyst is also a midline structure between the umbilicus and the anterosuperior surface of the bladder dome. It appears as an ovoid or rounded well defined, thin walled anechoic structure on ultrasound. When infected it changes in appearance to a thick walled structure with internal echoes with fluid-debris level.

- Bladder Diverticulum (**Fig. 13.31**) Congenital bladder diverticulum is rare as compared to the acquired variety. On ultrasound they appear as thimble shaped fluid containing structures with thin walls, protruding into the perivesical space. They communicate with the bladder through a wide or narrow orifice. A calculus within it is seen as an echogenic focus with shadowing and infection or hemorrhage suggested by presence of internal echoes or fluid-debris level.

- Duplication of bladder

  This is of three types:
  1. Type I—complete duplication with two separate bladders
  2. Type II—An internal complete or incomplete septum oriented in a sagittal or coronal plane.
  3. Type III—A transverse band dividing the bladder into two unequal cavities.

Exstrophy

In bladder exstrophy, ultrasound assesses the upper urinary tract for associated anomalies or features of obstruction.

Inflammatory Pathology of Urinary Bladder

Infectious Cystitis (Fig. 13.32)

This disease presents with bladder irritability and hematuria predominantly in women. In males it is associated with bladder outlet obstruction. *E. coli* is the most common offending organism. On ultrasound, it appears as diffuse bladder wall thickening and decreased bladder capacity. If changes are focal, pseudopolyps are difficult to differentiate from tumor.

Malakoplakia

This is a rare granulomatous infection seen more commonly in women in their 6th decade. It is seen in immunocompromised patients, or diabetics. Presentation is bladder irritability and hematuria. On sonography, single or multiple mucosal-based masses are seen commonly at the bladder base.

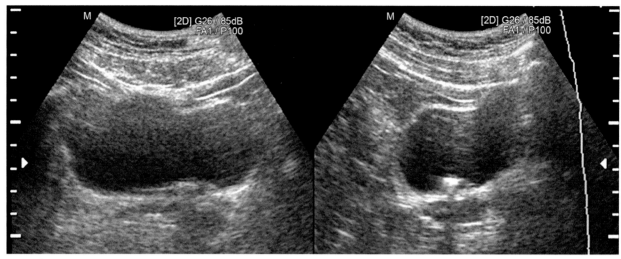

Fig. 13.30: A calculus at right vesicoureteric junction.

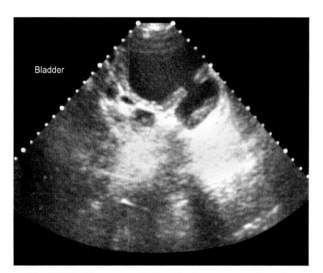

Fig. 13.31: Narrow neck diverticulum as seen from the posterior wall of urinary bladder with evidence of debris inside.

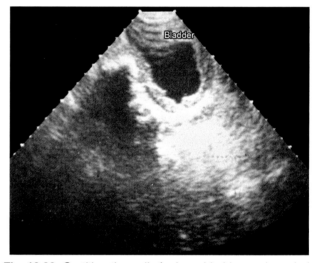

Fig. 13.32: Cystitis—the wall of urinary bladder are irregularly thickened.

Emphysematous Cystitis

This condition is seen in patients with diabetes and *E. coli* is a most common pathogen. Occasionally pneumaturia occurs with features of cystitis. Sonography demonstrates echogenic foci with ring-down or dirty shadowing within the bladder wall.

Chronic Cystitis

Sonographically the chronic inflammatory changes may be seen as cysts or solid papillary masses. These are difficult to differentiate from malignancy.

Vesical Calculus

Calculus in the bladder is easily visualized if the bladder is full. It appears as an echogenic focus casting a distal shadow. The echogenic focus is mobile and occasionally seen in the vesicoureteric junction or a diverticulum **(Figs. 13.33A to D)**.

Neurogenic Bladder

This is of two types:
1. Detrusor areflexia—caused by lower motor neuron lesions. On sonography, appears as a smooth, large capacity, thin-walled bladder. The bladder may extend high into the abdomen.
2. Detrusor hyperreflexia—upper motor neuron lesions. On ultrasound a thick-walled, vertical trabeculated bladder often with associated upper tract dilatation is seen. Large amount of post-void residual urine is present within a neurogenic bladder.

Bladder Tumors

Malignant (Figs. 13.34A to D)

- *Transitional cell carcinoma (TCC):* This is a common malignant tumor occurring more commonly in men

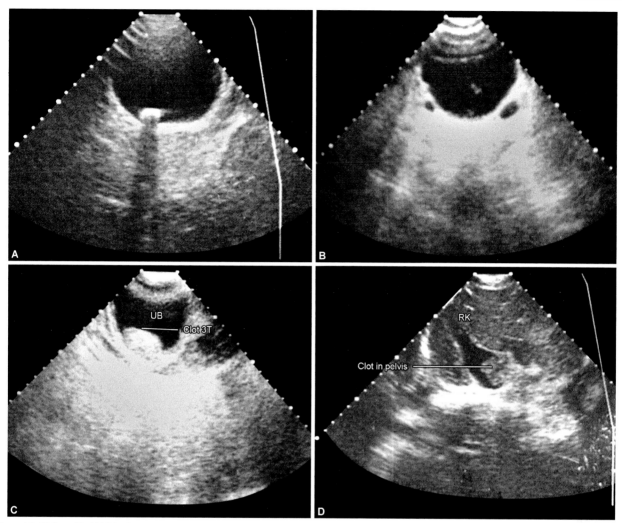

Figs. 13.33A to D: (A) Vesical calculus—an echogenic focus with distal acoustic shadowing seen in the urinary bladder; (B) The distended urinary bladder with echogenic strands inside it, both the lower ureters are dilated; (C) Clot in urinary bladder is seen as a large echogenic lesion in relation to the posterior wall of urinary bladder; (D) Clot is also seen in renal pelvis.

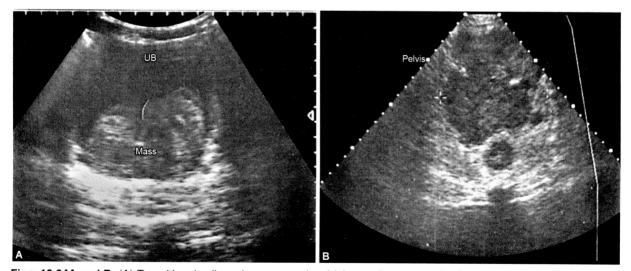

Figs. 13.34A and B: (A) Transitional cell carcinoma—a polypoidal mass is seen to arise from post wall of urinary bladder; (B) Carcinoma UB—a hypoechoic lesion is seen to occupy UB. The walls are not well seen.

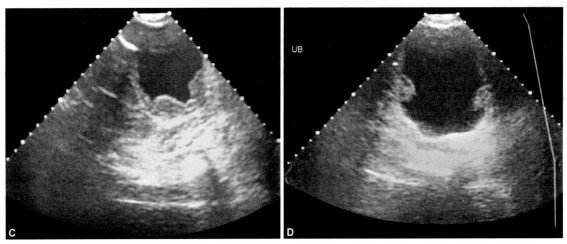

Figs. 13.34C and D: (C) Carcinoma—irregular wall thickening seen on posterior wall; (D) Multifocal carcinoma—transverse scan of UB showing nodular growth at two different regions.

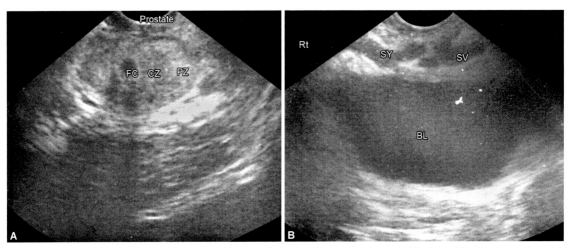

Figs. 13.35A and B: (A) Longitudinal and transverse scan showing Foley's catheter (FC) placed in the prostatic urethra in a case of BPH (CZ—central zone, PZ—peripheral zone); (B) Transrectal USG of prostate showing normal seminal vesicle.

(3:1) with a peak incidence in the sixth and seventh decade. They occur more frequently in the trigone and along the lateral and posterior walls. Patients present with hematuria, frequency, dysuria, and suprapubic pain. Sonographically it appears as focal, nonmobile mass attached to the bladder wall. The appearance is nonspecific and differentiated from a variety of causes like cystitis, adherent blood clot, invasive prostatic carcinoma, lymphoma, metastases, endometrioma, etc. The tumor may arise in a diverticulum attached to the bladder. Diverticular tumors appear as moderately echogenic nonshadowing mass.

Extension into the perivesical space, involvement of vesicoureteric junction or ureters and pelvic lymphadenopathy helps in staging the tumor.

- *Squamous cell carcinoma:* This is a rare but second most common tumor arising from the urothelium. It comprises 5 to 8 percent of all bladder tumors. Chronic infection, irritation and stones lead to squamous metaplasia and leukoplakia of the urothelium. On ultrasound, squamous cell carcinomas are large, solid, infiltrating mass lesions. An associated calculus is seen as an echogenic focus with distal acoustic shadowing. Adenocarcinomas are seen as bladder mass occasionally with evidence of calcification.
- *Lymphoma:* Most patients are between 40-60 years of age with women more commonly affected. On sonography, a bladder wall mass is seen usually covered by intact epithelium.
- *Metastasis:* Bladder involvement occurs in malignant melanoma, lung, breast, and gastric cancer. On ultrasound, a solid mass is seen in bladder wall.

Prostate (Figs. 13.35A and B)

Benign Hypertrophy Prostate (Figs. 13.36A to D)

Elderly males with symptoms of prostatism—urgency, frequency and hesitancy usually have an enlarged prostate gland. On sonography prostate is enlarged in size with a homogenous echotexture and well defined capsule. Median

CHAPTER 13: Abdomen: The Urinary Tract

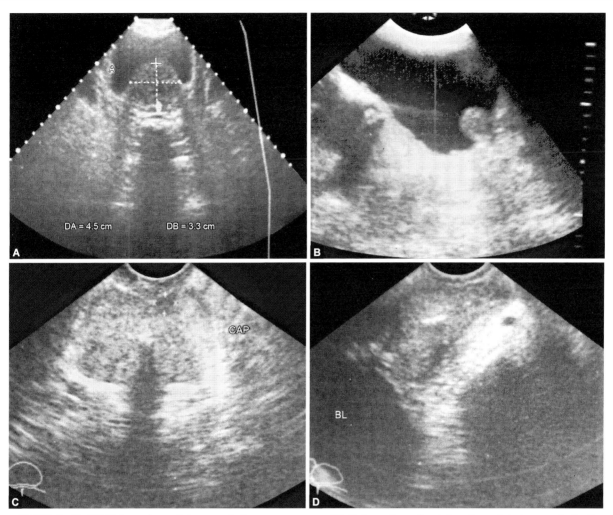

Figs. 13.36A to D: (A) Enlarged prostate seen in transverse scan; (B) Enlarged median lobe of prostate is seen indenting the bladder base. The bladder walls are irregularly hypertrophied suggestive of trabeculated bladder; (C) Transrectal ultrasound showing benign hypertrophy of prostate with focus of calcification in longitudinal (i) and transverse (ii) scan (shown in figure as (D)).

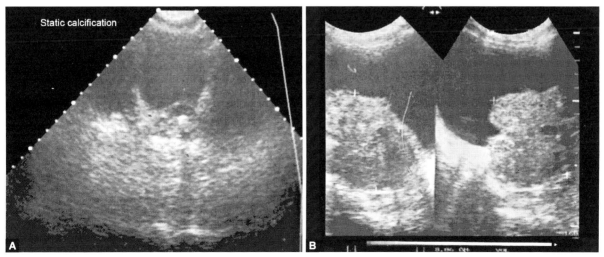

Figs. 13.37A and B: (A) Transverse scan of a normal sized prostate shows a dense echogenic focus with distal acoustic shadowing suggestive of calcification of corpora amylacea; (B) A large growth with heterogeneous echotexture and irregular margins seen in the region of prostate. The growth is invading the bladder. It was a case of post-prostatectomy.

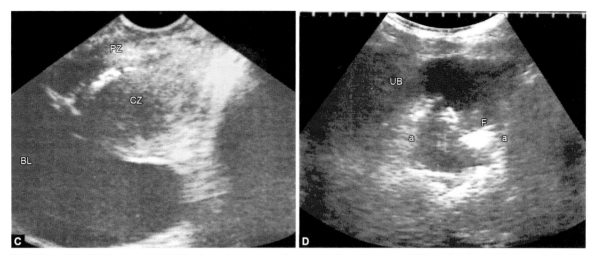

Figs. 13.37C and D: (C) Transrectal USG of prostate—showing prostatic enlargement. There is also evidence of calcification in central zone (CZ-central zone, PZ-peripheral zone, BL-bladder urinary); (D) Carcinoma prostate—transverse scan of prostate shows a predominantly hypoechoic enlarged prostate with a focus of calcification invading the bladder base: the interface between prostate and bladder base is lost.

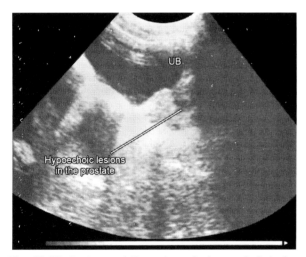

Fig. 13.38: Acute prostatism—irregular hypoechoic lesion seen in prostate in longitudinal scan.

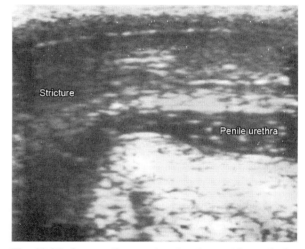

Fig. 13.39: Sonourethrography showing a stricture in the bulbar part of urethra.

lobe enlargement is seen as a protuberance into the bladder base while lateral lobes enlargement imparts a rounded shape to the prostate. Prostate enlargement is graded as 0 if weight is under 20 g, grade I if between 21 to 30, grade 2 if between 31 to 50 and grade 3 if above 51 gm. Corpora amylacea is seen as an echogenic focus while calcification if present is echogenic with distal acoustic shadowing. The bladder may show changes of cystitis seen as generalized wall thickening. Outflow obstruction also results in a trabeculated, thick walled urinary bladder. Small outpouchings, sacculations or diverticulum may be present. Post void scans show significant residual urine in the urinary bladder.

Prostatic Carcinoma (Figs. 13.37A to D)

The presence of malignancy cannot be easily ascertained from sonography including transrectal sonography, as the sonographic appearance of carcinoma of prostate is nonspecific. The lesion may be hypoechoic or hyperechoic with ill-defined outlines. The periprostatic region is still difficult to evaluate if the prostatic outline is irregular or indistinct, the possibility of local extension may be considered. Main use of transrectal ultrasound is in guiding biopsy from a suspicious site.

Inflammatory Diseases

- *Prostatic Abscess:* A hypoechoic area within the enlarged prostate on sonography suggests an abscess in a patient with symptoms of vague chromic ill health, perineal heaviness, pain and fever.
- *Prostatitis* **(Fig. 13.38)**: Acute prostatitis is seen in young patients. Per-rectal examination is very painful and on ultrasound, the gland appears enlarged and hypoechoic. Associated involvement of urethra can be best seen with sonourethrography **(Fig. 13.39)**.

14
CHAPTER

Abdomen: Adrenal Glands

INFECTIOUS DISEASES

Adrenals are most commonly affected by tuberculosis. US appearances vary with a stage of the disease. In the acute phase there is bilateral diffuse enlargement, often inhomogeneous. Chronic cases show atrophic and calcified adrenal glands.

AIDS—in 70% of patients who die with AIDS have focal or diffuse damage of adrenal glands by cytomegalovirus. These are usually hypoechoic masses, may be heterogeneous and gas containing if abscess formation occurs.

ADRENAL CYSTIC LESIONS

Most common adrenal cysts (50%) are endothelial in origin, more commonly lymphangiomatous than angiomatous. Pseudocysts secondary to hemorrhage are well known. Epithelial glandular cysts are rare. Even rarer are parasitic hydatid cysts. Cysts appear as oval-rounded well-defined anechoic lesions with posterior enhancement. Internal debris are often noted. Calcification may be found in pseudocyst or parasitic cysts.

ADRENAL TUMORS (FIG. 14.1)

Adrenal tumors cause focal enlargement of the adrenal glands. A round-oval focal mass 0.5 to 2 cm in size and with a lower reflectivity is suggestive of an adrenal tumor. Small lesions are homogenous **(Figs. 14.2A and B)** whereas larger ones are heterogeneous **(Fig. 14.3)** due to necrosis or hemorrhage. Adrenal tumors typically impress and displace the inferior vena cava (IVC) anteriorly and the kidney laterally and inferiorly.

- *Cortical adenomas*—are common and incidental findings or are detected as a part of endocrine neoplastic syndrome. These are small, homogenous tumors.
- *Carcinomas:* In children they are small, homogenous and produce steroids while in adults they are silent and therefore large and heterogeneous and commonly have invaded the adrenal vein and IVC. Nodal and blood-borne metastases are also common.
- *Myelolipoma:* A rare tumor, non-functional, containing fat and bone marrow elements. It is characteristically highly reflective due to fat.

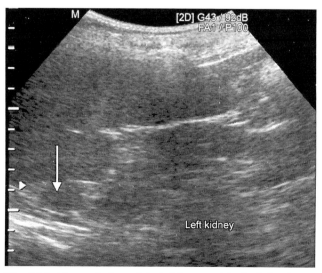

Fig. 14.1: Hypoechoic nodule (white arrow) in the left adrenal in a case of adrenal adenoma.

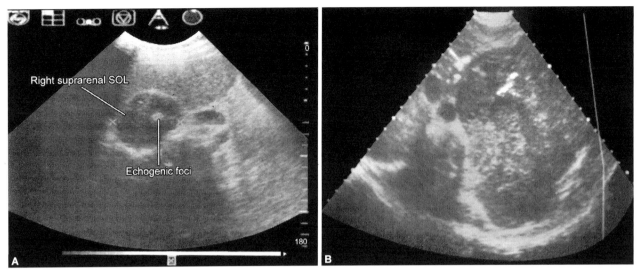

Figs. 14.2A and B: (A) A large hypoechoic mass lesion with uniform echogenicity with calcification seen in the right adrenal gland of a young female; (B) A large predominantly hypoechoic well-defined left adrenal mass lesion seen with evidence of calcification in it.

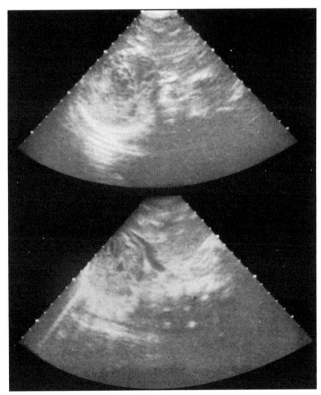

Fig. 14.3: Longitudinal and transverse scan of abdomen of a 6-month-old child with marked heterogenicity and areas of high reflectivity within it—neuroblastoma.

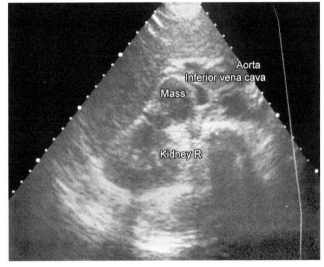

Fig. 14.4: Pheochromocytoma—a hypoechoic rounded well-defined lesion with uniform echogenicity is seen in the right adrenal gland.

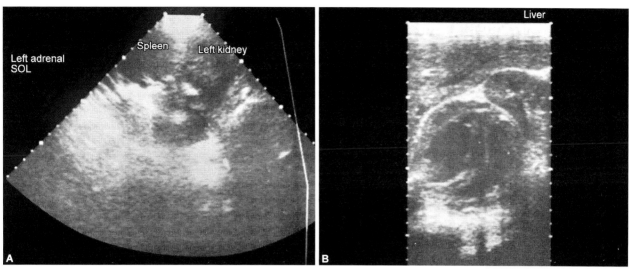

Figs. 14.5A and B: (A) Metastases—a hypoechoic mass with irregular outline is seen in the region of left adrenal in a case of bronchogenic carcinoma; (B) Adrenal metastases—a large heterogeneous mass seen in right adrenal gland. This is a typical appearance of large adrenal metastases.

- *Pheochromocytoma (Fig. 14.4):* These are uncommon tumors seen in 0.4 to 2% patients with hypertension, 10% of tumors arise in extra-adrenal site, 10% are malignant and 10% are multiple. Clinical feature is paroxysmal hypertension. Small tumors are oval to round, well-defined tumors of uniform reflectivity. Larger ones become heterogeneous due to necrosis and hemorrhage.

ADRENAL METASTASES (FIGS. 14.5A AND B)

Adrenals are the fourth most common site of metastases which commonly arise from bronchial and breast carcinomas or non-Hodgkin's lymphoma. Metastases are seen as rounded or oval, poorly reflective masses.

CHAPTER 15

Abdomen: The Retroperitoneum

AORTA (FIGS. 15.1A TO D)

- Congenital anomalies—in situs inversus all the abdominal contents are transposed so that the aorta lies on the right and appears normal.
- Atheroma—the normal thin, smooth endothelial lining of the aorta thickens and becomes irregular, often with calcification. The aorta may dilate and loses its normal tapering configuration and becomes tortuous.
- Aneurysm—is seen as a focal or diffuse dilatation of the aorta. An aneurysm with a true luminal diameter of 5 cm or more has a risk of rupture. US can demonstrate both the true lumen and the mural thrombus. US is also useful for serial measurement of the aneurysm, progressive expansion of more than 1 cm per annum is an indication for surgical intervention.
- Aortic dissection—gives a characteristic appearance of US "flapping" inner (media and intima) wall which has become separated from the outer (media-adventitia) wall. Color Doppler demonstrates separate vascular channels with different flow velocities.
- Aortic occlusions—absent pulsations in an anechoic aortic lumen suggest occlusion by aortic thrombus. Doppler confirms the diagnosis.
- Chronic aortic rupture—pulsating hematoma or periaortic collection is present.

Inferior Vena Cava (Fig. 15.2)

- Congenital anomaly—most common is left sided cava below renal level draining into a large left renal vein that crosses over the aorta to a normal upper vena caval segment.
- Pathological distention—not related to respiration is seen in congestive cardiac failure, cardiac tamponade or proximal inferior vena cava (IVC) obstruction.
- IVC obstruction—IVC is invaded in 10% renal cell carcinomas which is seen sonographically as a reflective material inside its lumen. Caval obstruction by a large mass compressing upon the IVC appears on US as proximal dilatation of IVC and lack of distention on valsalva.
- Thrombus—seen as a reflective material inside the IVC, though fresh thrombus is difficult to distinguish from blood.
- Filters—appear as highly reflective complex of linear echoes in the caval lumen.

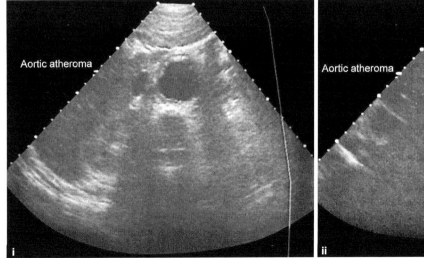
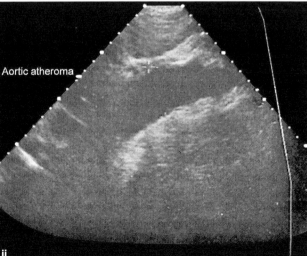

Fig. 15.1A: Dilated abdominal aorta in (i) transverse, and (ii) longitudinal scan with atherosclerotic plaques.

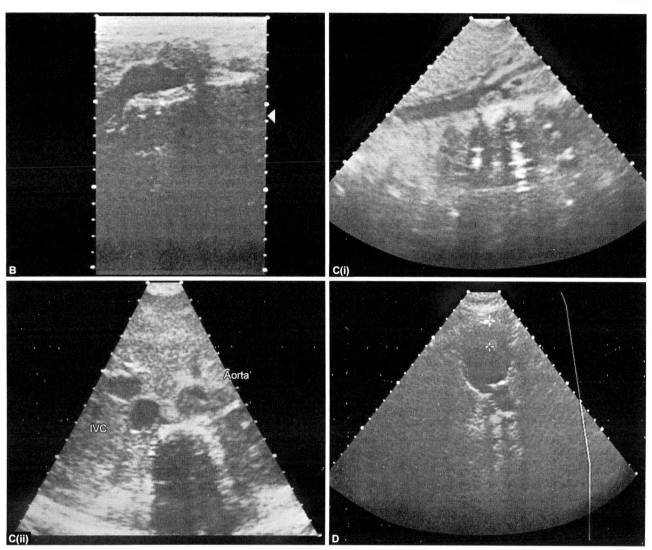

Fig. 15.1B to D: (B) Longitudinal scan of aortic aneurysm with atherosclerotic plaque; (C)(i) Longitudinal, and (ii) transverse scans of aorta showing a thrombus in the lumen just at the point of origin of superior mesenteric artery; (D) Transverse scan with aortic aneurysm with atherosclerotic plaque in anterior wall with small dissection in post wall.

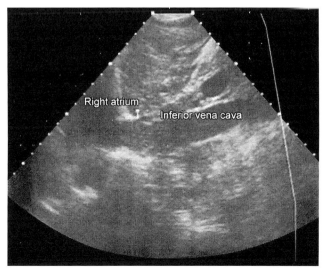

Fig. 15.2: A thrombus is seen inside the lumen just proximal to its entry into right atrium (RA).

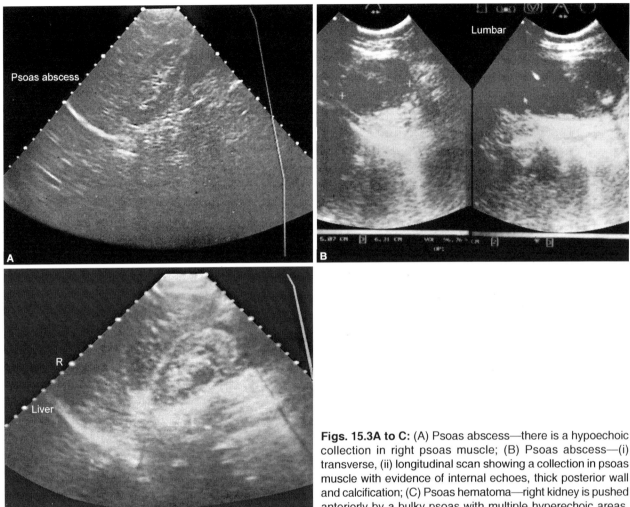

Figs. 15.3A to C: (A) Psoas abscess—there is a hypoechoic collection in right psoas muscle; (B) Psoas abscess—(i) transverse, (ii) longitudinal scan showing a collection in psoas muscle with evidence of internal echoes, thick posterior wall and calcification; (C) Psoas hematoma—right kidney is pushed anteriorly by a bulky psoas with multiple hyperechoic areas. The patient was a known case of hemophilia.

- IVC displacement—IVC can also be displaced anteriorly or posteriorly by enlargement of the adjacent structures, e.g., lymphadenopathy, adrenal masses, caudate lobe enlargement, etc.

RETROPERITONEAL FLUID COLLECTIONS (FIGS. 15.3A TO C)

US easily detects but fails to differentiate between types of fluid collections in the retroperitoneum. Unless US guided needle aspiration is done, various fluid collections are abscesses, hematomas, urinomas and lymphoceles.

- Abscesses are encountered in postoperative cases, extension from kidneys or spine or perforated retroperitoneal bowel. They appear as irregular thick walled collection with septae, internal debris or gas bubbles. (ii) Psoas abscess most commonly due to tuberculosis of spine is also seen in perirenal pathology, appendicitis. On US psoas outline is enlarged and bulging with diffuse hypoechogenicity or localized fluid collection in it.
- Hematomas vary from anechoic (fresh) to complex lesions. Chronic hematomas are multiseptate cystic spaces with reflective material which may layer or move. Psoas muscle is a site for spontaneous retroperitoneal hemorrhage in hemophilias. Differential diagnosis of psoas muscle enlargement is retroperitoneal tumor or hemihypertrophy.
- Urinomas and lymphoceles appear as anechoic fluid collections on US. Urinomas are limited to the perirenal space and found in postoperative cases or patients with obstructive uropathy.

RETROPERITONEAL FIBROSIS

It is an insidiously progressive proliferation of fibrous tissue, in the central and paravertebral regions, of unknown etiology. Thirty percent are related to inflammation, trauma or hemorrhage, primary or metastatic tumors or drug (methysergide) intake. It appears as ill-well defined, noncapsulated hypoechoic lesion encasing and displacing the adjacent structures. Minimal hydronephrosis due to ureteric obstruction may appear.

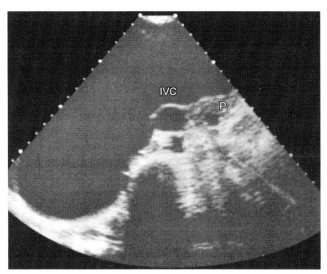

Fig. 15.4: A huge completely anechoic retroperitoneal cyst is seen in this transverse scan.

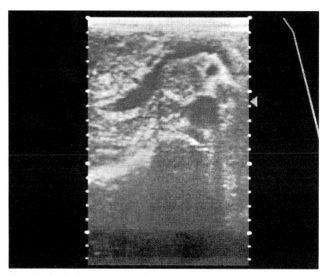

Fig. 15.6: A single rounded echogenic lumen seen anterior to the aorta. Superior mesenteric artery (SMA) is seen on the left side. Portal vein (PV) is anterior to the lymph node (LN). It was a metastatic LN from adenocarcinoma colon.

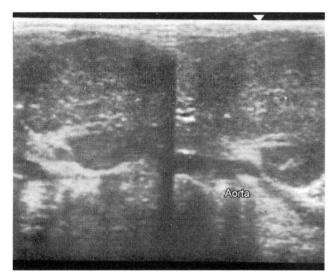

Fig. 15.5: A large ill-defined solid hypoechoic lesion seen anterior to the compressed aorta turned out to be a retroperitoneal sarcoma.

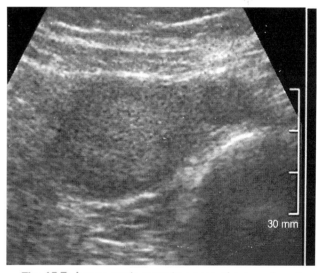

Fig. 15.7: A para-aortic mass in a case of extra-adrenal pheochromocytoma.

RETROPERITONEAL CYSTS (FIG. 15.4)

These are rare and are simple inclusion cysts arising from embryonic GI and GU tract, rest are acquired lymphatic, parasitic, traumatic or inflammatory cysts. Simple retroperitoneal cysts are smooth-walled echo-free regions with posterior enhancement. Abscesses and hematomas have internal echoes.

RETROPERITONEAL TUMORS (FIGS. 15.5 TO 15.7)

Most of these tumors arise in the kidneys or the adrenals. The rest are uncommon except lymphoma. An 80% of the primary retroperitoneal tumors are malignant. In adults most common tumors are liposarcoma, leiomyosarcoma and malignant fibrous histiocytoma. Rhabdomyosarcoma, neuroblastoma, ganglioneuroblastoma and teratomas occur in children.

Metastases are usually recurrence of a urological or gynecological malignancy. Abdominal pain is the most common presentation with the tumor palpable in 80% cases.

US features suggestive of a retroperitoneal location of a tumor are—anterior displacement or encasement of pancreas, kidneys, great vessels, ascending or descending colon or compression of iliopsoas or quadratus lumborum. US appearance is very variable from strongly or poorly refractive or mixed tumors with or without central anechoic

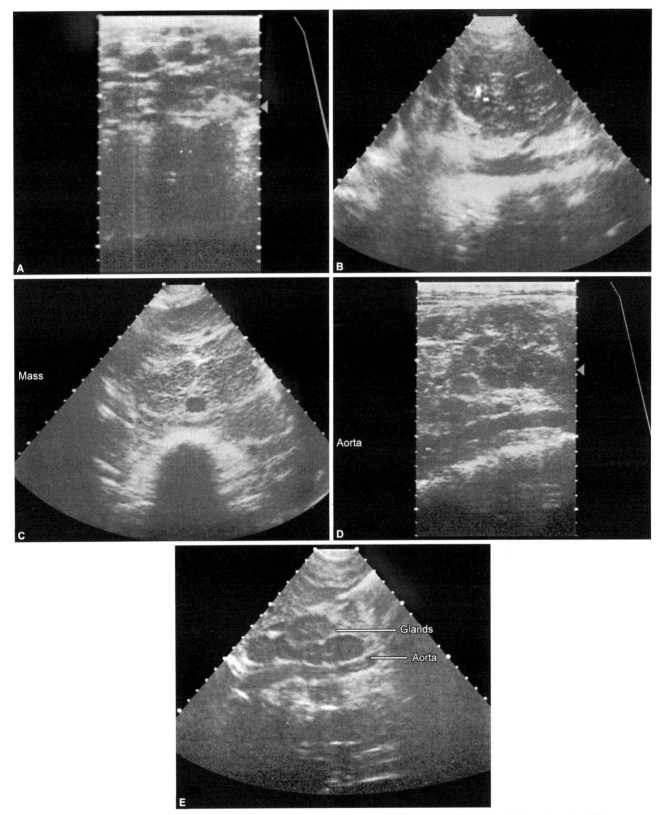

Figs. 15.8A to E: (A) Multiple small hypoechoic lesion seen around the aortic bifurcation; (B) Pre-aortic lymph node (LN) mass—a large well defined hypoechoic mass seen in the preaortic region in this longitudinal scan; (C) Conglomerate lymph nodes mass seen in the preaortic region; (D) Multiple hypoechoic nodular lesions with evidence of matting and necrosis suggestive of tubercular lymphadenopathy in para aortic region. (E) Discrete hypoechoic nodular lesions seen in preaortic region suggestive of lymph nodes. Fine needle aspiration cytology (FNAC) revealed lymphoma.

zones of necrosis. Malignant schwannoma or fibrous histiocytoma are anechoic or echo-poor lesions. A highly reflective tumor suggests liposarcoma. A solid mass of mixed echotexture with echopoor center suggests sarcoma. while a teratoma has a heterogeneous echopattern with solid, cystic, and calcified areas. A fat-fluid level may be found in teratomas.

Lymph Nodes (Figs. 15.8A to E)

Enlarged lymph nodes typically have a low and uniform reflectivity on ultrasound. Very large nodes may appear almost anechoic. Presence of calcification or lipid deposition appears as echogenic areas. Lymphadenopathy can occur in lymphoma, metastases or inflammatory disease and appear similar on US. Retroperitoneal lymphadenopathy occurs more commonly in non-Hodgkin's (40%) than Hodgkin's (25%) lymphoma. Various sonographic patterns are known:

- Discrete enlargement of individually identifiable nodes
- A homogenous confluent mass, enveloping and often elevating the great vessels
- Compression or displacement of adjacent organs by the nodal mass
- Rarely vascular invasion from malignant lymphadenopathy. The main differential diagnoses of lymphadenopathy are retroperitoneal fibrosis, neurofibromata, echopoor thrombus in an aortic aneurysm, adrenal masses on the right side or sometimes pancreatic mass.

16 CHAPTER

Abdomen: The Peritoneum

ASCITES (FIGS. 16.1A TO I)

Fluid within the peritoneal cavity is anechoic and easily visualized. The fluid is either transudate or exudate. Transudate is a clear fluid with no internal echoes or septations. The bowel loops are seen floating freely within it. Fluid enters the individual leaves. The mesentery is traceable till its root. Exudate may show floating echoes,

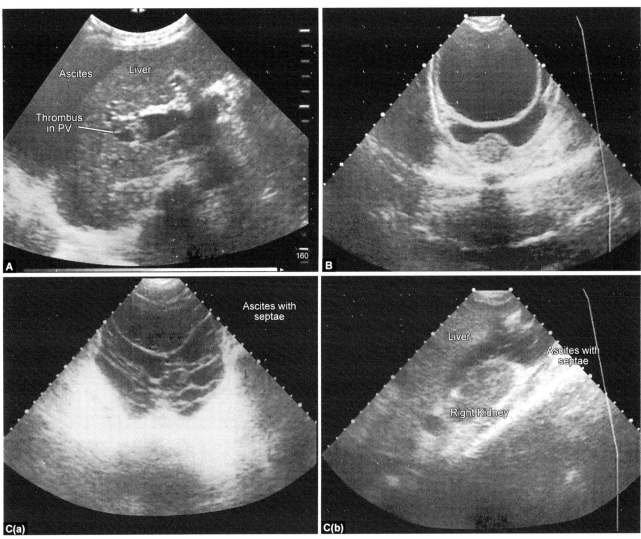

Figs. 16.1A to C: (A) Free fluid seen around the liver and thrombus is seen in the portal vein (PV); (B) Free fluid in uterovesical pouch; (C) Ascites with multiple thick internal septae seen in (a) pelvis and (b) hepatorenal pouch.

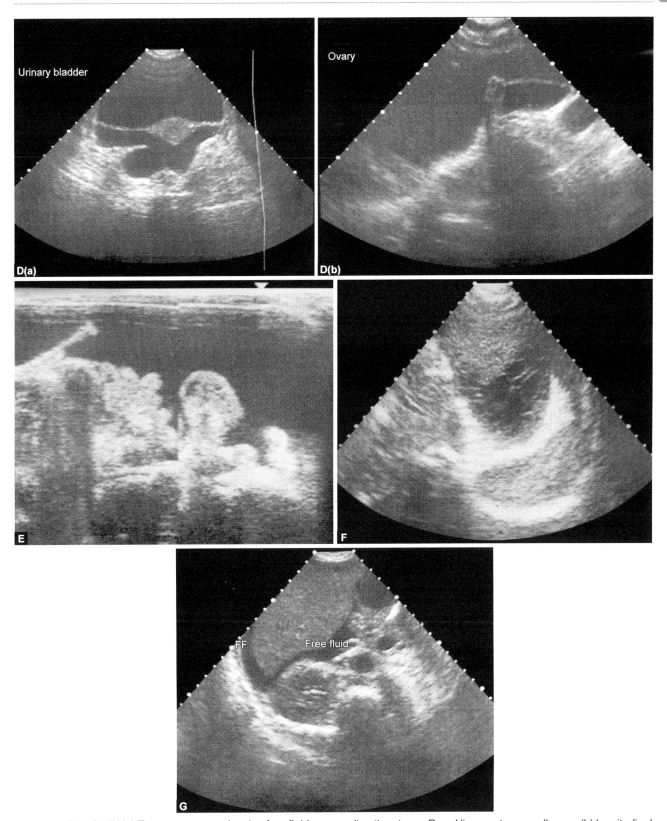

Figs. 16.1D to G: (D)(a) Transverse scan showing free fluid surrounding the uterus. Board ligaments are well seen, (b) longitudinal scan shows right and left ovaries with surrounding fluids; (E) Ascites outlining bowel loops; (F) Subdiaphragmatic collection fluid collections with multiple internal septae is seen below the diaphragm; (G) Free fluid is seen in the hepatorenal pouch and also around liver.

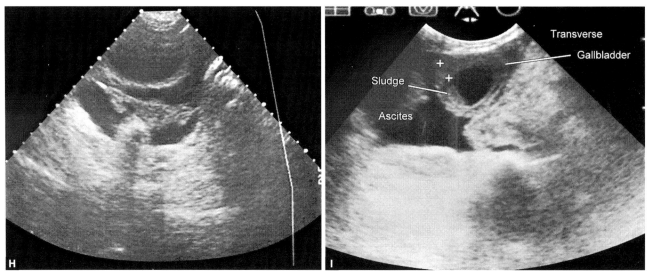

Figs. 16.1H and I: (H) Free fluid is seen in the uterovesical pouch and in the uterorectal pouch; (I) Gallbladder (GB) is thickened due to ascites. Note the sludge seen as a debris-fluid level inside the lumen of gallbladder.

septae or strands within it. Bowel loops are clumped together and the mesenteric leaves are not separable. In flank peritonitis echoes and numerous septations are seen with the fluid collection. The fluid collection in peritonitis may be generalized or localized. Collections are present in the dependent part of the abdomen, pelvis, flanks or subphrenic space if peritonitis develops due to bowel perforation. Air may be present in the peritoneal cavity and appear as bright echogenic foci with reverberation artifacts distal to it. Air may be found within the fluid collection as tiny bright specks or an air fluid level may be present. In malignant exudate peritoneal deposits or omental masses may be seen. Peritoneal deposits are seen as sessile or polypoidal lesions on the peritoneal surface of various organs or the dependent areas. Omental masses are usually complex masses with cystic and solid components. Sometimes peritoneal deposits in the pelvis mimic adrenal lesions.

MISCELLANEOUS FLUID COLLECTIONS

Fluid may collect secondary to bile leakage, trauma, bleeding due to any cause and infection. Depending upon the composition of the fluid it may range from clear, anechoic to an echogenic collection with evidence of shifting internal echoes on changing position. Patient's history is vital in deciding the type of collection as the US appearance of various types of fluids is overlapping.

Bilomas

These develop following biliary surgery, or perforation of the gallbladder due to acute distention or carcinoma. The collection is generally around the gallbladder and liver, is well localized and may be clear or have internal echoes.

Abscesses (Figs. 16.2 and 16.3)

These are localized collections with a variable US appearance. The possibility of an abscess is suggested by the presence of air in the lesion. Air appears as tiny echogenic specks with reverberation artefact or as an air-fluid level.

Hematoma (Fig. 16.4)

A fresh hematoma is highly echogenic and serially decreases in echogenicity to appear as an anechoic collection. The clinical data helps to differentiate it from abscess.

OTHER PERITONEAL LESIONS

Pseudomyxoma Peritonei

This is a peritoneal spread of a mucinous tumor from the appendix or ovaries. It appears fluid-like, with or without septations, with the clumped bowel loops posterior to the fluid collection.

Lymphocele

Loculated, elliptical clear fluid collections are seen following surgery in pelvis or retroperitoneum.

Peritoneal Metastases (Fig. 16.5)

Metastatic peritoneal deposits occur in primary malignancy of GB, ovary, stomach, colon or breast. US appearance of peritoneal deposits is variable—sheet-like masses, nodules

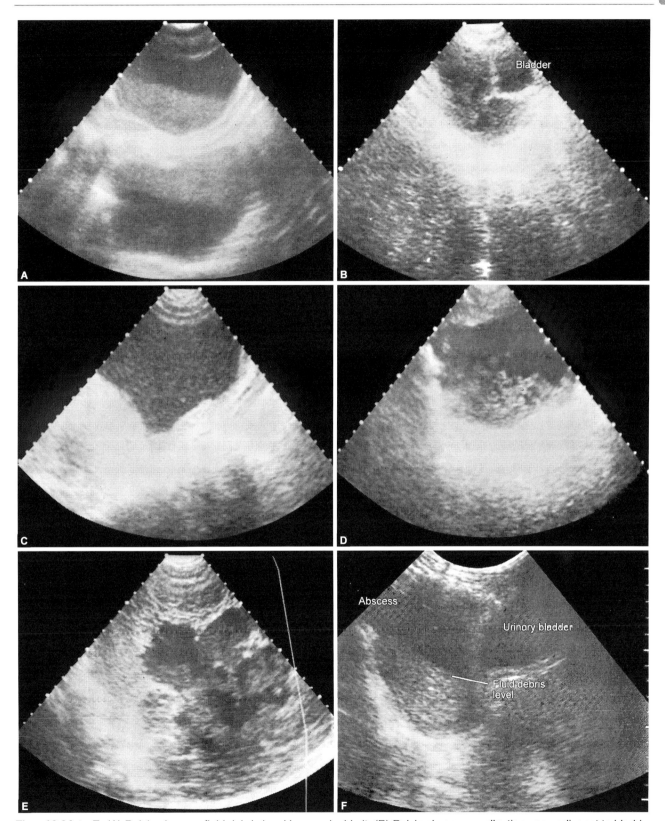

Figs. 16.2A to F: (A) Pelvic abscess-fluid debris level is seen inside it; (B) Pelvic abscess—collection seen adjacent to bladder with debris inside it. It was a postoperative case of acute appendicitis; (C and D) Infected ascites—free fluid with echogenic debris is seen on transverse scan; (E) peritoneal abscess—a large SOL with irregular thickened walls and heterogeneous echotexture is seen in the abdominal sac revealed thick pus; (F) Debris-fluid level seen inside a collection in the pelvis.

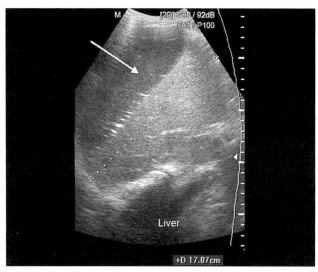

Fig. 16.3: Subphrenic abscess (white arrow) pushing the liver inferiorly.

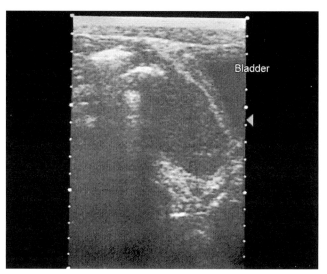

Fig. 16.4: Pelvic hematoma—in this case of blunt abdominal trauma. A collection is seen in the pelvis with internal echoes inside it.

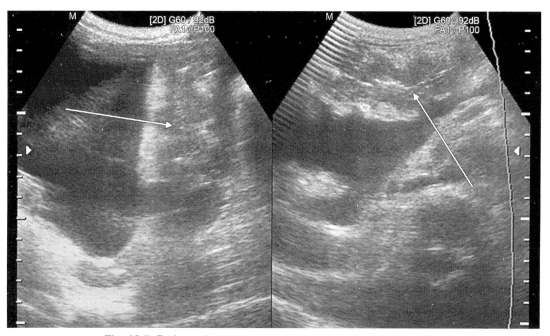

Fig. 16.5: Peritoneal metastases (white arrows) with gross ascites.

small or large or superficially located hypoechoic lesions. Small lesions are only picked up in the presence of ascites.

Peritoneal Mesothelioma

This is a differential diagnosis of all peritoneal lesions, especially in males. It can appear as fluid, sheet-like hypoechoic masses or nodular or globular opacities or form a thick layer separating the anterior abdominal wall from the underlying bowel loops.

CYSTIC PERITONEAL MASSES (FIGS. 16.6A TO F)

Cystic peritoneal lesions are peritoneal, mesenteric or omental cysts, hydatid disease, and pseudopancreatic cysts. These cystic lesions have quite similar US appearance and history helps to differentiate them. Sonographically, omental and mesenteric cyst often appear as unilocular cystic lesions that may be septated. A fat-fluid level may be seen. Mesenteric cysts are usually found in the root of the

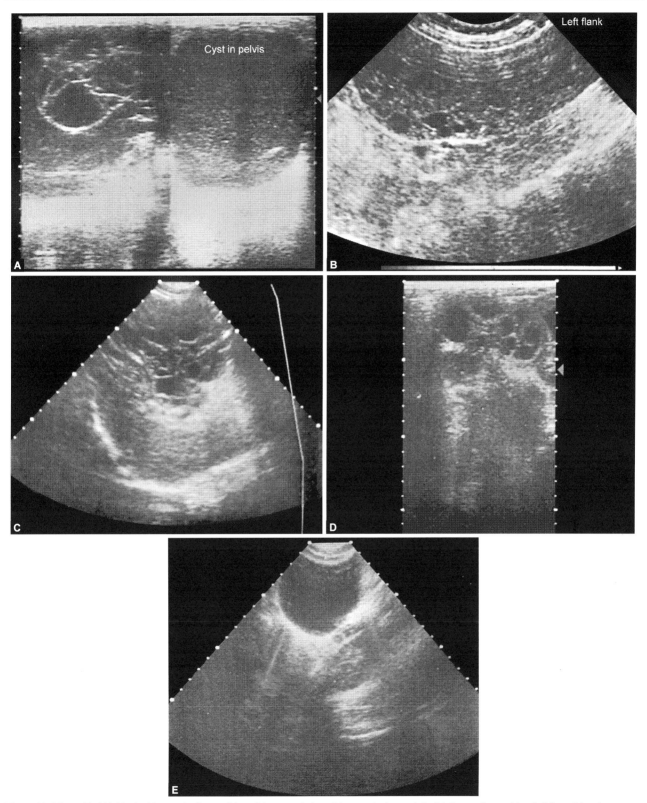

Figs. 16.6A to E: (A) Hydatid cyst in liver with evidence of daughter cyst. Associated intraperitoneal hydatid cyst is also seen in pelvis with internal debris; (B) Intraperitoneal hydatid—extends from the spleen to pelvis occupying whole of left flank. The lower pole of mass showed a rounded lesion with multiple daughter cyst in it; (C) Omental hydatid—a large hydatid with multiple daughter cyst in it; (D) Intraperitoneal hydatid—cyst with multiple daughter cyst inside it; (E) Mesenteric cyst—a large cystic anechoic SOL with thin wall seen displacing the bowel loops.

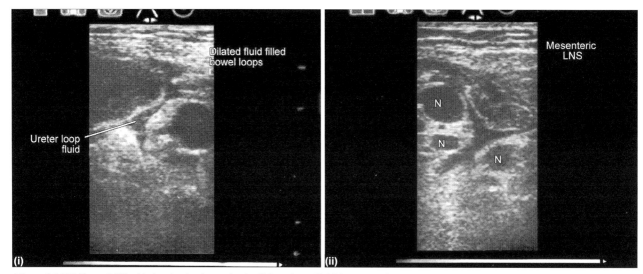

Figs. 16.6F (i) and (ii): Abdominal tuberculosis (i) interloop fluid between bowel loops, (ii) multiple hypoechoic well-defined lesion seen in the mesentery suggestive of lymph nodes (N).

mesentery while omental cyst occurs adjacent to the bowel. Hydatid cyst may appear as cyst within a cyst or multicystic lesions. Pseudopancreatic cysts are thick walled anechoic lesion with occasional septa and follow an episode of acute pain due to pancreatitis. Many times cyst aspiration and analysis of the fluid settle the diagnostic dilemma.

17
CHAPTER

Abdomen: The Uterus and Adnexa

UTERUS AND ADNEXA

Congenital Abnormalities (Figs. 17.1 and 17.2)

Congenital uterine abnormalities are present in 0.5% females and are associated with an increased incidence of spontaneous abortion. Arrested development of both the müllerian ducts results in uterine aplasia, while only of one side results in uterus unicornis, unicollis. The unicornuate uterus is suspected if on ultrasound the uterus appears small and laterally placed. Failure of fusion of müllerian ducts may be complete, resulting in uterus didelphys **(Fig. 17.3)** (Two vaginas, two cervices, and two uteri), or partial, which may result in either uterus bicornis bicollis (one vagina, two cervices and two uteri) or uterus bicornis unicollis (one vagina, one cervix, and two uterine horns), uterus arcuatus results in partial indentation of the uterine fundus.

Failure of resorption of the median septum results in septate or subseptate uterus.

Associated congenital renal abnormality especially renal agenesis and ectopia are detected on ultrasonography.

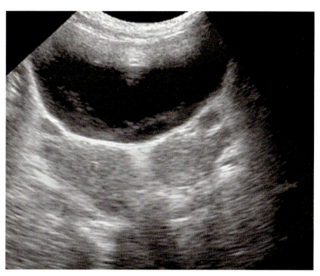

Fig. 17.2: A bicornuate uterus.

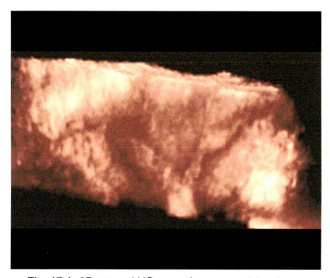

Fig. 17.1: 3D coronal US scan shows a septate uterus.

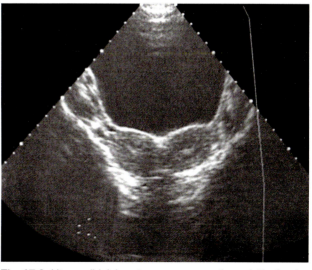

Fig. 17.3: Uterus didelphys, transverse scan through the fundus showing two separate endometrial echoes with intervening uterine musculature.

Most uterine abnormalities can be detected on sonography. Two endometrial echo complexes may be seen in the bicornuate or septate uterus. In didelphys and bicornuate variety the endometrial cavities are widely separated with a deep indentation on the fundal contour. A septate uterus has a normal outline and shape with the two endometrial cavities placed close together and separated by a thin fibrous echogenic septum.

Myometrial Abnormalities

Leiomyoma (Fibroid) (Figs. 17.4A to D)

Leiomyoma are the most common neoplasms of the uterus occurring in 20-30 percent females above 30 years of age. Although frequently asymptomatic, women with leiomyomas can present with pain and uterine bleeding. These may be subserosal, mural or submucosal in location. Sonographically, leiomyomas have variable appearances. The uterus may be enlarged with a globular outline and heterogeneous echotexture resulting from small diffuse leiomyomas. Localized leiomyomas are most commonly hypoechoic in echotexture and distort the external contour (if subserosal) or the endometrial echo (if submucosal). Many demonstrate areas of acoustic attenuation or shadowing. Calcification is seen in older females as echogenic foci with acoustic shadowing. Degeneration and necrosis are seen as areas of decreased echogenicity or cystic spaces within the fibroid.

Leiomyosarcoma

Leiomyosarcoma is rare and may arise in preexisting uterine leiomyoma. Sonographically picture is similar to degenerating fibroid with evidence of local invasion and distant metastases.

Adenomyosis (Figs. 17.5 to 17.7)

Middle aged females present with nonspecific symptoms of pelvic pain, dysmenorrhea and menorrhagia. This results

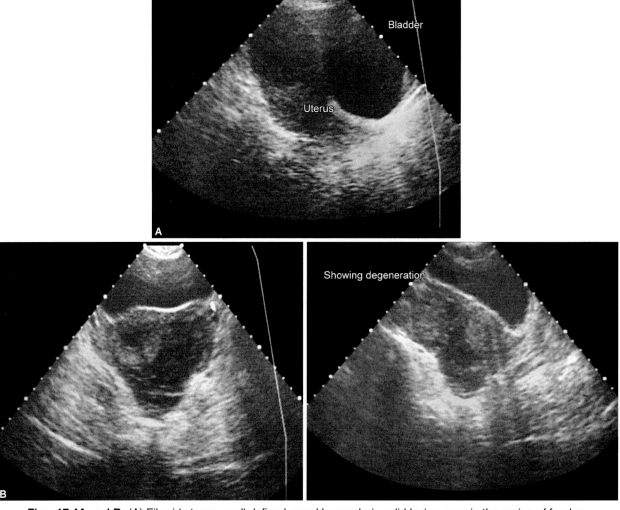

Figs. 17.4A and B: (A) Fibroid uterus—well-defined round hypoechoic solid lesion seen in the region of fundus; (B) Multiple uterine fibroids showing degeneration.

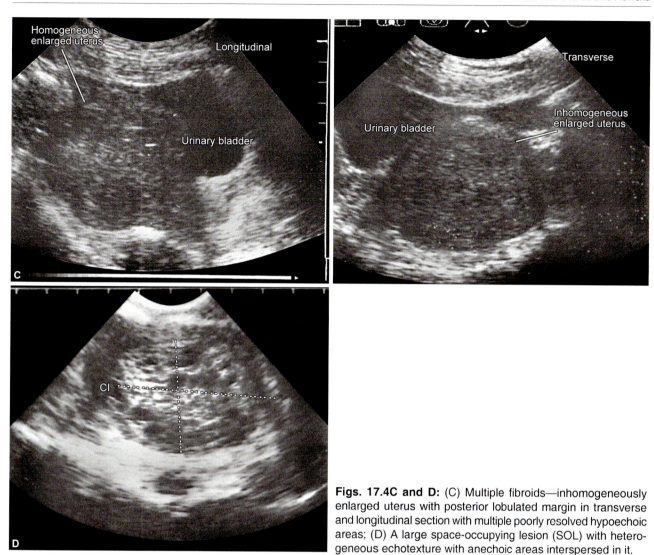

Figs. 17.4C and D: (C) Multiple fibroids—inhomogeneously enlarged uterus with posterior lobulated margin in transverse and longitudinal section with multiple poorly resolved hypoechoic areas; (D) A large space-occupying lesion (SOL) with heterogeneous echotexture with anechoic areas interspersed in it.

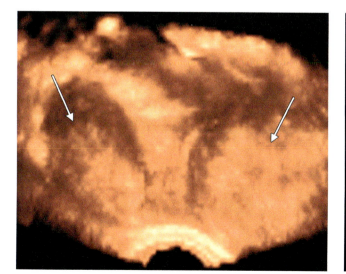

Fig. 17.5: 3D US scan shows adenomyomas on either side of the uterine fundus—white arrows (note homogeneous appearance with no distal shadowing.

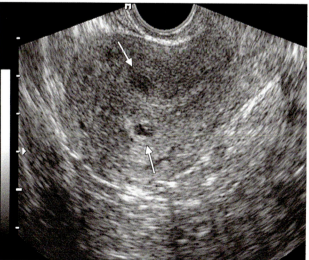

Fig. 17.6: Thick walled cystic adenomyotic lesions (white arrows) in subendometrial region.

from the presence of endometrial glands in the myometrium in diffuse or focal nodular forms; sonographically diagnosis is suggested by diffuse uterine enlargement with a normal contour, normal endometrium, normal myometrial echotexture or thickening of the posterior myometrium with a slightly more hypoechoic myometrium than normal. On transvaginal sonography it is seen as inhomogeneous hypoechoic or echogenic areas within the myometrium, having indistinct margins, and localized adenomyomas are seen as inhomogeneous areas of myometrium with indistinct margins and anechoic spaces on transvaginal sonography. Occasionally, adenomyomas may appear as well defined homogeneous masses in intramural or subserosal location with no evidence of any distal acoustic shadowing or calcification; distinguishing them from fibroids. Ill-defined cystic areas within the myometrium may result secondary to hemorrhagic collection within the adenomyotic cyst.

Abnormalities of Endometrium

Hydrometra and Hematometra (Figs. 17.8A and B)

Acquired causes of these conditions are cervical stenosis resulting from endometrial or cervical tumors or post-irradiation fibrosis. Patients are middle aged or elderly females with clinical features of the underlying cause and a pelvic lump. Sonographically, a distended, fluid filled endometrial cavity containing echogenic material is seen. Pyometra is caused by superimposed infection. It has a similar ultrasound picture with clinical features suggestive of infection.

Endometrial Hyperplasia (Figs. 17.9 and 17.10)

Hyperplastic endometrium develops due to unopposed estrogen hormone replacement therapy, i.e., post- or perimenopausal females. It presents as abnormal uterine bleeding. Women of reproductive age group with persistent anovulatory cycles, polycystic ovaries disease or estrogen producing tumors (like granulosa cell tumors and thecomas of the ovary) may also have a hyperplastic endometrium. Sonographically a thick, echogenic, endometrium with well-defined margins is present. Small cysts may be seen as anechoic spaces within the endometrial echo.

Endometrial Atrophy

Majority of the females presenting with postmenopausal bleeding have endometrial atrophy. On sonography a thin (less than 5 mm) endometrium is seen.

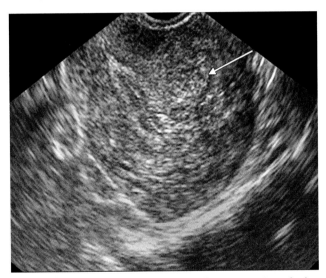

Fig. 17.7: An ill-defined echogenic adenomyomatous lesion in the myometrium with mass effect on the endometrial echo complex (white arrow).

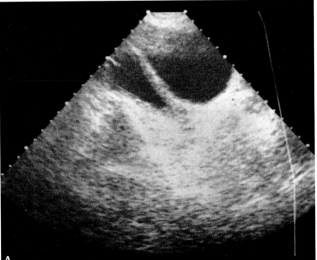
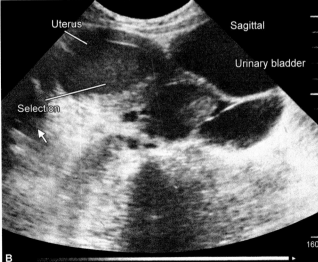

Figs. 17.8A and B: (A) Uterine cavity filled with low level echoes in a case of pyometra with cervical stenosis; (B) Hematometra with hematosalpinx—uterine cavity is distended with fluid showing low level echoes. Dilated fallopian tube is showing low level echoes, septal and echogenic clot inside it.

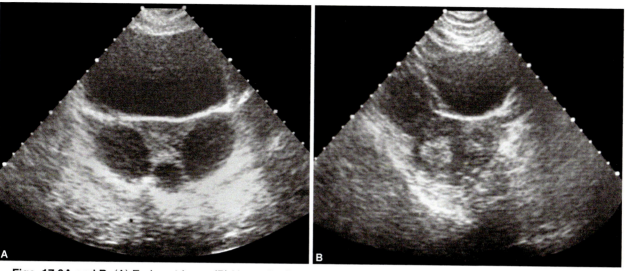

Figs. 17.9A and B: (A) Endometrioma; (B) Hyperplastic endometrium in uterus with cystic lesion in left ovary—ectopic pregnancy cannot be ruled out in such case.

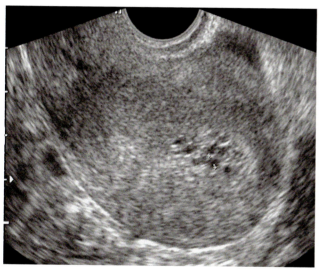

Fig. 17.10: Cystic endometrial hyperplasia.

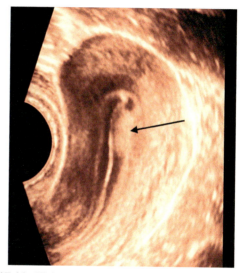

Fig. 17.11: 3D longitudinal US scan shows an endometrial polyp (black arrow).

Endometrial Polyp (Fig. 17.11)

Endometrial polyps are common lesions and most frequently occur in perimenopausal and postmenopausal women. Most are asymptomatic, but may present with uterine bleeding. In menstruating females they present with intermenstrual bleeding or infertility. Occasionally, a polyp may have a long stalk and protrude into the cervix or the vagina. On sonography, polyp appears as nonspecific endometrial thickening, which may be diffuse or localized. They may appear as focal, rounds, echogenic mass within the endometrial cavity. Cystic areas may be seen inside a polyp as anechoic spaces.

Endometrial Carcinoma (Fig. 17.12)

Carcinoma of the endometrium is a common gynecological malignancy. Most cases occur in postmenopausal women and the most common clinical presentation is uterine bleeding. Sonographically, a thickened endometrium is considered malignant until proved otherwise. The thickened endometrium may be well-defined, uniformly echogenic or of inhomogeneous echotexture with ill defined margins. Associated hydrometra or hematometra may be present. Intactness of the subendometrial halo (the inner layer of myometrium) usually indicates superficial invasion, whereas obliteration of the halo is indicative of deep invasion, lymphadenopathy and distant spread of the malignancy is also demonstrated on ultrasound.

Endometritis

Women of reproductive age group following delivery, dilatation and curettage or pelvic inflammatory disease may be affected by this disease. On ultrasound, endometrium

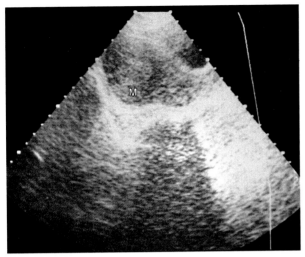

Fig. 17.12: Choriocarcinoma seen as echogenic mass in fundus involving the myometrium posteriorly.

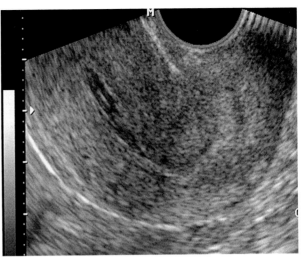

Fig. 17.13: Multiple synechia in the uterine cavity in an infertile female.

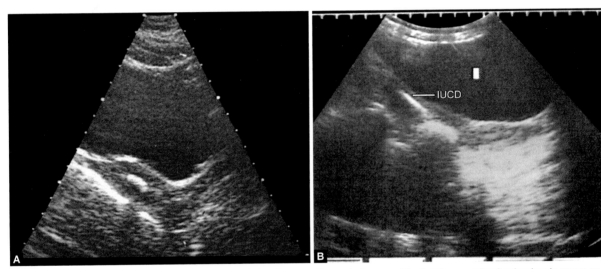

Figs. 17.14A and B: (A) Foreign body in uterus; (B) A linear echogenic focus with distal acoustic shadowing is seen outside the uterine cavity representing misplaced intrauterine contraceptive device (IUCD).

may appear thickened, irregular with or without presence of fluid in the endometrial cavity. Gas, if present is seen as echogenic foci with distal reverberation artifacts.

Endometrial Adhesions (Fig. 17.13)

This disease entity may present with infertility or recurrent abortions. Sonographically adhesions are seen as irregularities or hypoechoic bridge-like band within the endometrium. This is appreciated best in the secretory phase or when fluid is present in the endometrial cavity. A normal endometrium does not rule out presence of adhesions.

Intrauterine Contraceptive Device (IUCD) (Figs. 17.14A and B)

Sonographically these appear as highly echogenic linear structures in the endometrial cavity in the body of the uterus. Acoustic shadowing is usually demonstrated from the echogenic focus. Eccentric position of the device suggests myometrial penetration.

Retained Products of Conception (Fig. 17.15)

Following delivery or abortion secondary postpartum hemorrhage or prolonged bleeding per vaginum suggests retained products. Sonographically, an echogenic mass in the endometrial cavity is seen. A heterogeneous mass may also be seen.

Ectopic Pregnancy (Fig. 17.16)

Presence of pregnancy outside the normal uterine location is termed ectopic. The infertile women of known tubal disease, cases of tubal surgery, pelvic inflammatory disease or intrauterine contraceptive devices are at increased risk of ectopic pregnancy. Patients are of reproductive age group and present with pain, abnormal bleeding, missed

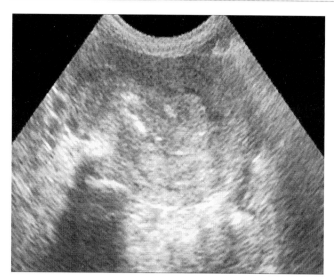

Fig. 17.15: Retained products of conceptus in a postabortal uterus.

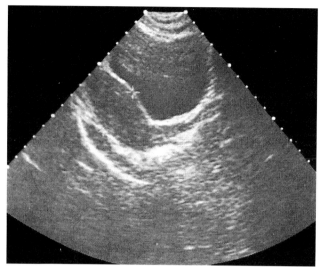

Fig. 17.17: A small conical cervix is seen consistent with hypoplastic cervix.

Cervical Polyp

Polyps usually present with cervical bleeding. They are sonographically seen as an echogenic, well-defined mass.

Cervical Carcinoma (Fig. 17.19)

Patients of cervical carcinoma present with post-coital bleeding or watery blood mixed discharge per vaginum. Sonography reveals a heterogeneous mass in the cervical region. Posterior wall of the bladder or the lower ureters may be involved causing hydronephrosis. Pelvic lymphadenopathy if present is also detected on ultrasound.

OVARY

Non-neoplastic Cysts (Figs. 17.20A to I)

Functional cysts—are the most common cause of ovarian enlargement in a young woman.

Follicular Cyst

These are usually asymptomatic, unilateral and detected incidentally in women of reproductive age groups. On ultrasound, they appear as well defined, anechoic cystic structures with in the ovary with evidence of posterior enhancement. Their size ranges from 2.5 to 20 cm.

Corpus Luteal Cyst

Failure of resorption of corpus luteum results in corpus luteal cyst. These are also found in women of reproductive age group and present with pain. These are usually unilateral and more prone to hemorrhage and rupture. On ultrasound it appears as a unilocular, anechoic, rounded-oval structure with well defined walls and posterior acoustic enhancement.

Hemorrhage in to a functional cyst has a variable appearance on sonography. Acute hemorrhagic cyst is

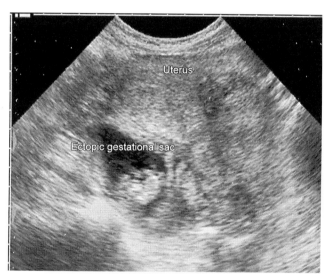

Fig. 17.16: Ectopic pregnancy in the adnexa with no intrauterine gestational sac.

menstrual period, or finding of a tender pelvic mass. Sonographic documentation of an adnexal mass and/or pelvic intraperitoneal fluid in a woman with measurable circulating HCG and no evidence of an intrauterine pregnancy substantially suggest an ectopic pregnancy. Prominent endometrial echoes or a gestation-sac like structure (echogenic rim surrounding fluid collection) in the uterine cavity is present. A complex or an echogenic ring-like adnexal mass with or without free fluid in the cul-de sac and with or without internal echoes is seen.

Abnormalities of Cervix

Nabothian Cysts (Figs. 17.17 and 17.18)

These are common, incidental finding seen as cystic structures in the cervical region. They may be single or multiple and vary size from a few mm to 4 cm.

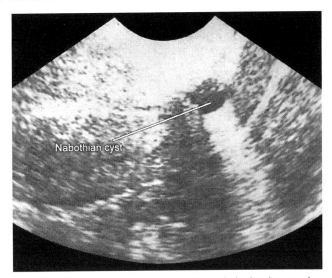

Fig. 17.18: Nabothian cyst—a small cystic lesion is seen in cervix in this longitudinal transvaginal scan of uterus.

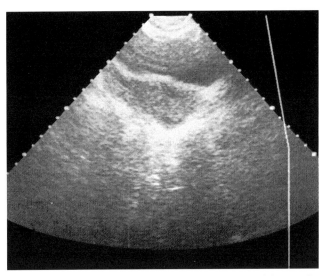

Fig. 17.19: Carcinoma cervix—longitudinal scan of the cervix shows an irregular growth. Base of the bladder is not involved.

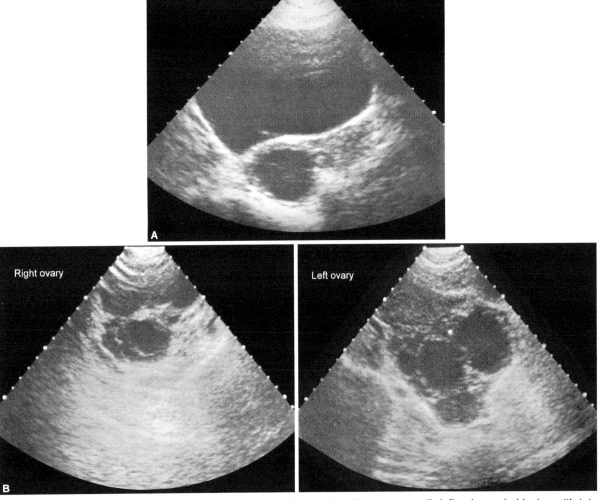

Figs. 17.20A and B: (A) Functional ovarian cyst with internal hemorrhage is seen as well-defined rounded lesion with internal echoes inside it; (B) Theca lutein cyst seen on follow-up case of hydatidiform mole. Bilateral adnexal lesions are showing multiseptate appearance.

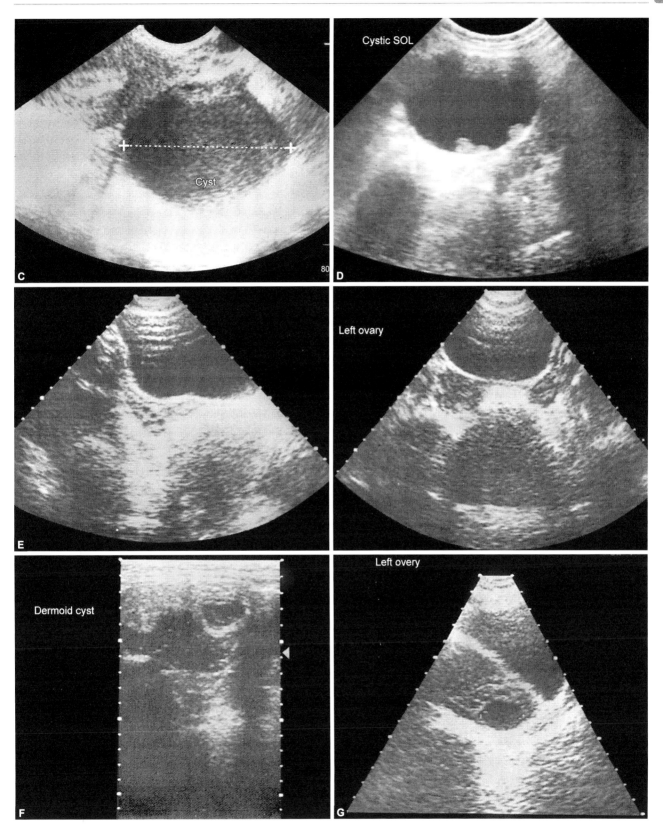

Figs. 17.20C to G: (C) Hemorrhagic cyst of ovary well-defined rounded hypoechoic cystic lesion with low level echoes and forming a level seen on the left of scan; (D) An adnexal cystic SOL with multiple small nodules seen in its wall; (E) Polycystic ovary; (F) Dermoid cyst—a complex mass lesion in right adnexa with solid and cystic areas. Multiple linear hyperechogenic interfaces floating in the mass; (G) Mature follicle in a normal ovary.

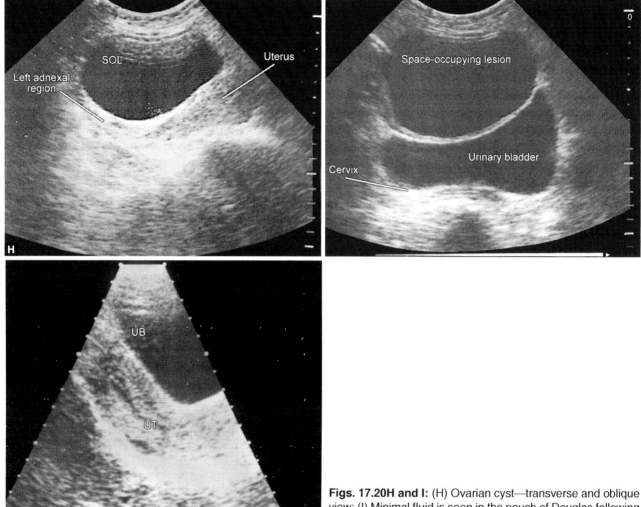

Figs. 17.20H and I: (H) Ovarian cyst—transverse and oblique view; (I) Minimal fluid is seen in the pouch of Douglas following follicular rupture.

usually hyperechoic with clot lyses-a reticular-type pattern containing internal echoes and septations is present. A fluid-filled level may be seen. Presence of echogenic fluid in cul-de-sac represents leaking or ruptured hemorrhagic cyst.

Theca Luteal Cyst

These cysts are found in patients with gestational trophoblastic disease or in ovarian hyperstimulation syndrome associated with high levels of human chorionic gonadotrophin. On ultrasound, bilateral multilocular, large cystic structures are seen. They may undergo hemorrhage, rupture or torsion.

Parovarian (Paratubal) Cysts

These cysts may occur at any age, most commonly in the third and fourth decade of life. 10% of all adnexal masses are parovarian cysts. They are found in the broad ligament and are usually mesothelial or paramesonephric in origin.

On ultrasound a variable sized cyst usually located superior to the uterine fundus is found. A normal, ipsilateral ovary is found close to the cyst. Hemorrhage, rupture or torsion are complications of these cysts.

Peritoneal Inclusion Cysts

These cysts are predominantly found in premenopausal women with a history of previous abdominal surgery, trauma, pelvic inflammatory disease or endometriosis. Presentation is with pain and/or a pelvic mass. Peritoneal inclusion cysts are formed by accumulation of peritoneal fluid within the adhesions with entrapment of the ovaries. On ultrasound, a multiloculated cystic adnexal mass with an intact ovary with septations and fluid are present. Echoes may be present in the cyst.

Endometriosis (Fig. 17.21)

Presence of functioning endometrial tissue outside the uterus (in ovary, fallopian tube, broad ligament, posterior cul-de-sac etc.) is termed endometriosis. It has two forms—a diffuse and localized form. Women of reproductive age group are commonly affected and present with dysmenorrhea, dyspareunia and infertility. The localized form consists of a discrete mass called as endometrioma or chocolate cyst. On sonography, a well-defined, unilocular or multilocular, predominantly cystic mass containing diffuse homogeneous, low-level, internal echoes is seen. Occasionally a fluid-filled level may be seen. This appearance may be confused with a hemorrhagic functional cyst. A hemorrhagic functional cyst presents with acute pelvic pain and may resolve or show a decrease in size, whereas, endometriomas present with chronic symptoms and show little change in size or internal pattern.

Polycystic Ovarian Disease (PCOD) (Fig. 17.22)

Polycystic ovarian disease (PCOD) is a common cause of infertility. PCOD is a complex endocrinological disorder resulting in chronic anovulation. Sonographic findings are those of bilaterally enlarged ovaries containing multiple small follicles and increased stromal echogenicity. The ovaries are rounded in shape and the follicles are usually located peripherally. According to the consensus definition, polycystic ovaries are present when (a) one or both ovaries demonstrate 12 or more follicles measuring 2-9 mm in diameter, or (b) the ovarian volume exceeds 10 cm^3. Only one ovary meeting either of these criteria is sufficient to establish the presence of polycystic ovaries.

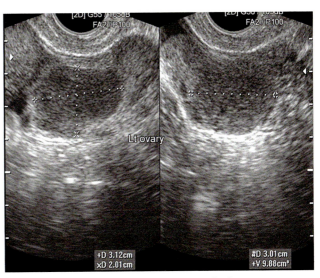

Fig. 17.21: An endometriotic cyst in the ovary.

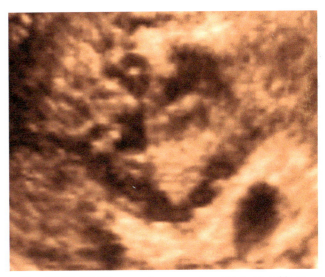

Fig. 17.22: 3D US scan shows a polycystic ovary with an echogenic stroma.

Neoplasms (Figs. 17.23A to J)

Ovarian neoplasms are histologically classified into four types:

Serous Cystadenoma and Cystadenocarcinoma

Thirty percent of all ovarian neoplasms are serous tumors. Half to two-thirds of all the benign neoplasms and half of all the malignant neoplasms are of serous origin. Serous cystadenomas usually occur in the fourth and fifth decades, whereas cystadenocarcinoma occur in perimenopausal and postmenopausal women. Sonographically, serous cystadenomas are usually large, thin-walled, unilocular cystic masses that may contain thin septations with occasional papillary projections. Serous cystadenocarcinomas are larger tumors, multilocular in appearance with multiple papillary projections arising from the cyst wall and thick septae. Echogenic solid material may fill up the loculations. Ascites is frequently seen.

Mucinous Cystadenoma and Cystadenocarcinoma

These are the second most common ovarian neoplasms and majority are benign constituting 20-25% of all benign ovarian neoplasms, and mucinous adenocarcinoma make up 6 to 10 percent of all primary malignant ovarian neoplasm.

Sonographically mucinous cystadenomas are large cystic masses with multiple thin septae and low-level echoes in the dependant portion. Mucinous cystadenocarcinoma are similar to serous cystadenocarcinoma on sonography. Rupture of the tumor into the peritoneal cavity causes pseudomyxoma peritonei.

Endometroid Tumor

These are the second most common epithelial neoplasms. They are seen as cystic masses containing papillary projections or a solid mass with hypoechoic and echogenic areas representing necrosis and hemorrhage respectively.

Clear Cell Tumor

Sonographically, these appear as a complex predominantly cystic mass.

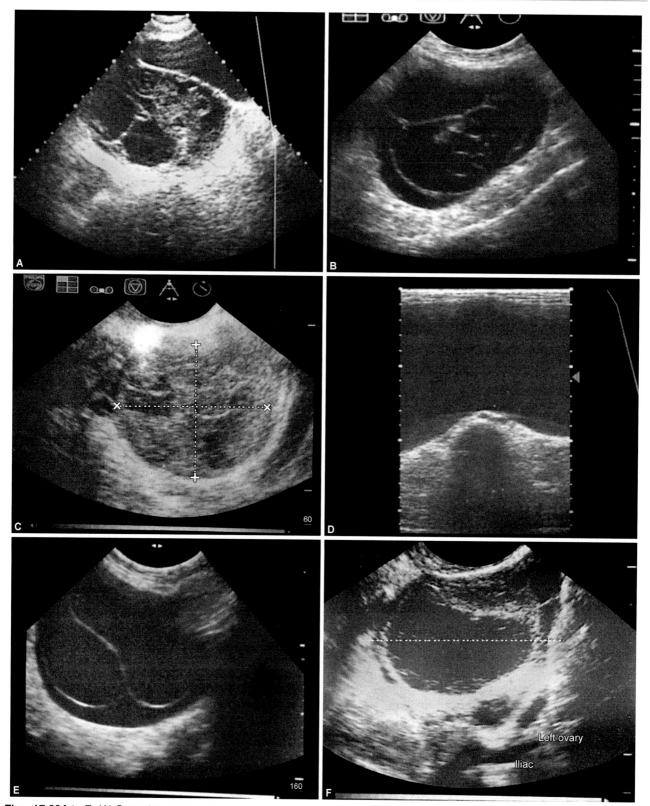

Figs. 17.23A to F: (A) Cystadenocarcinoma—large complex mass with cystic and solid areas and multiple septae in right adnexa; (B) Mucinous cystadenoma large anechoic lesion with multiple septae in right adnexal region; (C) Solid ovarian mass lesion suggestive of ovarian malignancy; (D) Serous cystadenoma—large thin wall anechoic lesion in left adnexal region; (E) Serous cystadenoma—large anechoic lesion with thin septae in right adnexal region; (F) Mucinous cystadenoma—large multiseptate cystic lesion in left ovary.

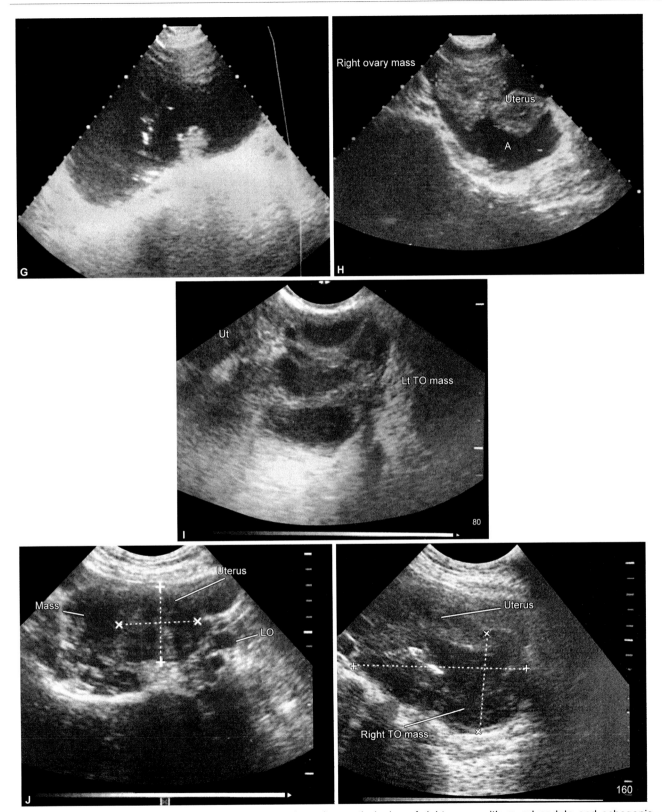

Figs. 17.23G to J: (G) Malignant ovarian mass—an irregular cystic lesion of right ovary with mural nodule and echogenic branching septae; (H) Transverse scan of pelvis shows heterogeneous, predominantly echogenic ovarian mass surrounded by free fluid; (I) Multiseptate complex heterogeneous tubo-ovarian (TO) mass is seen in transverse section; (J) Tubercular tubo-ovarian mass—longitudinal and transverse scan of pelvis showing normal left ovary (LO) and a complex adnexal mass on right side with heterogeneous echotexture. The mass blends with posterior uterine wall. Also evidence of calcification is seen in mass.

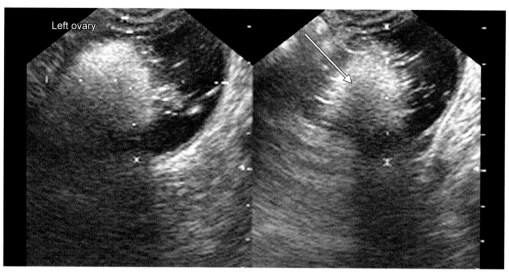

Fig. 17.24: Cystic teratoma with an echogenic dermoid plug (white arrow).

Brenner Tumor or Transitional Cell Tumor

This is an uncommon neoplasm seen as a hypoechoic solid ovarian mass. Calcification may be present in the outer wall.

Germ Cell Tumors

Germ cell tumors are the most common ovarian malignancies in children and young adults. The 95% are benign cystic teratomas, rest are dysgerminomas and endodermal sinus tumors. A malignant germ cell tumor appears as a solid ovarian mass on ultrasound.

Cystic Teratoma (Fig. 17.24)

These account for 15 to 25 percent of all ovarian neoplasms. A cystic teratoma is virtually always benign and is also called dermoid cyst and is seen more commonly in the active reproductive years. Occasionally this tumor is found in postmenopausal women, where the risk of malignant transformation is higher. On ultrasound the appearance of cystic teratoma varies from anechoic to hyperechoic. It may be seen as a predominantly cystic mass with an echogenic mural module (dermoid plug), which frequently casts an acoustic shadowing. A lesion with ill-defined acoustic shadowing that obscures the posterior wall of the lesion may be seen. A fat-fluid level or a hair-fluid level may be apparent.

Sex Cord-stromal Tumors

This group include granulosa cell tumor, Sertoli-Leydig cell tumor, thecomas, and fibromas. This accounts for 5 to 10% of all ovarian neoplasms. These occur in the post menopausal age group except Sertoli-Leydig cell tumor which occurs in women under 30 years of age and presents with features of masculinization. Granulosa cell tumors and thecomas present with clinical signs of estrogen production. Fibromas are relatively asymptomatic sonographically, these tumors are predominantly solid or solid with echogenicity similar to uterine fibroids. Larger granulosa cell tumors are multiloculated and cystic resembling cystadenomas sonographically. Ascites is present in 50% fibromas larger than 5 cm.

Metastatic Tumors

5–10% of ovarian neoplasms are metastatic in origin, mainly from breast and gastrointestinal tract malignancy. On ultrasound usually solid, bilateral ovarian masses are found. In case of necrosis they have a predominantly cystic appearance.

Table 17.1 summarizes different types of tumors and their incidence.

It is important to differentiate benign from malignant ovarian tumors on ultrasound **(Table 17.2)**.

FALLOPIAN TUBE (FIGS. 17.25A AND B)

Pelvic Inflammatory Disease (PID)

This common gynecologic condition affects women of reproductive age group. It is usually due to sexually

TABLE 17.1: Different types of tumors and their incidence.

Type	Incidence	
I. Surface epithelial stromal tumors	65–75%	Serous cystadenoma/carcinoma mucinous cystadenoma/carcinoma Endometrioid carcinoma, clear cell carcinoma
II. Germ cell tumors	15–20%	Transitional cell tumor Teratoma Dysgerminoma Yolk sac tumor
III. Sex cord-stromal tumors	5–10%	Granulosa cell tumor Sertoli-Leydig cell tumor Thecoma and fibroma
IV. Metastatic tumors	5–10%	

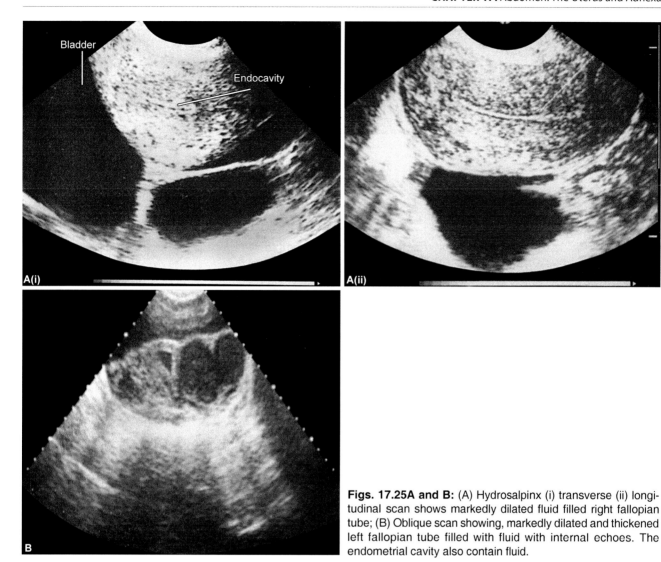

Figs. 17.25A and B: (A) Hydrosalpinx (i) transverse (ii) longitudinal scan shows markedly dilated fluid filled right fallopian tube; (B) Oblique scan showing, markedly dilated and thickened left fallopian tube filled with fluid with internal echoes. The endometrial cavity also contain fluid.

TABLE 17.2: Difference between benign and malignant tumors.

Features	Benign	Malignant
1. Size	Small, usually < 6 cm	Large, usually > 10 cm
2. External contour	Thin wall well-defined borders	Thick wall Ill-defined or irregular borders solid or complex.
3. Internal characteristic	Purely cystic or thin septations	Thick (> 2 mm) septations or irregular septations. Papillary projections or echogenic solid nodules.
4. Associated findings		Ascites, peritoneal implants, liver metastases.

transmitted disease (gonorrhea, chlamydia), tuberculosis, spread from an adjacent inflammatory lesion (appendicular abscess) or post-abortion complication. Presence of an intrauterine contraceptive device increases the changes of PID. Patients present with pain, fever, pelvic tenderness, vaginal discharge, abnormalities in menstruation or infertility (especially in case of tuberculosis). A spectrum of sonographic findings are present according to the stage of the disease. Endometrial thickening or fluid indicates endometritis. Pus may be seen in the cul-de-sac as echogenic material. Periovarian inflammation appears as enlarged ovaries with multiple cysts and indistinct margins. Dilated fallopian tubes appear as complex predominantly cystic masses. Pyosalpinx is seen as tubular or funnel-shaped cystic structure with internal echoes or pus-fluid level. In hydrosalpinx no internal echoes are seen. A tubo-ovarian mass appears as a complex mass incorporating the ovary. A tubo-ovarian abscess appears as a complex multiloculated mass with septations, irregular margins and internal echoes, debris-fluid level or gas seen as echogenic with reverberation artifacts. Posterior acoustic enhancement is present in case of an abscess.

18
CHAPTER

Pediatric Abdomen

BILIARY SYSTEM

Neonatal Jaundice

Mild physiological jaundice occurs in 90% of newborn, usually between the second and eighth day of life. If the jaundice is noted within 24 hours or the bilirubin exceeds 200 mmol/L, if it persists after 8 days, an underlying pathology is looked for. Conjugated hyperbilirubinemia may be 'medical' in origin but also raises the possibility of a structural defect of the biliary system including:
- Extrahepatic biliary atresia
- Choledochal cyst
- Biliary hypoplasia
- Inspissated bile syndrome
- Choledocholithiasis
- Bile duct stenosis
- Spontaneous perforation of bile duct.

Obstructive jaundice in childhood is most likely to be associated with choledochal cyst, biliary calculi, and rarely bile duct tumors, pancreatic mass, lymphadenopathy and subhepatic benign masses of pancreatic or bowel origin may obstruct the common duct.

Biliary Atresia

Congenital extrahepatic biliary atresia occurs in 1 per 10,000 live births and if untreated, gives rise to secondary biliary cirrhosis and death with in the first two years of life. The etiology is an aggressive inflammatory process which damages and destroys the biliary tree and gives rise to apparent atresia. The 25% of babies with biliary atresia have an associated congenital anomaly like intestinal malrotation, situs inverses abdominus, polysplenia, preduodenal portal vein or abnormalities of inferior vena cava. On sonography, 70% of the gallbladder are found to be small with thickened wall and irregular shape. There is failure to detect the intrahepatic bile ducts, and common hepatic ducts. Ultrasound finding of a known associated anomaly may be the strongest evidence for the diagnosis.

Choledochal Cyst

Choledochal cysts are congenital cystic dilatation of the common bile duct and a large majority present in childhood, usually with recurrent jaundice. The classic and most common form of choledochal cyst is a large spherical subhepatic cyst. Patients with this type of cyst may present in the neonatal period as well. The cyst is echo-free. An associated pancreatic disease should be ruled out since it is liable to occur due to abnormal insertion of the pancreatic and biliary duct into the ampulla.

Rhabdomyosarcoma

A rare differential diagnosis of choledochal cyst is rhabdomyosarcoma of the common bile duct which often has a similar clinical presentation. On sonography, common bile duct is dilated and filled with structured echoes.

Inspissated Bile Duct Syndrome

This syndrome is responsible for a minority of cases of neonatal jaundice. On sonography the common bile duct is dilated up to the lower end and may be associated with dilatation of the gall-bladder which may also contain inspissated bile or frank calculi seen as echogenic bile or echogenic foci with acoustic shadowing, respectively.

Spontaneous Perforation of Bile Duct

This rare condition occurs in cases of distal common bile duct obstruction due to inspissated bile or calculi. Patients present between two and eight weeks with jaundice and ascites. On ultrasound a subhepatic fluid collection which usually contains structured echoes and ascites are found.

GALLBLADDER

Primary disease of gallbladder is rare in children.
- Calculi—seen as echogenic focus with distal shadowing may be seen in children with metabolic disorders, hemoglobinopathies (sickle cell anemia).
- Acute cholecystitis—is rare in pediatric patients and may be of acalculous variety. Cystic duct obstruction by parasites such as ascaris should be considered.
- Hydrops—occasionally the gallbladder may be found to be distended in children with acute upper quadrant pain with no fever, leukocytosis or hyperbilirubinemia. On ultrasound a tense, distended gallbladder with no

evidence of calculi or bile duct dilatation is seen. This is a benign self-limiting condition.

LIVER

Congenital Abnormalities

Cardiac malpositions in children are associated with abnormalities of position of liver and spleen. Mirror image dextrocardia is most common form. There is complete inversion of cardiac chambers with apex towards, right, and situs inversus, with liver towards the left and stomach and spleen on the right side of abdomen.

Liver is usually right sided in cases of dextroversion with situs solitus. Liver is midline in cases of polysplenia or asplenia.

Congenital cysts of liver are uncommon and are derived from the biliary tree and may occur in any lobe. These may be associated with renal and pancreatic cysts.

Diffuse Parenchymal Liver Disease

Hepatomegaly and a generalized alteration in the normal reflectivity are features of diffuse parenchymal disease of the liver.

- *Acute hepatitis:* In this condition sonography shows an enlarged liver with a normal or diffuse echo poor pattern with accentuation of the periportal echoes. Acute hepatitis is caused by a number of causes—viral infection viz. hepatitis A and B, Ebstein Barr virus, cytomegalovirus, drugs, toxins and Reye's syndrome. Ultrasound also helps to exclude a surgical cause of jaundice by excluding biliary tree dilatation.
- *Hepatomegaly with a homogeneous increase in reflectivity and attenuation occurs in numerous conditions:* Reye's syndrome, malnutrition, obesity, steroids, metabolic liver disease (glycogen storage disease, Wilson's disease, Gaucher's disease, etc). All these condition cause a fatty liver.
- Chronic liver disease with cirrhosis and fibrosis is sonographically seen as increased parenchymal reflectivity which may be non-uniform with a nodular pattern. The liver may be enlarged or small with an irregular surface. Periportal fibrosis appears as periportal increased echogenicity. The caudate lobe is enlarged relative to the rest of the liver. The various conditions giving this sonographic appearance are cystic fibrosis, later stages of metabolic liver disease, hepatic fibrosis in renal cystic disease, biliary atresia, etc.

Hepatic Calcification

Calcification in the liver may be seen with congenital infections, toxoplasmosis, rubella, cytomegalovirus, and herpes simplex. It also follows granulomatous infections like tuberculosis. Hepatic masses like hepatoblastoma, hemangiomas and teratomas may show evidence of calcification. Metastatic neuroblastoma may also calcify in the liver. Sonographically highly echogenic focus with distal acoustic shadowing is present.

Hepatic Abscess

In children presenting with fever, hepatomegaly and upper abdominal pain sonography is done to exclude liver abscesses. Liver abscess may be pyogenic or amebic. On ultrasound they have a variable appearance. Honeycombed abscesses are more commonly pyogenic whereas those sharply defined with a peripheral halo and homogeneous appearance are amebic abscesses.

Portal Hypertension

Portal hypertension follows intrahepatic or extrahepatic obstruction to the portal system.

Extrahepatic Obstruction

It follows thrombosis of portal vein and is seen in infants with a history of neonatal sepsis and dehydration or neonatal umbilical venous catheterization. It may occur as a complication of appendicitis in older children or follow splenectomy. Cases present with splenomegaly and variceal bleeding. On ultrasound multiple collateral develop in the porta hepatis. Collaterals may be seen at other places like splenorenal, ligamentum teres and around the spleen.

Intrahepatic Obstruction

Chronic liver disease with cirrhosis causes features of portal hypertension.

Hepatic Neoplasms

Benign Hepatic Neoplasms

These comprise about a third of all primary liver tumors in childhood. The majority are mesenchymal in origin and include hemangiomas, hemangioendothelioma and mesenchymal hamartoma.

- *Hemangiomas:* Benign vascular tumors of the liver may be solitary or multiple. They are divided into cavernous and capillary lesions. The commoner ones are capillary hemangiomas and hemangioendotheliomas. They are usually symptomatic and present with an abdominal mass or congestive cardiac failure or rarely thrombocytopenia due to platelet trapping. Sonographically these appear as clearly defined lesions with a reflectivity less than that of the liver. Very occasionally focal calcification may be seen. The celiac axis and common hepatic artery are dilated with prominent draining hepatic veins.
- *Mesenchymal hamartoma:* This is a well-defined large liver tumor which usually presents in the first two years of life and is slightly more common in males. Sonography demonstrates a large, discrete, solitary mass

which is predominantly cystic with numerous septa. The lesion is typically found in the right lobe.

Malignant Hepatic Neoplasm

Five percent of the pediatric tumors and two-thirds of the hepatic tumors are malignant tumors. These are of four types—hepatoblastoma, hepatocellular carcinoma, fibrolamellar carcinoma and the mesenchymoma.

- *Hepatoblastoma:* This malignant tumor occurs in children is up to three years of age and is associated with hemihypertrophy, Beckwith-Wiedemann syndrome and familial polyposis coli. On ultrasound solitary or multiple lesions with poorly-defined walls and slightly more reflective than normal liver, occasionally with calcification are found in the liver. Venous invasion may occur.
- *Hepatocellular carcinoma:* This tumor occurs in children with two peaks of incidence at 1 year and 13 years of age. Some cases occur in children with pre-existing cirrhosis, there is a very high risk of occurrence of hepatocellular carcinoma in patients with hereditary tyrosinemia. Sonographically, this tumor is indistinguishable from hepatoblastoma. Poorly defined reflective mass is seen. Lesions are multiple in some cases, invasion of the hepatic and portal veins and inferior vena cava may occur.
- *Fibrolamellar carcinoma:* A rare variant of hepatocellular carcinoma usually affecting older children. A well defined reflective mass is present.
- *Mesenchymoma:* Also called as undifferentiated sarcoma of the liver, presents in older children (peak age 11 years) and is solid and reflective, but most appear as multiseptate cystic lesions.

Metastases

Secondary deposits from Wilm's tumor, neuroblastoma, teratoma, lymphoma and leukemia may occur. Wilms' tumor produces solitary or multiple reflective metastases in the liver. Disseminated neuroblastoma with liver involvement appears as gross hepatomegaly with a diffuse irregular texture with nodules of decreased reflectivity. Calcification may be present in the lesions. Lymphoma and leukemia produce hepatosplenomegaly with a diffuse, homogeneous increase in echogenicity throughout the liver, focal echo-poor lesions or a liver with normal echo pattern.

SPLEEN

In both polysplenia and asplenia, liver lies in the midline of the abdomen. Associated abnormality of abdominal vasculature like absent inferior vena cava or its continuation into the azygos or hemiazygos veins may be seen.

A preduodenal portal vein may be found. Ectopic spleen—no spleen is detected in its usual position and the patients present with intermittent abdominal pain due to torsion around the splenic pedicle of a malpositioned spleen.

Accessory spleen is seen on ultrasound as a rounded mass near the splenic hilum with a similar echotexture as the normal spleen.

Hepatomegaly and splenomegaly may be seen in the neonate with congenital infections like rubella, toxoplasmosis, cytomegalovirus, herpes and syphilis. Foci of calcification may be present within the liver.

Other causes of splenomegaly are:
- Chronic hepatic disease, with portal hypertension—spleen appears more reflective.
- Lymphoma and leukemia
- Hemolytic anemias
- Gaucher's disease, glycogen storage disease, mucopolysaccharidoses
- Viral infections
- Splenic masses—splenic masses are rare in childhood
- Congenital or epidermoid cysts occasionally present in childhood. On sonography they appear as a well-defined cystic an echoic posteriorly enhancing lesion with or without evidence of wall calcification.

URINARY TRACT

Congenital Anomalies of Urinary Tract

Renal Duplication

A common congenital anomaly of the urinary tract is duplication of the collecting system, which may be partial or complete. In complete duplication, two pelvis and two separate ureters drain the kidney. The upper moiety ureter inserts ectopically, inferior and medial to the site of normal ureteral insertion. Its orifice may be stenotic or associated with a ureterocele resulting in obstructive dilatation of the pelvicalyceal system of upper moiety. The lower moiety is usually affected by reflux. Sonographically a duplex collecting system is diagnosed by separation of the central echo complex into two parts by a column of normal renal parenchyma. A dilated collecting system of the upper moiety may be seen. The ureterocele is seen as a cyst like structure within the bladder. Unobstructed but dilated pelvicalyceal system of the lower moiety suggests the presence of vesicoureteric reflux.

Hydronephrosis

Dilatation of the renal collecting system is a common problem in the pediatric patient. Dilatation may be due to obstruction, reflux, or abnormal muscle development.

Ureteropelvic Junction (UPJ) Obstruction

A hydronephrotic kidney is the most common neonatal abdominal mass. Obstruction is commonly encountered at the UPJ, secondary to a functional stricture which results in failure to initiate a normal peristaltic wave within the ureter. This results in a dilated collecting system, whereas the ureter is normal in caliber. Sonographically a grossly hydronephrotic kidney appears as a cystic mass, reniform in shape in the renal fossa. The dilated pelvis is seen as a larger medially placed cyst communicating with smaller cysts placed around it, representing the dilated calyces. The ureter is not visualized. This condition is found more commonly in males with more frequent involvement of the left kidney.

Ureteral Obstruction

Obstruction can be encountered anywhere along the course of the ureter. It may be extrinsic cause by a mass (such as lymphadenopathy, abscess, etc.) or intrinsic due to stone or blood clot. Obstruction at the vesicoureteric junction can occur due to primary megaureter or ureteroceles.

Primary megaureter: A segment of the distal ureter is devoid of muscle and narrowed by an increase in fibrous tissue. Sonographically there is a variable degree of dilatation of the intrarenal collecting system and the ureter proximal to the narrow segment of distal ureter.

Bladder Outlet Obstruction

Bilateral hydronephrosis is frequently caused by obstruction at the level of bladder or bladder outlet.
- *Neurogenic bladder:* Sonographically it appears as a thick walled and/or dilated bladder with bilateral dilatation of collecting system and ureters.
- *Posterior urethral valves:* On ultrasound an enlarged bladder with thick irregular walls suggests bladder outlet obstruction. A dilated posterior urethra suggests the presence of posterior urethral valves. Bilateral upper urinary tracts are dilated.

Prune Belly Syndrome

Prune belly or abdominal muscle deficiency syndrome includes congenital absence or deficiency of abdominal musculature, large hypotonic dilated tortuous ureters, a large bladder, a patent urachus, dilated posterior urethra and cryptorchidism.

Vesicoureteric Reflux

This is a common cause of nonobstructive hydronephrosis in infants and children. Reflux can be unilateral or bilateral and of different grades. When the reflux of urine is up to the pelvicalyceal system with resultant dilatation of the collecting system, US helps in diagnosing this entity. US reveal unilateral or bilateral hydronephrosis with a hydroureter in the absence of an obstructive lesion in the urinary tract.

MEDICAL RENAL DISEASES

Acute Tubular Necrosis

This is the most common cause of reversible acute renal failure. The various etiological factors are dehydration, sepsis, drugs, hypotension, etc. On sonography no findings may be evident, but some cases show bilateral renal enlargement with enlarged well-defined pyramids or increased cortical reflectivity with preservation of corticomedullary differentiation.

Medullary Sponge Kidney

This is probably a developmental anomaly leading to dilatation of the distal collecting tubules in the medullary papillae. Children present with symptoms of renal calculus like pain and hematuria, but initially the patients are asymptomatic. Ultrasound may show early nephrocalcinosis as increased echogenicity of the renal pyramids. No shadowing is evident in the early stage of the disease but later highly echogenic medulla with distal acoustic shadowing is seen.

Nephrotic Syndrome

Nephrotic syndrome presents with albuminuria, hypoalbuminemia, and swelling. It may be caused by primary renal or systemic conditions and is seen in the younger children. Acute poststreptococcal glomerulonephritis predominates in the older children. On ultrasound normal sized kidneys may be seen or both the kidneys may demonstrate enlargement. The cortical reflectivity is increased with preservation of corticomedullary differentiation.

Renal Vein Thrombosis

Renal vein thrombosis (RVT) is relatively common in the neonate and may result from hemoconcentration especially due to dehydration. Adrenal hemorrhage may be associated with it. On ultrasound, in the acute phase the kidney is enlarged with patchy increase in cortical reflectivity. Some corticomedullary differentiation may still be evident. The kidneys ultimately become smaller and less echogenic than in the acute stage, ultimately returning to normal echotexture but small in size.

Nephrocalcinosis

Nephrocalcinosis is characterised by the presence of calcium deposits in the renal parenchyma when associated with metabolic disease it is most prominent in the medulla, especially at the corticomedullary junction.

Cortical nephrocalcinosis may be a consequence of cortical necrosis for example in a child who had renal vein thrombosis as a neonate.

Medullary nephrocalcinosis is usually associated with hypercalciuria, hypercalcemia, distal renal tubular acidosis, hypervitaminosis D, etc. On ultrasound medullary nephrocalcinosis is seen as a highly reflective rim around the sides and tip of medulla or as more intense rim with some infilling of the medulla or as echogenic medulla with shadowing or as a solitary focus of intense echoes at the tips of the pyramid casting acoustic shadows.

KIDNEYS

Cystic Renal Diseases of Children

Medullary Cystic Disease

This disease of unknown pathogenesis occurs due to progressive renal tubular atrophy. The childhood form is an autosomal recessive disorder. On sonography small echogenic kidneys with medullary cysts are present.

Autosomal Recessive Polycystic Kidney Disease

Autosomal recessive polycystic kidney disease (ARPCK) presents with renal abnormality in the younger patients (neonatal, infantile) and older patients (juvenile) have predominantly hepatic abnormality due to associated periportal fibrosis. Sonography shows massively enlarged, echogenic kidneys with lack of corticomedullary differentiation. In the intrauterine period these findings are present with hypoplastic lungs and oligohydramnios.

Multicystic Dysplastic Kidney

Also called as renal dysplasia, it characterises small, malformed non- or poorly functioning kidneys. Males and females are equally affected, 30% cases have contralateral pelviureteric junction obstruction. Sonography demonstrates multiple, non-communicating cysts with absence of both normal renal parenchyma and normal renal sinus. Focal echogenic areas if present represent primitive mesenchymal tissue or tiny cysts.

Tumors

Multilocular Cystic Nephroma

This is an uncommon benign neoplasm composed of multiple, non-communicating cysts contained within a well-defined capsule. Occasionally bilateral lesions are found. Males less than four years of age and females between 4 and 20 or 40 and 60 years are affected. Most children present with an abdominal mass.

Mesoblastic Nephroma

This is the most common renal tumor diagnosed in early infancy. It is usually found in children less than three month of age and sonographically presents as a solid mass with occasional cystic areas with in it.

Wilms' Tumor (Nephroblastoma) (Figs. 18.1A and B)

This tumor is a malignant renal tumor and the second most common tumor of childhood after neuroblastoma. It may be polar in location or replace the whole kidney. Sonography shows an encapsulated, heterogeneous lesion replacing a part or the entire kidney. The lesion could be hypo, iso or even moderately hyperechoic. Necrosis if present is seen as irregular anechoic areas within the lesion. Involvement of the renal vein and inferior vena cava may occur. The contralateral kidney should be evaluated since the lesion may be bilateral.

Metastatic Involvement

Lymphoma and leukemia can spread to the kidneys by blood route.

Lymphoma—focal parenchymal involvement is seen on ultrasound as solitary or multiple homogeneous, hypoechoic

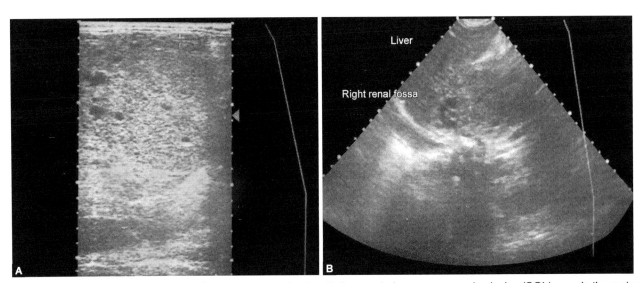

Figs. 18.1A and B: (A) Wilms' tumor—a homogenous predominantly hyperechoic space-occupying lesion (SOL) seen in the region of lower pole of right kidney; (B) Postoperative case of Wilms' tumor showing recurrence of the tumor seen as a heterogeneous echotexture mass lesion with anechoic areas right representing necrosis in it.

nodules. Diffuse involvement causes disruption of the normal renal architecture with usually a hypoechoic appearance. Leukemic renal involvement sonographically shows bilateral diffuse renal enlargement with a coarsened echopattern or a diffuse decrease in echogenicity with distortion of the central sinus echo-complex. Focal involvement is with solitary or multifocal hypoechoic nodules.

Adrenals

Adrenal Hemorrhage

The large adrenal gland of the neonate undergoes a marked reduction in size following birth. The vessels in the primitive adrenal cortex are prone to hemorrhage. Hemorrhage occurs in stressful conditions like birth trauma, anoxia and systemic illness and infants present within two to seven days of birth. Right adrenal gland is more commonly involved with up to 10% cases having bilateral involvement. On sonography, the adrenal hematoma is usually echo-free and becomes more reflective due to fibrin strand formation as resolution occurs. The hematoma may resolve, calcify or remain as a residual adrenal cyst.

Congenital Adrenal Hyperplasia

Congenital adrenal hyperplasia is an autosomal recessive disorder due to an inborn error of metabolism in the enzymatic production of cortisol. Deficiency in hormone results in over production of adrenocorticotropic hormone. The two most common syndromes are virilizing form also called as adrenogenital syndromes and salt loosing form. In adrenogenital syndrome female children present with ambiguous genitalia. Sonography shows adrenal gland enlargement in these cases and presence of a uterus establishes the gender of the baby with ambiguous genitalia.

Neuroblastoma (Figs. 18.2A and B)

This is the second most common abdominal malignancy in childhood and is seen most frequently during the first

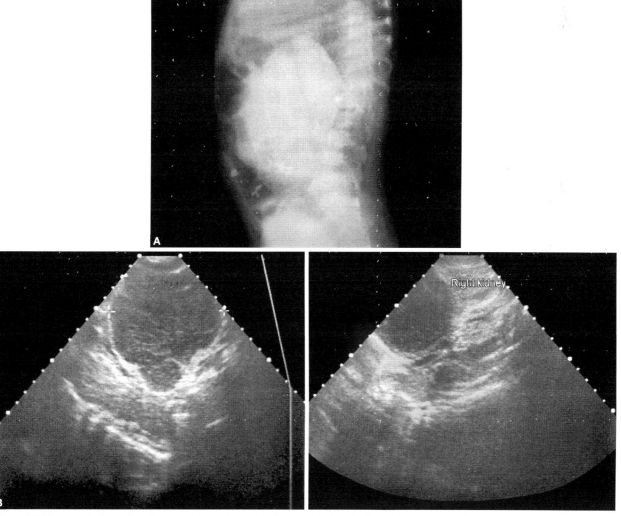

Figs. 18.2A and B: Neuroblastoma—a large hypoechoic mass lesion in the region of adrenal gland which is displacing the kidney anteriorly and inferiorly (A) IVP; and (B) USG.

four years of life. Two-thirds of neuroblastomas occur in the abdomen and 65% of these are suprarenal. Patients present with general debility, weight loss, fever and abdominal mass. Three fourths have metastases at the time of presentation. Ultrasound examination reveals a poorly defined echogenic mass which displaces the normal kidney and characteristically crosses the midline, infiltrating the retroperitoneal tissues and surrounding the aorta and inferior vena cava (IVC). Necrosis and calcification seen as hypoechoic areas and echogenic foci with distal shadowing, respectively, may be seen in the tumor mass. The main differential diagnosis is Wilms' tumor which is renal in origin, encapsulated and thus well defined, homogenous lesion not crossing the midline.

Wolman's Disease

Wolman's disease is a rare autosomal recessive lipid storage disease due to deficiency of liposomal acid lipase. Most patients die within six months of birth. There is marked hepatosplenomegaly and massive adrenal gland enlargement. The adrenal glands demonstrate diffuse punctate calcification.

GASTROINTESTINAL TRACT

Esophagus

Gastroesophageal Reflux

On ultrasound gastroesophageal (GE) junction is visualized by examining the patient with sagittal images in supine position. Regurgitation of fluid from the stomach into the retrocardiac portion of the esophagus suggests reflux.

Stomach

Hypertrophic Pyloric Stenosis (HPS) (Fig. 18.3)

Ultrasound demonstrates gastric muscle thickening the hallmark of HPS as a hypoechoic layer just superficial to the more echogenic mucosal layer of the pyloric canal. In transverse section it appears as a sonolucent "doughnut" muscle width of 3 mm or more is diagnostic of HPS. Pyloric canal length equal to or greater than 1.2 cm and no peristalsis through the pylorus are additional diagnostic points. Active gastric peristaltic waves end abruptly at the margin of the hypertrophied muscle with absence of normal opening of the pylorus.

Gastric Diaphragms

Gastric diaphragm or web, are congenital membranes extending across the gastric antrum. Sonographically they appear as echogenic band across the distal gastric antrum.

Bezoar

Lactobezoars are the most common form of bezoars in children, occurring predominantly in infants fed with improperly reconstituted powdered milk. A fluid filled stomach reveals lactobezoars as a solid, heterogeneous, echogenic intraluminal mass on ultrasound. Trichobezoars is seen in older children and on US appears as a characteristic arc of echogenicity that obscures the mass.

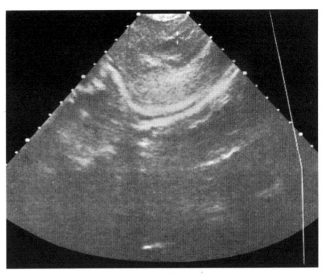

Fig. 18.3: Infantile hypertrophic pyloric stenosis. The total length of the canal is 24 mm. The diameter of the antrum is 15 mm. The muscle thickness is 10 mm.

Duodenum and Small Bowel

Congenital Duodenal Obstruction

Various causes of congenital duodenal obstruction are duodenal atresia with or without associated annular pancreas, duodenal stenosis, duodenal diaphragms, congenital band associated with midgut volvulus. The newborn or infant presents with bilious vomiting. With sonography, characteristically dilated duodenal bulb, stomach and even distal esophagus may be readily demonstrable. Severe duodenal stenosis may mimic atresia. In mid gut volvulus, a churning peristalsis of the duodenal C-loop is seen with characteristic tapering of the distal, twisted end. In this condition abnormal position of superior mesenteric vein and artery can be identified because they are rotated out of normal position as a result of volvulus.

Small Bowel Obstruction

On ultrasound multiple loops of fluid distended small bowel showing hyperperistalsis are seen.

Intussusception

Most cases of intussusception occur between 6 months and 4 years of age. Clinical presentation is intermittent colicky pain, vomiting and passage of blood per rectum. Ileocolic type is the most common variety and on ultrasound it appears as an oval, pseudokidney mass with central echoes on longitudinal scan and a sonolucent doughnut or target configuration on cross-sectional scans. Multiple concentric rings may be seen on coronal scans.

GASTROINTESTINAL MASSES

Duplication Cyst

Gastrointestinal (GI) duplication is the most common abdominal mass of GI origin in the neonate. It occurs more frequently in the small bowel, at the terminal ileum. Ultrasound will demonstrate a well-defined cystic mass with double layered wall, having both mucosal and muscular layer. Occasionally debris may be present in the cyst due to hemorrhage.

TERATOMA

Abdominal teratoma may be attached to the stomach or located in the retroperitoneum. Sacrococcygeal region is the most common location. Majority are benign with a potential for malignant change. US will demonstrate a well-defined mass with solid and cystic areas. Calcification appears as echogenic focus with distal acoustic shadowing. A fat-fluid level may be seen in the cystic components.

Omental and Mesenteric Cysts

These present as a freely mobile abdominal mass in a child. US demonstrates a thin walled, mobile loculated fluid collection without internal echoes. If the cystic mass is large it may be mistaken for ascites. The lesion is usually unilocular but septae may be seen in it.

PANCREAS (FIGS. 18.4A AND B)

Congenital Disorders

Hereditary Pancreatitis

This is an autosomal dominant condition which presents in childhood with chronic pancreatitis. US demonstrates a variable sized pancreas with altered echotexture, irregular margin, calcifications and ductal changes.

Cystic Fibrosis

Pancreatic insufficiency and pancreatitis are features of cystic fibrosis. US reveals changes of chronic pancreatitis with fine granular calcification seen as tiny echogenic foci with or without shadowing.

Pancreatic Masses

Pancreatic tumors are extremely uncommon in children, but insulinomas and enlargement of the pancreas in Beckwith-Wiedemann syndrome may be encountered sporadically.

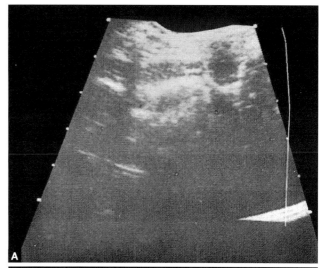

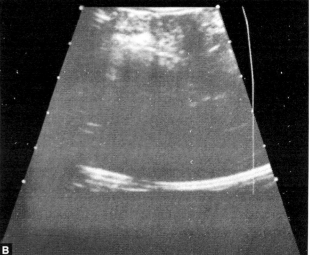

Figs. 18.4A and B: (A) Umbilical cyst—a small anechoic rounded space-occupying lesion (SOL) seen in the region of the umbilicus; and (B) Umbilical granuloma—small defined hypoechoic solid SOL with areas of calcification seen at the umbilicus.

Pancreatic Pseudocyst

Attacks of subacute or chronic pancreatitis result in pseudocyst formation. In children the most common form of pancreatitis is traumatic followed by viral pancreatitis. US demonstrates a cystic, echolucent lesion in a typical location, with or without sonographic findings of pancreatitis.

PERITONEUM

Meconium Peritonitis

Meconium peritonitis occurs due to aseptic chemical inflammation of the peritoneum in cases of prenatal bowel perforation. Intestinal stenosis or atresia and meconium ileus are the most common causes, accounting for 65%

cases. Extravasated meconium causes an intense foreign body reaction leading to fibroadhesive peritonitis that may calcify over time. A fibrous wall may develop around the mass of spilled meconium. On ultrasound it appears as a diffuse echogenicity throughout the abdomen described as a "snow storm" appearance or as a walled off echogenic mass. Calcified peritoneal thickening appears as scattered linear echoes with or without acoustic shadowing.

Pelvic Masses (Fig. 18.5A)

Large pelvic masses in neonate and children often present as an abdominal mass.

Hydrocolpos or Hydrometrocolpos

This accounts for 15% of the abdominal masses in newborn girls. Obstruction of the vaginal (imperforate hymen, stenotic or atretic vagina) results in accumulation of mucous secretions in the vagina and/or the uterine cavity. On sonographic examination hydrocolpos appears as a large tubular cystic mass posterior to the urinary bladder and extending inferior to the pubic symphysis. Low-level echoes inside the fluid represent mucous secretion. A similar condition is found in postpubertal girls but menstrual blood instead of mucous secretion fills up the dilated vagina. This is called as hematocolpos.

Ovarian Masses

- Benign—The majority of the cystic ovarian lesions are benign.
- Dermoid **(Fig. 18.5B)**—a dermoid is the most common benign cystic lesion and is freely mobile on a pedicle and thus more prone to torsion. On US a fat-fluid level is diagnostic of a dermoid.
- Malignant ovarian lesions—Malignant ovarian lesions are rare and appear as solid lesions on US.

Dysgerminoma

This is the most common malignant germ cell tumor of the ovary in childhood. They are found before puberty. On US it appears as a large, solid, encapsulated, rapidly growing mass containing hypoechoic areas. Retroperitoneal lymph nodes may be present as a result of metastatic involvement.

Embryonal Carcinoma

This is a less common malignant germ cell tumor. Choriocarcinoma is extremely rare in children. Both are rapidly growing and appear as solid neoplasms with evidence of direct extension, lymph nodes and peritoneal seedlings.

Epithelial Tumors

These include serous and mucinous cystadenoma or cystadenocarcinoma and represent 20% of ovarian tumors in children. On US they are predominantly cystic masses with septa of variable thickness. It is difficult to differentiate benign from malignant lesions.

Rhabdomyosarcoma

Rhabdomyosarcoma is the most common malignant tumor of the uterus, vagina, bladder, and prostate in childhood. They present as solid masses which are echogenic on ultrasound. Evidence of direct extension of the tumor may be present by presence of poorly defined margins.

RETROPERITONEUM

The most common pathology of the retroperitoneum is the presence of a mass whether solid or cystic. The origin

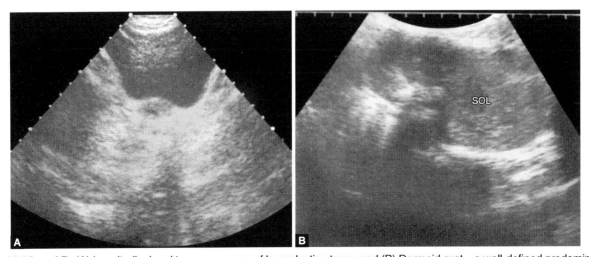

Figs. 18.5A and B: (A) Longitudinal and transverse scan of hypoplastic uterus; and (B) Dermoid cyst—a well-defined predominantly hypoechoic space-occupying lesion (SOL) is seen in the pelvis with evidence of echogenic focus with acoustic shadowing.

of the mass can be renal or non-renal, mainly from the adrenal glands. Pancreatic pseudocyst also present as retroperitoneal collection.

Solid Masses

- *Lymphadenopathy:* Retroperitoneal lymphadenopathy is most commonly seen in lymphoma.
- *Lymphoma:* Its sonographic appearance is variable. Most commonly, discrete hypoechoic masses or anechoic masses are seen both anterior and posterior to the great vessels. Occasionally a hypoechoic mantle of tissue is formed surrounding the aorta. Extranodal lymphoma is also typically hypoechoic, it may be the result of spread from the nodes or arises de novo in the retroperitoneal space.
- Metastases to the retroperitoneal lymph nodes appear as lymph node enlargement, with a more echogenic and heterogeneous appearance.

TUMORS

Teratoma

Teratoma is a germ cell tumor may be attached to the stomach or located in the retroperitoneum. The majority are benign with a potential of malignant transformation with increasing age. On sonography a well defined heterogeneous mass with solid and cystic areas is seen. Calcification may be present as echogenic focus with distal acoustic shadowing. A fat-fluid level may be apparent in the cystic component of the tumor.

Rhabdomyosarcoma

Rhabdomyosarcoma is the most common primary retroperitoneal tumor occurring in the pediatric populations. On sonography it appears as a hypoechoic mass.

Neuroblastoma

Other retroperitoneal tumors found in children are neuroblastomas and ganglioneuroblastomas. Majority of the neuroblastomas arise in the adrenal medullary tissue. Neuroblastomas are one of the most common tumors of childhood with 80% occurring in children less than five years of age. On ultrasound, an ill-defined, heterogeneously echogenic mass with evidence of necrosis and calcification is seen which often crosses the midline.

Retroperitoneal Cysts

These rare lesions may be simple inclusion cysts or cysts of embryonic gastrointestinal and genitourinary tract. Sonographically they appear as simple cysts with smooth well-defined walls and echofree lumen and increased through transmission.

Lymphangioma

Lymphangioma may be seen in children and are multiseptate in appearance.

Retroperitoneal Fluid Collections

These may be abscesses, hematomas, urinoma or lymphoceles.

Psoas Abscess

Psoas abscess is a common pediatric problem most commonly secondary due to a tuberculous bacterial spondylitis. It may present as a palpable tender abdominal mass or occasionally as a lump in upper thigh. It appears as a hypoechoic collection inside the psoas muscle with evidence of posterior enhancement and internal echoes. When extensive it may be track down to the hip joint as well.

Hematomas

Retroperitoneal hematoma may be seen in association with trauma and hemophilia, perirenal hematomas follows renal trauma while hematoma in posterior pararenal space or psoas muscle are more likely to occur spontaneously in patients of hemophilia. On ultrasound a fresh hematoma appears anechoic, while a chronic one has a complex multiseptate appearance containing reflective material.

THORAX

Pleural Space

The pleural space can be assessed by a direct intercostal approach or the abdominal approach through the liver and spleen. The pleural space is located within 1 cm of depth from the rib interface when scanned by a direct intercostal approach. The air filled lung, covered by visceral pleura, is a potent reflector of the ultrasound beam producing a bright, linear interface which moves with respiration ("gliding sign"). When imaged from the abdomen, the diaphragm appears as a bright, curving, echogenic line that moves with respiration. The normal diaphragm is 5 mm thick. When the lung above the diaphragm is air filled, the curved diaphragm-lung interface acts as a specular reflector. A mirror image reflection of the liver or spleen seen above the diaphragm is a definitive evidence of the presence of air-filled lung and absence of pleural fluid above the diaphragm.

Pleural Fluid

Direct intercostal approach can detect even minute amount of pleural fluid using a high resolution linear-array transducer. Ultrasound signs of pleural fluid are:

- Hypoechoic fluid separating the visceral and parietal pleura

- Floating echogenic particles
- Moving septations within the pleural space
- Moving lung suspended within fluid.

Abdominal approach-sonographic signs of pleural fluid are:
- Hypoechoic fluid above the diaphragm
- Visualization of the inside of thorax through the fluid collection
- Absence of mirror image reflection of liver or spleen above the diaphragm
- Large fluid collection causing inversion of diaphragm.

The sonographic appearance of pleural fluid is helpful in differentiating transudate from exudate. Anechoic pleural fluid may be either a transudate or an exudate. Echogenic fluid, fluid containing floating particles, septations or fibrin strands, or associated pleural nodule or pleural thickening greater than 3 mm represents an exudate. Pleural fluid associated with lung infections, malignancy, trauma or collagen vascular disorders are exudative in nature. While effusion caused due to a cardiac pathology like congestive heart failure, or conditions which cause hypoalbuminemia like nephrotic syndrome, cirrhosis result in transudative pleural collection.

PLEURAL THICKENING

Diffuse Pleural Thickening

This usually indicates pleural fibrosis (pleural peel) or pleural malignancy. Diffuse pleural fibrosis more commonly involves the visceral pleura and causes restriction of ventilation. It may be caused by an exudative pleural effusion, hemothorax or empyema. Associated calcification favors tuberculosis or empyema. Metastatic disease to the pleura may cause diffuse lobulated pleural thickening or multiple discrete pleural masses. Sonographically is seen as solid, smooth or lobulated pleural tissue displacing the air-filled lung away from the chest wall. It becomes more obvious when pleural fluid is present.

Pleural Plaques

Focal pleural thickening usually indicates fibrosis occurring due to a variety of causes like pneumonia, asbestos exposure, trauma or chemical pleurodesis. On ultrasound smooth, elliptical, hypoechoic pleural thickening is evident. Plaques due to asbestos exposure are usually present on the parietal pleura.

Pleural Masses

- *Pleural metastases:* In older patients this is a common cause of pleural effusion. Common malignant tumors causing metastatic pleural implants are lung, breast and gastrointestinal cancer. Sonographically, pleural metastasis as a cause of pleural effusion is suggested by solid nodules, circumferential pleural thickening, nodular pleural thickening, pleural thickening > 1 cm, and pleural thickening involving the mediastinal parietal pleura.
- *Pleural mesothelioma:* 80% cases are associated with asbestos exposure. Sonographic findings are:
  – Diffuse pleural thickening, often nodular and irregular
  – Calcification in the pleura
  – Pleural effusion
  – Focal pleural mass
  – Rib destruction in advanced disease.

Pneumothorax

Free air in the pleural space produces a linear highly reflective interface as the pleural lung interface but does not move with respiratory motion.

Lung Parenchyma

Consolidation

Consolidation causes filling up of the air filled spaces with fluid. The highly reflective aerated lung is converted into a firm, dense, solid mass with good sound transmission. Sonographically consolidated lung appears hypoechoic than liver and spleen, is wedged shaped, with presence of branching air bronchogram. Air in the bronchi is seen as highly reflective branching pattern with reverberation artifacts. Sonographic fluid bronchogram appear as branching tubular fluid filled structures. The consolidated lung is poorly defined centrally, while has a sharp peripheral definition. Visualization of the intrapulmonary arteries and veins is possible in a consolidated lung. The diseased portion of the lung moves with respiration.

Atelectasis

Atelectasis refers to the absence of air in all or part of the lung alveoli causing volume loss and crowding of blood vessels. It may be caused by obstruction of the bronchi or due to pleural effusion. Sonographically it appears as wedged echogenic lung having sharp borders defined by visceral pleurae. There is decreased volume of the affected lung, crowding of bronchi and pulmonary blood vessels, sonographic fluid bronchogram with presence of appropriate motion with respiration. When atelectasis is due to bronchial obstruction sonographic air bronchogram are absent.

Lung Tumors

Lung tumors abutting the pleural surface are seen sonographically as hypoechoic masses with well-defined deep margin. Lesions larger than 5 cm appear isoechoic with the lung parenchyma. There is evidence of posterior enhancement as the tumor mass is a better transmitter of ultrasound beam. Pleural involvement causes absence of linear lung surface reflection echo. There is no evidence of tapered edges on sonographic air bronchograms. A cavitory lesion has hyperechoic walls with central echolucent areas. Calcification if present is seen as echogenic focus with distal acoustic shadowing. Absence of movement with respiration indicates invasion of the chest wall resulting in fixation of the peripheral tumor.

Centrally located lung tumors are seen only when associated with peripheral lung consolidation. Tumors with surrounding consolidation appear as a mass within hypoechoic fluid filled lung.

Lung Abscess

Localized area of necrosis of the lung tissue results in an abscess. Primary lung abscess are caused by septic emboli, aspiration or necrotizing pneumonias. Secondary lung abscess are caused by lung carcinoma, pulmonary sequestration, bronchoesophageal fistula, etc.

Most lung abscesses abut the pleura and can be visualized on ultrasound. Sonographic findings are an irregular, thick echogenic walled hypoechoic cavity with air echoes or air-fluid level in it. Differentiation from empyema is difficult. Empyema are in the pleural space, and have smooth walls of regular thickness with compression and displacement of underlying lung parenchyma. In empyema only the internal wall and visceral pleura shows motion with respiration.

Mediastinum

Ultrasound is best for seeing the superior and anterior mediastinum but is not useful in evaluating posterior mediastinal and paravertebral region. US guided needle biopsy of a pathological mediastinal lesion can also be carried out. Mediastinum can be scanned by suprasternal, right and left parasternal and posterior paravertebral approach.

Lymphadenopathy

Sonographically visualized lymph nodes are always pathologically enlarged due to an inflammatory or neoplastic process. Inflammatory lymph nodes appear as hypoechoic rounded discrete or matted structures. Neoplastic nodes are also hypoechoic when small (< 2 cm), and complex when large. Calcification in lymph nodes appears as echogenic focus with distal acoustic shadowing. Lymphoma characteristically causes coalescence of multiple lymph nodes into a large, homogenous, solid mass. When on therapy they decrease in size and become more echogenic.

Solid Masses

Main role of ultrasound in mediastinal ultrasound is to differentiate solid from cystic and vascular lesions, and guide biopsy procedures for accurate diagnosis of the lesion. Extension of thyroid gland into the mediastinal space is easily recognised by its continuity with the thyroid gland. In the neck various solid mediastinal masses are:
- Thymus normal or hyperplastic
- Thymic tumors—thymoma, thymolipoma
- Lymph nodes—granulomatous, neoplastic, lymphoma
- Retrosternal thyroid-adenoma carcinoma
- Germ cell tumors-teratoma
- Neurogenic tumors-neurofibroma
- Primary tumors from esophagus, tracheal/bronchial tumors, mesenchymal tumors.

Vascular Lesions

Real-time ultrasound accurately and noninvasively establishes the vascular origin of different masses in the mediastinum. Color Doppler is an imaging supplement to diagnose vascular masses. The main causes are:
- Arterial—Tortuous bracheocephalic artery
  - Aortic aneurysm
  - Sinus of valsalva aneurysm
  - Right-sided aortic arch.
- Venous—Dilated SVC
  - Esophageal varices
  - Dilated azygus/hemiazygous.

Cystic Masses

Twenty percent of the primary mediastinal masses are cystic. US clearly differentiates cystic from solid vascular lesions and is also used to characterize wall thickness, septations, vascularity, internal appearance, location, and relationship to the adjacent structures.

The main differential diagnosis is as follows:
- Thymic origin—thymic cyst, cystic degeneration in thymoma or thymic lymphoma
- Germ cell tumors—dermoid cyst
- Thyroid origin—cystic degeneration in adenoma or carcinoma, adenomatous hyperplasia
- Bronchogenic cyst
- Pleuropericardial cyst.

19
CHAPTER

Intracranial Sonography

Since the advent of high resolution ultrasonography this noninvasive, nonionizing means of imaging has become an important tool in the assessment of pathologies of infant brain and spine:

The common indications for infant brain sonography include:
- Hydrocephalus
- Intracranial bleeding
- Hypoxic damage
- Congenital anomalies
- Intracranial infections.

NORMAL ANATOMY

Sagittal section: The angled sagittal sections on each side of the brain will show the lateral ventricles shaped like an inverted U. Solid thalamus and caudate nucleus are identified below the ventricle separated from it by the echogenic caudothalamic groove. Angling the transducer further, demonstrates the entire lateral ventricle containing the echogenic choroid plexus.

Coronal section: Coronal sections are obtained by angling the transducer from anterior to posterior side. The anterior sections show anterior most tips of frontal horn of lateral ventricle, interhemispheric fissure and orbits. As the transducer is angled posteriorly the frontal horns, bodies of lateral ventricles, corpus callosum forming the roof of lateral ventricles are visualized. The next scan shows communication of lateral and third ventricle. Normal third ventricle is very thin slit like structure in the midline, situated between the two thalami.

Posterior scan shows cerebellum and quadrigeminal cistern, bodies of lateral ventricles superiorly and temporal horns inferiorly. Cerebellar vermis appears as midline pie-shaped area of echogenicity occupying the lower third of brain. Further posteriorly the occipital lobes are visualized.

AXIAL SECTIONS

The first most inferior section shows heart-shaped pedicle and shows arterial pulsation of circle of Willis.

The next section shows thalamus and central linear echo of falx cerebri. The superior most section shows the walls of lateral ventricles. The ventricles and the corresponding hemisphere can be measured at this level.

HYDROCEPHALUS (FIGS. 19.1A TO F)

Hydrocephalus is the dilatation of ventricular system resulting from interference in the flow of cerebrospinal fluid, between its origin in choroid plexus and its absorption.

Most commonly this dilatation occurs following obstruction at the level of aqueduct or with Arnold-Chiari malformation. But failure of absorption, as after meningitis and excessive production of cerebrospinal fluid (CSF) by choroid plexus produce the same features.

Ultrasonography is the initial modality used for evaluation of babies with head measurement more than 90 percentile.

The posterior horn tends to dilate first. Serial scans are taken to assess the progression of dilatation.

Normally, the ratio of ventricular diameter to hemispherical diameter should be less than 1:3. If the ratio is greater it represents hydrocephalus.

Aqueduct stenosis is seen as dilatation of lateral and third ventricle with normal aqueduct and fourth ventricle. The diagnosis should be made early to present massive dilatation and subsequent damage to brain parenchyma.

INTRACRANIAL HEMORRHAGE (FIGS. 19.2A AND B)

Intracranial hemorrhage (ICH) is the leading cause of serious mortality and morbidity in the neonate, especially in premature infants. Neonatal ICH occurs most commonly in developing, immature brain and is therefore most common in premature infants less than 32 weeks gestational age. The risk factors include prematurity, low birth weight, male sex, multiple gestation, trauma at delivery, prolonged labor.

ICH in premature neonates has been divided into four grades.
1. Grade I—Subependymal germinal matrix hemorrhage.
2. Grade II—Germinal matrix hemorrhage and intraventricular hemorrhage without ventricular dilatation.

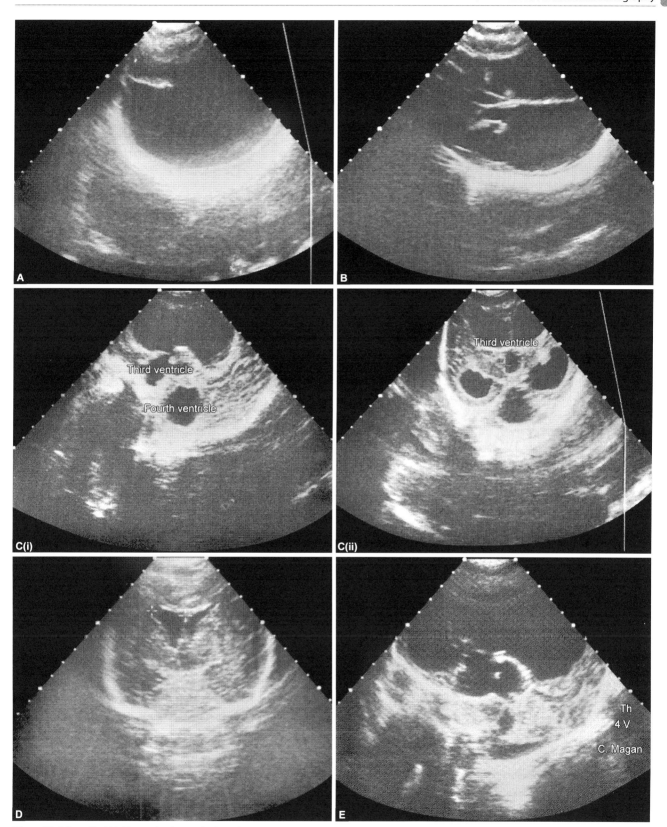

Figs. 19.1A to E: (A) Gross hydrocephalus showing disrupted septum pellucidum. A thin rim of cortex is left behind; (B) Bilateral lateral ventricles appear dilated. Normal septum pellucidum is seen; (C) Communicating hydrocephalus; (D) Frontal horn of right lateral ventricles appears dilated. Left is normal suggestive of asymmetrical hydrocephalus due to obstruction at foramen of Monro; (E) Communicating hydrocephalus—ventricular system is dilated and cisterna magna is prominent.

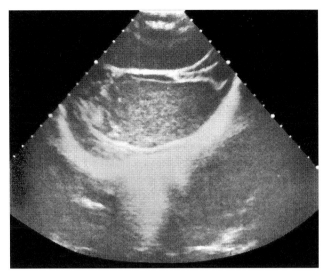

Fig. 19.1F: Infected hydrocephalus—showing internal echoes.

3. Grade III—Germinal matrix hemorrhage and intraventricular hemorrhage with ventricular dilatation.
4. Grade IV—Intraparenchymal hemorrhage with intraventricular hemorrhage.

SONOGRAPHIC APPEARANCE

The germinal matrix is a highly cellular and vascular area lying beneath the ependyma of lateral ventricle. The most prominent portion of germinal matrix lies between the thalamus and caudate nucleus just anterior to caudothalamic notch. The germinal matrix usually involutes by 34 weeks and being very susceptible to hypoxic damage is the usual site of ICH in premature infants.

Germinal matrix hemorrhage appears as a uniformly echogenic mass inferolateral to the frontal horns, at a level just posterior to the foramen of Monro. The hemorrhage may occur unilaterally or bilaterally. Larger hemorrhages cause focal compression of inferolateral margin of the ventricle. As the hemorrhage resolves, the focal echogenic lesion decreases in size and echogenicity. Frequently, the hemorrhagic lesion undergoes central liquefaction resulting in well defined subependymal cyst.

Intraventricular hemorrhage appears as bright echoes within the ventricular lumen. If the ventricle is not dilated, the clot may be difficult to identify. The presence of bright echoes within the frontal, occipital horn or a blood-CSF level may be the only sign of grade II bleed. In grade III and IV bleeding with ventricular dilatation, the entire ventricle is filled with blood, forming a cast of the ventricle. As the hemorrhage resolves, the intraventricular clot gradually decreases in size and echogenicity due to internal liquefaction. As the blood absorbs, ventriculomegaly may resolve spontaneously, persist or progress.

Intraparenchymal hemorrhage is the most severe grade of ICH in premature baby. As the clot retracts a porencephalic cyst forms at the site of the original hemorrhagic parenchyma and communicates with the dilated ipsilateral ventricle.

Hypoxic-ischemic Encephalopathy (Figs. 19.3 and 19.4)

Major neurological and developmental deficits in the infants and young child are the result of prenatal hypoxic ischemic injury to the brain.

In the preterm infant, germinal matrix-intraventricular hemorrhage is the most common manifestation of hypoxic brain injury. However, if there is a significant ischemic component in the insult, then infarction may result. Periventricular leukomalacia and periventricular hemo-

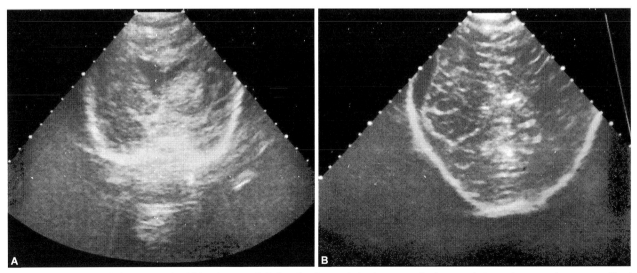

Figs. 19.2A and B: (A) Intracerebral bleed—a well-defined echogenic lesion seen in the caudate region causing mass effect on frontal horn; and (B) Subdural effusion—small amount of fluid is seen in the right subdural space.

rrhage manifestations are the primary manifestation of hypoxic-ischemic encephalopathy (HIE) in premature infant.

Periventricular leukomalacia (PVL) is coagulation necrosis of the deep white matter and occurs in two common sites: the external angle of the frontal horns near the foramen of Monro and the level of optic radiation adjacent to the trigone. The earliest sonographic abnormality in PVL consists of bilateral coarse, globular or broad bands of echodensity in the periventricular white matter. Secondary petechial hemorrhages can occur within areas of PVL.

Periventricular hemorrhagic infarction is an area of hemorrhagic necrosis in the periventricular white matter. It is usually large asymmetric lesion that coexists with large IVH. The appearance of periventricular hemorrhagic infarction is unilateral or bilateral, asymmetrical, globular or triangular fan-shaped echodensity radiating from the external angle of lateral ventricle. These echodensities evolve into cysts with time.

Congenital Anomalies of Brain (Fig. 19.5)

Corpus Callosum Agenesis: It forms in 3rd or 4th fetal months. Primary complete agenesis occurs prior to the 12th gestational week as a result of vascular or inflammatory insult. Secondary dysgenesis may occur later in gestational life as a partial or total destruction of a previously well formed corpus callosum.

Sonographic appearance in agenesis of corpus callosum include complete absence of the normally seen sonolucent band with a resultant radial arrangement of the medial cerebral sulci around the roof of the third ventricle, narrowed, pointed and widely separated frontal horns with relatively dilated occipital horns.

Chiari Malformation

Type I chiari malformation consists of inferior displacement of tonsil and cerebellum without displacement of fourth ventricle or medulla. The Chiari II malformation is the most commonly seen in neonates and infants and this complex includes a small posterior fossa, elongation of pons and IVth ventricle and downward displacement of medulla, IVth ventricle and cerebellum into the cervical spinal canal. These infants present as newborn with obvious spina bifida and meningomyelocele. Most often, there is variable degree of hydrocephalus with worsening following the closure of back defect.

Cystic Abnormalities of Posterior Fossa

Differentiation of various cystic abnormality of posterior fossa is important.

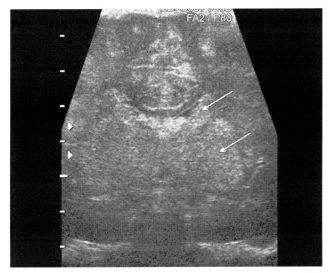

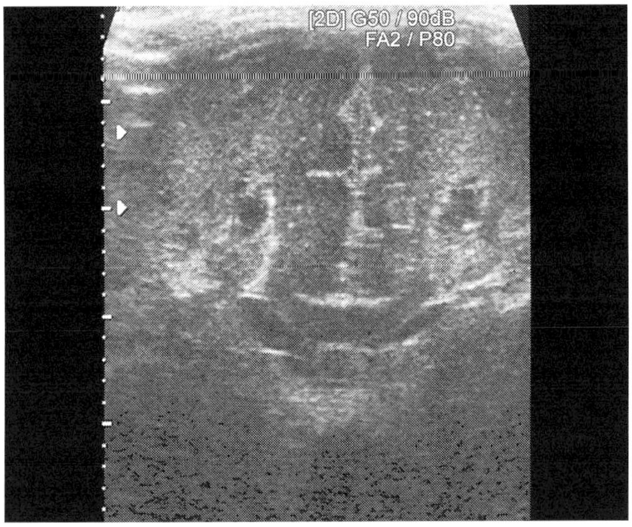

Fig. 19.3: Bilateral echogenic basal ganglia (white arrows) s/o hypoxic-ischemic encephalopathy (HIE).

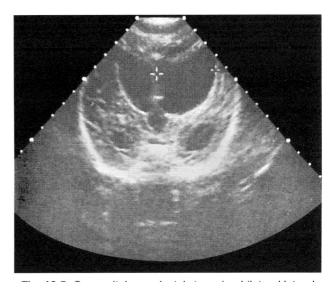

Fig. 19.4: Periventricular cystic changes s/o leukomalacia, a sequelae to HIE.

Fig. 19.5: Congenital aqueductal stenosis—bilateral lateral ventricles appear dilated with funnel-shaped third ventricle.

Dandy-Walker syndrome is characterized by a large posterior fossa cyst continuous with IVth ventricle, hypoplastic cerebellar hemisphere and absent or rudimentary vermis. There is variable degree of dilatation of lateral and third ventricle and hypoplastic cerebellar hemisphere is displaced anteriorly. Dandy-Walker cyst must be differentiated from mega cisterna magna, a trapped fourth ventricle and arachnoid cyst.

Intracranial Infections (Figs. 19.6 to 19.8)

Neonatal and infantile meningitis is a very serious illness. In the neonate, group B *Streptococcus* and *E. coli* are the most common causative agent.

After the neonatal period, H.influenza, *S. pneumoniae* and *N. meningitidis* are the most common cause of meningitis.

Perinatal intracranial infections may occur secondary to viral or protozoan agents like cytomegalovirus, Toxoplasma *gondii*, rubella and herpes simplex virus.

The sonographic feature of perinatal meningitis is nonspecific for a particular causative organism and is related to inflammation, edema and vasculitis common to all cerebral infection. Sonographically, the abnormalities detected are echogenic sulci, extra-axial fluid collection, hydrocephalus, ventriculitis, abnormal parenchymal echogenicity, abscess, encephalomalacia, and calcification.

In meningitis, there is an increase in echogenicity of the cortical sulci and widening of sulcal echoes which is attributed to accumulation of inflammatory exudates. The exudates may accumulate in subarachnoid space also and result in extra axial fluid collection. The extra-axial collection cause widening of interhemispheric fissure and displacement of the brain away from cranial vault. Ventricular enlargement may occur early or late in the course of the the illness. In the acute stage, due to cerebral edema, the ventricles may appear slit-like. Ventricular dilatation however, can also occur in the acute stage. The dilatation is thought be the result of communicating hydrocephalus following arachnoiditis.

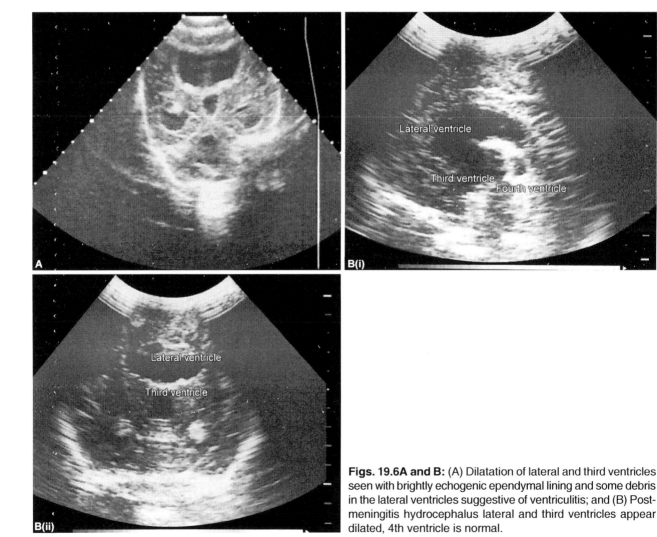

Figs. 19.6A and B: (A) Dilatation of lateral and third ventricles seen with brightly echogenic ependymal lining and some debris in the lateral ventricles suggestive of ventriculitis; and (B) Post-meningitis hydrocephalus lateral and third ventricles appear dilated, 4th ventricle is normal.

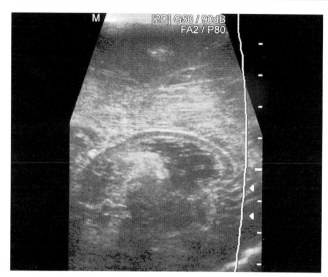

Fig. 19.7: Septations within the lateral ventricle s/o ventriculitis.

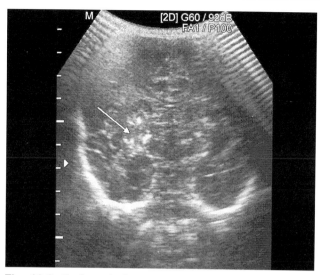

Fig. 19.8: Periventricular linear and punctate calcifications (white arrow) in a case of congenital cytomegalovirus (CMV) infection.

Focal or diffuse areas of abnormal parenchymal echogenicity are associated with meningoencephalitis. The increase in echogenicity is thought to be secondary to edema, cerebritis and/or infarction.

Abscess formation is an uncommon complication of infantile meningitis. On ultrasound, the abscess appears as a well-circumscribed lesion with a thick echogenic wall and a relative hypoechoic center. In the end stage of meningoencephalitis, multicystic encephalomalacia, appearing as anechoic areas of cystic degeneration develops in the previously abnormal echogenic parenchyma.

Sonographic Imaging of Neonatal Spine (Figs. 19.9A and B)

Ultrasound is primarily used as an initial noninvasive screening examination and is usually supplemented by AP and lateral radiographs.

Spinal Dysraphism

The most common application for infant spinal ultrasound is in overt or suspected spinal dysraphism.
Spinal dysraphism includes:
- All forms of spina bifida in which there is incomplete fusion of the neural tube, meninges, vertebral column or skin.
- Failure of separation of the germinal layers, e.g., a deep dermal sinus.
- Abnormal growth of ectopic cell rest, e.g., dermoid or epidermoid cyst.
- Disturbance of growth of an otherwise normal tissue, e.g., an intraspinal or intramedullary lipoma.

In overt dysraphism, there is externally obvious incomplete closure of the bony elements of spinal canal with posterior protrusion of all or part of spinal canal contents. The overt forms can be a simple meningocele, myelocele or meningomyelocele.

In simple meningocele there is an extension of dura and arachnoid but no neural tissue protrudes out. In myelocele, a midline plaque of neural tissue is present lying exposed to the skin surface. Myelomeningocele is a myelocele which has been elevated above the skin surface by expansion of subarachnoid space anterior to it.

In myelocele the anatomy is readily visible and neural tissue is vulnerable making direct ultrasound inadvisable. However, the spine above and below the lesion should be examined. There may be associated hydromyelia, diastematomyelia or intracanalicular lipoma.

In meningocele and myelomeningocele, the epithelialized sac should be imaged sonographically to determine the contents and presence or absence of neural tissue. A transfontanellar ultrasound examination should be undertaken to diagnose and monitor hydrocephalus which is associated with 98% of cases of spinal dysraphism. Sonography is also useful in evaluation of postoperative spine. Tethering of the cord to the scar tissue, tight constricting ring cord compression by inclusion dermoids or lipomas or ischemia due to vascular compromise are some of the causes of neurological deterioration following surgery which can be diagnosed on ultrasound.

In occult dysraphism there is dysraphic state with normal skin covering. Occult spinal dysraphism includes simple meningocele, diastematomyelia, dorsal dermal sinus, and spinal lipomas, etc.

Simple meningocele is a fluid filled dorsal sac and is directly continuous with the spinal canal. Sonographically, it is echo-free and does not contain any neural tissue.

Spinal lipomas are masses of fat and connective tissue and have a connection with leptomeninges or spinal cord.

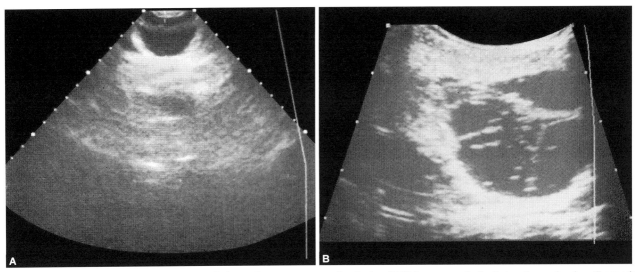

Figs. 19.9A and B: (A) Meningocele—anechoic cystic space-occupying lesion (SOL) seen posterior to lumbar spine in a 6-month-old female child; and (B) Myelomeningocele—cystic SOL with internal septae seen posterior to lumbar spine in one year old female. The patient also had hydrocephalus.

Spinal lipomas are of three types: intradural lipomas, lipomeningomyelocele and lipomas of filum terminale.

Intradural lipomas sonographically appear as highly reflective intradural or extra medullary mass. Lipomyelomeningocele are large subcutaneous masses, in which highly reflective fat is seen on ultrasound traversing from subcutaneous plane into the spinal canal through a posterior spina bifida. The subarachnoid space and cord bulge through spina bifida into subcutaneous tissue. In lipomyelocele, the cord remains intracanalicular and meninges do not bulge. The lipoma which is echogenic, is tethered to the cord which is low and often eccentrically positioned, within spinal canal. Those lipomas with a large area of direct interface with the sinal cord often termed as leptomyelolipoma. Lipoma of filum terminale is seen sonographically as a low lying cord with a complex highly reflective mass in the filum.

Diastematomyelia: It is a sagittal partial or complete clefting of the spinal cord into two hemicords each containing a central canal. At the level of diastematomyelia, two hemicords lying side by side or sometimes ventrodorsal may be seen sonographically. Reunion of two hemicords may be sometime seen caudally. It may be associated with hydromyelia.

Hydromyelia: It is CSF distention of central canal of spinal cord. It may be focal or may extend the full length on ultrasound imaging, the cord is widened and central echogenic lines separate as the central distend with CSF.

Tethered Spinal Cord

A conus terminating low in the spinal canal below L_{2-3} indicates a tethered cord unless the child has had a meningomyelocele repaired in which case the cord remains low after initial closure and diagnosis of tethering is more difficult. The tethered lumbar cord is usually eccentric, often dorsal within the spinal canal. Cord oscillations are often diminished at or above the point of tethering.

Midline lumbosacral skin abnormalities can herald an occult tethered spinal cord, e.g., subcutaneous lipoma, hair tuft, sinus tract, dimple, hemangioma, pigmented navi and skin tract. Spinal cord tethering can have a variety of pathologic causes, including intraspinal lipoma, thick filum terminale, diastematomyelia, and dermatosinus.

CHAPTER 20

Eye and Orbit

Pathological conditions in which assessment of the globe cannot be made by direct ophthalmoscopy should undergo high resolution sonography of the globe. Some of the important diseases encountered in practice are discussed below.

CONGENITAL DISEASES

Anophthalmia

It is also called agenesis of eye. Normal development of eyeball and orbit does not take place. A small cystic mass with rudimentary orbital fat is seen in such anomalies. The shape of the orbit is deformed and normal anatomic landmarks of orbit and eye are absent.

Congenital Exophthalmos

This is a feature of Crouzon's disease. The eye is protruded out and appears to be diseased. However, sonography shows normal proptosed eye and no retrobulbar pathology.

Persistent Hyperplastic Primary Vitreous (PHPV) (Fig. 20.1)

Patient presents with leukocoria or white reflex usually unilateral. It is not surgically correctable. Microphthalmia is usually seen with a thick echogenic membrane in posterior segment (vitreolenticular). Rarely a thick band is seen from posterior surface of membrane, in PHPV to optic disc. It may result into retinal detachment. This band may contain hyaloid artery.

Congenital Cataract

US gives information about the posterior segment, e.g., any retrolenticular membrane in this condition.

VITREOUS EXAMINATION (FIGS. 20.2A TO F)

Vitreous Hemorrhage

Causes are trauma, diabetic retinopathy, macular degeneration, with occlusion, retinal tear and intraocular tumors.

In small, subtle hemorrhage low intensity echoes are seen on high gain settings. In fresh hemorrhage, dense echogenic collection is seen in posterior segment. Layering of collection and pseudomembranes may also be seen. Posterior vitreous detachment (PVD) takes place with vitreous hemorrhage.

Asteroid Hyalosis

It is a senile degenerative condition of unknown etiology. It is unilateral in 75%. Bright-echogenic dots showing considerable movement are scattered throughout vitreous—represent calcium soaps.

Posterior Vitreous Detachment (PVD)

The posterior hyaloid may be separate completely from posterior pole—seen as an echogenic undulating membrane. It may remain attached at optic disc giving a tunnel-shaped appearance. Undulating movement and after movement differentiate it from retinal detachment. PVD is usually smooth, but may be thick when blood is layered posteriorly.

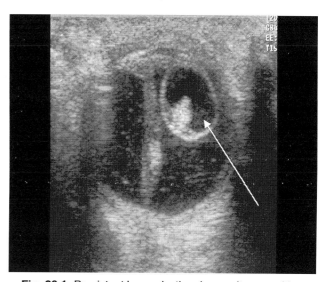

Fig. 20.1: Persistent hyperplastic primary vitreous with a vitreal cyst (white arrow).

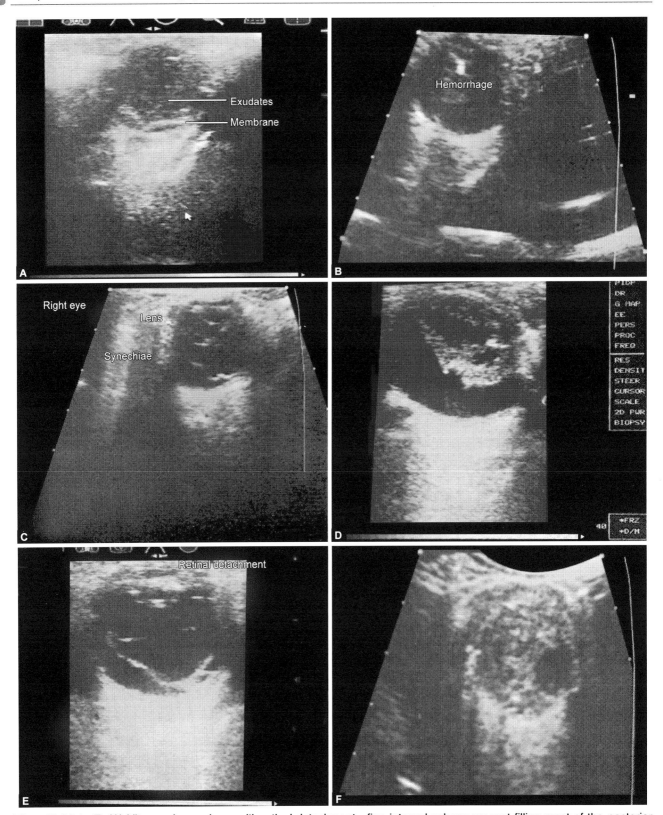

Figs. 20.2A to F: (A) Vitreous hemorrhage with retinal detachment—fine internal echoes present filling most of the posterior chamber and with a V shaped membrane in its posterior aspect; (B) Vitreous hemorrhage seen as fine internal echoes in the posterior chamber; (C) Vitreous synechia; (D) Vitreous detachment with organized vitreous hemorrhage; (E) Echogenic mass seen in relation to the posterior capsule of the lens with a echogenic strand extending up to retina; and (F) Left eye shows an echogenic mass with a cystic area and foci of calcification.

Posterior Hyphema

Subvitreal hemorrhage layers out with its surface showing a smooth, echogenic dense membrane. With movements of eye or change in position of patient, this hyphema changes in position.

RETINA (FIGS. 20.3A TO D)

Retinal Tears

Usually show flapping movement. Small tears may be associated with vitreous hemorrhage. Focal retinal tears are usually seen in superior fundus.

Retinal Detachment (RD)

It produces a bright, continuous, folded membrane appearance. When total or complete, the detached retina remains adherent at optic disc and ora serrata. RD exhibits a more tethered, restricted after movement than highly mobile posterior vitreous detachment. Mobility of retina can vary, however—fresh, bullous detachments and those with large tears may be very mobile, whereas long-standing detachments of proliferative vitreoretinopathy may be quite stiff. An RD with subretinal hemorrhage produces echoes in subretinal space and a hyphema like appearance as subretinal blood does not clot. Configuration of retinal detachment may vary from shallow, flat and smooth membrane, bullous, folded membrane; funnel-shaped membrane open, or closed—concave, triangular or T-shaped. Longstanding RD may develop retinal cysts, become partially calcified and cholesterol debris may accumulate in subretinal space.

Tractional retinal detachment may be caused by traction exerted on retina by vitreous membranes or bands secondary to vitreous hemorrhage (in diabetic retinopathy,

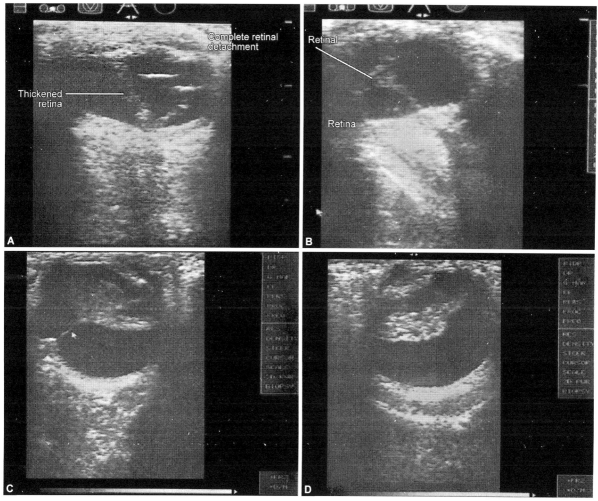

Figs. 20.3A to D: (A and B) Retinal detachment-transverse scan through eye shows V shaped membrane attached posteriorly to the optic nerve; (C) Echogenic mass is seen in relation to the posterior surface of the lens and the retina with a linear strand connecting them—retinal fibroplasia with retinal detachment in a 6-month-old child; and (D) An echogenic mass is seen in the posterior compartment with a thin linear strand extending up to retina and causing mild tractional retinal detachment.

trauma, endophthalmitis, etc). Common types of traction detachments are (i) tent-like (ii) table-top like (plateau).

Retinoschisis

A thin, dome-shaped, smooth membrane that does not insert into optic disc is seen inferotemporally. It may be unilateral or bilateral. It differs from RD by its more smooth, focal and thin character.

CHOROID

Choroidal Detachment (CD) (Fig. 20.4)

It presents as smooth, dome-shaped thick echogenic membrane in the periphery, showing little or no movement. Extensive CD along 360° produces classical 'kissing bullae' appearance.

TRAUMA

Sonography can assess the extent of damage. Severe blunt trauma can cause compression of eyeball and expansion and rupture of globe at equator (in upper nasal quadrant commonly).

Anterior Segment Trauma (Fig. 20.5)

Sonography can display, blood clot, depth of anterior chamber, moderately dense post-traumatic cataract, subluxation of lens, etc.

Posterior Segment Trauma

Vitreous hemorrhage, PVD, retinal detachment, and retinal tears can be detected.

Posterior Scleral Rupture

Sclera in area of rupture shows moderately irregular contour and low echogenicity. Indirect signs include (i) vitreous incarceration into fundus with vitreous hemorrhage and PVD (ii) thickening or detachment of surrounding retina or choroid (iii) hemorrhage in episcleral space (iv) vitreous traction towards site of incarceration.

FOREIGN BODIES (FIG. 20.6)

Metals, glass, and stones are highly reflector and picked easily on US. They may cast acoustic shadowing. Track of traveling foreign body may be identified. Entry or exit sites of foreign body may cause vitreous incarceration. Air bubbles are also seen in the globe as highly reflective spots which show rapid movements with change of posture.

Objects of low density, e.g., wood, cotton, fiber, or organic materials can be missed on US.

If foreign body is lying near sclera, CT cannot identify, if it is lying just within or outside the globe, unlike US.

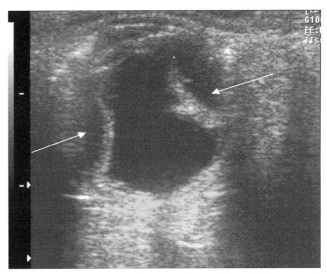

Fig. 20.4: Choroidal detachment at the periphery (white arrows).

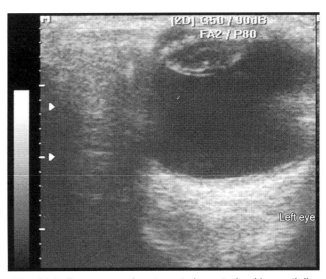

Fig. 20.5: Post-traumatic cataract characterized by partially hypoechoic lens.

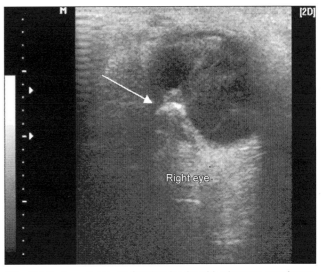

Fig. 20.6: An echogenic foreign body with vitreous exudates.

ENDOPHTHALMITIS

It is characterized by dense opacities in posterior segment. Thick echogenic exudative collection is seen. Diffuse thickening of retinochoroid layer as well as retinal detachment can occur.

INTRAOCULAR TUMORS

Tumors must have an elevation of 8 mm before it can be detected by US.

Retinoblastoma (Figs. 20.7A to C)

It is most common in children up to six years. Frequently presents as white reflex or cat eye reflex. It can be unilateral or bilateral, focal or multifocal. Endophytic tumor grows toward vitreous and exophytic toward choroid.

They appear to have smooth, dome-shaped appearance, when small and heterogeneous echotexture, when large. Calcification is the hallmark of retinoblastoma. US can detect retrobulbar extension of tumor. US can monitor response of tumor to treatment. Differential diagnoses are coats disease, PHPV, retrolental fibroplasia, and toxocariasis.

Ocular Melanoma (Fig. 20.8)

It is most common tumor in adults. The 80% arise from choroid and 15% from ciliary body occurs in 5th and 6th decades.

They present typically with dome-shaped, collar-button appearance with smooth surface. It has low reflectivity, homogeneous texture. Calcification is rare. Large tumor can attenuate sound beam resulting in decreased reflectivity of tumor base called 'acoustic hollowing' choroidal excavation may be seen. Associated exudative retinal detachment, vitreous hemorrhage, scleritis can occur.

Choroidal Metastases

Metastatic deposits in choroid are more common than primary malignancies. CA bronchus in males and CA breast in females metastasize to choroid posterior pole. Commonly bilateral single or multiple low undulating masses with a broad base. Choroidal thickening may occur.

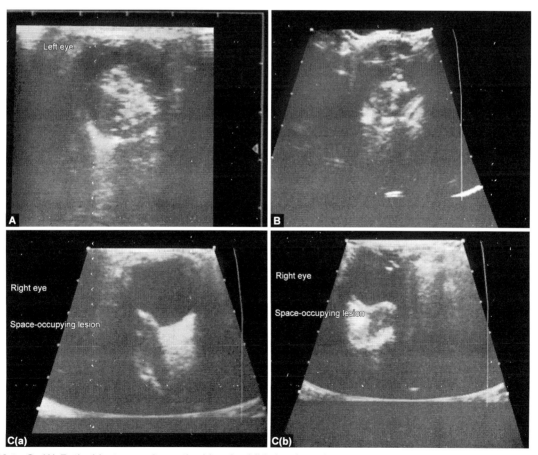

Figs. 20.7A to C: (A) Retinoblastoma—6-month-old male child showing a heterogeneous echotexture mass in the left eye with multiple dense echogenic and anechoic areas; (B) Retinoblastoma—transverse scan of left eye in a 3-year-old female child showing a solid intraocular mass attached posteriorly with areas of calcification in it; and (C) Pseudotumor—(a) longitudinal, (b) transverse scan shows well-defined, spindle shaped hypoechoic solid mass with foci of calcification in the lateral rectus muscle.

ORBITAL DISEASES (FIGS. 20.9A TO D)

Orbital Trauma

Retrobulbar hematoma can be identified giving a mixed echo-complex appearance. US is useful to monitor regression of hematoma.

Muscle Hypertrophy

It is common in thyrotoxicosis. Medial rectus muscle is taken as standard and thickness of more than 4 mm is suggestive of Graves' disease. Typically enlargement involves muscle belly. Other features include increased orbital fat and orbital edema.

Vascular Masses

Hemangiomas (cavernous type) are seen as highly reflective echogenic mass in retrobulbar space. Arteriovenous fistulae can be diagnosed by Doppler examination. Orbital varices-exaggerate with bending of head and Valsalva maneuver. Lymphangiomas—seen in children or young adults present as multiseptate masses.

Orbital Lymphoma

It is one of the three major causes of proptosis usually non-Hodgkin's lymphoma (NHL). US shows a complex, elongated or oval mass in retrobulbar space usually bilateral.

Orbital Cysticercosis

A well-defined cystic mass is seen in belly of the muscle. Echogenic nidus representing scolex is seen within cyst near inner wall. US can be used for studying response to therapy.

Hydatid Cysts

Not uncommon. They are seen as thin-walled, well-defined cystic masses with thin septa at times.

Rhabdomyosarcoma

It is most common primary orbital tumor in childhood. It presents as rapidly increasing exophthalmos. Commonest location is in superonasal quadrant of orbit. It is seen as medium to low echo-complex mass. Orbital walls may be eroded. Differential diagnosis is from lymphomas and pseudotumors.

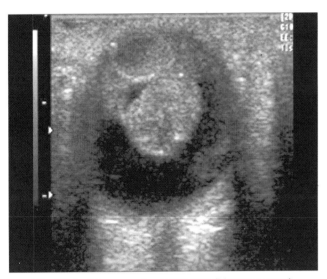

Fig. 20.8: A large ocular melanoma (biopsy proven).

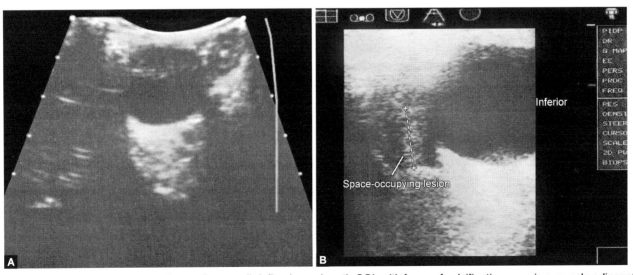

Figs. 20.9A and B: (A) Orbital cysticercosis—a well-defined round cystic SOL with focus of calcification seen in a muscle adjacent to eyeball; (B) Follow-up case of Hodgkin's lymphoma showing a well-defined round hypoechoic SOL adjacent to the eyeball FNAC—confirmed lymphomatous origin.

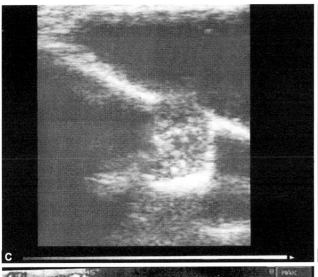
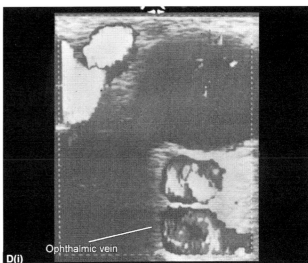
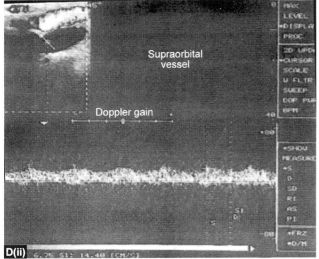

Figs. 20.9C and D: (C) Epidermoid cyst—a large SOL with predominant cystic areas with internal debris is seen anterosuperiorly to the eyeball. The lesion is seen to extend intracranially and causing bone destruction. The intracranial part is predominantly solid with foci of calcification in it. The eyeball is not involved. FNAC confirmed case; and (D) There is evidence of dilatation of superior ophthalmic vein and dilated vessels in the super-orbital region and within extraconal compartment. The dilated vessels on duplex showed an mixed arteriovenous turbulent signal.

Optic Nerve Tumors

Meningiomas, gliomas, neurilemmomas can occur. Gliomas are smooth, fusiform or ovoid masses which replace normal optic nerve.

Optic Neuritis

Optic nerve is enlarged due to fluid collection in perineural sheath. A 30% test is useful to differentiate it from optic nerve tumor. Patient is asked to fix primary gaze position and rotate his eye 30° towards probe. Fluid redistributes along nerve sheath as nerve stretches and swelling subsides. It persists in tumor of optic nerve.

Orbital Metastases

It is common in neuroblastoma (40%). It is also seen in Ewing's sarcoma, Wilms' tumor and leukemia.

Dermoid Cyst

It presents either superotemporally or superonasally. It may be present within lids, at orbital rim, near outer canthus, on conjunctiva, or within orbit. Commoner in children. Usually heterogeneous in echotexture because may contain keratin, sebaceous materials, hair follicles or inflammatory cells.

Periorbital Abscess

It present as painful swelling pushing eyeball. Thick-walled low level echo collection with weak sound transmission. US-guided aspiration is possible.

Mucoceles

These are usually seen as low-reflective, homogeneous, cystic masses in superonasal quadrant causing outward and downward displacement of globe.

21

CHAPTER

Thyroid

THYROID LESIONS

Goiter (Figs. 21.1A to D)

This is the generic term which refers to diffuse enlargement of thyroid gland. Ultrasound more accurately measures the dimensions of the gland. The normal dimensions of lateral lobe are: 5–8 cm (craniocaudally), 1–2.5 cm (AP) and 2–4 cm (transverse).

Sonographic Appearance

- *Simple (Colloid goiter) goiter:* The thyroid becomes enlarged. The parenchymal echogenicity varies, it may be similar to that of a normal gland or coarsely increased
- *Graves' disease:* Thyroid becomes diffusely enlarged. The echotexture is equivalent to the normal gland or rarely, less than normal. Color Doppler imaging reveals an overall increase in the color signal and pulsatility during systole (thyroid inferno)
- *Multinodular goiter:* The thyroid gland is asymmetrically enlarged and displays an inhomogeneously reduced echotexture with coarse, bright, linear echoes scattered throughout. The latter alterations are produced due to calcification and scar tissue. Inspissated colloid and shrunken follicles are visualized sonographically as multiple hypoechoic nodular with variable sizes.

THYROIDITIS

Thyroiditis denotes diffuse inflammation of the gland.

SONOGRAPHY

Hashimotos' thyroiditis (Fig. 21.2): Thyroid is asymmetrically enlarged with a parenchymal echotexture that is inhomogeneously decreased compared to normal. Foci of mixed/increased echogenicity are dispersed throughout the gland (fibrosis and scarring), multiple small hypoechoic nodules may be imaged within the thyroid parenchyma.

Thyroid cyst (Figs. 21.3 and 21.4): Congenital thyroid cysts are very rare. A true cyst will sonographically lack internal echoes, posses a thin well-defined posterior wall and demonstrate through transmission of sound with posterior wall enhancement. However, presence of mucinous material in the thyroglossal cyst may give rise to homogeneous, low level internal echoes.

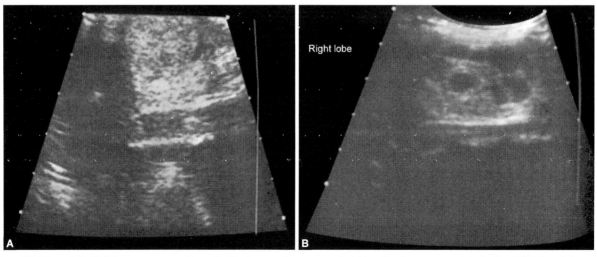

Figs. 21.1A and B: (A) Transverse and longitudinal scan shows a well-defined echogenic nodule in the left lobe of thyroid; (B) Goiterous nodule seen as multiloculated cystic space-occupying lesion (SOL) in the right lobe of thyroid.

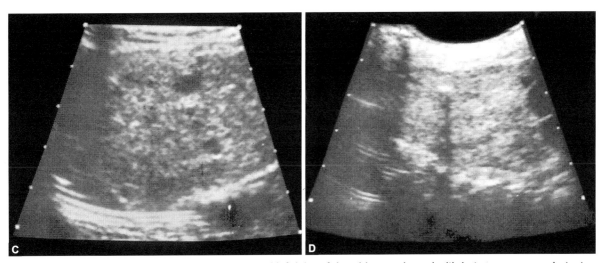

Figs. 21.1C and D: (C) multinodular goiter—isthmus and left lobe of thyroid are enlarged with heterogeneous echotexture and multiple cystic areas, (D) multinodular goiter—longitudinal scan showing small hyperechoic nodules with the peripheral halo. One nodule shows evidence of calcification.

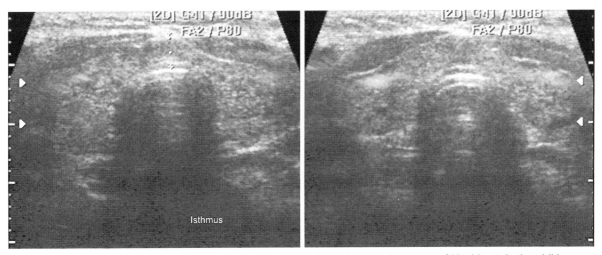

Fig. 21.2: Enlarged thyroid with inhomogeneous parenchymal pattern in a case of Hashimoto's thyroiditis.

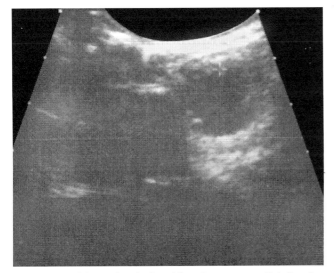

Fig. 21.3: Hemorrhagic thyroid cyst seen as well defined cystic lesion with internal echoes.

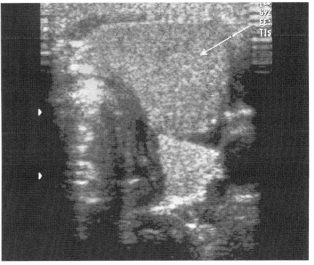

Fig. 21.4: A thyroglossal cyst at the superior pole of left thyroid lobe (white arrow).

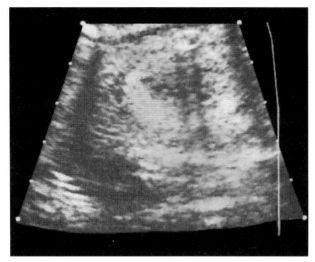

Fig. 21.5: Thyroid adenoma—a well-defined hypoechoic lesion is present in an enlarged right lobe of thyroid with a cystic necrotic area anteriorly. A focal scar is also seen in the lesion.

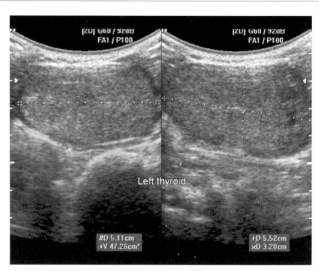

Fig. 21.7: A classical follicular adenoma of thyroid (FNAC proven).

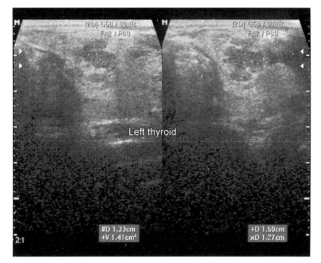

Fig. 21.6: A well-defined colloid adenoma (FNAC proven).

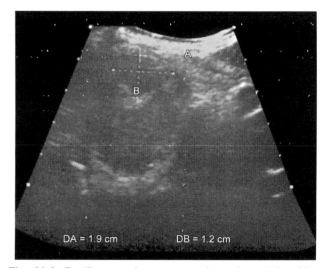

Fig. 21.8: Papillary carcinoma—an echogenic nodule with a thin uneven peripheral halo and a central hypoechoic area and a focus of calcification is seen. Fine needle aspiration cytology confirmed the diagnosis.

Thyroid adenoma (Figs. 21.5 to 21.7): This is the most common benign, solitary, solid thyroid mass. On ultrasound, it is visualized as a hypoechoic nodule, which is fairly well defined. When hemorrhage/ischemic necrosis occur, this nodule becomes sonographically complex with a grainy echogenicity. Occasionally coarse foci of echogenicity may be seen. A well-defined sonolucent rim measuring approximately 1 to 2 mm is visualized sonographically around the solitary follicular enhancement.

Thyroid malignancies (Fig. 21.8): Papillary carcinoma is more common than follicular carcinoma of the thyroid. Papillary carcinoma is more common in the 4th/5th decade in females. It is frequently a solitary lesion but can be multiple. It commonly metastasizes to lymph nodes.

Follicular carcinoma occurs in older women. It tends to invade the surrounding vessels and shows distant metastasis to the lungs and bones.

Medullary carcinoma may be encountered sporadically or show a familial tendency (MEN IIa and MEN IIb syndromes). It arises from C-cells of thyroid. On ultrasound, both benign and malignant thyroid neoplasms possess similar sonographic features. Thyroid malignancies are commonly solitary, solid masses although they may be multifocal. Echotexture may be hypoechoic to hyperechoic. They have irregular, ill-defined margins with punctate microcalcifications.

The neck lymph nodes should also be scanned carefully for evidence of any metastatic lesion.

CHAPTER 22

Small Part Ultrasound

BREAST

Breast ultrasound is an important adjunct to screen-film mammography in the evaluation of breast disease. The indications of sonography include:
- To differentiate solid from cystic lesions.
- To differentiate palpable masses in women who are pregnant and lactating.
- As the primary modality for the imaging of breast in women of less than 30 years of age.
- To evaluate asymmetric density on mammogram.
- To provide guidance for interventional procedures such as cyst aspiration, fine needle aspiration and biopsy.

Specific Conditions

Cysts: Breast cysts **(Figs. 22.1A to C)** are common in women in the perimenopausal years of 35–50 years of age. The most important contribution of breast sonography is confident diagnosis of cyst.

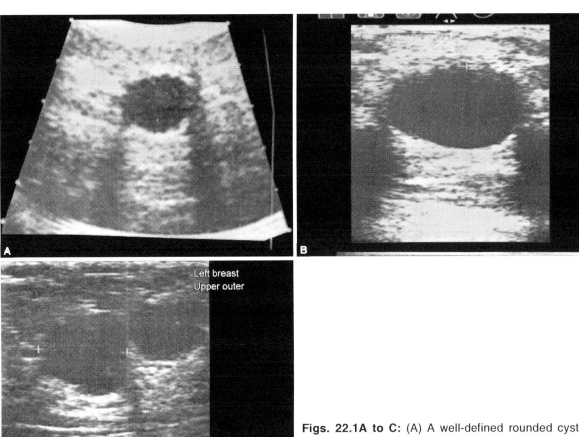

Figs. 22.1A to C: (A) A well-defined rounded cystic space-occupying lesion (SOL) with scattered internal echoes with posterior acoustic enhancement; (B) Simple cyst—anechoic well-defined cysts seen in breast; and (C) Two well-defined anechoic cysts with posterior acoustic enhancement seen adjacent to each other.

The diagnostic criteria are strictly applied for accurate diagnosis of simple cyst. It should be anechoic, round or oval sharply marginated (especially posteriorly), no internal echoes should be present and cyst should demonstrate acoustic enhancement posteriorly.

When cyst is not under tension, it may alter shape when pressure is applied. Any nonpalpable lesion that may represent a cyst but does not fulfill the sonographic criteria must be aspirated under sonographic guidance.

For appropriate diagnosis of cysts, focal zone placement must be appropriate and gain and power setting must be adjusted for each unit and reset for each patient. Varying the transducer pressure on the lesion and altering patient positioning may be necessary to demonstrate features of a cyst in lesions deeply seated in the breast.

Benign Solid Lesions

Fibroadenoma (Figs. 22.2A to D): It is a commonly occurring palpable mass lesion seen in young women under the age of 35 years. These lesions have mixed histological elements (fibrous and epithelial) and have little of any malignant potential.

Fibroadenomas are hypoechoic well-defined lesions with smooth, sharp often lobulated margin. They are oriented with long axis parallel to the skin. The pattern of acoustic enhancement varied most often demonstrating slight enhancement or no attenuation. Calcifications may be detected within the mass. Unlike microcalcifications of malignancy the calcific foci in these lesions are large enough to interrupt ultrasound beam resulting in intratumoral shadowing.

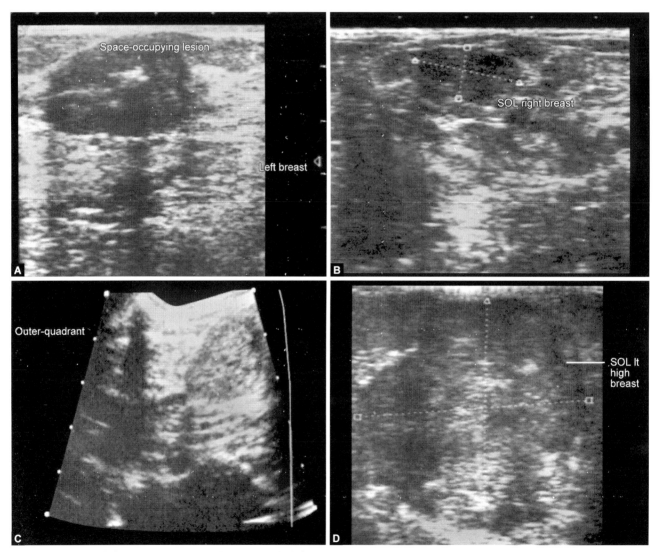

Figs. 22.2A to D: (A) Benign breast neoplasm—a well-defined homogeneously hypoechoic space-occupying lesion (SOL) with a dense focus of calcification; (B) Benign breast lump—well-defined hypoechoic lesion with irregular wall; (C) Fibroadenoma—well-defined SOL of homogeneous echotexture as a mobile lump in right upper outer quadrant; and (D) Giant fibroadenoma large mass occupying most of breast with well-defined margin and slightly heterogeneous echotexture.

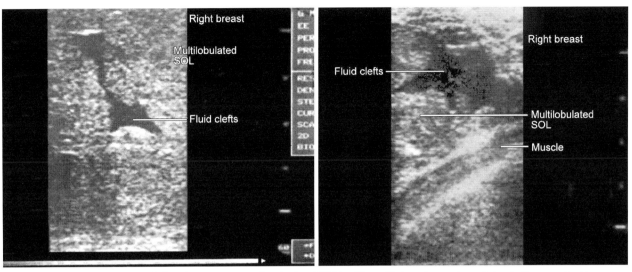

Fig. 22.3: A large well-defined space-occupying lesion (SOL) with multiple echogenic nodules in it separated by fluid clefts are seen.

The features of fibroadenoma which aid in differentiating them from carcinoma include sharp margination, mobility of the mass, its compressibility, tendency of long axis parallel to skin and lack of posterior shadowing.

Other benign solid lesions include papilloma, adenomata which are usually situated close to the nipple and surrounded by rim of fluid (due to intraductal location); Hamartomas—which show uneven internal echo pattern with well-defined margins. Lipomas are surrounded by thin fibrous tissue capsule and show low to medium level echoes.

Large benign solid masses seen in younger patients are giant fibroadenomata and, in older patients, Phylloides tumor **(Fig. 22.3)**. The giant fibroadenoma is well-defined with an even internal echo pattern. The phylloides tumor is similar but shows additional features of calcification and fluid clefts.

Malignant Neoplasms

Carcinoma **(Figs. 22.4A and B)** of the breast is one of the leading causes of cancer in women.

The principal sonographic features of malignant mass lesion include: (a) marginal irregularity, (b) irregular shape, (c) hypoechogenicity relative to fibroglandular tissue, (d) long axis of the mass perpendicular to skin, and (e) an echogenic rim of variable thickness (possibly representing tumor, extension, desmoplasia, compressed breast tissue or edema), (f) posterior acoustic shadowing or attenuation.

There may be additional features of trabecular distention, tissue plane distortion, skin thickening and microcalcification.

The majority of malignant breast masses are less echogenic than fibroglandular tissue and cancers may even be more hypoechoic than fat lobules. With high resolution ultrasound border characteristics can be assessed sonographically. Spiculations, extension of lesion along the ducts and fine (1–2 mm) microlobulations are highly suggestive of malignancy. Acoustic shadowing, which occurs due to fibrous response to the tumor is seen in 40–60% of tumors. Other conditions which may show acoustic shadowing include postsurgical and traumatic scarring, fat necrosis, calcified fibroadenoma, sclerosingadenosis and air containing abscess.

Microcalcifications are unreliably shown as small intense echoes with no attenuation. Skin thickening and edema may signify inflammatory breast carcinoma but is also seen in other benign conditions like breast abscess, irradiations therapy, congestive heart failure.

Sometimes carcinoma is diffuse and may give rise to two appearances. First, the breast plate is largely replaced by poorly reflective tissue which does not produce any shadowing. This may be indistinguishable from diffuse benign breast change and fine needle aspiration biopsy may be required for confirmation of diagnosis. The second presentation of diffuse carcinoma is seen when there is widespread involvement of lymphatics by cancer or following axillary dissections. The skin is thickened and dilated lymphatics may be detected in subcutaneous tissue.

Ultrasound examination of axilla may demonstrate nodal involvement in breast cancer.

Miscellaneous Conditions

Fat necrosis: Fat necrosis cause great difficulty in diagnosis. There are two main features: attenuation, which may be very marked and widespread and focal lesion, which is poorly defined echo poor masses which may contain fluid spaces. The attenuation pattern of fat necrosis makes it very difficult to differentiate from carcinoma.

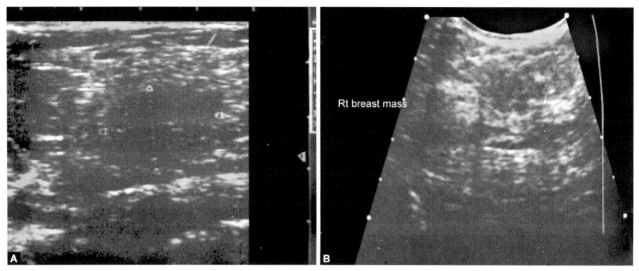

Figs. 22.4A and B: (A) Hypoechoic SOL with ill-defined lateral margins fine needle aspiration cytology (FNAC) confirmed infiltrating duct carcinoma; and (B) breast carcinoma—hypoechoic SOL with ill-defined walls seen in right breast.

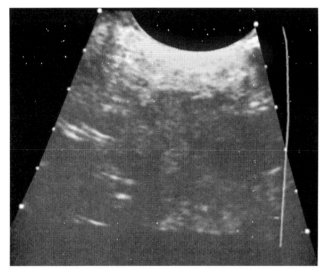

Fig. 22.5: Breast abscess—SOL with ill-defined margins with internal echoes in outer quadrants of left breast. Superficial fat is thickened and echogenic.

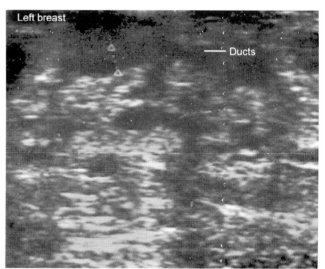

Fig. 22.6: Dilated ducts are seen in left breast.

*Abscess (**Fig. 22.5**):* An abscess may produce a number of echo poor areas in a larger area of disordered breast tissue. One feature of an abscess is variable attenuation from portions of the inflamed breast. The diagnosis must be confirmed by aspiration of pus from focal regions of liquefaction.

Galactoceles: These are cystic masses that contain milk. They occur during or after lactation. Sonographically, galactoceles appear as echogenic lesions and cystic masses with less through transmission than expected for cysts.

Plasma cell mastitis: It represents focal or more generalized attenuation with disruption of tissue planes in the breast.

*Duct ectasia (**Fig. 22.6**):* It is diagnosed on ultrasound when the duct caliber exceeds 3 mm.

Scrotal Ultrasound

Benign Intratesticular Lesions

*Cysts (**Figs. 22.7A to C**):* Testicular cysts are incidentally discovered in 8–10% of population. Intratesticular cysts are simple cysts filled with clear serous fluid varying in size between 2 to 18 mm. They are well-defined, anechoic lesions with thin, smooth walls, and posterior acoustic enhancement on ultrasound.

Epidermoid cysts: These are believed to be mesodermal development of a teratoma. Sonographically, they are well-defined, solid, hypoechoic masses which are internally hyperechoic occasionally.

Testicular abscesses: These are usually a complication of epididymo-orchitis. Other causes are mumps, smallpox, influenza, typhoid, osteomyelitis, and appendicitis,

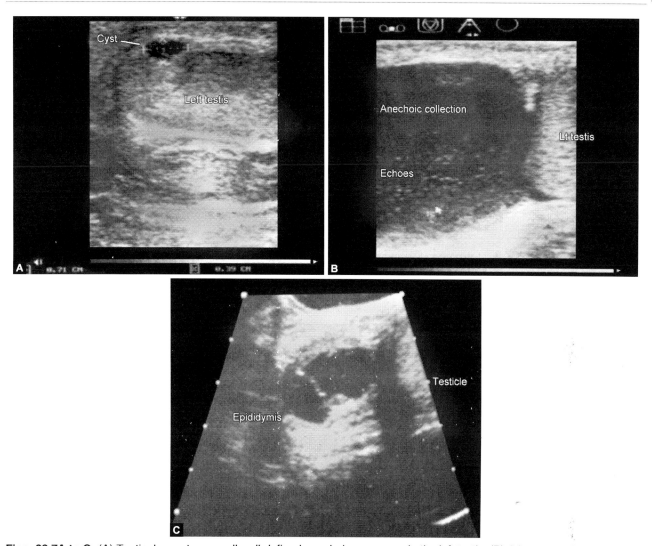

Figs. 22.7A to C: (A) Testicular cyst—a small well-defined anechoic area seen in the left testis; (B) A large anechoic collection with coarse internal echoes superior to left testis-spermatocele; (C) Anechoic simple cyst with thin septa seen in the region of head of the epididymis. Note the absence of internal echoes.

etc. Sonographically, an enlarged testicle containing a predominantly fluid filled mass with hypoechoic/mixed echogenic areas is visualized.

Infarction: Testicular infarction may result from neglected testicular torsion, trauma, leukemia, and polyarteritis nodosa (PAN). Sonographic appearance depends on the age of infarction. In the early stage, testicular infarction is seen as a focal hypoechoic mass/as a diffusely hypoechoic testicle of normal size. Later on, the entire testicle often decreases in size showing hyperechoic areas that represent fibrosis or dystrophic calcification.

Malignant Tumors (Figs. 22.8A to C)

Germ cell tumor: Pure seminoma accounts for 40 to 50 percent of all germ cell tumors. The peak incidence is in the 4th or the 5th decades. Sonographically, a seminoma demonstrates predominantly hypoechoicechotexture without cysts or calcification. Seminomas have the most favorable prognosis of the malignant testicular tumors.

Embryonal cell carcinoma: This is the second most common testicular germ cell neoplasm. This occurs in the younger age group (peak incidence in second and third decades). They are small but more aggressive than seminomas. The infantile form is the yolk sac tumor which is more common before two years of age. Sonographically, this tumor is more inhomogeneous and poorly marginated than seminomas. Invasion of tunica may cause distortion of testicular contour. Cystic areas of degeneration and echogenic areas representing calcification are commonly visualized.

Teratomas: These comprise 5–10% of primary testicular neoplasms. Sonographically, teratomas are well-defined, markedly inhomogeneous masses containing cystic and solid areas of various sizes. Dense echogenic foci with acoustic shadowing are quite common due to focal

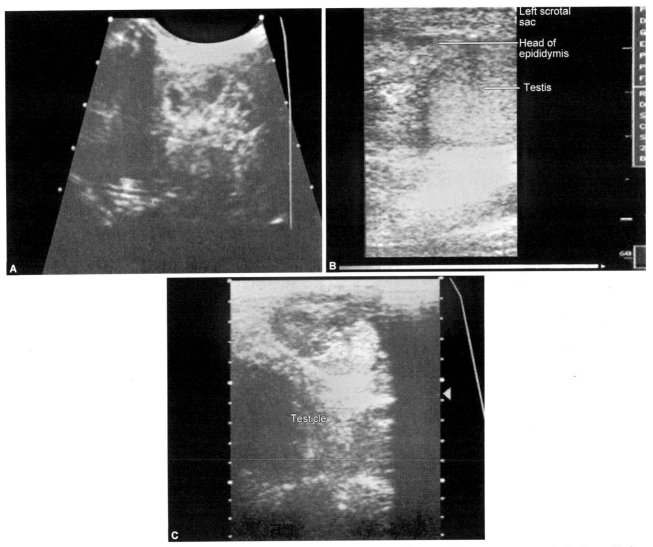

Figs. 22.8A to C: (A) Testicular malignancy—right testis is replaced by a solid mass of heterogeneous echotexture with few hypoechoic, anechoic and hypoechoic areas; (B) A heterogeneous predominantly echogenic SOL is seen in the left scrotal sac superior to testis in a case of left inguinal hernia; (C) Testicular malignancy—hypoechoic mass arising from superior pole of right testis.

calcification, cartilage, immature bone, fibrosis, and noncalcific scarring.

Choriocarcinoma: This is the rarest germ cell tumor. Peak incidence is in the second and third decades. It is highly malignant and metastasizes early. Sonographically, a mass of mixed echogenicity containing areas of hemorrhage, necrosis and calcification is visualized.

Stromal tumors: The majority are Leydig cell tumors occurring between the ages of 20 and 50 years. Sonographically, these are small, solid, and hypoechoic. Cystic degeneration is occasionally visualized.

Testicular metastases: Malignant lymphoma and leukemia are the most common metastatic testicular tumors. Majority of malignant lymphomas are homogeneous, hypoechoic, and diffusely replace testis.

Extratesticular Lesions

Hydrocele **(Figs. 22.9A to D):** Serous fluid, blood, pus/urine may collect in between the parietal and visceral layers of tunica vaginalis. Sonography can detect a potential cause of hydrocele and permits visualization of testes when palpation is hampered. Sonographically, anechoic collections with increased sound transmission are visualized surrounding anterolateral aspects of the testes. Low level to medium level echoes may be seen moving freely in hydroceles. Hematocele and pyocele contain internal septations and loculations.

Varicocele **(Figs. 22.10A and B):** This is an abnormal collection of dilated, tortuous and elongated pampiniform plexus veins. Sonographically, varicocele appears as multiple serpiginous anechoic structures more than 2 mm

CHAPTER 22: Small Part Ultrasound

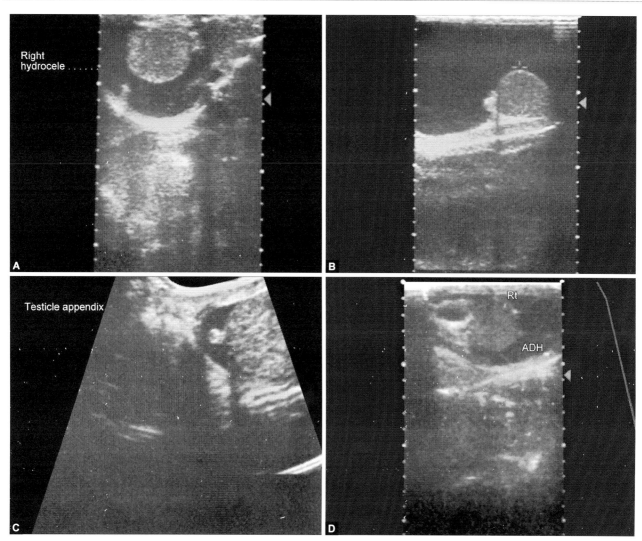

Figs. 22.9A to D: (A) Transverse section of right scrotal sac showing hydrocele; (B) Gross hydrocele; (C) Appendix testis with hydrocele; (D) Hydrocele with epididymitis (tubercular)—the epididymis is swollen and shows a hypoechoic area in it. Hydrocele shows multiple strands in it.

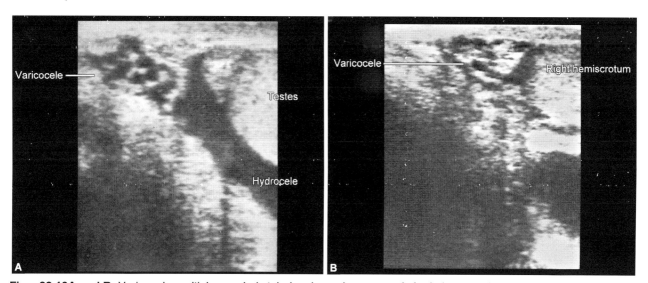

Figs. 22.10A and B: Varicocele-multiple anechoic tubular channels are seen in both the scrotal sacs. Hydrocele is also seen on the left side.

in diameter. These are seen to decrease in size when the patient lies supine and the scrotum is elevated. Color Doppler can visualize the slow blood flow in the dilated veins. Venous flow can be augmented with patient in upright position or during Valsalva maneuver.

Epididymo-orchitis (Figs. 22.11A to C): The common causative organisms are *Escherichia coli, Pseudomonas, Gonococcus,* and Chlamydia. The peak age incidence is 40 to 50 years. Sonography demonstrates thickening and enlargement of epididymis. The echogenicity is usually decreased with coarse echotexture which is often inhomogeneous. The orchitis may be evident as focal or generalized hypoechogenicity of the testicle which might be enlarged.

Testicular Torsion

Torsion is more common in children and seen in only 20% postpubertal males with an acute scrotum. Prompt diagnosis is necessary since torsion requires immediate surgery to preserve the testis. Testicular salvage rate is 80–100% if surgery is performed within 5–6 hours of onset of pain, and only 20% if surgery is delayed for more than 12 hours.

In acute phase testicle becomes enlarged, inhomogeneous and hypoechoic as compared to contralateral normal testis. Common extratesticular findings include an enlarged epididymis containing foci of increased and decreased echogenicity, skin thickening and reactive hydrocele formation.

Pulsed wave and color flow Doppler examination of the spermatic cord and testicular vessels have been used to differentiate torsion from epididymo-orchitis. The presence of normal or increased blood flow within the testicle would exclude the diagnosis of acute torsion. The diagnosis of testicular ischemia depends on unequivocal demonstration of normal blood flow in normal, contralateral asymptomatic testicle. Recently power mode Doppler sonography has increased the ability to detect, the slower blood flow within the smaller caliber vessels seen in testes.

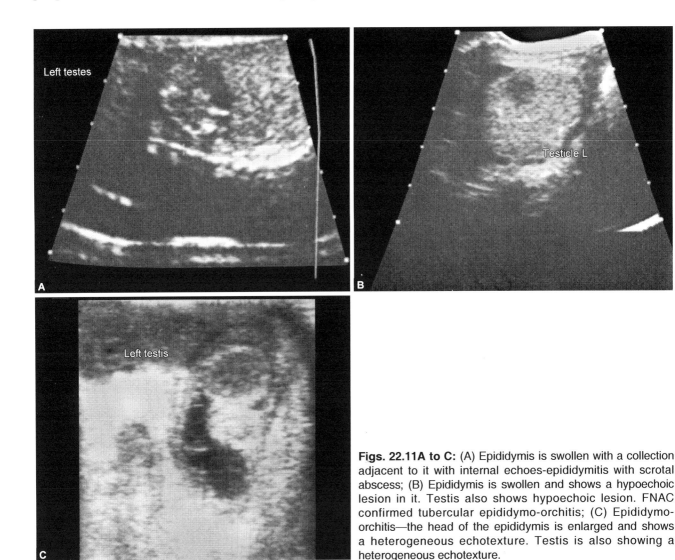

Figs. 22.11A to C: (A) Epididymis is swollen with a collection adjacent to it with internal echoes-epididymitis with scrotal abscess; (B) Epididymis is swollen and shows a hypoechoic lesion in it. Testis also shows hypoechoic lesion. FNAC confirmed tubercular epididymo-orchitis; (C) Epididymo-orchitis—the head of the epididymis is enlarged and shows a heterogeneous echotexture. Testis is also showing a heterogeneous echotexture.

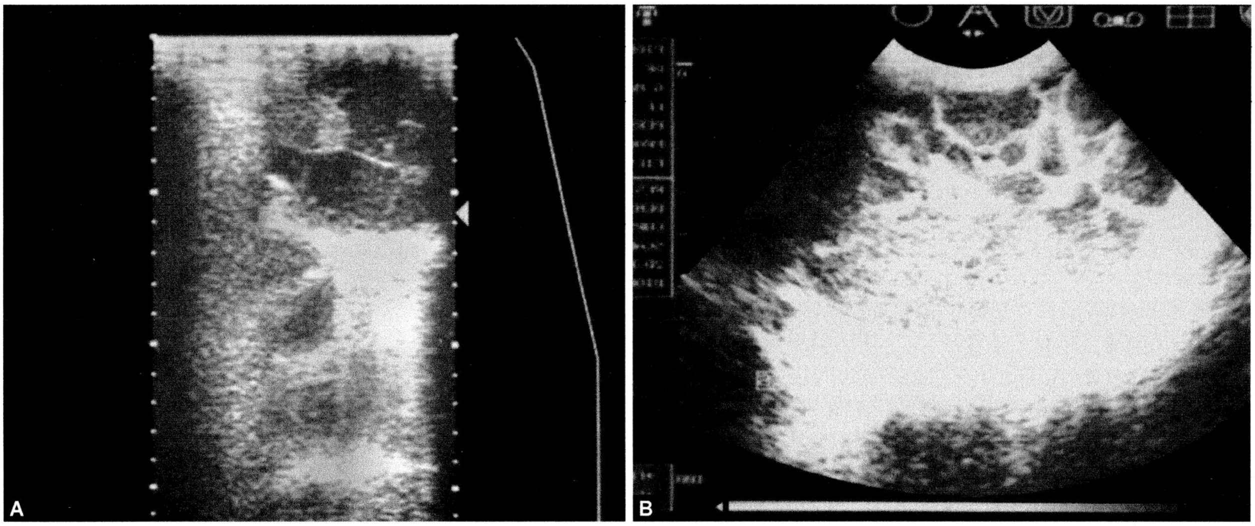

Figs. 22.12A and B: (A) Organized scrotal hematoma; (B) Multiloculated collection with internal echoes seen in the left scrotal sac pushing the testis to one corner—organized hematoma.

Trauma (Figs. 22.12A and B)

Prompt diagnosis of a ruptured testis is of utmost importance because 90% testicles can be saved if surgery is performed within the first 72 hours. Clinical diagnosis is often impossible because of marked scrotal pain and swelling. Sonographic features include focal areas of altered testicular echogenicity corresponding to areas of hemorrhage or infarction, and hematocele formation. A discrete fracture plane may be seen (in 17%). Testicular contour is irregular. Use of Doppler may aid in separating normal vascularized testis from a complex intrascrotal hematoma.

Cryptorchidism (Figs. 22.13A and B)

The majority (80%) of undescended testes are palpable, lying at or below the level of inguinal canal. Because of the superficial location, sonography of undescended testes should be performed with a high frequency transducer and a stand-off pad to avoid reverberation artifacts. Sonographically undescended testis is often smaller and slightly less echogenic than normally descended testes. A specific diagnosis of undescended testes can be made if mediastinum testis (an internal echogenic band) is identified. A large lymph node or pars infravaginalis gubernaculi (PIG) which is the distal bulbous segment of gubernaculum testes may be mistaken for testes, but neither of these contain internal echogenic band. If testes remain undescended PIG persists distal to undescended testes, usually in scrotum as a hypoechoic, cordlike structure of echogenicity similar to testes.

Complications of cryptorchidism are infertility and cancer. The undescended testes are 48 times more likely to undergo malignant change than normally descended testis. The most common malignancy is seminoma.

THORAX

Ultrasonography, till date, has not been much exploited for the evaluation of diseases of the chest because of the basic inability of ultrasound waves to 'see through' air and bone medium. Due to this limitation and the ease of getting a chest X-ray and even CT exam, coupled with the 'familiarity', the clinicians feel with chest X-rays, USG, is almost unheard of as a diagnostic tool in the field.

However, as has been proved in the past couple of years, USG has a role in management and diagnosis of chest diseases in specific clinical setting, i.e.

- Evaluation of chest wall lesions by high frequency probes, e.g. chest wall abscess, cartilaginous cap of osteochondroma, osteomyelitis of bones of chest wall, etc.
- Pleural lesions.
- Pulmonary, mediastinal and hilar regions seen through the window of pleural effusion or that of the consolidated lung.
- Mediastinal lesions seen through the heart from suprasternal notch, parasternal regions, intercostal, and subcostal areas. Ultrasound can be used as a primary diagnostic-modality, can be used as an adjunct to other imaging and can be used as guidance for intervention for diagnosis and treatment.

DIAGNOSTIC

- Pleural Effusion **(Figs. 22.14 A to L)**
  – Minimal pleural effusions (US is much more sensitive than radiography for diagnosing minimal pleural effusion).
  – A typical pleural collections which are mistaken for other parenchymal or mediastinal lesions on X-rays.

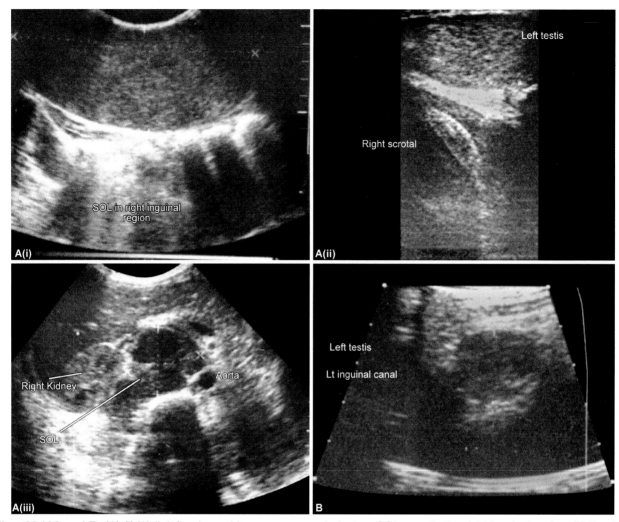

Figs. 22.13A and B: (A) (i) Well-defined round homogeneous echotexture SOL seen in the right inguinal region, (ii) the right scrotal sac is empty and left testis is normal in position, (iii) there are para-aortic lymph nodes. Excision biopsy from the lesion revealed seminoma testis, (B) left ectopic testis lying in the inguinal canal.

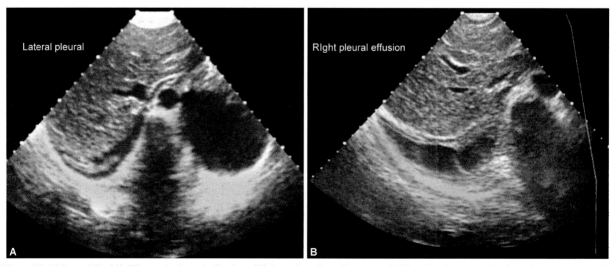

Figs. 22.14A and B: (A) Bilateral pleural effusion; (B) Loculated multiseptate fluid collection seen in the pleural cavity with associated pleural thickening.

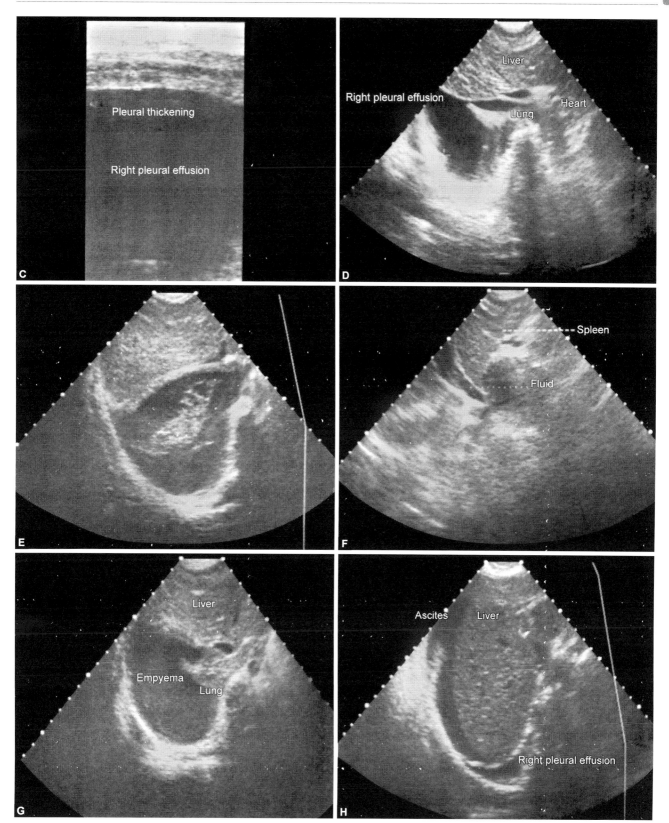

Figs. 22.14C to H: (C) Thickened pleura seen along with pleural effusion; (D) Transverse epigastric scan shows fluid in right pleural cavity with collapsed lung seen inside it; (E) Free fluid seen in right pleural cavity with collapsed lung inside note the inverted diaphragm; (F) Minimal pleural fluid seen in left costophrenic angle; (G) Empyema-free fluid in right pleural cavity with internal echoes in it with pleural thickening; (H) Ascites with right pleural effusion.

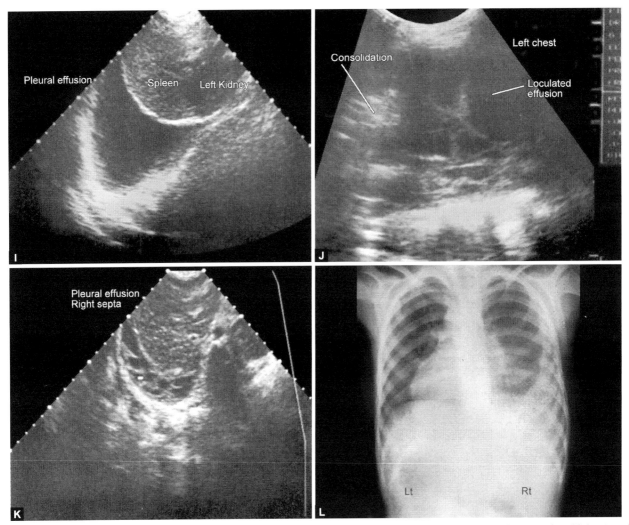

Figs. 22.14I to L: (I) Free fluid in left pleural cavity; (J) A loculated collection in left pleural cavity with evidence of multiple strands in it, pleural thickening and adjacent consolidated lung with air bronchogram in it; (K) Multiseptate fluid collection seen in right pleural cavity in the case of infected pleural effusion; (L) Chest X-ray shows evidence of blunted right CP angle suggestive of right pleural effusion.

- Encysted/loculated pleural effusions.
- Presence or absence of associated pleural masses.
- Evaluation of a radiographically opaque hemithorax Differentiation of pleural, pulmonary, and mediastinal components leading to the opacity in the hemithorax and the final pathology can often be seen on ultrasonography.
- Chest wall lesions.

ADJUNCT IN THE DIAGNOSIS

As it adds to the information already obtained by some other modality like X-ray chest.
- Type of pleural effusion—A pleural collection seen on ultrasonography can be of variable echogenicity, leading us towards the etiology of the effusion.
  - *Anechoic:* All transudates are anechoic. However, all anechoic collections are not transudates. About 1/3rd of exudates collection tends to be anechoic in the beginning.
  - *Hypoechoic:* Usually exudative effusion. It may be seen in late stages of hemothorax.
  - *Echogenic:* Hemothoraces or empyemata.
  - *Presence of debris:* Debris usually represents settled down pus cells, blood cells, etc. giving fluid-fluid levels at times.
  - *Septations:* They represent a process of loculation and fibrosis, occurring in a pleural effusion.
    Clean, thin septae with minimal debris most often represent tubercular pleural effusion while pyogenic pleural effusions like empyemata are usually seen to be having thick and shaggy septations with echoes in the collection.
  - *Pleural nodules/masses:* May represent mesotheliomas, metastatic nodules or tuberculomata depending on the clinical setting.

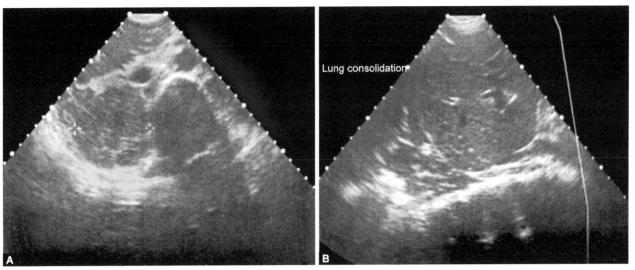

Figs. 22.15 A and B: A predominantly hypoechoic solid mass lesion seen in right lower lobe of lung; and (B) Consolidation—seen as a homogeneous hypoechoic lesion with air bronchogram in right lower lobe of lung.

- *Evaluation of lung obscured by pleural effusion on X-ray:* In this setting, the pleural effusion gives a window to the evaluation of the underlying lung.
    - Consolidation **(Figs. 22.15A and B)** shows air/fluid bronchogram pattern.
    - Collapsed lung appears like a collapsed tongue of tissue moving with respiration in a pleural effusion.
    - An abscess **(Fig. 22.16)** developing in the consolidated lung can be readily identified.
    - Evaluation of lesions of lung parenchyma **(Figs. 22.17A to F)**
- *Evaluation of a mass leading to distal consolidation:* This is another setting when a patient comes, with an unresolving consolidation and a hilar or mediastinal mass is picked up on USG which is the actual cause of the consolidation in the distal lung. Of course, the mass requires further evaluation by bronchography/CT for a final diagnosis.
- *Evaluation of intrathoracic masses in children:* Easy differentiation of cystic and solid masses can be made on USG in such cases. Position of the mass especially in cases of mediastinal masses and their differentiation from normal structures like thymus can be readily obtained by USG in a couple of minutes. The lack of radiations and noninvasiveness of USG are added attractions in case of a pediatric patient.
- Evaluation of cardiac lesions **(Figs. 22.18A to E)**.

Aids in Intervention

Guidance of FNA, diagnostic pleural aspirations, therapeutic pleural taps especially in loculated pleural effusions, guidance for I/c tube placement which can all be done easily and actually are being done widely and using USG.

Another field where use of USG is being exploited in diagnosing chest diseases is case of critically ill patient, i.e. trauma patients and patients in ICU who often need serial portable chest skiagrams to evaluate day to day change in their lesion. Portable chest X-rays in these settings are usually substandard in quality with the added inability to position the patient as required. Portable USG has found to be able to provide most of the 'clinically useful' information which would affect management.

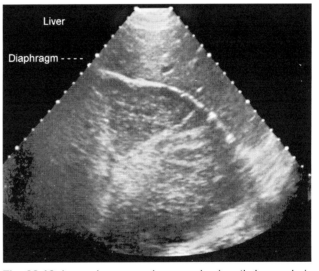

Fig. 22.16: Lung abscess—a large predominantly hypoechoic SOL with internal septae and posterior enhancement is seen in lower lobe of right lung. Aspiration revealed pus. Inversion of diaphragm is seen.

Other advantages adding to the attractions of USG.
- Cost
- Flexibility
- No radiation
- Good guidance tool
- Possibility of repeated evaluations
- Ability to detect abdominal lesions associated with/causative of the chest lesions, e.g. liver abscess leading

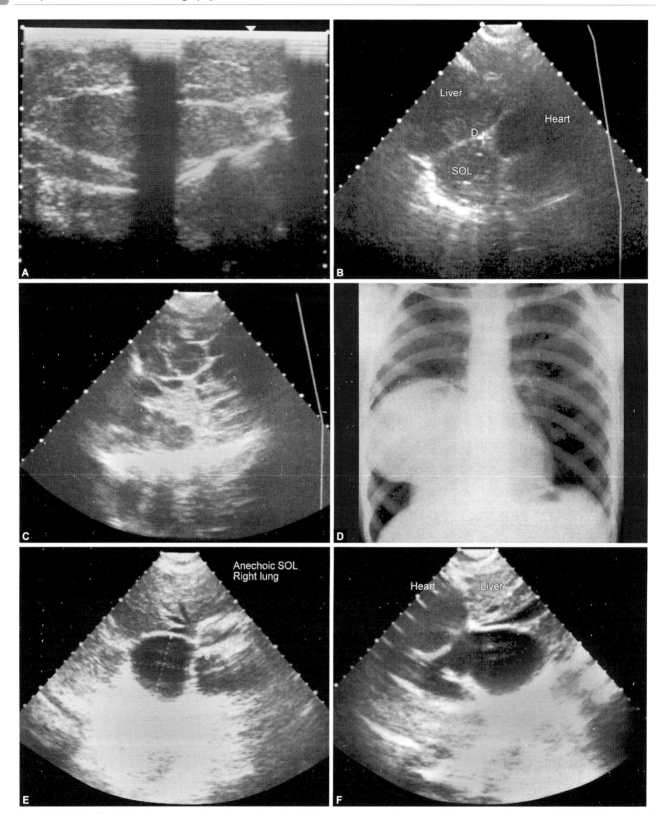

Figs. 22.17A to F: (A) Axillary scan showing predominantly hypoechoic solid mass with echogenic septae in it FNAC revealed adipocysts—lipoma; (B) Lung sequestration—predominantly hypoechoic SOL with air bronchogram in it is seen in right lower lobe of lung adjacent to the heart in this case of nonresolving pneumonia in 16 years old patient; (C) A classical hydatid cyst seen in lower lobe of right lung; (D) Chest X-ray of the same patient. Lung hydatid seen as anechoic cystic lesion in transverse; (E) and longitudinal; (F) Scan of lung.

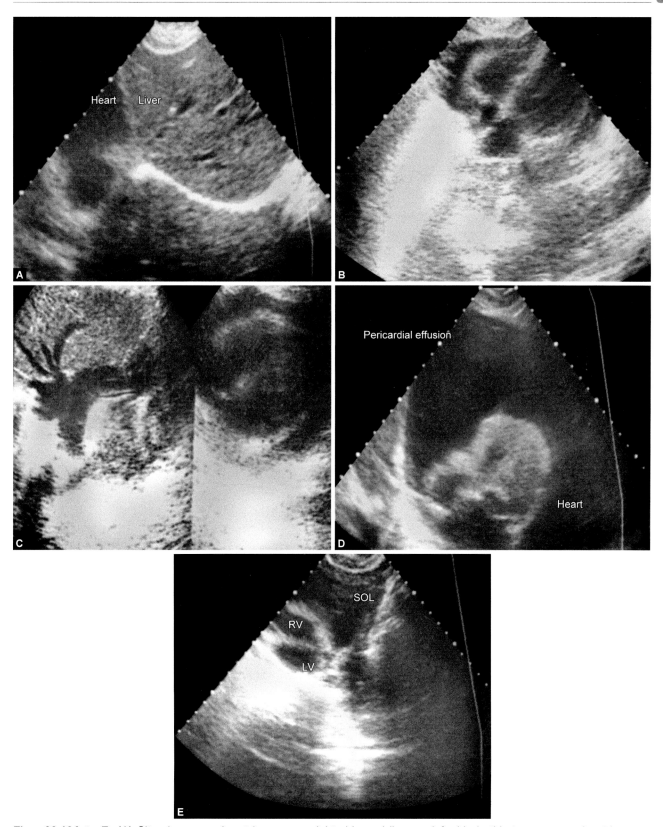

Figs. 22.18A to E: (A) Situs inversus—heart is seen on right side and liver on left side in this transverse epigastric scan; (B) Minimal pericardial effusion; (C) Dilated IVC in a case of pericardial effusion; (D) Gross pericardial effusion. The patient presented with signs and symptoms of cardiac tamponade; (E) Pericardial abscess—anechoic collection seen in relation to right atrium and right ventricle in the longitudinal and transverse gray scale scan and Doppler image. Aspiration revealed pus.

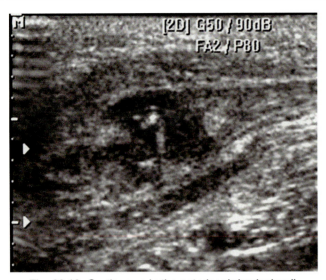

Fig. 22.19: Cysticercus in the anterior abdominal wall.

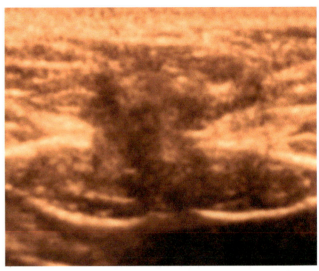

Fig. 22.20: Anterior abdominal wall hernia with herniation of properitoneal fat.

to pleural effusion—abdominal tuberculosis associated with tubercular pleural effusion.

Limitations

- Pneumothoraces/hydropneumothoraces are missed or underestimated.
- Limited information about mediastinal, hilar, and proximal airway lesions.
- Restricted field of view as opposed to a global view presented on X-rays with which the clinicians are familiar.
- Operator dependence.

Anterior Abdominal Wall Ultrasound (Figs. 22.19 to 20.21)

High resolution US of the anterior abdominal wall lesions is useful in a number of clinical entities and yields significant clinical information. It reveals the size, nature, and extent of lesion. It is useful in detecting infective and inflammatory lesions along with their extent. It is useful in the evaluation of the anterior abdominal wall hernias.

Musculoskeletal Ultrasound

Tendon tears: In complete tears, the two tendon fragments are separated by a gap of variable length and echogenicity. This corresponds to the hematoma which is subsequently replaced by granulomatous tissue. A bone avulsion may also be visualized as a brightly echogenic focus with acoustic shadowing.

Rotator cuff tears **(Figs. 22.22A to E)**: The diagnostic criteria for rotator cuff is the nonvisualization of the rotator cuff retracted under the acromion process. Focal thinning and discontinuity are the other two criteria. The presence of

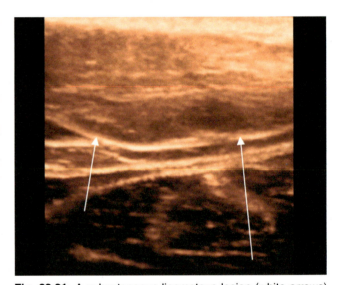

Fig. 22.21: A subcutaneous lipomatous lesion (white arrows) in the anterior abdominal wall in a case of benign lipomatosis of the skin.

foci of increased echogenicity in the cuff is the least reliable indicator of rotator cuff tear.

Meniscal tear **(Figs. 22.23A to C)** are one of the most common lesions of the knee joint. Tears are more common in the medial than lateral. The menisci are well evaluated of USG. The normal menisci are seen as homogeneously echogenic triangular structure with apex of triangle pointed towards middle of the joint. The tear is seen as an irregular hypoechoic area in the echogenic menisci.

Patellar tendon tears: This result in a small well-defined, hypoechoic hematoma which is located in the midline (best seen on transverse scans).

Achilles tendon tears: Mostly it ruptures in the midportion of the tendon, about 2–3 cm from calcaneal attachment. In complete tears, the gap between the 2 fragments is variable, and the hematoma may extend along the tendon over a long distance. The tendon fragments show jagged margins, resembling a frayed loupe.

Tendinitis: In acute tendinitis, the tendon is swollen, its echogenicity is decreased, and its contours are blurred. Minute calcifications can be demonstrated on sonography.

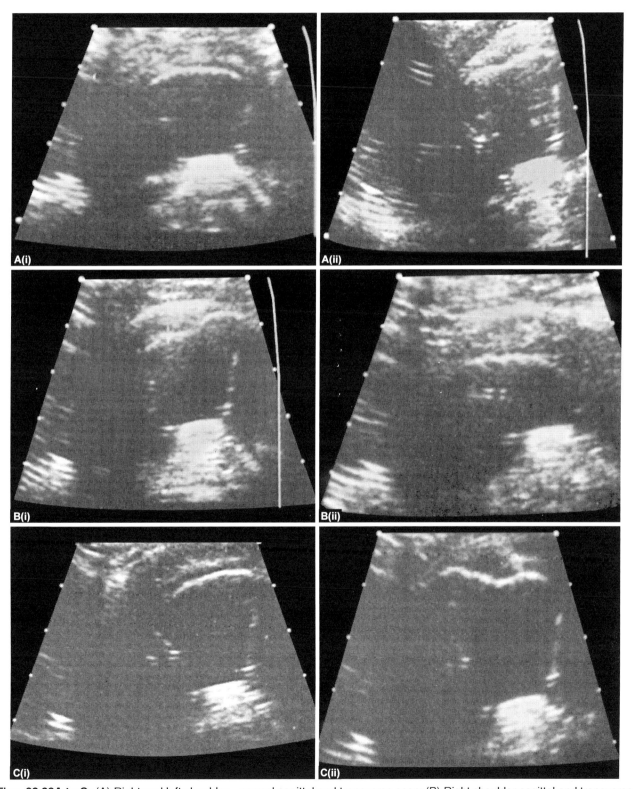

Figs. 22.22A to C: (A) Right and left shoulder—normal sagittal and transverse scan; (B) Right shoulder sagittal and transverse scans show swelling and edema of rotator cuff; (C) Right shoulder shows evidence of partial tear of rotator cuff.

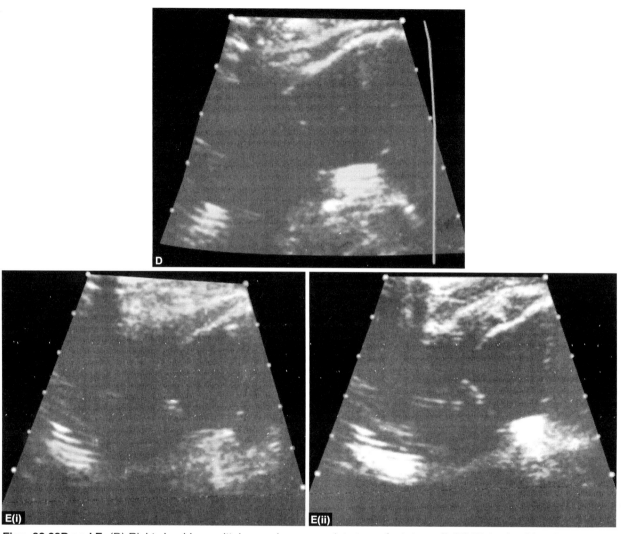

Figs. 22.22D and E: (D) Right shoulder sagittal scan shows complete tear of rotator cuff; (E) Right shoulder shows partial atrophy of rotator cuff.

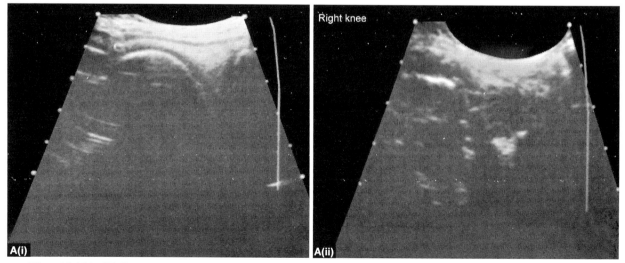

Figs. 22.23A: (A) (i) Ultrasonogram shows normal knee joint, (ii) tear of anterior horn of lateral meniscus is seen.

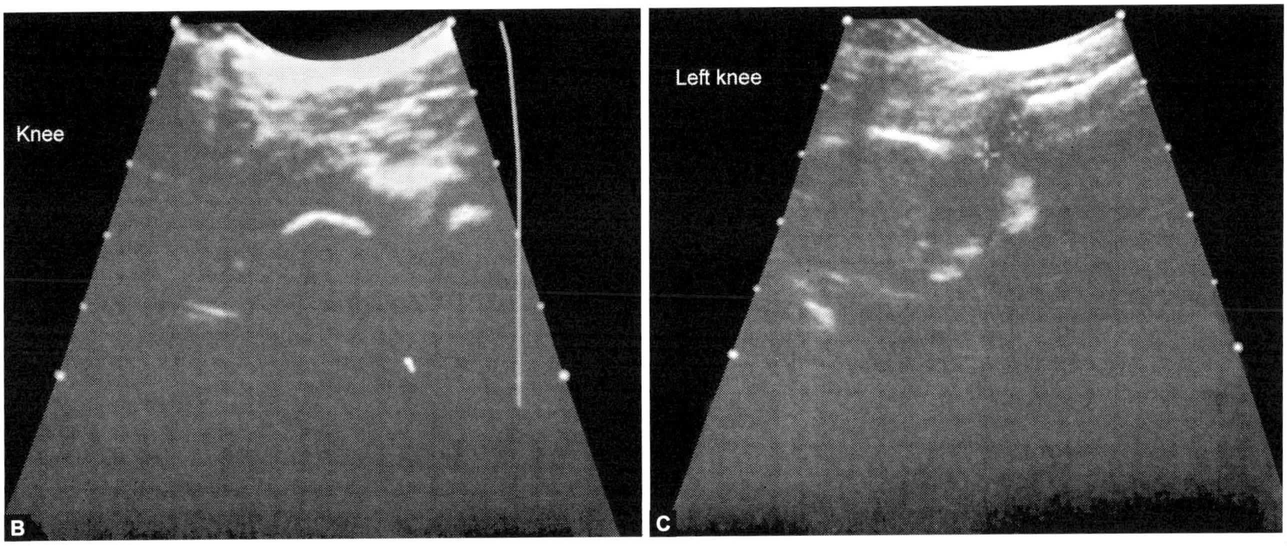

Figs. 22.23B and C: (B) Right knee shows synovial effusion; (C) Tear of posterior horn of medial meniscus is seen.

Bursitis: This may be isolated or associated tendinitis. Subdeltoid, olecranoid, patellar, and calcaneal bursae are involved most frequently. Sonography demonstrates a swollen rounded, fluid-filled bursa with ill-defined margins. In chronic bursitis, the bursa may exhibit a complex appearance, while calcification gives rise to hyperechoic foci with shadowing.

Ultrasound of Joint Lesions

Joint effusions **(Figs. 22.24A and B):** Sonography demonstrates intra-articular fluid collections. Septic effusion may contain debris. Sonography is ideal for guiding aspiration of small effusions.

Synovial cysts **(Fig. 22.25):** These develop from joint spaces/adjacent bursae. Popliteal cysts typically appear as fluid filled collections, often wrapping around the gastronemius-semimembranous bursa. Inflamed cysts may contain echogenic fibrinous debris. In patients with rheumatoid arthritis, the cysts may be filled with pannus and mimic solid masses. A ruptured cyst may be diagnosed as fluid dissecting into the calf.

Bones and Soft Tissues (Figs. 22.26A to E)

Trauma: In neonates and children, sonography can demonstrate fractures and dislocations of unossified epiphysis. Bone formation at fracture site can be visualized and monitored easily on sonography.

Osteomyelitis: Sonographically, it is visualized as fluid collection abutting the bone. It can also be seen as a detached sequestrum (brightly echogenic with acoustic shadowing) lying at a variable distance from the bone. It can also distinguish osteomyelitis born cellulitis and abscess.

Sonographic Evaluation of Pediatric Hip (Figs. 22.27A to F)

During first few months of life, ossification around hip joint is only partial and ultrasound can directly image the cartilaginous femoral head and visualize its relationship with acetabulum.

Congenital Dislocation of the Hip

In neonates, sonography has become the technique of choice to examine hips.

Graf in 1980 developed a set of measurements on coronal scanning for diagnosis of congenital dislocation of the hip (CDH). These lines are drawn about the acetabulum. The first, baseline, connects the osseous acetabulum convexity to the point of insertion of joint capsule to perichondrium. A second inclination line joins osseous convexity to labrum acetabulare. The third, acetabular roof line connects lower edge of acetabular roof medially to osseous convexity.

Two angles are then measured; one between acetabular roof line and baseline (alpha) measures "osseous acetabular convexity." A small acetabular angle indicates a shallow bony acetabulum. The second angle (Beta) is measured between baseline and line of inclination and gives an indication of additional coverage of femoral head by cartilaginous coverage.

In normal hip	α is more than $60°$ and β is less than $55°$.
In subluxation	α is less than $44°$ β is more than $77°$.

Coronal images are used to evaluate the position of femoral head within the acetabulum. If acetabular cup accommodates less than one-third of femoral head then

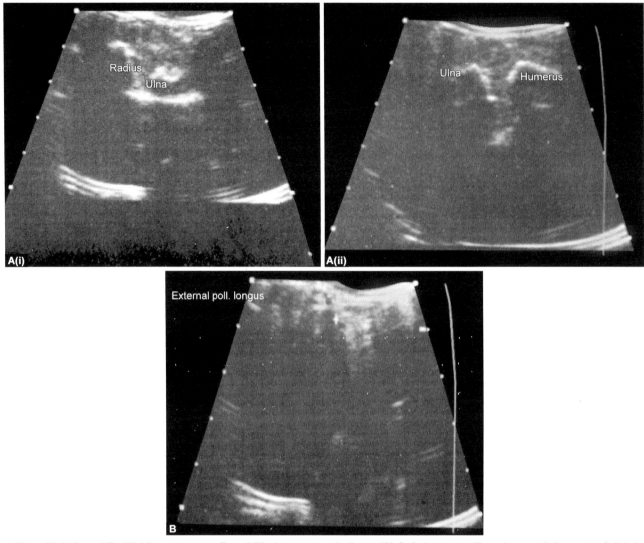

Figs. 22.24A and B: (A) Ultrasonogram (i) and (ii) shows normal elbow; (B) Soft tissue swelling along radial aspect of distal forearm (left), with minimal collection along adductor pollicis longus tendon-synovitis.

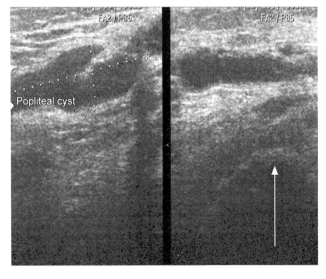

Fig. 22.25: Irregular anechoic popliteal cyst, femoral condyle is indicated by white arrow.

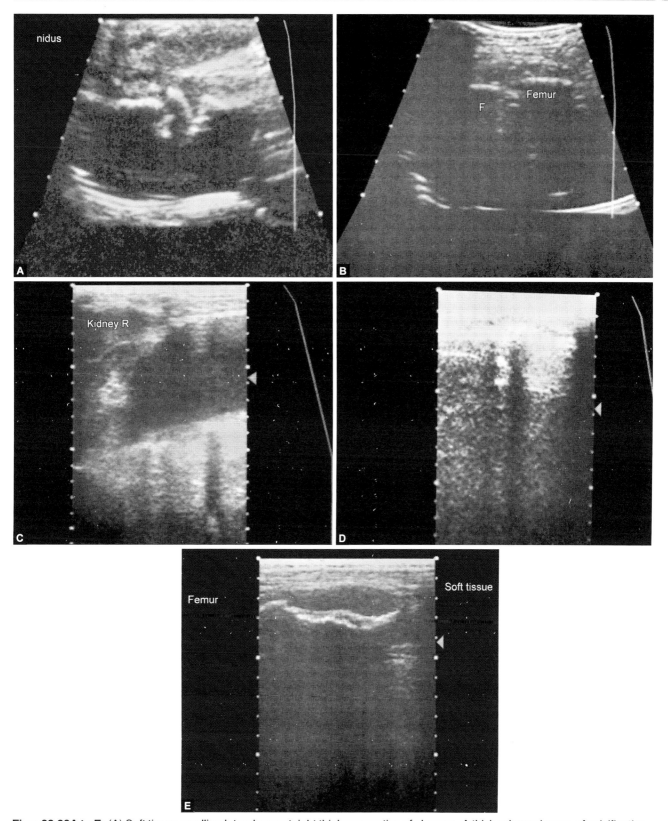

Figs. 22.26A to E: (A) Soft tissue swelling lateral aspect right thigh suggestive of abscess. A thick echogenic area of calcification-chronic osteomyelitis; (B) Ultrasonogram shows fracture right femur; (C) A hypoechoic collection is seen medial, posterior and inferior to right kidney in paravertebral gutter-psoas abscess; (D) A hypoechoic lesion seen in mid thigh anteriorly with c/o calcification-cysticercosis; (E) Longitudinal scan of right thigh showing hypoechoic area adjacent to bone with cortical irregularity—osteomyelitis.

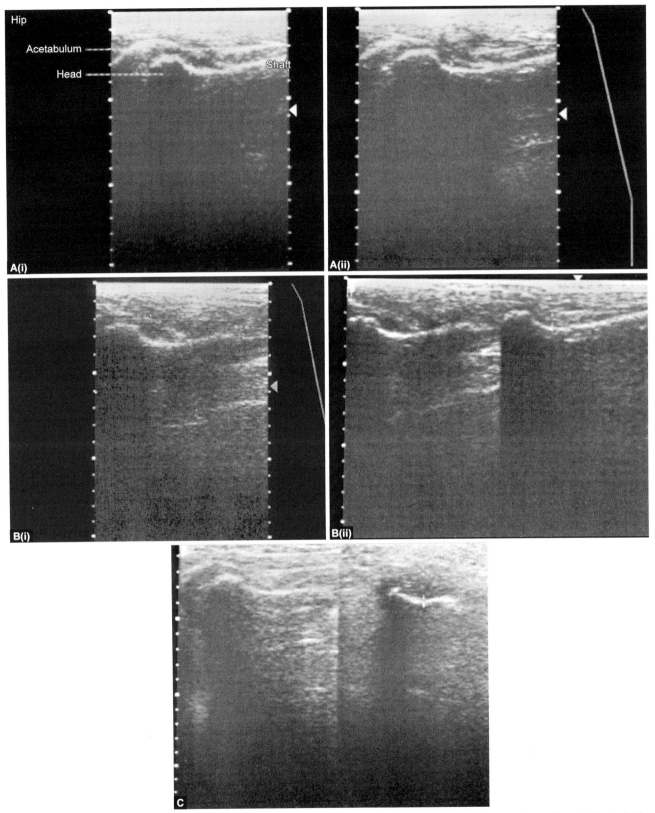

Figs. 22.27A to C: (A) Right hip shows hypoechoic collection—TB hip. Left hip is normal; (B) Right hip septic arthritis. Left hip normal; (C) Septic arthritis—right side with destruction of head of femur.

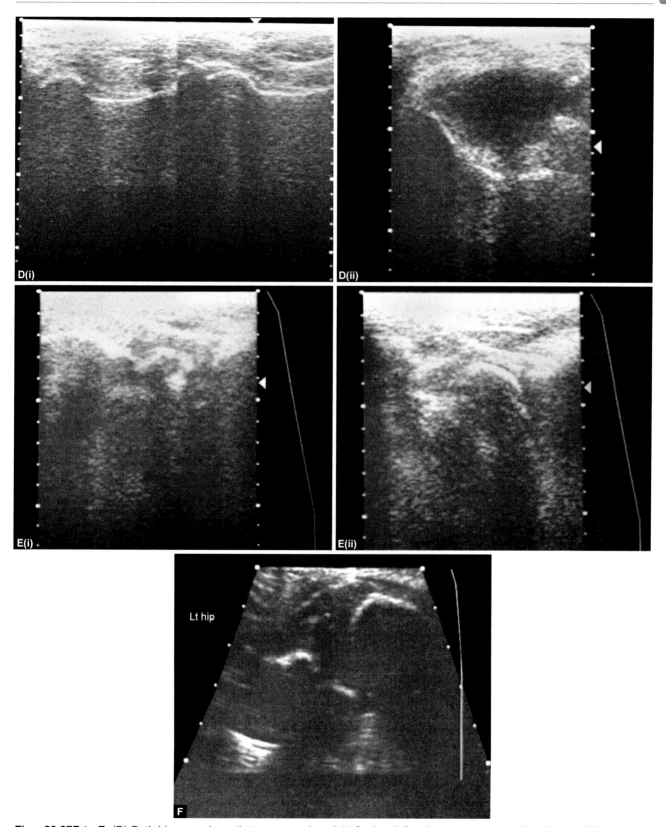

Figs. 22.27D to F: (D) Both hip normal—patient presented as right flexion deformity abscess in right iliac fossae; (E) Right hip normal. Left hip shows avascular necrosis (Perthes' disease); (F) Ultrasound left hip shows dislocation of left hip.

TABLE 22.1: Classification of hip dysplasia on the basis of ultrasonographic measurements.

Character	Type I (normal)	Type II (dysplasia)	Type III (subluxation)
Alpha angle	>60°	44°–60°	<34°
Beta angle	<55°	55°–77°	>77°
Percentage coverage	>58%	58–33%	<33%

acetabular dysplasia is definitely present. If one-half to one-third of head is accommodated, acetabular dysplasia must be suspected.

In addition, shape of acetabular rim and roof is assessed. In all pathological hips, the lateral bony rim is rounded or has bony defects.

In complete dislocation, position of limbic cartilage is important since it may be interposed between femoral head and acetabulum.

Table 22.1 gives the classification of hip dysplasia on the basis of ultrasonographic measurements.

Joint Effusion

The hip is commonly evaluated for joint effusion in children, the causes may be septic arthritis, transient synovitis, traumatic hemarthrosis, Perthes' disease, rheumatoid arthritis. Ultrasonography can delineate clearly the presence and the nature of fluid. Anterior approach along the plane of neck is used. The joint capsule is lifted and becomes convex. Comparison with the opposite hip is always useful. If the fluid is completely hypoechoic, it is likely to be transudate. If the fluid is dense and echogenic, it is an exudate or hematoma. Increased echogenicity of fluid and thick capsule (more than 2 mm) suggest septic arthritis. An anterior synovial space of more than 3 mm with asymmetry of more than 2 mm with opposite side is taken as abnormal (effusion). It is idiopathic (more common) or secondary to number of conditions. Among them sickle cell anemia, gout, renal osteodystrophy, exogenous steroid use, Cushing syndrome, Gaucher's disease and rarely repeated pregnancy.

Perthes' disease: It is a self limiting osteonecrosis of the femoral head epiphysis and commonly occurs between 3 and 10 years in boys. Ultrasound assessment shows widening of anterior joint space, and fragmentation. It not only helps in measuring the growth and development, i.e. size of femoral head but also helps in detecting progress of lesions.

Trauma: Trauma in a growing child may involve growth plate and result in growth disturbances. Ultrasound examination may show fluid (blood) within the joint.

23
CHAPTER

Ultrasound Examination of the Peripheral Arteries

EQUIPMENT AND DOCUMENTATION

Real time imaging should be conducted at the highest clinically appropriate frequency. A linear or curved array transducer in the range of 5–7.5 MHz should be used. There should be a permanent record of the ultrasound (US) exam. Images of all appropriate areas, between normal and abnormal should be recorded. Appropriate velocity parameters should be recorded as well, within the site at which velocity signals are obtained clearly indicated. Variations from normal size or flow dynamics should be accompanied by measurements. All relevant images should be clearly labeled by text characters, preferably in capitals indicating the name of the artery and its position. All images should be labeled with the examination date, patient identification, image location, and orientation.

Technique (Figs. 23.1 to 23.8)

The patient is positioned supine with the head slightly elevated. The leg being examined is abducted and externally rotated with the knee flexed. Acoustic gel applied in the region of the groin and a 5 MHz frequency used to start the examination.

Thigh: The transducer is placed in the groin resembling a transverse orientation. The transducer position is actually guided by manual palpation of the femoral pulse. The sonographer starts the initial positioning of the transducer right over the maximum pulsation of the femoral artery. The vessels visualized are the common femoral artery (CFA) and common femoral vein (CFV). The CFA is lateral to the vein within good arterial pulsation, compression of the CFV can be performed to distinguish it from the artery, after the CFA is seen, the probe is angled superiorly in the long axis of the artery, to visualize the most proximal part of the CFA. Next the transducer is moved inferiorly over the CFA to the point where the CFA bifurcates into the profound femoral (PF) and superficial femoral artery (SFA). The SFA is anterior whereas the PF is posterior. Generally only the beginning of the PFA can be visualized. The rest of the artery is not easily visualized, as it is deep seated. The SFA is superficial and is easily rolled on the medial aspect of the thigh. The transducer is gently moved along the long axis of the SFA till the level of the adductor canal just above the knee.

The popliteal artery is a continuation of the SFA. To image the popliteal artery the patient is turned prone and again after palpation of the popliteal artery in the knee posteriorly, the transducer is placed in the appropriate location. Start with a transducer scan, with the popliteal artery and popliteal vein are seen side by side with the artery deeper than the vein. The transducer is moved superiorly along the posterior thigh and then along the posterior part of the knee inferiorly till the trifurcation of the popliteal artery is seen just below the knee, in the upper leg.

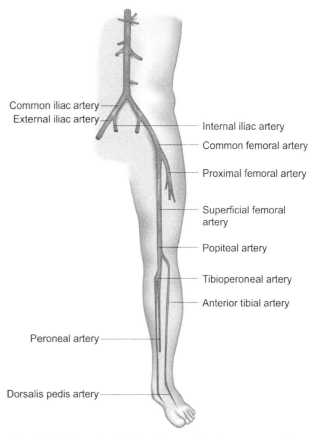

Fig. 23.1: Normal arterial anatomy of the leg-common iliac artery (CIA)

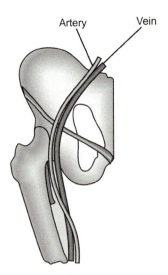

Fig. 23.2: The femoral vein is medial to the artery in the groin but is lateral to the artery in the popliteal region.

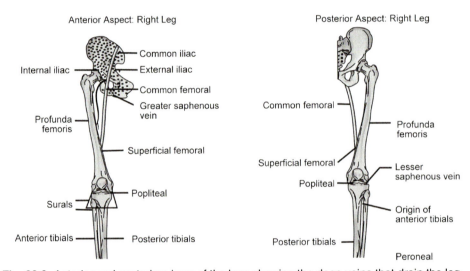

Fig. 23.3: Anterior and posterior views of the legs showing the deep veins that drain the leg.

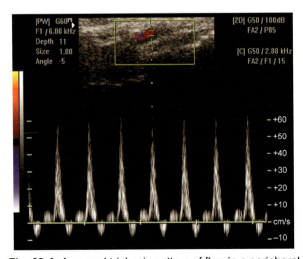

Fig. 23.4: A normal triphasic pattern of flow in a peripheral artery.

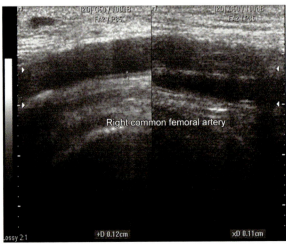

Fig. 23.5: Thickening of the intima media complex in the right femoral artery s/o atherosclerotic changes.

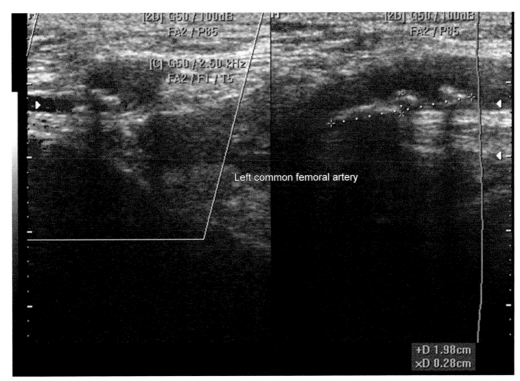

Fig. 23.6: A large, calcified atherosclerotic plaque in the left common femoral artery.

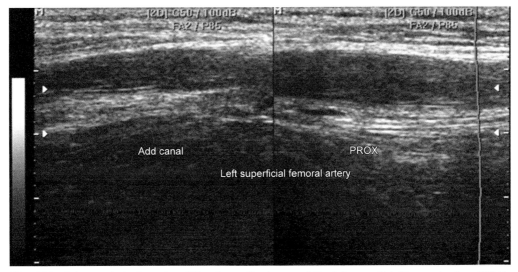

Fig. 23.7: A hypoechoic thrombus filling the entire lumen of the left superficial femoral artery (SFA).

Lower leg: The branches of the popliteal arteries are again best visualized from the posterior approach. The popliteal artery divides into two. Anterior tibial (AT) and tibioperoneal trunk (TP). The AT runs along the lateral aspect of the leg accompanied by a pair of veins. The posterior tibial (PT) is easily examined from its distal location. The artery is palpated just above the medial malleolus and examined by placing the probe directly over the artery.

Pulsed Doppler technique: The anterior artery (CFA and its branches) is examined with Doppler color and spectral. At appropriate intervals the pulsed Doppler sample volume is placed in the center of the artery being examined and using an angle of 60° the waveform is assessed for direction of flow, peak systolic velocity (PSV), and spectral broadening. All Doppler calculations at proximal, mid and distal artery segments are recorded **(Fig. 23.9)**. If B mode image abnormalities are seen without a change in Doppler velocity, this is recorded showing the image abnormality and the corresponding Doppler waveform. All Doppler waveforms which are abnormal, should be repeated flow of several views to avoid an error in calculations.

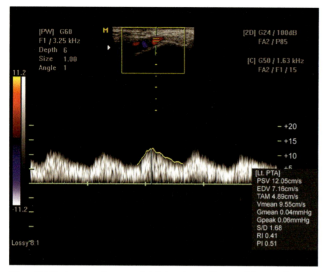

Fig. 23.8: Loss of normal triphasic pattern with continuous forward diastolic flow in posterior tibial artery in a case of Buerger's disease.

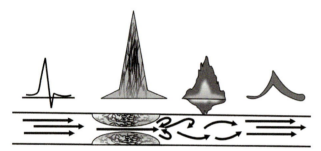

Fig. 23.9: Doppler spectral changes in the presence of hemodynamically significant stenoses.

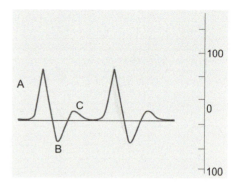

Fig. 23.10: Normal triphasic waveform: (A) Systolic upstroke; (B) Early diastolic reverse flow; (C) Diastolic forward flow.

TABLE 23.1: Relationship of diameter of vessel with waveform.

Classification	Features
Normal	Triphasic waveform. No spectral broadening
1–19% DRL	Triphasic waveform. Spectral broadening
20–49% DRL	Reverse flow component diminished spectral broadening prominent. PSU increases from 30–100%. Distal waveform remain normal
50–75% DRL	Monophasic waveform with loss of reverse flow extensive spectral broadening PSV increase >100%
75–99% DRL	End diastolic velocity >100 cm/cc monophasic waveform with loss of reverse flow extensive spectral broadening. Distal waveform monophasic with reduced systolic velocity
Occlusion	No flow detected. Preocclusive "thumb" heard just proximal. Distal waveform monophasic
DRL	Diameter reducing lesion

Peak systolic velocity increase—comparing the maximum velocity at the stenosis to that just proximal

The normal lower extremity arterial waveform is triphasic within a marked systolic up stroke, early diastolic reverse flow and end diastolic forward flow **(Fig. 23.10)**.

Figure 23.9 for (1) stenosis (2) narrowing (3) beyond narrowing.

For a complete lower extremity arterial evaluation scanning begins in the upper abdominal aorta. The aorta is followed distally to its bifurcation, and the iliac arteries are examined separately at each groin. Each lower extremity is examined individually starting at the CFA. Recordings are made at standard locations **(Table 23.1)**.
- Aortic bifurcation
- Internal and external iliac artery
- Common femoral artery
- Superficial femoral artery
- Proximal mid and distal SFA
- Popliteal artery till its bifurcation.

Anatomy of Venous System

Upper Extremity Veins

The upper extremity is drained by superficial and deep venous system. The superficial veins are primary route of drainage in contrast to the lower extremity where the deep veins form the primary route.

Deep venous system: The deep veins are paired structures and accompany the corresponding arteries. The subclavian vein and the internal jugular veins join behind the sternal end of clavicle to form brachiocephalic vein. The subclavian vein has a pair of valves 2 cm from its termination. It is anterior and inferior to the subclavian artery and is posterior to the clavicle. The external jugular vein is its prominent tributary. The subclavian vein becomes axillary vein at the upper border of first rib. The axillary vein lies medial and inferior to axillary artery and the medial end of brachial plexus lies between artery and vein. The axillary vein becomes brachial vein at the lower border of teres major. The brachial vein is duplicated in most individuals and it drains the basilic vein. The radial and ulnar veins become confluent on anterior aspect of the elbow to form brachial vein. The radial and ulnar veins are paired, they are formed by superficial and deep palmer venous arch on radial and the ulnar aspect respectively. The radial veins are smaller than ulnar veins. Paired anterior and posterior interosseous veins drain in to the ulnar veins.

Superficial venous system: It consists of cephalic vein, basic vein and its tributaries. The cephalic vein joins the subclavian vein at the distal end of the clavicle. It pierces the clavipectoral fascia before draining into the subclavian vein. It passes between the clavicular portion of the pectoralis major and the deltoid muscle and here it is accompanied by the deltoid branch of thoracoacromial artery. From here it emerges into subcutaneous tissue and continues along the lateral margin of upper extremity up to the wrist and form lateral portion of dorsal venous arch of hand and courses along the medial aspect of the forearm and arm. In the upper arm it pierces the deep fascia and then continues medial to the brachial artery to the interior border of teres major muscle, where it joins the brachial veins.

Anatomy of Lower Extremity Veins

The veins of lower extremities comprise of deep, superficial and perforating veins. The deep venous system is more important as most of the venous return from lower extremity is channeled through the deep system. The bicuspid values direct the flow from superficial to the deep venous system. The valves are more numerous in the deep venous system and the distal vein.

Deep Venous System (Figs. 23.11 and 23.12)

Inferior vena cava (IVC) and iliac vein: The IVC is formed by the confluence of the common iliac veins at the L_5 level and it has no valves. The common iliac veins are formed at the sacroiliac junction by confluence of external iliac vein and internal iliac vein. The right common iliac vein is shorter, nearly vertical and ascends behind the lateral to the artery. The left common iliac vein is longer and more oblique than right. It is first medial to the corresponding artery and then behind the right common iliac artery. It is crossed anteriorly by the root of the sigmoid colon and the superior mesenteric vessels. On the right, the external iliac vein lies first medial to the artery, but as it passes upwards, it gradually includes behind it. On the left, it lies medial to the artery.

Femoral venous system: At the inguinal ligament, CFV continues into the external iliac vein and it is medial and posterior to the common femoral artery. The great saphenous vein joins CFV. At it's antero-medial aspects about 3 cm below the inguinal ligament. The CFV is formed by the confluences of the superficial femoral vein (SFV) and profunda femoral vein 4 to 12 cm below the inguinal ligament. The SFV continues into thigh till the adductor canal in adductor muscles. It is bifid in 25% of cases.

Popliteal and calf veins: The popliteal vein is formed at the lower border of popliteal muscle by the confluence of pairs of posterior tibial vein (PTV), peroneal vein (PV) and the anterior tibial vein (ATV). In the proximal part it lies posterolateral as it passes between the gastrocnemius heads, it lies anteriorly and further distally it lies medial to the artery. Twenty-five percent

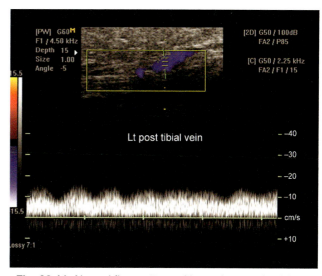

Fig. 23.11: Normal flow pattern with respiratory phasicity in the deep vein of leg.

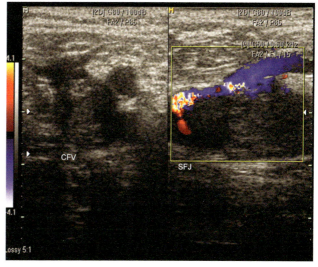

Fig. 23.12: Thrombosis of common femoral vein (CFV) with partial occlusion of saphenofemoral junction (SFJ) as confirmed on the color Doppler image.

of the popliteal veins are bifid. The gastrocnemius veins are one or more sizable veins which drain into the popliteal vein. The short saphenous vein drains into the popliteal vein 3–7.5 cm. above the knee joint. It continues into the subcutaneous tissue in middle of the calf posteriorly. The posterior tibial veins are formed by the confluence of superficial and deep plantar veins beneath the flexor retinaculum. The posterior tibial veins pass in the fascial plane between superficial and deep muscles of posterior compartment of calf. The posterior tibial veins are joined by the peroneal veins in the proximal one-third of calf prior to entering the popliteal vein. The soleal veins are baggy sinusoidal veins with no valves and form the arcades between posterior tibial and peroneal veins. The anterior tibial vein courses along the anterior aspects of the interosseous membrane, while the peroneal veins course on the posterior aspect of interosseous membrane.

Superficial venous system: The main components of superficial venous system are the great saphenous vein and the short saphenous vein. The great saphenous is the longest vein in the body. It courses along the medial aspect of lower extremity starting at the anterior aspect of the medial malleolus and drain into the common femoral vein below the inguinal ligament. The short saphenous vein is formed at the lateral aspect of the ankle. It runs subcutaneously in the middle of the calf posteriorly and drains into the popliteal vein.

Equipment: A linear array 7–10 MHz frequency transducer is preferred. Imaging and flow analysis are currently performed with duplex sonography usually range gating. Color flow imaging can be used to facilitate the examination. Adequate documentation should be done of all normal and abnormal areas. A record of abnormal flow dynamics is made. Variations in size should be accompanied by measurements. All images should be appropriately labeled.

Technique

The study is performed in the supine position with the affected limb mildly flexed and turned laterally. This allows the upper middle portion of the thigh to be examined without moving the patient. Identification of the SFV is essential. The FV **(Figs. 23.13A to C)** is located by palpating the SFA and placing the transducer just medial to it. The SFV is identified as a vascular channel within thin walls which are compressible on pressure from the transducer. After identification CFV **(Fig. 23.14)** of the vein is compressed in the transverse position. A normal vein flattens out whereas a clot filled vein does not change. Compression is best demonstrated in the transverse view, if done only in the longitudinal plane, the transducer can slip off the clot and give erroneous results. Comparison with the healthy vein of the opposite side is always useful.

Next the Doppler cursor is placed within the femoral vein and the audio-signal from venous flow appreciated. This is a low pitched phasic signal and distinctly different from the shotty signals of arterial flow. At this point of time it is important to assess patency of the system above the FV. This is done by asking the patient to perform a valsalva maneuver. The patient takes in a full inspiration, holds it and contracts the abdominal muscles. In the ordinary language, the patient is instructed to lean down as in passing stools and then holding his/her breath. At this point of time there is complete loss of venous flow in the SFV. The patient is then instructed to breathe on normally, at this point flow in the SFV is seen again. The next important test to be performed is the augmentation test. With the transducer on the vein, the lower thigh is squeezed medially. This leads to a sudden peak or spurt of flow in the SFV. The vein is thus followed along the medial aspect of the leg to the popliteal fossa to look for a clot.

Popliteal Vein

The popliteal vein is found behind the medial aspect of the knee joint. Popliteal vein can be evaluated in the

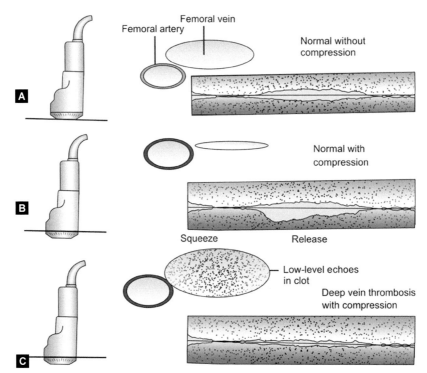

Figs. 23.13A to C: The femoral vein: (A) The normal femoral vein shows good venous flow without compression; (B) With compression, the femoral vein collapses, and there is no flow. On release, flow will be seen; (C) with deep vein thrombosis, the vein will not compress. There is no flow, and low level echoes can be seen within the clot.

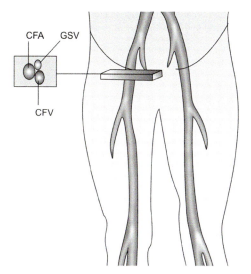

Fig. 23.14: In the groin, the common femoral vein (CFV) lies medial to the common femoral artery (CFA). The greater saphenous vein (GSV) arises from the femoral vein in the groin.

prone or sitting up position. Augmentation is done as and when required. The posterior tibial and peroneal veins are examined throughout their length in the longitudinal and transverse planes.

Venous Thrombosis-B Mode Features

The venous distention is out of proportion to the size of the corresponding artery. The walls of the two veins are ill-defined. The lumen is filled with anechoic or hypoechoic material which usually occludes the vein. Recent thrombus is anechoic and appears more black as the thrombus becomes chronic, its echogenicity increases and more bright. The thrombosed vein loses its compressibility. In a chronic thrombus, the echogenicity of the thrombus increases, the distention of the vein is less, the thrombus becomes more adherent and eventually there is recanalization of the vein. The residual lumen can be, evaluated easily on color flow imaging.

Doppler features: There is no flow in the vein spontaneously or on augmentation on color flow imaging. Proximal to the thrombus augmentation is absent and flow is decreased. Distal to the thrombus flow is continuous and Valsalva response is absent.

Acute Deep Vein Thrombosis

A typical clot expands the vein which is filled with low level echoes. The vein will not be compressible. There will be no flow with color.

Chronic Deep Vein Thrombosis

A chronic thrombus increases in echogenicity and decreases in size. The affected vein has a normal caliber although it still contains echogenic clot which partially blocks the vein.

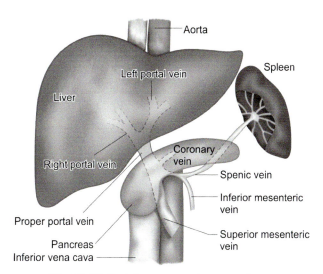

Fig. 23.15: Portal venous system—anatomy.

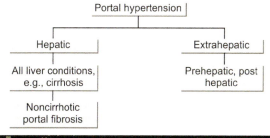

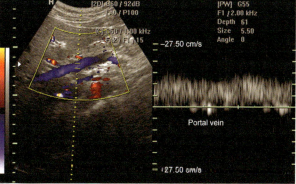

Fig. 23.16: Normal pattern of flow in the portal vein with respiratory variations.

Imaging and Doppler of the Portal Venous System

Before proceeding to imaging of the portal venous system it is essential to know the portal venous anatomy **(Fig. 23.15)**.

Ultrasonography and Doppler of Normal Veins (Figs. 23.16 and 23.17)

Differentiation of portal veins from hepatic veins should be clear and generally this is simple. Peroneal veins are more or less transversely oriented and converge to the porta hepatis. Also, the walls of the portal vein are thick and echogenic.

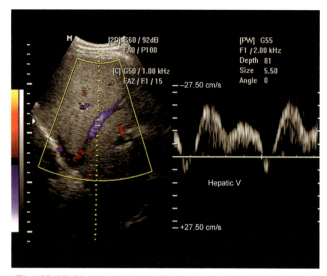

Fig. 23.17: Normal pattern of blood flow through the hepatic veins.

The normal portal flow is low velocity with some change in quiet respiration. Normal flow in the PV is towards the liver or hepatopetal. Hepatic veins have echopoor walls and are oriented longitudinally. Converging towards the inferior vena cava flow in these is pulsatile and there is an alternate forward and reverse flow component. Flow direction in the hepatic veins is hepatofugal.

The hepatic artery is recognized by low resistance arterial signals. The most common condition in the Indian context which requires imaging is portal hypertension. At this point it is important to know the basic disease process and how to investigate further.

Portal hypertension is basically an increase in the hydrostatic pressure of the PV. Normal pressure is 5–10 mmHg. An increase to more than 15 mm Hg in the PV is considered symptomatic.

Extrahepatic Portal Hypertension

In extrahepatic portal hypertension, color doppler study is the initial screening modality of choice. Sonography shows stenosis of the hepatic veins which often have thick echogenic walls with reversed flow in the hepatic veins, or the flow of blood which should have been away from the liver and towards the IVC now gets reversed. This reversal of flow is diagnostic of Budd Chiari syndrome.

Prehepatic Portal Hypertension

The most common cause of portal hypertension in this group is portal vein thrombosis or occlusion. This is frequently related to infection of the umbilical vein. Ultrasound is very specific in the diagnosis of portal vein thrombosis. The PV may be expanded measuring more than 13 mm with the presence of echogenic material within the lumen of the portal vein since the portal vein is patent in the majority of patients, the fact that you cannot see a patent portal vein at the liver hilum suggests PV thrombosis. At this moment CDs has the advantage over spectral flow as the presence of flow and its direction can be easily assessed by CDs in real-time.

Cavernous transformation of the PV, which means that a bunch of collaterals has opened up is recognized as multiple tubular vessels in the porta hepatis, the superior mesenteric vein (SMV) and the splenic vein may also be dilated.

Hepatic Portal Hypertension

Ultrasonography can depict variceal collaterals, splenomegaly, as well as identify under lying diseases causing portal hypertension. Duplex patterns which have to be carefully evaluated in portal hypertension are:
- PV diameter
- PV, SV, SMV, response to respiration
- Portal flow direction
- Velocity waveform
- Splenic size

A portal vein diameter of more than 13 mm is indicative of PH. The velocity also decreases and the direction of flow becomes biphasic or to and fro and ultimately reverses to hepatofugal.

Technique/Portal Vein

The portal vein has echogenic walls and branches towards the diaphragm. Imaging is performed in a plane perpendicular to the right costal margin. The patient is turned to the left lateral decubitus position to provide a good acoustic window. The portal vein is easily seen as an anechoic tubular structure with bright echogenic walls in the region of the porta hepatis. On Doppler the normal PV shows a monophasic flow pattern as the flow of blood is towards the liver.

Caution: A poor angle can create the impression of hepatofugal flow, suggesting a fake diagnosis of portal hypertension.

Lower frequency transducers are often necessary to get adequate penetration for Doppler examination of the adult abdomen. A 2.25 MHz transducer will increase the Doppler sensitivity greatly with little degrading effect on the resolution.

Renal Artery Doppler (Fig. 23.18)

Patients are referred for renal artery evaluation because of uncontrolled hypertension, decrease in renal function and or abdominal bruits. Patients who have had a renal transplant also require repeated evaluation of the renal arteries in the postoperative period as a regular follow up.

Scan Protocol and Technique

Imaging of the renal arteries is performed with a 3.5 MHz imaging transducer which allows adequate imaging of the aorta and the renal vessels.

CHAPTER 23: Ultrasound Examination of the Peripheral Arteries

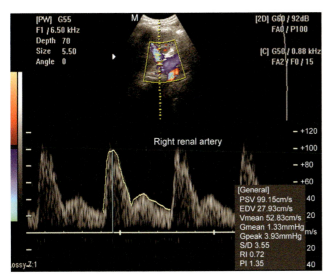

Fig. 23.18: Normal pattern of flow through the renal artery at the hilum in a case of renal hypertension (PSV close to 100 cm/sec and RI >0.7).

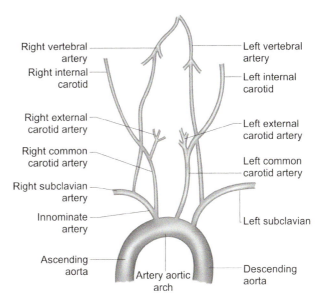

Fig. 23.19: Anatomy of major blood vessels supplying the brain.

The patient should be well-hydrated and the examination begins in the supine position. Identify the superior mesenteric artery (SMA) in the midline and rotate the transducer to the transverse plane. Using the SMA as the landmark, move distally to see the left renal vein as it crosses from the left to the right between the anterior to the aorta and posterior to the SMA. Immediately below the left renal vein, to the right of the aorta and right renal vein (RRA) will be seen in its long axis as it passes under the vena cava and proceeds to the right kidney.

If the color Doppler in the system is set so that flow towards the transducer is red, blood flow in the renal arteries will be away from the transducer and will appear blue.

Obtain Doppler spectra at the renal origin, in the mid renal artery and in the distal RRA. Move back to the aorta and slightly distal to the RRA origin to visualize the left renal artery. The left renal artery is frequently more difficult to visualize, partly due to bowel gas.

If the origins of the renal arteries are not well visualized from the anterior approach, turn the patient into the lateral decubitus position. The renal arteries can frequently be visualized using this flank approach. The renal artery is followed from the kidney back to the aorta. The left renal artery is visualized when the patient is on the right side and the RRA is seen when the patient is on the left side.

Interpretation

Normal renal artery signals are of low resistance and have continuous flow in diastole, similar to the carotid and celiac arteries. Although the arterial narrowing of renal artery stenosis is rarely visible with US, there may be Doppler evidence of narrowing. At the site of stenosis there is little flow in diastole, much turbulence and abnormal systolic diastolic ratio.

Ostial renal artery stenosis is difficult to visualize. It becomes important to get a good spectral trace distal to the stenosis in this condition. The acceleration time, i.e. the time required to gain the peak is increased. The duration of the ascent segment in systole is a sensitive way of assessing renal artery stenosis. This pattern is also called the tardus parvus phenomenon.

Role of Duplex Ultrasonography in Carotid Artery Disease

Vascular Supply of the Brain

It would be worthwhile to briefly recapitulate the cerebrovascular anatomy **(Fig. 23.19)**. The right common carotid artery originates from the innominate artery, while the left carotid artery originates from the aortic arch. The common carotid artery slightly widens before bifurcation into internal and external carotid arteries. This widened area is called carotid bulb.

Indications for Doppler Cerebral Vascular Examination

Presently the various indications of Doppler ultrasonography are as follows:
- Transient ischemic attacks (TIA), i.e. ischemic neurological deficit which resolves completely within 24 hours.
- *Recurrent ischemic neurological deficit (RIND):* Ischemic neurological deficit which lasts more than 24 hours but which resolves completely. Both transient ischemic attack (TIA) and reversible ischemic neurologic deficit (RIND) are significant risk factors for stroke
- Transient mono-ocular blindness (Amaurosis Fugax). Its etiology is usually an embolic interruption of retinal arterial blood flow

- Dizziness, which may be generalized or position dependent
- *Cervical bruits:* A cervical bruit is a significant risk factor for cerebrovascular disease. It is not clear, however, that a cervical bruit is a significant risk factor for stroke
- Surveillance for plaque progression.

Examination Protocol

Patients are examined in the supine position. Exposure of the neck is facilitated by hyperextension of neck, patients dropping the ipsilateral shoulder as far as possible and neck slightly turned to the opposite side. Since the carotid arteries are superficial, a high frequency imaging probe (7.5 MHz) is used. The study is performed both in horizontal and transverse plane. As per universally accepted convention, the longitudinal images are oriented with the patients head on the left side of the screen. This is achieved by keeping the index mark of the transducer in such a direction that the head is directed to the left side. Transverse images are oriented as if viewed from the patients' feet, hence the patients' right appears on the left side of the image.

Step in carotid examination technique: The examination is performed from various transducer positions namely anterolateral, posterolateral, anterior (roughly right angles to the longitudinal plane), and horizontal planes.

Step 1: The examination begins with either a longitudinal or horizontal plane preferably the former. The common carotid artery (CCA) is profiled at the level of clavicle and the transducer is gradually moved cephalad keeping CCA in view. The probe is pivoted clockwise or anti-clockwise, so that CCA is fairly horizontal on the screen with vessel wall open at both the ends. As the probe is moved cephalad, attempt is made to see the carotid bifurcation **(Fig. 23.20)**. Contrary to expectations, visualization of the bifurcation may not be seen in about 50% of the cases. Furthermore, visualization of bifurcation, internal and external carotid arteries in the same longitudinal plane is a rarity. The internal and external carotid arteries are then individually identified. Their differentiating features are listed in Table 23.3. As the carotid bifurcation and the internal carotid artery (ICA) are most commonly involved in a disease process, hence stress is placed on their study and the ICA should be followed as cephalad as possible by using a posterolateral approach. During this step of examination any plaques or narrowing are looked for. Document the site, extent and internal plaque characteristics, together with degree of luminal narrowing by color flow mapping and spectral Doppler. Normally the β-mode imaging, color flow mapping and spectral Doppler examination continue simultaneously to save time of examination.

The transverse scan examination helps in (a) reaffirming the plaques and luminal narrowing (b) when there is difficulty in profiling the ICA or external carotid artery (ECA), the probe is brought cephalad and the two branches can be seen as circular vessels **(Figs. 23.21A and B)**.

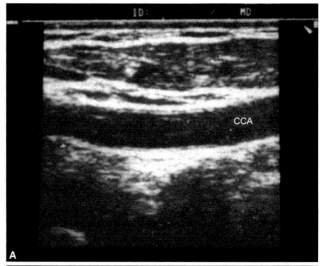

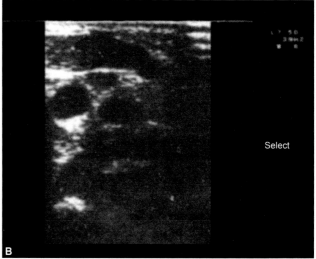

Figs. 23.21A and B: Transverse scan showing right internal carotid artery (RICA) and external carotid artery (ECA) depicted in a circular manner. PL-plaque.

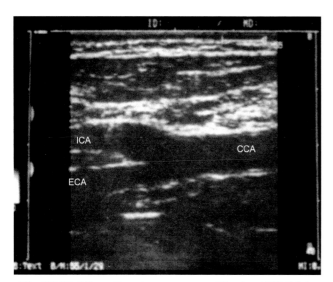

Fig. 23.20: Bifurcation of common carotid artery (CCA) into internal and external carotid arteries (ICA) and (ECA).

TABLE 23.2: Different velocities according to the percentage of stenosis.

Diameter stenosis (Category)	Peak systolic velocity (cm/sec)	Peak diastolic velocity (cm/sec)	Systolic velocity ratio (ICA/CCA)	Diastolic velocity ratio (ICA/CCA)
0% (Normal)	<110	<40	<1.8	<2.6
1–39% (Mild)	<110	<40	<1.8	<2.6
40–59% (Moderate)	<130	<40	<1.8	<2.6
60–79% (Severe)	>130	>40	>1.8	>2.6
80 v 99% (Critical)	>250	>100	>3.7	>5.5
100% (Occlusion)	NA	NA	NA	NA

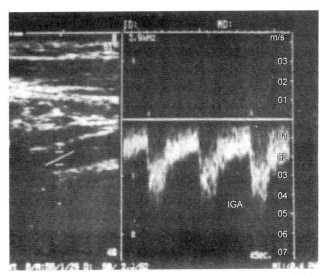

Fig. 23.22: Doppler waveform of internal carotid artery (ICA) showing gradual upstroke and slow diastolic slope. Doppler flow in diastole seen with an end diastolic velocity of 0.2 m/sec.

Keeping the branches in view, the probe is gradually rotated to the longitudinal plane and vessel identified by the features mentioned in **Table 23.2**.

Doppler Characteristics or Normal Carotid Arteries

The spectral Doppler tracing is analyzed for peak systolic velocity, end diastolic velocity, the pattern of systolic and diastolic slope, with window, i.e. "the clear area" that displays no Doppler frequencies, the ICA/CCA systolic and diastolic velocity ratio.

Internal Carotid Artery

The ICA feeds the brain and the eyes. The brain demands a large blood supply, because it is a highly vascular structure. Because of the numerous blood vessels, a high velocity flow is required to perfuse the brain, hence, a low resistance flow. The ICA flow is characterized by Doppler flow in diastole and systole **(Fig. 23.22)**, gradual upstroke and slow diastolic slope, high flow velocity.

External carotid artery: The ECA feeds the face and the scalp. The number and size of the branches of ECA produce a high resistance flow. The flow is of low velocity, flow is mainly in systole, there is rapid systolic upstroke **(Fig. 23.23)** abrupt diastolic slope, very narrow window and hardly any diastolic flow.

Common carotid artery: It is also a low resistance type of flow characterized by rapid systolic peak **(Fig. 23.24)**, gradual diastolic deceleration slope and presence of antegrade diastolic flow. These are less marked as compared to ICA flow.

The ICA/CCA systolic velocity ratio is normal if less than 1.8 and the diastolic velocity ratio is less than 2.6.

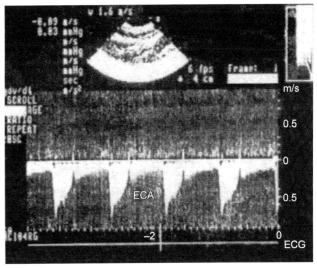

Fig. 23.23: Doppler spectrum of external carotid artery (ECA) showing a high resistance type of flow with rapid systolic upstroke and brisk diastolic slope with very minimal diastolic flow.

Interpretation of Common Pathological Lesions

Carotid Plaques

These are atherosclerotic and echogenic materials that encroaches upon the arterial lumen. They should be evaluated both in longitudinal and transverse scans. These should be evaluated for:
- Extent and thickness.
- Resultant degree of luminal narrowing.
- Its composition.

Plaque extent and thickness: As a general rule the extent of the plaque is better seen in longitudinal plane while the

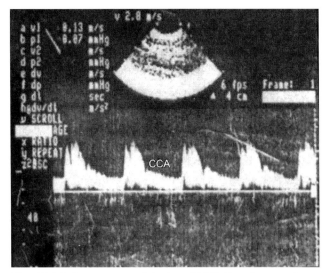

Fig. 23.24: Common carotid artery (CCA) Doppler waveform.

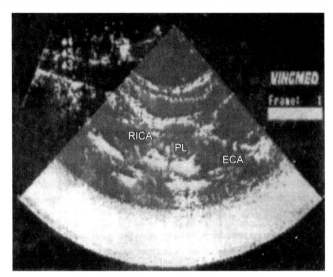

Fig. 23.25: Hyperechoic plaque (PL).

plaque severity and resultant degree of luminal narrowing is much better determined by transverse imaging. A false-positive diagnosis can be made if there is off diameter oblique scanning, imaging a curving vessel or abnormal gain settings.

Plaque composition: Sonography has great potential to assess internal composition of the plaque and its surface characteristics. The plaque can be subdivided as:

Hypoechoic: These contain large amount of lipid material, and are less echogenic than the sternomastoid muscle.

Moderately echogenic: This plaque is more echogenic than the sternomastoid muscle but less echogenic than the arterial adventitia.

Hyperechoic: It is brighter than or as bright as the adjacent wall **(Fig. 23.25)**. Calcified areas are present in these plaques. Multiple scan planes should be utilized for the diagnosis. Their extent, severity and echogenicity should be determined.

Assessment of Carotid Stenosis

Carotid stenosis is assessed by two techniques: (a) determination of percent stenosis by B-mode imaging (b) assessment of Doppler and color flow mapping technique which is more accurate.

Percent stenosis: This is the actual calculated percent reduction in the vessel lumen. This is represented either as diameter stenosis or area stenosis. The diameter stenosis is the percent reduction in the vessels original diameter and is calculated as:

$$\frac{\text{Diameter of residual lumen}}{\text{Diameter of original lumen}} \times 100$$

Diagnostic criteria of stenosis by Doppler technique: Assessment of severity of carotid luminal narrowing by

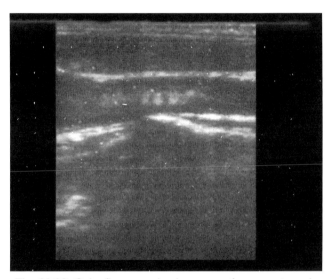

Fig. 23.26: Color flow mapping in a case of severe stenosis of left internal carotid artery (LICA) showing turbulence.

Doppler technique has high degree of sensitivity and specificity which exceeds 90% for various degrees of stenosis. Both color flow mapping (CFM) and Doppler are used simultaneously. Any significant flow limiting stenosis is immediately evident by CFM as a turbulent (mosaic colored) flow **(Fig. 23.26)**, while Doppler provides a quantitative information. Color flow mapping has the advantage of picking up a stenotic lesion of less than 60% while Doppler velocity changes are minimal for that grade of diameter stenosis. Hence, Doppler spectral analysis is a highly accurate method for assessment of stenosis exceeding 60% decrease in diameter.

Assessment of carotid Doppler signals: Before discussing this important aspect it would be worthwhile to remember certain basic fundamentals. The vessel should be open at both ends by manipulation of the probe. The angle of incidence, i.e.

the angle at which an ultrasound beam strikes an interface should be below 70° and as close as possible to 50-60°. The Doppler sample volume should be placed at the center of the stream or point of maximum flow. The recording of the signals in CCA should be at least one cm below the bulb area. In the ICA, it is at the point of fastest velocity. This may occur at the distal most end of the vessel, or it may actually occur in the bulb area, since stenosis in the bulb directly affects ICA flow. If ICA velocities are uniform, obtain the ICA sample from a point at least one cm distal to the origin. In the ECA, flow velocity is recorded at least one cm distal to the origin.

Doppler flow patterns at different points in a stenotic lesion: Basically there are two types of flow—Laminar which is the flow in a non diseased state and the flow velocities and direction are symmetrical, while a turbulent flow (found in stenotic lesions) has multiple velocities and flow directions with spectral broadening (wide window).

As regards flow pattern, the flow is laminar proximal to a stenotic lesion, as this segment may be normal. Within a stenotic zone, there may be some increase in velocity, but flow may remain laminar with some spectral broadening. The diastolic velocity may be more increased. In the immediate post stenotic area, frank turbulent flow is present with significantly increased velocities. This may be restricted to within 1.0 cm of stenotic lesion, unless stenosis is very severe.

Quantitative Doppler for severe stenosis evaluation: As mentioned earlier, Doppler spectral analysis is a very accurate method to measure extent of carotid obstruction. This is measured by analysing the flow velocity patterns in the stenotic segments.

Doppler measurement: In a carotid stenotic lesion, four measurements are routinely made:
- Peak systolic velocity
- Peak end diastolic velocity
- ICA/CCA systolic velocity ratio
- ICA/CCA diastolic velocity ratio.

Peak systolic velocity: This is a reliable Doppler parameter for assessing the severity of carotid stenosis. Studies have shown that up to about 50-60% of stenosis the rise in systolic velocities may be minor, while beyond it, the velocities increase significantly **(Fig. 23.27)**.

Peak end diastolic velocity: The diastolic velocity remains normal up to about 50% diameter reduction. Beyond this, the diastolic velocity increases in proportion to degree of luminal narrowing. There is sharp increase beyond 70% obstruction. This Doppler parameter is very reliable in detecting high grade Carotid Stenosis.

ICA/CCA systolic and diastolic velocity ratios: Various factors like heart rate, BP, cardiac output, peripheral resistance, and contralateral carotid obstruction can affect the carotid systolic and end diastolic velocities in patients with carotid stenosis. However, velocity ratios are less prone to these physiological variables. The systolic velocity ratio is determined as follows. The internal carotid (stenotic zone) peak velocity is divided by the peak velocity of CCA

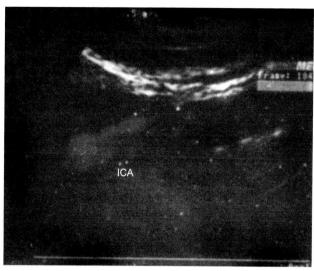

Fig. 23.27: Doppler waveform of the patient shown in Figure 23.26. A very high velocity systolic (>5 m/sec) and diastolic flow (>1.0 m/sec) seen indicative of critical stenosis of ICA.

TABLE 23.3: Differences between internal and external carotid arteries.

Internal carotid artery	External carotid artery
• Imaged by sliding the probe towards earlobe	• Imaged by pointing the probe towards angle of mandible
• Larger size	• Smaller size
• No extracranial branches	• Extracranial branches
• Posteriorly situated	• Anteriorly situated
• On color flow mapping, flow is persistent throughout cardiac cycle though undulating	• Flow flickers off and on because flow disappears or almost ceases during diastole
• Doppler characteristics show low resistance flow pattern	• High resistance flow pattern

determined in any normal segment proximal to the stenosis. A systolic ratio more than 1.8 indicates a 60% stenosis **(Table 23.3)**. The end diastolic ratio is similarly determined and the severity is based as shown in **Table 23.3**, i.e. ratio more than 5.5 indicates very severe stenosis **(Figs. 23.28A to N)**.

Criteria of Total Occlusion

- Absence of arterial pulsation distal to the block
- Lumen filled with echogenic material
- Subnormal vessel size in chronic occlusion
- Absence of Doppler flow signals
- Abnormal CCA Doppler signals characterized by rapid systolic upstroke with loss of normal diastolic flow pattern.

Limitations of Cerebrovascular Sonography

Though Duplex sonography of carotid vessels gives significant diagnostic information but there are certain limitations to this study.

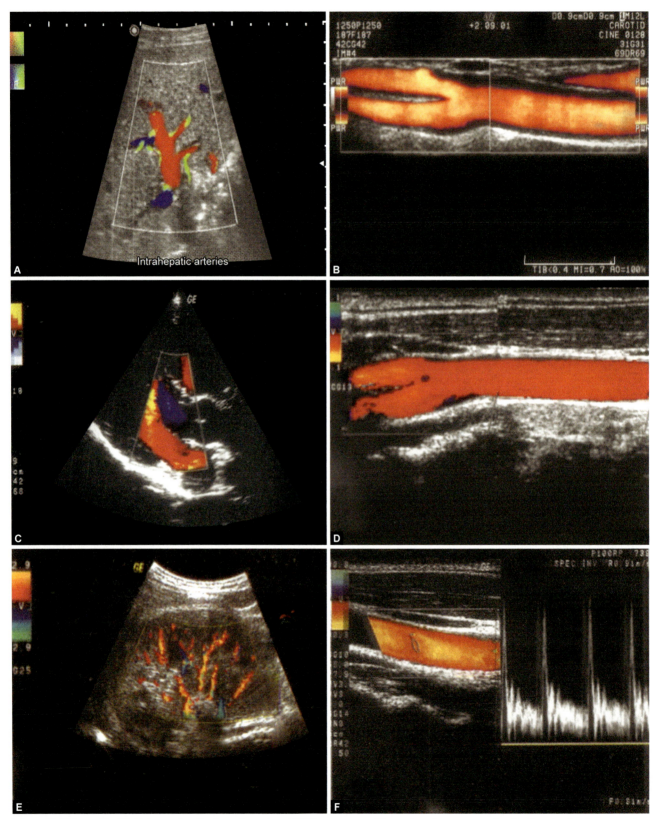

Figs. 23.28A to F: (A) Using pulsatile flow detection (PFD), you can differentiate between pulsatile flow in the liver arteries (green) and non-pulsatile flow in the portal vein at one glance; (B) Maximum resolution power Doppler imaging clearly and easily differentiate the vessel wall from the lumen in this carotid artery; (C) Plax view—heart; (D) Carotid artery; (E) Renal perfusion; (F) Spectral Doppler on CCA.

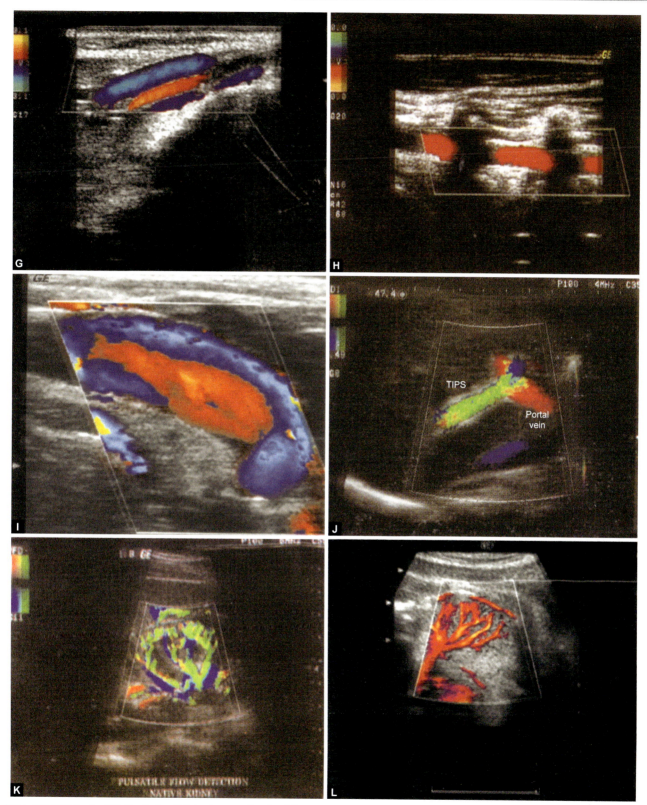

Figs. 23.28G to L: (G) Posterior tibial artery and vein; (H) Vertebral artery; (I) Right common carotid artery origin; (J) Pulsatile flow detection (PFD) clearly demonstrates the different hemodynamic flow states in the portal vein and TIPS shunt; (K) Pulsatile vs. nonpulsatile flow states can quickly be differentiated with the use of pulsatile flow detection, demonstrated in this normal native kidney; (L) The minute branching of vessels in the fetal lung revealed with power Doppler imaging renders unsurpassed color resolution.

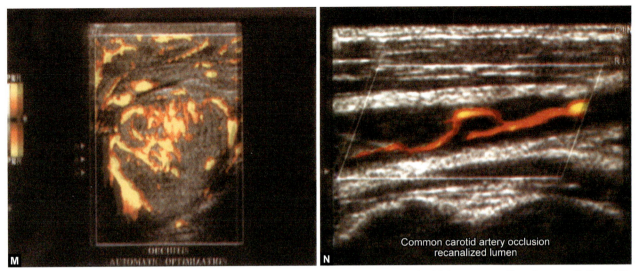

Figs. 23.28M and N: (M) Auto optimization applies optimal settings to demonstrate the highest power Doppler sensitivity, adding a higher degree of confidence to every examination; (N) Superb sensitivity is depicted in this study of a common carotid artery occlusion with a recanalized lumen.

- Limited accessibility of examination due to short, thick neck
- Inability to follow the vessels sufficiently after the bifurcation
- Lack of technical skill and interpretive experience may lead to false positive or false negative findings
- Only the cervical portion of carotid and vertebral arteries are accessible to direct imaging while the intracranial vessels are mainly accessible to Doppler study.
- Artifacts may be misdiagnosed as plaques. Nonvisualization in various scan planes and non pulsatility exclude artifacts
- Interrogating a flow perpendicular to the transducer may suggest a "no flow" situation
- Increased flow acceleration at tortousities and branchings may be misdiagnosed as increased velocity due to stenosis.

24
CHAPTER

Intraoperative and Laparoscopic Sonography

Intraoperative ultrasonography (IOUS) is a dynamic and rapidly growing imaging technique providing important real time information to the radiologist and the surgeon. It identifies and characterizes the lesions seen on preoperative imaging and discovers new lesions not detected by preoperative imaging or surgical inspection and palpation. Intraoperative ultrasonography is usually the final imaging procedure with the ultimate goal being to correlate preoperative images, surgical inspection and palpation, and IOUS findings, to determine the most appropriate surgical procedure. The technique offers the potential for reducing operative complications, shortening operative time and possibly extending the range of surgical procedures influence. A-mode IOUS was used in the early 1960s for evaluating the biliary system for calculi. Image quality was not ideal and interpretation was difficult. However, a number of technical advances have made IOUS both practical and useful. Smaller, dedicated IOUS have been developed and equipment advances have allowed real-time images of high quality to be produced with ease in the operating room. Although IOUS accounts for a small percentage (> 1%) of ultrasound examinations, its rate of growth has been rapid and the number of IOUS examinations has increased by more than 200% during the past five years. Recent advances in ultrasound technology especially color Doppler imaging offer greater role for this technique usefulness. Continued growth of IOUS is expected as more surgeons become aware of its usefulness and as laparoscopic ultrasound techniques and intraoperative ultrasound-guided tumor ablation techniques are improved. IOUS allows the use of high frequency, high resolution probes to be used directly on the surface of the origin being examined as technical problems in routine ultrasonography such as shadowing from overlying bony structures and bowel and sound attenuation in the body walls are not present. This allows high resolution images of high quality to be obtained allowing superb lesion detection, localization and characterization.

For the radiologist, the most important and significant drawback of IOUS is the time away from the radiology department. Depending on the complexity of the case, the radiologists and the ultrasound equipment can be out of the department for 30-60 minutes or longer. The surgeon should notify the radiologist 20-30 minutes before the actual scanning is to be done to allow sufficient time for equipment transportation and preparation and for the radiologist to scrub in. Time invested in the operating room is well-spent if the radiologist has a high level of scanning skills and experience, so that patient care is significantly improved.

Equipment: Requirements are a transportable good quality ultrasound system, high frequency transducer and some forms of image recording facilities. Equipment should be regularly cleaned and kept dust-free prior to entry to OT. Dedicated intraoperative transducers are small and of a high frequency. Their small size allows the transducer to be cradled in the examiners hand and easily maneuvered into small spaces.

The ultrasound transducers used in the operating room must have sterile surfaces.

Some ultrasound transducers can be gas sterilized (ethylene oxide). However, the high temperatures used can potentially damage the transducer; therefore some manufacturers do not recommend this technique. The manufactures that allow gas sterilization are usually very specific in their recommendations. Sterilization with low concentration ethylene oxide typically requires this and is followed by 10 hours of rest and aeration. Consequently the transducer can be used only once a day. Transducers can also be sterilized by immersion in liquid (2% glutaraldehyde), which also requires a significant delay before the ultrasound transducer can be used again. In addition, some surgeons do not allow any glutaraldehyde to come in contact with visceral surfaces or in the peritoneal cavity. Therefore, the sterilization method must be chosen in consultation with the surgeon. This can be a problem if the transducer must be used in consecutive intraoperative cases. In many practices, the ultrasound transducer is covered by a sterile latex/plastic sleeve. Gel must be applied into the sleeve to couple the transducer to the sleeve. As the potential for tearing drape on rough bony margins like craniotomy which, ideally the head must be draped with at least two layers of protective covering. Great care must be taken to be certain that no air bubbles are present between the head of the transducer and the sterile sleeve covering it. This method allows several uses of the same intraoperative probe on the same day. However, the sleeve-draped transducer is slightly more cumbersome to use than is the non-draped sterile transducer. Intraoperative ultrasonography has its main applications in cranial, spinal and abdominal organs.

INTRAOPERATIVE CRANIAL SONOGRAPHY

Intraoperative cranial sonography allows rapid and accurate localization of abnormality; it defines the exact extent of the disease process and also characterizes the cystic and solid elements within the lesion; without causing any risks of radiation. In addition, the ability to image both the normal and the abnormal structures during surgery enables precise guidance for biopsy and interventional procedures and also provides direct observation of the site of intervention immediately following the procedure.

Technique: Intraoperative cranial sonography is generally done under general anesthesia (GA). The selection of the burr hole/trephine site is made on careful conjunction with the preoperative CT/MRI. The isocenter of the lesion is identified on scan topogram and measurements are derived to localize the burr hole site. Transducer is covered with 2 layers of sterile transducer drapes with intervening sterile gel and scan head is touched gently to the duramater/ or brain cortex. Experience has shown that there is little difference in image quality whether scanning on duramater/cortex. Saline draped onto the surface of brain acts a coupling agent (sterile gel is not used). If necessary, the wound itself can be filled with saline creating a natural fluid path for scanning.

The most difficult aspect of using intraoperative sonography is being oriented to the slices generated during surgery. Because the ultrasound sections are generated at surgical site, the orientation of the images almost never corresponds to the standard anatomic sections. The inability to recognize the normal anatomy because of these strange perspectives can cause significant frustration in an operation theater. To avoid this, the radiologist is generally advised to follow:

- Begin scanning at frequency low enough to traverse the entire brain (3 MHz)
- Find choroid plexus, lateral ventricles, falx, and tentorium. By identifying these, the operator can produce a slice that corresponds to a standard anatomic plane
- Place transducer in the center of surgical field, rotate, and do not slice the scan head to obtain standard anatomic sections.

Once a recognisable section has been produced, slide the scan head maintaining the same orientation, from one edge of the craniotomy to the other. After this, rotate by 90° and scan the normal anatomy.

- Avoid random scanning

- Only after a complete familiarity with the field and its relationship to cranium, the slices has been obtained, should the search for lesion begin. Once orientation is understood, a 5 MHz transducer may be used to interrogate the lesion

  A correctly placed craniotomy almost always places the area of interest within the near field of transducer (within 6 cm)

- 5 MHz or greater frequency probe may be used for providing surgical guidance.

Indications

- Primary indication for IOCUS is identification and localization of intracerebral tumors biopsy and/or excision. Cortical and subcortical lesions are amenable to this technique. High frequency transducers provide excellent spatial and contrast resolution enabling avoidance of eloquent areas during biopsy. Before sonography surgeons had to approach the mass by the most direct or often shortest paths. If this path transgressed is in viable portion of the brain, like motor strip, the lesion was labeled inoperable. Using ultrasound, the surgeons can approach from any number of oblique directions. Because of the increased flexibility, rapid localization of tumors and increased precision in tumor removal, USG has led to significant decrease in morbidity and mortality with brain surgeries. However, deeper seated, midline and posterior fossa lesions are best managed by CT/MRI (especially brainstem) guided biopsy
- Other indications include drainage and monitoring of abscesses, guidance for placement of shunts and other catheters such as Ommaya reservoir for intracavitary instillation, of chemo/radiopharmaceutical agents, localization of posttraumatic foreign bodies and bone fragments.

INTRAOPERATIVE SPINAL ULTRASOUND

Intraoperative spinal ultrasound (IOSUS) is a relatively new technique which enables the contents of the spinal canal to be safely examined in real-time during the course of operation for precise localization and characterization of normal and abnormal structures.

Intraoperative spinal ultrasound is usually employed in cases requiring a posterior spinal approach with the patient in prone position. Anterior scanning is possible, following a corpectomy, however the scanning conditions are less favorable. Choice between a sector and linear array transducer is partly dependent upon the size of the surgical access created. High frequency transducers (7–10 MHz) should be employed. The draped transducer is gently introduced into the operating site which is filled with sterile saline which acts both as an acoustic stand off and as a compliant. The fluid in the operating site should be sucked out and replaced with fresh saline, if excessive hematoma accumulates and blood attenuates the ultrasound beam and degrades the image. The operator manipulates the transducer obtaining transverse and longitudinal plane images. The equipment console operator shows select suitable focusing or magnification to view the appropriate area and adjust gain settings appropriately.

Indications include evaluation of spinal tumors, cysts herniated discs, canal stenosis, spine fracture, inflammatory masses, congenital anomalies, locate foreign bodies, and to guide procedures like biopsies drainage and shunt placements. Color Doppler imaging may help assess cerebrospinal fluid (CSF) movements alone, during and after surgery.

Limitations IOSUS is limited by the field of view which is determined by the extent of laminectomy performed structures under unresected bone are not seen. A laminectomy which measures at least 1.5 × 1 cm is necessary for adequate visualization of the canal and its contents. A laminectomy of this size does not affect spinal stability and in most cases does not require added resection. Intraoperative spinal ultrasound (IOSUS) cannot be however, used in microsurgery for disc disease due to small sized laminectomy. Other structures which will interfere include calcified duramater and gel foam in large quantities

INTRAOPERATIVE AND LAPAROSCOPIC SONOGRAPHY OF ABDOMEN

Technique: The combination of curvilinear transducer and dedicated IOUS proper may be used when a large organ such as liver is scanned. The curvilinear transducer demonstrates a global perspective of the relationships of large tumors and key structures. The dedicated IOUS transducer can then be used to detect small, occult masses. With experience, the familiar vascular landmark within the liver are easily recognized. Knowledge of portal and hepatic venous anatomy allows the radiologist to assist in a complete and safe surgical resection. Ideally the radiologist review preoperative images before surgery. After the review, the radiologist knows the location of the suspected malignant masses and indeterminate lesions that need further characterization. Radiologist experienced in IOUS scrubs in and scans the organ of interest. To avoid confusion, one must try to scan from the patients' right side as if performing a routine ultrasound examination. The normal moisture on the surface of the organ to be evaluated can provide acoustic coupling. Warm-saline poured into the peritoneal cavity can be used as stand off agent during a search for surface lesions. The entire organ should be scanned along with the adjacent structures such as regional LNS. When a mass is localized, it should be characterized and its relationship to vascular structures carefully delineated.

HEPATOBILIARY SYSTEM

Applications of Intraoperative Liver Sonography

- Detection of occult and nonpalpable masses
- Determination of the relationship of the mass to vessels
- Definition of lobar and segmental liver anatomy
- Characterization of small hepatic masses, e.g. cystic/solid
- Guidance for cryoablation, biopsy or drainage.

INDICATIONS FOR INTRAOPERATIVE BILIARY SONOGRAPHY

- Identification of biliary calculi
- Identification of biliary neoplasms
- Localization of the common bile duct (CBD) and its relationship to other structures.

Indications for evaluation of pancreas: Intraoperative ultrasound may be used to evaluate complications associated with chronic pancreatitis, including pseudocyst, abscesses and secondary involvement of gastrointestinal tract (GIT), biliary tract or abdominal vessels.

- Used to provide guidance for biopsies and drainage
- Location of islet-cell neoplasm.

Indications for Intraoperative Sonography of Kidneys

- To locate occult, nonpalpable tumors
- To characterize indeterminate renal masses
- To delineate the boundaries of the renal mass
- To guide partial nephrectomy
- Renovascular abnormalities like residual renal artery or anastomotic stenosis, thrombosis/occlusion of the graft or renal artery, intimal flap/dissection, extrinsic compression or kinking of the renal or graft artery.

LAPAROSCOPIC SONOGRAPHY

The latest development in IOUS has been application of specially designed probes that can be inserted through the standard laparoscopic probes that are typically no more than 10–11 mm in size. Because these laparoscopy probes are at some distance from the intra-abdominal organs, the laparoscopic ultrasound (LUS) probes must be mounted on long thin shaft. The earliest reports of LUS used A mode ultrasound for diagnosis of intra-abdominal pathology, although this was of limited usefulness. Miniaturization techniques were then applied, allowing for a substantial decrease in probe size, thus making laparoscopic real-time ultrasound feasible. The extremely small sized catheter mounted transducers which were originally developed for intravascular ultrasound, are used laparoscopically.

Probe Features

- Center frequency ranging from 5–7.5 MHz
- Long rigid shaft of at least 15–20 cm in length
- Real-time grayscale as well as Doppler color flow capability
- Linear/curvilinear array transducers with crystal length ranging from 1 to 3 cm
- Sterile sheaths designed for each individual-probe. It is important to observe the insertion of the LUS probe under direct visualization using the fiberoptic laparoscope. Split screen presentation of both the laparoscopic and real-time ultrasound images on same monitor is convenient and requires only an inexpensive beam filter.

GOALS OF LAPAROSCOPIC ULTRASOUND

- To detect and characterize all possible lesions and to accurately localizes these lesions to lobes and segments and to assess relationships to vascular and biliary structures.
- To guide biopsy and aspirations and to guide minimally invasive ablation techniques.
- Reports have been slated to its use to localize renal stones in patients undergoing laparoscopic nephrolithotomy and in evaluation of hydrosalpinx.

Limitations

- Because the probe sizes are necessarily small, the amount of time required to completely image an organ is substantially longer than imaging with standard IOUS probes (for example complete assessment of the liver might take less than 5 min using 10 probes, but would take 15–20 minutes with LUS examination).
- Since the probe pivots on a single point in space (i.e. the entry laparoscopic port), there is limitation to the freedom of motion of the scanhead such that it is impossible to maintain the probe in standard transverse or longitudinal orientations. This can cause disorientation and also some difficulty in ensuring that the image planes overlap one another.

Three-dimensional Ultrasound (Figs. 24.1 to 24.13 and Flowchart 24.1)

3D reconstruction of sonograms has been performed sporadically for the last 10 years. Although these attempts

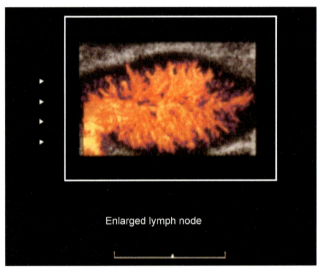

Fig. 24.2: 3D Symmetrical velocity imaging provides a excellent visualization of the vascular architecture in this inflammatory lymph node.

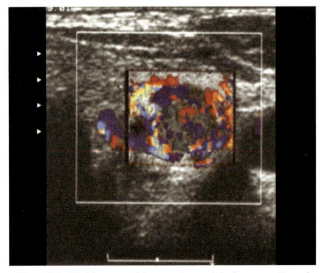

Fig. 24.1: 3D View provides a unique global perspective of anatomic structures as demonstrated in this thyroid nodule.

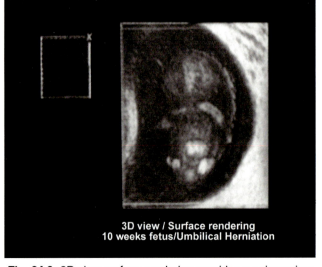

Fig. 24.3: 3D view surface rendering provides a unique view of normal umbilical herniation in this 10-week fetus.

CHAPTER 24: Intraoperative and Laparoscopic Sonography

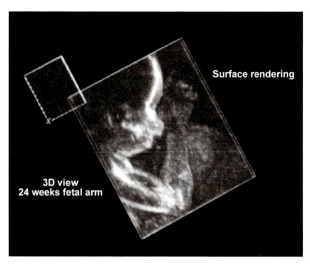

Fig. 24.4: 3D view surface rendering demonstrates an exceptional view of a fetal arm at 24 weeks.

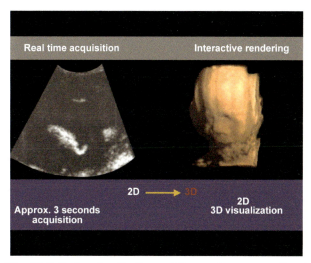

Fig. 24.5: Better visualization on 3D scan than conventional 2D scan in approx 3 seconds aquisition time.

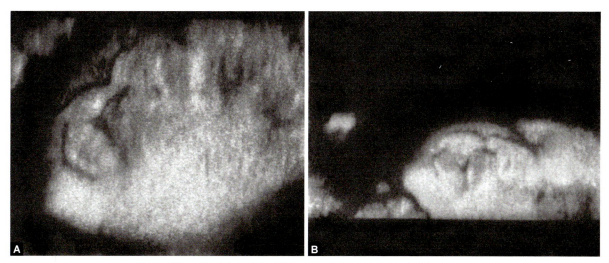

Figs. 24.6A and B: 3D image of face showing left lip.

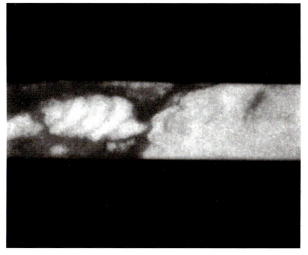

Fig. 24.7: 3D scan showing umbilical cord.

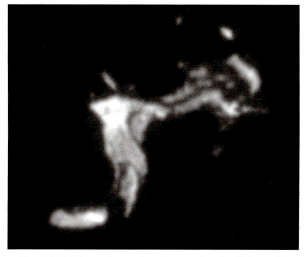

Fig. 24.8: Three-dimensional scan showing fetus—36 weeks—umbilical cord using Power-Doppler.

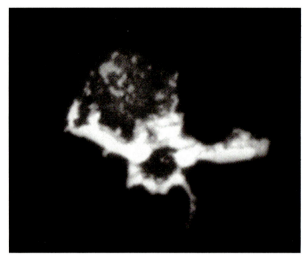

Fig. 24.9: Three-dimensional—transcranial Power-Doppler using contrast agent (Levovist, Schering AG)—angioma.

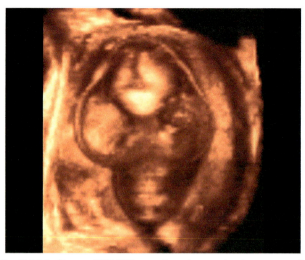

Fig. 24.11: Coronal 3D US scan in color mode shows a cystic hygroma arising from the fetal neck.

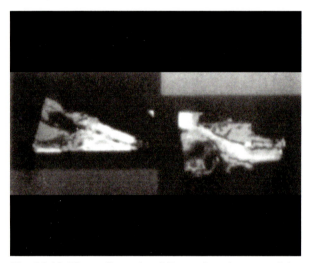

Fig. 24.10: Three-dimensional Power-Doppler scan of the vena-cava—occluded.

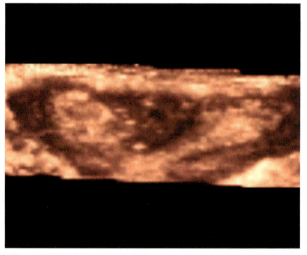

Fig. 24.12: Coronal 3D US scan in color mode shows a septate uterus.

showed great promise, they were constraint by the limitations of the available computing power. With the availability of greater computing power, at reasonable prices, a resurgence of interest in 3D sonographic techniques is occurring. Advantages of 3D sonography include:

- Real-time acquisition of images with total volume acquisition, generally during a single breath hold.
- Acquisition of a single volume and its subsequent reconstruction and viewing at a work station, allows images to be acquired and quickly, freeing the remainder of the examination time to view selected areas under real-time 2D visualization.
- Potential for accurate cardiac gating of image acquisition has important implications for visualization of the heart and blood vessels, i.e. its use to assess abnormal motion of the walls of the blood vessels. Addition of color flow information makes assessment of blood flow and its various parameters more extensive.

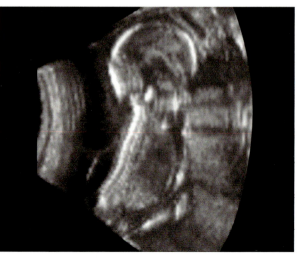

Fig. 24.13: Sagittal 3D US scan in gray scale mode shows the entire skull and spine including CVJ.

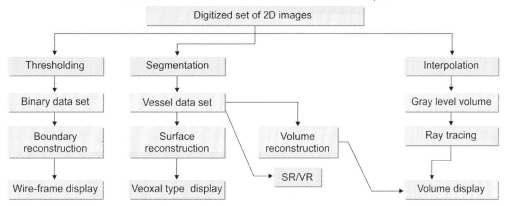

Flowchart 24.1: Overview of reconstruction techniques.

- Innovative methods of transducer localization and image display, offer real advantages in certain situations, such as intraoperative imaging.
- The examinations are more standardized than conventional 2D sonography and are readily repeatable, which reduce operator dependence and increases utility on follow up examination.

However, problems with 3D sonography do exist, including the following:

- Sonography contains more mottle than comparable CT and MRI images and this is not altered by 3D reconstruction
- The volume imaged depends on the physical characteristics of the transducer used and each transducer will need a specially built assembly for 3D acquisition with the mechanical method of localization.
- Inability to image through air/bone.

Physical Principles

Acquiring the sequence is the critical step in the process for two reasons. First because the sequence of acquired tomographic images will be assembled into a 3D image, the acquisition geometry must be known precisely to avoid distortions and the images must be acquired to avoid patient motion. Secondly, the mechanism that manipulates the transducer or localizes its position in space must not interfere with the usual sonographic examination.

Localizing the 3D volume may be done with mechanical localizers, dedicated 3D probes and remote localizers.

Mechanical Localizers

With this approach, the operator can scan the patient/cause the transducer to be moved under motor control, while its position and angles are automatically and simultaneously recorded. This approach has been used extensively for echocardiography for measurement of ventricular volume. However, mechanical tracking can be difficult to carry out on curved surface such as the female breast/3rd trimester abdomen.

Dedicated Mechanical 3D Probes

In this approach, either a mechanical 2D probe or a linear array probe is mounted on a hand hold assembly that allows the translation or rotation of the transducer by a stepping motor under computed control. Due to the need for additional motors, such probes are often more bulky and hence, more cumbersome to use than the conventional transducers. However, this is not to such a degree where it constitutes a major problem. This approach has been used successfully for the heart, kidney, eye, prostate, and breast. A variation on this approach is the use of a motorized rotating transducer mounted on the end of a catheter and introduced into the vasculature for intravascular imaging. Withdrawal of the catheter and transducer through the vessel allows collection of a stock of 2D images for forming a 3D volume.

Remote Localizers

This approach makes use of either optical, acoustic or magnetic remote localizers to measure the two transducer position and angle in space. To scan the patient, the operator manually moves the hand-hold transducer, while the remote localizer monitors its movement. This approach allows the operator to move the transducer in the usual manner without-constraints thereby offering great flexibility of movement and allowing the operator to scan large and small volumes using a hand hold probe.

Surface and Volume Rendering

Once the 3D volume is defined and a set of 2D images have been acquired (and digitized for computer manipulations), the 3D data set needs to be displayed. Two main ways for viewing 3D data exist—one is formed surface rendering and the other is called volume rendering.

Clinical Uses of 3D Ultrasound

Gray scale 3D imaging: By far, the most common approach to 3D ultrasound is based on digitizing the B-mode videosignal directly to produce gray scale 3D images.

Fetus

Three-dimensional sonography has the potential to provide cleaner visualization of ribs and spine, which may assist the clinician in (i) understanding fetal anatomy more easily and with more confidence as in fetal spine which is otherwise difficult to see in completeness, (ii) determining the extent of abnormalities more clearly, (iii) showing anomalies which have not been previously detected with 2D sonography.

Three-dimensional sonography has the potential to enhance identification of spinal and thoracic abnormality like scoliosis, spinal disruption, hemivertebra, butterfly vertebral, and ribs abnormality. Three-dimensional ultrasound has been reported to be better than 2D ultrasound for fetal ankle evaluation and for assessment of micrognathia and cleft palate and lips. The diagnosis of cardiac abnormality is likely to be improved with 3D images. Three-dimensional ultrasound might also play a role is increasing the accuracy of volume determinations for evaluation of growth retardation. Additionally, a possible benefit of 3D imaging is reduction of the exposure of the fetus to ultrasound waves by acquiring all the data needed in a single 3D volume. It also allows the image to be interpreted and reviewed separately from the performance of the study and to be viewed at different angles, planes, etc.

However, 3D imaging of the fetus is technically challenging. Fetal movement is a major problem which ideally requires data acquisition times of <5 sec. Furthermore, the 3D volume to be interrogated, can be very large, especially, later in pregnancy.

Eye and Orbit

With 3D ultrasound, orbital tumors can be evaluated with greater accuracy than before and their relationship to the globe, optic nerve and ocular mass can be determined without the risks of ionizing radiations and use of contrast media (as with CT). In addition, it is less expensive and less time consuming than MRI. 3D images can be more accurate than radially acquired images for precise calculation of tumor volumes and follow up of therapeutic response.

3D ultrasound may provide a method whereby the eye and its surrounding structures can be evaluated in patients with congenital malformations or deformities (e.g. coloboma), disorders of ocular mobility like strabismus and in dealing with complex vitreal disease.

Prostate

Three-dimensional transrectal sonography, may allows precise volumetric analysis of prostate and may prove to be better than 2D ultrasound in staging prostatic cancers and may allow more accurate follow up of tumor volume. Three-dimensional transrectal ultrasound may reduce operator dependency, reduce the examination time, increased patient comfort, and acceptability and better reproducibility.

Kidney and Liver

Three-dimensional imaging may prove to be beneficial especially in (i) imaging of intrarenal neoplasia, in solitary kidneys where organ sparing operations are necessary and 3D imaging has ability to depict the relationship of the tumor to vasculature, collecting system and capsule, (ii) imaging of renal transplants with the ability of 3D ultrasound to visualize regional perfusion, early changes of rejection may be possibly detected. Additionally, accurate assessment of renal volume and changes in volume with time may also help in defining rejection.

The use of 3D imaging is speculative, although initial sonograms of the biliary tree do show some potential imaging of the abnormal biliary tree in 3D and imaging of liver vasculature with color flow in 3D may help locate intrahepatic tumor before lobar/segmental resection.

Heart and Vascular System

Three-dimensional reconstruction may provide accurate definition of the size and features of individual atherosclerotic plaques which will allow assessment of therapies for atherosclerosis and hypertension. Moreover, the spatial relationship between the different cardiac structures and calculation of ventricular volumes is better with 3D ultrasound. Data acquisition is cardiac gated and is either performed transthoracically or transesophageally. Additional, 3D intravascular imaging is a new and exciting technique which provides visualization of luminal and transmural vessel morphology.

Color 3D Imaging

The technically most advanced system for CD 3D imaging was developed by PICOT and coworkers. They used a 5 MHz linear array transducer mounted in a motor driven, handhold translation assembly to image flow in carotid artery. The system is also capable of acquiring multiple images at several points during the cardiac cycle to form a set of 3D reconstructions, which can then be viewed in a cine loop fashion. This ability is S/T referred to as 4-D US imaging.

The clinical applications of color 3D imaging include visualization of cardiac jets due to valve defects and display of vasculature in an area suspected of containing a mass. Other areas where 3D imaging has been attempted are prostate (to monitor tumor flow after radiation therapy) and brain (to evaluate major brain arteries).

3D power Doppler imaging may allow detection of high velocity flow and areas of segmental infarction and abnormal vessel architecture known to occur in most tumors. Currently, we cannot adequately image these vessels noninvasively with any other imaging technique. It is postulated that this technique will provide improved detection of vessels with diameters of < 2 mm, when combined with sonographic contrast enhancement. This technique is however, not yet a commercial reality, but is less expensive and has a shorter examination time.

25 CHAPTER

Intravascular Ultrasound: Current Concepts

INTRODUCTION

Angiography has been an indispensable reference tool for vascular imaging, especially during interventional procedures. Angiography remains the gold standard for vascular imaging due to advancement in catheter technology, digital imaging systems, and contrast technology. Nonetheless, significant limitations exist between pathologically proven specimens and angiography such as differentiation between thrombotic episodes, embolic occlusions and atheromatous plaques; all of these appear as an interruption in the flow of contrast within the vessel. Angiography provides two-dimensional (2D) longitudinal images of patent vessel lumens. However, no information is provided regarding the vessel wall, morphology of plaque, etiology of stenoses, occlusions or perivascular structures. Intraobserver and interobserver variations also may tend to make angiographic interpretations less accurate.

This led to the quest for development of an alternative modality, like intravascular ultrasound (IVUS) **(Fig. 25.1)**. Several characteristics inherent to ultrasound imaging offer potential advantages in the evaluation of vascular diseases. intravascular ultrasound refers to the acquisition of cross-sectional images of the target vessel by an ultrasound probe placed on the tip of endoluminally positioned catheter.

Historical Aspects

Omoto R (1967) and Bom et al. (1970) used intraluminal ultrasonographic imaging for obtaining more detailed information of the cardiac chambers because of limitations of external ultrasonography at that time. Later additional studies comparing IVUS with angiography reported superiority of IVUS in calculation of luminal dimension and cross-sectional area in elliptical lesions.[1] Nissen et al. in 1990 also reported superiority of IVUS in measurement of coronary artery dimensions, degree of stenosis, detection of arterial dissections and intimal flaps.[2] Considerable engineering ingenuity and advances in catheters and ultrasound technology have permitted the marriage of miniaturized ultrasound transducer on catheters usually ranging from 3 to 9 French.

Limitations of Catheter Angiography

Angiography provides detailed longitudinal information about vessels, but is limited in its ability to assess the vessel wall. Intravascular ultrasound permits 2D axial imaging of the vessel, providing information about the luminal surface as well as the other histologic layers. Post-processing can permit three-dimensional reconstruction of imaged segments, further enhancing the quality of the acquired information. It requires no ionizing radiation and no injections of fluids, and there is no inherent time limit on imaging. Additionally, the information is digitized and may be suitable for quantitative analysis, such as diameter, area, and percentage stenosis calculation, as well as useful in attempting tissue characterization.

Technical Consideration of Intravascular Ultrasound

Two types of systems have been developed for intravascular applications: mechanically rotating devices and electronic array devices **(Fig. 25.2)**. Typically IVUS catheters use a frequency ranging from 20 to 40 MHz. These high frequencies allow greater lateral and axial resolution, at the expense of lesser tissue penetration due to energy dissipation at the higher frequencies.

Three-dimensional (3D) computer enhanced reconstruction of IVUS images is achievable. The 3D images are obtained by performing a slow pull back of the IVUS

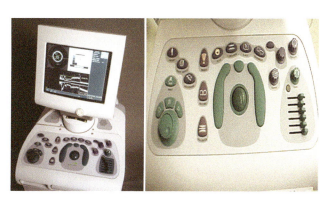

Fig. 25.1: Boston Scientific Galaxy™ System (BSC).

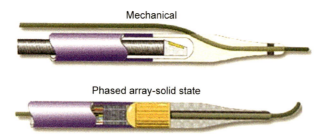

Fig. 25.2: Transducer types.

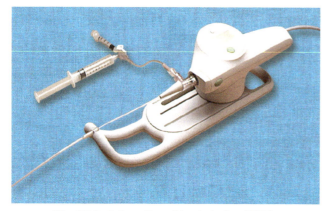

Fig. 25.3: Automatic pull back device (BSC).

catheter at a uniform speed. Images are acquired during the pull back at a rate of approximately six images per second (**Fig. 25.3**). Uniform geometric sampling can be achieved with constant pull-back speed. The system processes image sets up to 255 slices. The 3D images are obtained online during the procedure with minimal delay. This added information provides further insight into vessel wall, plaque, and lumen characteristics. Recently, a new forward-viewing IVUS catheter has been described that provides faster 3D reconstruction.

Most IVUS catheters are braided polyethylene and require sheaths for introduction. The lower MHz transducers usually require larger catheters and therefore large sheaths. Penetration is extremely important in large vessels such as the aorta where a 30-MHz probe may be of little benefit, as it will not penetrate to the wall of the aorta. 20 MHz probe generally penetrates up to 2 cm from the catheter.

Intravascular Ultrasound Evaluation of Vascular Anatomy

Intravascular ultrasound is uniquely capable of providing insight into the structure and composition of the normal arterial wall because of its ability to provide transmural information.

Normal Arterial Wall

The three histologic layers of the arterial wall can be identified clearly and have distinctive ultrasonic characteristics due to difference in acoustic impedance of these layers.[3-5] The wall of the artery is composed of the intima, internal elastic lamina, media, external elastic lamina, and adventitia. The intima consists of a monolayer of endothelial cells. The outermost layer, i.e. the adventitia is collagen-rich and is thus bright in appearance with an indistinct outer margin due to surrounding soft tissues. The intima is hyperechoic with a varying coarse and smooth echogenic pattern. In normal arteries, it is quite thin but can thicken significantly if intimal hyperplasia develops. The internal elastic lamina is seen as the innermost thin echogenic layer.[6] The actual thickness of the intimal layer may be overestimated because of its high echogenicity, making distinction difficult from mild intimal proliferation.[7] The echogenicity of the media varies in muscular and elastic arteries in view of varying amount of smooth muscle, collagen and elastin content respectively. Hence, media of elastic arteries such as aorta, subclavian, carotid and iliac arteries is echo-reflective, resulting in a two-layered appearance.[8]

Calcium

Calcium within the wall of a vessel produces acoustic shadowing, a typical sonic characteristic. Generally, this calcium is deep to the intima and does not result in degradation of the image.

Flowing Blood

Flowing blood has a characteristic speckled pattern and is easily identified during real time examination with pulsations of the cardiac cycle.

Classically, the muscular arterial wall is easily identified by a characteristic three-layered appearance. The inner layer is hyperechoic and represents the intima and internal elastic lamina. The intima itself is not resolvable as a thin cell layer with current technology.[6] The media is identified as a thin anechoic band with the more hyperechoic thicker adventitia on the external aspect of this layer. The large elastic arteries, such as the aorta, are visualized less clearly because the high amounts of elastin in the media increases the reflection of echoes from this layer.

Veins are recognized by a thin hyperechoic wall with no discernible separation of wall layer due to the lack of an organized thick media as seen in arteries. A very hyperechoic wall usually characterizes synthetic bypass grafts with little sound-through transmission because of the lack of ability of high megahertz transducers to penetrate the synthetic material (e.g. Dacron, PTEE).

Stents filters and other metallic objects such as needles are characterized easily by their focal intense hyperechoic appearance.

Intravascular Ultrasound in Disease States

Plaque Morphology

Intravascular ultrasound can help delineate the type of vascular disease present (atherosclerotic or non-

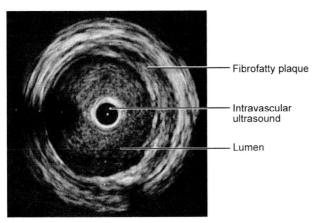

Fig. 25.4: Eccentric fibrofatty plaque.

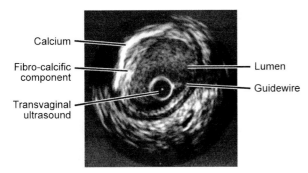

Fig. 25.5: Calcified plaque.

atherosclerotic), its severity and the degree of luminal obstruction.[4] On the basis of the quantitative analysis of the reflective intensity of the ultrasound signal, attempts to characterize the components of the atherosclerotic plaque have been undertaken because such information has practical implications regarding the success or failure of interventional vascular procedures.[9] Typically lipid collections are echolucent and can be easily identified within an atheroma; fibrous tissue and collagen are strong echo reflectors and are therefore visualized as an echogenic, speckled-to-homogeneous bright structures **(Fig. 25.4)**. Calcium, which is the strongest echo-reflector, produces intense bright areas within the plaque, associated with a dropout of peripheral echoes due to the intense reflection of the ultrasound signal.[10] **(Fig. 25.5)** Furthermore, atherosclerotic plaques are to a variable degree covered by a denser fibrous cap that appears as a reflective structure during ultrasound imaging at the arterial wall interface.[3,11]

In addition, IVUS demonstrates the distribution of plaque within the vessel. In atherosclerotic arterial disease, following the initial plaque formation and subsequent compensatory vessel dilatation, up to 70% of coronary and peripheral plaques are eccentrically positioned and elliptical in shape.[4] Uniplanar angiography is likely to inaccurately determine cross-sectional area stenosis unless the diseased segment has maintained a circular shape.[12] The use of biplanar angiographic techniques can lessen the error, although the degree of stenosis is generally underestimated. Intravascular ultrasound provides accurate cross-sectional area measurements and precise calculation of percentage of stenosis. In studies in which near circular lumens were evaluated, good correlation existed between angiography and IVUS in determining dimensions. In severely diseased arteries with eccentric lumens, IVUS is more accurate than angiography for making precise measurements.[6]

Characterization of Thrombi

The ability to detect thrombi with IVUS is directly related to the thrombus composition. Thrombi consisting solely of platelet-rich plasma cannot be detected. As the content of red cells within the thrombus increases, there is a concomitant increase in the echogenicity.[13] A linear correlation between the amount of red blood cells in the thrombus and the intensity of the speckled ultrasonic signal was demonstrated by Frimerman et al.[13] The intensity of reflection is brighter for a more recent thrombus than for organized older clots.[10] This speckled ultrasonic appearance is not specific to thrombus; it can also be seen with soft plaques composed mainly of loose connective or fibromuscular tissue.[5] Studies by Alibelli-Chemarin et al. demonstrated that IVUS can correctly identify thrombus in 63% of patients with a recent infarction.[14] Siegel et al. found that IVUS has a specificity of 95% in identifying thrombus, with a sensitivity of 57%.[6]

Thrombus: Thrombus is echogenic and may be difficult to distinguish from a noncalcified fibrous plaque or stagnant blood. It however, has a typically scintillating or sparkling pattern on real time US examination. The presence of micro channels and an echodensity of less than 50% of the adventitia are important clues to its correct identification.[6]

False lumen: A false lumen may occur spontaneously or commonly following endovascular interventions. Mistaking a false lumen for true lumen can have serious consequences if the former is selected for stent or stent-graft placement (as in aortic dissections) IVUS may help in such situations by recognition of the characteristic three layered appearance of true lumen identification of side branches taking off from the true lumen identification of side branches taking off from the true lumen and by the slow flowing, more echogenic blood within the false lumen. In addition, flush injections of contrast may at times reveal the echogenic patterns of the contrast to "hang up" and take longer to evacuate from the false lumen compared to the true lumen.[15]

Aneurysm: A true aneurysm is differentiated histologically from a false aneurysm by the presence of media in the former. Intravascular ultrasound can detect the presence of hypoechoic media to distinguish the two entities, although at times the media may be very thinned out.

Nonspecific aortoarteritis: S Sharma et al. had reported the IVUS imaging findings in Takayasu's arteritis. The intima is relatively unaffected and remains thin. There is an increase in the echogenicity and thickness of the media. The adventitia is also similarly affected with diffuse periarterial fibrosis. Due to these changes, the characteristic three-layered appearance may not be seen at places. In addition, the lesions can be complicated by the presence of calcification. The compliance of the aortic wall is lost in the involved segments on real time imaging. These changes are seen even in the angiographically "normal" segments of the vessel, emphasizing the diffuse nature of the disease. This observation has important therapeutic implications. Correct demonstration of normal segments helps in choosing the sites for placement of proximal and distal anastomosis in bypass grafting at surgery and for optimal positioning of the balloon catheter or stent and interventional radiological treatment. Intravascular ultrasound helps in making this decision and has the potential to improve the long-term results of the above treatment methods.[15]

Interpretation and Application

Significant investigative research has validated qualitative and quantitative information obtained with IVUS. These studies demonstrate high accuracy in measurements obtained with IVUS, thus validating information such as percent stenosis, vessel diameters, and circumferences. Qualitatively the layers of the normal vessel wall are easily identifiable; plaque composition, thrombus characteristics, and vessel wall composition may be assessed; and the data are reproducible.[3,6,11]

CLINICAL APPLICATIONS

Benanati[16] has divided the applications of IVUS into four large groups:
1. Diagnostic adjunct.
2. Therapeutic adjunct.
3. Real time therapeutic monitoring.
4. Therapeutic tool.

Intravascular Ultrasound as a Diagnostic Adjunct

A widely used role for IVUS is in confirming angiographic information. Pre-interventional planning may be facilitated by accurate IVUS information. Vessel size is often estimated by obtaining measurement from angiograms. Accuracy is diminished because of factors such as magnification.[17] Exact sizing is critical when trying to select the appropriate atherectomy catheter and balloons. Many institutions have used IVUS to confirm suspicious angiographic findings in the aorta. Aortic transection secondary to trauma and aortic dissections are readily diagnosable with IVUS imaging and IVUS may be used in a complementary manner when angiography is equivocal.[18]

This may be especially beneficial, for example, in trying to distinguish a prominent ductus bump from a subtle transection; the implication being major cardiothoracic surgery if a transection is present. Intravascular ultrasound may be the modality of choice to evaluate perivascular disease processes. Intravascular ultrasound is an excellent tool for evaluating intravascular tumor growth. Renal, adrenal, and hepatocellular carcinomas may have venous invasion. If venography is equivocal or if renal function is impaired thus making iodinated contrast undesirable, intravascular ultrasound should be considered as an excellent imaging option. Intravascular ultrasound also may be used as an adjunct in evaluating disease processes such as coarctation of the aorta and Takayasu's arteritis.[19]

Intracardiac sonography is feasible using 12.5 MHz transducers, which will allow good resolution of the cardiac chambers. Potentially, diagnosis of congenital defects, valve abnormalities, and intra-cardiac masses may be evaluated in addition to the assessment of wall motion and valve function.[19] Pulmonary IVUS is also feasible. Normal pulmonary artery anatomy has been described by IVUS as having a smooth thin inner wall with poor media and adventitia visualization because of air in the surrounding lung.[19] Pulmonary hypertension causes the arterial wall to thicken and become irregular.

Qualitative assessment of plaque and vessel wall allows wall compliance assessment and tissue characterization. For example, aortic changes such as aneurysmal dilatation secondary to Marfan's syndrome are related to elastin content and structure. Preliminary work done by Recchia et al.[20] has suggested that IVUS can sensitively detect abnormalities in aortic elastin and thus may be a tool for both diagnosis of Marfan's syndrome and for monitoring the syndrome over time. Intravascular ultrasound has been shown to be superior to angiography in assessment of plaque progression and regression.

Intravascular Ultrasound as a Therapeutic Imaging Adjunct

Because of the additional time and cost as well as the larger sheath requirements justification for using IVUS necessitates that the additional information gained actually alter outcomes, determine endpoints, or influence the choice of interventional modality [precutaneous transluminal angioplasty (PTA), atherectomy, stent, and lysis]. Prior to intervention, IVUS provides accurate vessel measurements, allowing for proper sizing of the devices to be used. Evaluation of the lesion may influence the therapeutic modality. Identification of thrombus, for example, would mandate fibrinolysis as opposed to angioplasty or atherectomy. During intervention, endpoints determination may have a direct impact on long-term patency. Intravascular ultrasound yields specific information that benefits each type of interventional modality. Pretreatment IVUS may influence treatment strategies in up to 44% of cases making the extra time required to perform the procedure cost-effective. Predicting restenosis on the basis of information obtained with IVUS after intervention may have a dramatic impact on treatment strategies.[21]

PERCUTANEOUS TRANSLUMINAL ANGIOPLASTY

Accurate determination of balloon size is enhanced by using IVUS to measure vessel diameters. In addition, the ability to evaluate circumferential compromise of a vessel lumen by plaque allows for a greater appreciation of the true hemodynamic compromise. Angiographic evaluation of stenoses relies only on diameter measurement. This has been shown to grossly underestimate the extent of plaque and the degree of luminal compromise [a 50% diameter stenosis corresponds to a 75% area stenosis].[17,18] In addition, angiographic measurements assume that vessel measurements proximal and distal to the lesion represent normal diameter. Intravascular ultrasound evaluation frequently demonstrates diffuse concentric plaque lining the vessel and thus rendering angiographic measurements inaccurate[2,20] [this may be especially true in the superficial femoral artery, a vessel long recognized as having diffuse atheromatous involvement] **(Fig. 25.6)**. Intravascular ultrasound measurements of vessel diameters are larger than those measured with angiography. If larger balloon sizes create larger lumens, this information may influence decision making because long-term patency may improve with larger post-treatment vessel lumens. They also may decrease cost of the procedure or at least offset the cost of having used IVUS.

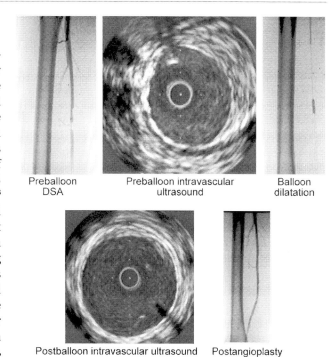

Fig. 25.6: Superficial femoral artery.

The ability to assess the vessel after intervention influences decisions concerning endpoints and need for further treatment. Typically, after PTA, a dissection is present in the vessel wall. Failure to recognize this dissection with IVUS implies that inadequate PTA has occurred and even though lumen area may be increased, elastic recoil is likely.

The degree of dissection present is variable, ranging from eccentric plaque fracture with large central patent lumens to complete circumferential plaque fracture with severe compromise of vessel lumen. When the latter is encountered, it is best to proceed to stent deployment in the dissected area to avoid acute closure **(Fig. 25.7)**. Intravascular ultrasound is able to demonstrate the pulsatility of the intimal flap and the compliance, or lack of compliance, in the post-PTA vessel segment.

When abrupt closure complicates PTA, IVUS is capable of discerning severe dissection (requiring prolonged inflation or stent placement) versus thrombosis (requiring fibrinolysis or embolectomy). Angiography even when performed in multiple projections, consistently underestimates the degree of residual stenosis when compared to IVUS.[1] IVUS is helpful after PTA when pressure gradients still exist despite a satisfactory angiogram. Vessel interrogation with IVUS frequently uncovers stenoses not appreciated angiographically.

ATHERECTOMY

Intravascular ultrasound may play a larger role with atherectomy than with any of the other interventional procedures. Long-term results of peripheral atherectomy have been somewhat disappointing compared to initial enthusiastic results reported when this modality was first introduced. Reason for success and failure of atherectomy procedures may be explained on the basis of IVUS-derived information. Under sizing the atherectomy catheter implies that residual plaque will be left behind in the vessel and the final vessel diameter will be sub-optimal. An oversized device may shave or cut into the media and adventitia, putting the vessel at risk for rupture or pseudoaneurysm. In addition, cutting deep to the intima may cause accelerated cellular proliferation and onset of intimal hyperplasia.[22]

Angiography significantly underestimates the amount of residual stenosis. Angiograms with near normal angiographic appearance (stenosis <10%) have been documented by IVUS as residual stenosis of 60–70%. Intravascular ultrasound frequently demonstrates the eccentricity of the atherectomy cuts. IVUS demonstrates that circumferential compression causes eccentric vessel narrowing because the more compliant (less diseased) portions of the vessel compress more easily than the less compliant (more diseased) segments. This explains why significant atheroma remains after multiple passes with this device and why significant plaque remains despite the presence of media in histologic specimens.

STENT DEPLOYMENT

With the applications for stents expanding both in the coronary and peripheral circulation, the need for more precise information regarding vessel size, plaque

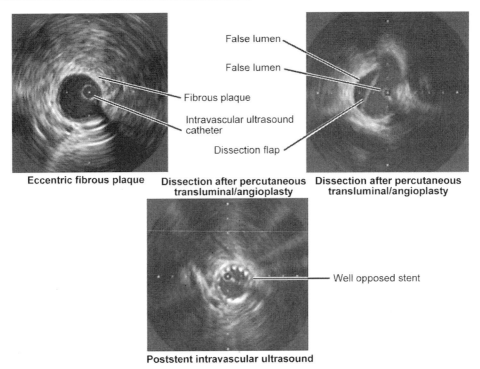

Fig. 25.7: Intravascular ultrasound before and after coronary artery stenting.

characteristics, and the relationship of the expanded stent to the vessel wall is required. Intravascular ultrasound provides accurate information that impacts the size of stent expansion. Studies have shown that angiography underestimates the residual narrowing after stent deployment.[23] Intravascular ultrasound helps appreciate the under expansion of the stent and it demonstrates incomplete apposition of the struts to the vessel wall. Dilatation is routinely performed with larger balloons until the stent struts are completely opposed to the luminal wall. This information is not obtainable using angiography. Ideal stent placement results in integration of the stent into the vessel wall. Once this occurs, an endothelial layer covers the stent preventing thrombus from forming on the stent. This layer may not develop or may be delayed in developing if thrombus is allowed to form between the stent and the vessel wall. The stent struts are easily recognized by their bright, evenly spaced, and hyperechoic appearance. In time, a thin hypoechoic layer, representing a neo-intima, may be appreciated within the stent.

STENT GRAFTS

Intravascular ultrasound plays two major roles in stent graft or endovascular graft procedures: sizing of the proximal and distal neck, which determines the diameter of the proximal and distal graft; and intra-procedure evaluation of the stent struts or hooks to determine if the graft is properly expanded **(Fig. 25.8)**. Measuring the diameter of the proximal and distal grafts is critical because if the graft device is designed too small, leaking into the aneurysm sack will be inevitable. These measurements cannot be accurately obtained angiographically.

CAVAL FILTER AND OTHER VENOUS INTERVENTIONS

Evaluation of caval filters and associated thrombus has been performed yielding information that may complement or obviate cavography. While it is not common to study filters after deployment, there may be a need when questions concerning filter migration, recurrent pulmonary embolism, caval thrombosis, or filter tilting arise. If technical problems arise during deployment, careful assessment of the filter hooks may be achieved using IVUS. Identification of renal veins is not difficult with IVUS, making the entire procedure of filter deployment possible with IVUS monitoring.[24,25]

Intravascular ultrasound also has been used to evaluate changes in vessel diameter with positional changes such as in patients with thoracic inlet syndrome. Dramatic IVUS images are obtained by changing the patient's arm position while the catheter is positioned at the thoracic inlet. Intravascular ultrasound also has been used to evaluate changes in hepatic vein size and transjugular intrahepatic portosystemic shunt (TIPS) size during changes in respiration.

REAL TIME MONITORING OF THERAPEUTIC PROCEDURES

Percutaneous fenestration of aortic dissection has been accomplished successfully using IVUS as the primary imaging modality to guide the needle fenestrations. Because

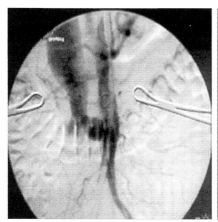
Digital subtraction angiography showing infra-renal aorto-caval fistula

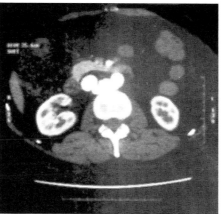
Contrast enhanced computed tomography abdomen at level of fistula

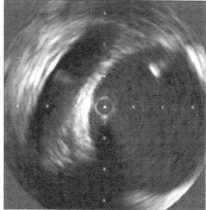
Arteriovenous/Fistula on IVUS

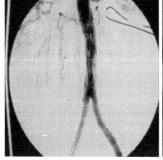
Postgraft angio with residual narrowing

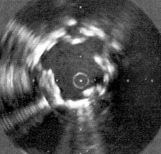
Incomplete inflation

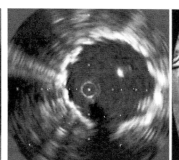
Postballoon dilatation on IVUS and DSA

Fig. 25.8: Aortocaval fistula.

of the high-resolution axial information, IVUS is ideally suited for this application. Angiography is practical because of the need for real-time assessment and because it provides information about the lumen that the catheter does not.[26] The hyperechoic needle is seen as an intensely hyperechoic foci that may be monitored as it passes from one channel to another. Intravascular ultrasound also assists in providing information concerning which branch vessels arise from true or false lumens.[27] It is superior to angiography in identifying entry and re-entry points in the thoracic and abdominal aorta. Assessment of this information is superior with IVUS when compared to angiography and transesophageal echocardiography.

Future Directions

Integration of the IVUS transducers with other interventional catheters is already underway and should greatly enhance the use of IVUS as a diagnostic adjunct. Hybrids of IVUS and interventional catheters that are currently being evaluated include laser hybrids, atherectomy hybrids, and balloon angioplasty hybrids.[28] Fine positioning of the atherectomy catheter using online real time IVUS might help to ensure adequate removal of plaque without shaving of disease-free segments of vessel.[29]

Intravascular ultrasound in conjunction with PTA catheters could conceivably provide real-time images of plaque fracture or recoil, thus influencing inflation pressures and inflation times. Intravascular ultrasound also has been used in conjunction with thrombectomy catheters to guide percutaneous procedures. With Doppler capabilities, IVUS can provide online hemodynamic evaluation of lesions. Doppler changes recording during catheter passage across a lesion may dictate whether treatment is indicated or whether treated segments require further intervention.

Ultrasound also may be used as a therapeutic modality. Ultrasonic probes are being evaluated as tools for pulverizing plaque and thrombus. This concept has potential application in rapid declotting of bypass or access grafts. This potential could decrease the cost of lysis procedures and would greatly reduce the time of procedures.[30]

Continued improvement in transducer design and technology will allow for better resolution and penetration of ultrasound waves. Reliability of transducers and catheters has improved dramatically in the past five years. Improvement in catheter design to allow for more trackable and steerable catheters will greatly expand the use of IVUS because it will allow catheter guidance in tortuous vessels and branch vessels that are currently difficult to select.

Recent Advances of Intravascular Ultrasound

Borges AC et al. studied the relationship between hemodynamics and morphology in pulmonary hypertension by intravascular ultrasound. The authors stated that intravascular ultrasound imaging of the pulmonary arteries was a reliable method of quantifying vessel diameter, luminal area and pulsatility. Simultaneous measurement of flow velocity and its response to vasodilators allowed the relationship between morphology and functional compromise to be studied, especially endothelial dysfunction.[31]

Sharma S et al. in 1998 evaluated the IVUS imaging appearances of the aorta and the iliac artery in atherosclerosis and concluded that IVUS shows typical alterations in the wall morphology in atherosclerosis. It better demonstrates vascular calcification and thrombus. The detection of mural changes will improve our understanding of the pathogenesis of this disease and will help in better planning of interventional therapeutic techniques.[15] They also described current trends and future applications of intravascular ultrasound in 2003.

Aquilla S et al. in 1999 did experimental studies in Canines and concluded that intravascular sonography is a novel technique for visualizing the ostium (neck) of an aneurysm. It provides complete morphologic delineation of the size of the aneurysm's ostium and the relationship of the ostium to adjacent arterial branches–information that is not obtainable with the use of any other currently available imaging technique. In conjunction with digital subtraction angiography (DSA), intravascular sonography opens another window to monitor and control endovascular therapeutic procedures.[32]

Early clinical experience with color 3D IVUS in peripheral interventions was described by Irshad K et al. in 2001, who demonstrated Chroma Flow-enhanced IVUS; where blood flow inside the vessel lumen was seen as color on images, which is helpful in distinguishing echolucent disease from luminal blood flow. They also advocated its use in peripheral interventions in patients with renal failure or allergy, avoiding the use of contrast media.[33]

Buckley CJ et al. in 2002 advocated that intravascular ultrasound scanning improves long-term patency of iliac lesions treated with balloon angioplasty and primary stenting. Long-term follow up of treated patients shows outcomes that are comparable with direct surgical intervention. Intravascular ultrasound significantly improved the long-term patency of iliac arterial lesions treated with balloon angioplasty and stenting by defining the appropriate angioplasty diameter endpoint and adequacy of stent deployment.[34]

Saket RR et al. in 2004 demonstrated the feasibility of using IVUS-guided method to create transintimal arterial communications for subintimal recanalization with controlled re-entry in chronic total occlusions and for aortic flap fenestrations in aortic dissections. The authors concluded that this approach can improve the technical success rate, reduce the time of the procedure, and minimize potential complications.[35]

REFERENCES

1. Tabbara MR, White RA, Cavaye DM, et al. In vivo comparison of intravascular ultrasound and angiography. J Vascular Surg. 1991;14:496-504.
2. Nissen SE, Gurley JC, Grines CL, et al. Comparison of intravascular ultrasound and angiography in quantification of coronary dimensions and stenoses in man: Impact of lumen eccentricity. Circulation. 1990;82 (Suppl III):440.
3. Gussenhoven EJ, Essed CE, Lancee CT, et al. Arterial wall characteristic determined by intravascular ultrasound imaging: an in vitro study. J Am Coll Cardiol. 1989;14:947-52.
4. Waller BF, Pinkerton CA, Slack JD. Intravascular ultrasound: a histological study of vessels during life- the new gold standard for vascular imaging. Circulation. 1992;85(6):2305-10.
5. Pandian NG, Kreis A, Weintrasub A, Kumar R. Intravascular ultrasound assessment of arterial dissection intimal flaps and intra-arterial thrombi. Am J Card Imaging. 1991;5:72-77.
6. Siegel RJ, Ariani M, Fishbein MC, et al. Histopathological validation of Angioscopy and intravascular ultrasound. Circulation. 1991;84:109.
7. Porter TR, Sears T, Xie F, et al. Intravascular Ultrasound study of angiographically mildly disease coronary arteries. J Am Coll Cardiol. 1993;22:1858-65.
8. Ge J, Erbel R, Gerber T, et al. Intravascular ultrasound imaging of angiographically normal coronary arteries: a prospective study in vivo. Br Heart J. 1994;71:527-78.
9. Waller BF, Miller J, Morgan R, et al. Atherosclerotic plaque calcific deposits: an important factor in success or failure of transluminal coronary angioplasty. Circulation 1988;78(suppl II):II-376.
10. Tobis JM, Mahon DJ, Goldberg SL, et al. Lessons from intravascular ultrasonography: observations during interventional angioplasty procedures. J Clin Ultrasound. 1993;21:589-607.
11. Gussenhoven WJ, Essed CE, Frietman P, et al. Vascular echocardiographic assessment of vessel wall characteristics. A correlation with history. Int J Card Imaging. 1989;4:105-16.
12. Soward AL, Essed CE, Serruys PW. Coronary arterial findings after accidental death immediately after successful PTCA. Am J Cardiol. 1985;56:794-95.
13. Frimerman A, Miller HI, Hallman M, et al. Intravascular ultrasound characterization of thrombi of different composition. Am J Cardiol. 1994;73:1053-57.
14. Alibelli-Chemarin MJ, Puel J, et al. Identification of thrombus by intravascular ultrasound.
15. Sharma S, Mahawar RM, Gupta H, et al. Initial experience with intravascular ultrasound imaging of the aorta in atherosclerosis. Indian Journal of Radiology and Imaging. 1998;8(1):27-31.
16. Benanati JF. Intravascular ultrasound: the role in diagnostic and therapeutic procedures. Radiol Clin North Am 1995;33(1):31-50.
17. Glagor S. Weinserberg E, Zarins CK, et al. Compensatory enlargement of human atherosclerotic arteries. N Engl J Med 1987;316:1371-75.

18. Harrison DG, White CW, Hiratzka LF, et al. The value of lesion cross-sectional area determined by quantitative coronary angiography in assessing the physiologic significance of proximal left anterior descending coronary arterial stenosis. Circulation. 1984;69:1111-19.
19. Williams DM, Simon HJ, Marx MV, et al. Acute traumatic aortic rupture: intravascular US findings. Radiol. 1992;182:247-49.
20. Recchia D, Kouchoukos NT, Bosner MS, et al. Quantification of abnormal aortic elastin content and organization in Marfan syndrome with ultrasonic tissue characterization [abstract]. Circulation 1993;88:31-19.
21. Gorge G, Erbel R, Schuster S, et al. Intravascular ultrasound in diagnosis of acute pulmonary embolism. Lancet. 1991;337:623-24.
22. Ehrlich S, Hoyne J, Mahon D, et al. Unrecognized stenosis by angiography documented by intravascular ultrasound. Cathet Cardiovasc Dign. 1991;3:198-201.
23. Waller BF, Pinkerton CA, Orr CM, et al. Morphological observations late (>30 days) after clinically successful coronary balloon angioplasty. Circulation. 1991;83(I):28.
24. Nakamura S, Colombo A, Gaglione A, et al. Coronary stenting guided intravascular ultrasound [abstract] Circulation. 1993;88:32-11.
25. Marx MV, Taushcer JR, Williams DM, et al. Evaluation of the inferior vena cava with intravascular US after Greenfield filter placement. J of Vasc Interv Radiol 1991;2:261-68.
26. McCowan TC, Ferris EJ, Carver DK. Inferior vena caval filter thrombi: evaluation with intravascular US. Radiology 1990;177:783-88.
27. Waller PJ, Dake MD, Mitchell RS, et al. The use of endovascular techniques for the treatment of complications of aortic dissection. J Vac Surg. 1993;18:1042-51.
28. William DM, Joshi A, Dake MD, et al. Aortic cobwebs. An anatomic marker identifying the false lumen in aortic dissection imaging and pathologic correlation. Radiology. 1994;190:167-74.
29. Crowley RJ, Hamm MA, Joshi CD, et al. Ultrasound guided therapeutic catheters: recent developments and clinical results. Int J Card Imaging. 1991;6:145-46.
30. Yock PG, Fitzgerald PJ, Jang YL et al. Initial trials of a combined ultrasound imaging/mechanical atherectomy catheter [abstract]. J Am Coll Cardiol. 1990;15:17A.
31. Borges AC, Wensel R, Opitz C, Bauer U, et al. Relationship between haemodynamics and morphology in pulmonary hypertension. A quantitative intravascular ultrasound study. Eur Heart J. 1997;18(12):1847-48.
32. Aquilla S. Turk, Charles M. Strother, Daniel I. Crouthamel and James A. Zagzebski Definition of the Ostium (Neck) of an Aneurysm Revealed by Intravascular Sonography: An Experimental Study in Canines American Journal of Neuroradiology; 1999:20:1301-08.
33. Irshad K, Reid DB, Miller PH, et al. Early clinical experience with color three-dimensional intravascular ultrasound in peripheral interventions. J Endovasc Ther. 2001;8(4):329-38.
34. Buckley CJ, Arko FR, Lee S, et al. Intravascular ultrasound scanning improves long-term patency of iliac lesions treated with balloon angioplasty and primary stenting. J Vasc Surg. 2002;35(2):316-23.
35. Saket RR, Razavi MK, Padidar A, et al. Novel intravascular ultrasound-guided method to create transintimal arterial communications: initial experience in peripheral occlusive disease and aortic dissection. J Endovasc Ther. 2004;11(3): 274-80.

26
CHAPTER

Perendoscopic Ultrasound

PERENDOSCOPIC ULTRASOUND/ ENDOSCOPIC ULTRASONOGRAPHY/ ENDOULTRASONOGRAPHY

Endoscopic ultrasonography is no longer considered a new technology. Approximately 15 years have passed since endoultrasonography was first introduced and in the interval the test has become established for staging of gastrointestinal and pancreatic malignancies. The first publication on its clinical use came in 1980 by D Magno and Strohm.

Technique

Endoultrasonography (EUS) relies on the complex combination of an ultrasonic probe and a flexible endoscope. The endoscope is made up of optic fibers which enable the operator to zero in on the lesion to be ultrasonically scanned; a mechanical device aids the focusing of the probe on the lesion; and an operative canal enables air to be aspirated or water to be injected in order to improve the acoustic coupling and comfort to punctures. The probe emits high frequency of 7-12 MHz. Two types of echoendoscope (EE) are currently employed. With mechanical EE's, the transducer rotates in a plane perpendicular to the axis of the endoscope, covering a circular field of 360° around the probe; this yields circumferential sections of the digestive tract. The transducer is attached at the distal end of the endoscope. Rotation takes place around a flexible mechanical axis. Since there is only one transducer with a fixed focus of about 2 cm, mechanical maneuvering is required to bring the distance between the transducer and the lesion into the range necessary for focus. Such rotatory mechanical devices (e.g. OLYMPUS) are most popular EUS instruments available and are most frequently employed in digestive pathology. Dedicated devices are now available, echogastroscopes offering oblique views (60°), echoduodenoscopes with lateral views and large diameter echocoloscopes with axial views. However, with these, biopsy is practically impossible to achieve since the needle is perpendicular to the ultrasonic beam.

In the other type of EE, the probe is linear array, yielding longitudinal sections of the digestive wall. Such electronic devices (e.g. Pentax) may be attached to conventional ultrasound machines. Another advantage is their electronic focusing, which yields optimal resolution at different depths, a Doppler facility is available. Since the needle is parallel to ultrasonic beam, and can be mechanically moved, puncture is easier. However, since these do not demonstrate anatomic landmarks as clearly, they are less widely used for digestive examinations.

Examination Technique

Endoultrasonography (EUS) carried for digestive evaluation proceeds through the following steps: Circumferential exam of the digestive wall along a whole digestive segment; identification of the multilayer pattern of the wall; evaluation of juxta-digestive anatomic structures including lymph node (LN). At the first stage, endoscopy enables one to move the probe forward under optical monitoring; sonography is performed secondarily while extracting EE. Sometimes further forward movement is required with bending maneuvers and if necessary, repositioning of patient. Pancreatic/biliary examinations rely on particular landmark sections obtained through the stomach and duodenum. Such sections yield complete evaluation of pancreas, biliopancreatic area and common bile duct (CBD).

Intraluminal air may impede endosonography. Degassed water improves the acoustic coupling of the probe either by direct injection or within balloon.

Preparation is similar to that for conventional ultrasound. The examination is carried on the fasting outpatient after light sedation. Pancreatic and biliary examinations are longer and may require neurolept analgesia. Rectal examination requires mere cleansing enemas.

Endoscopic Ultrasonography: Indications

Diagnostic

- Upper gastrointestinal (GI) tract
    - Esophagus
        - Cancer staging
        - Submucosal tumors
        - Varices in portal HT
        - Postoperative cancer surveillance

Less accepted

Indications: Achalasia and Barrett's esophagus

- Stomach
  - Cancer staging
  - Lymphoma staging
  - Submucosal tumors
  - Varices
  - Large gastric folds
  - Mediastinal and perigastric LN assessment
  Less accepted
  Indications: Ulcers and polyps
- Duodenum
  - Cancer staging
  - Submucosal tumors
  - Varices
- Retroperitoneum
  - Pancreas—cancer staging
    - Pancreatitis—diagnosis and staging
    - Pseudocysts
- Biliary tree
  - Cancer staging
  - CBD stones—diagnosis and treatment
- Lower GI tract
  - Colon/rectum
    - Cancer staging
    - Submucosal tumors
    - Sessile polyps
    - Inflammatory bowel disease
- Heart
  - Diseases around the aortic root, dissections and atrial and mitral valve diseases.

Interventional/Therapeutic

- Guided fine needle aspiration cytology which has maximum role in diagnosis of pancreatic cancer and in nodal staging of gastrointestinal, pancreatic and pulmonary malignancies
- Endoultrasonography guided paracentesis to sample pleural and ascitic fluid seen with EUS (and often not seen on abdominal ultrasound permitting early diagnosis of malignant ascites)
- Endoultrasonography guided cyst gastrostomy for pseudocysts
- Endoultrasonography guided botulinum toxin injection into the lower esophageal sphincter in patients with achalasia
- Endoultrasonography guided coeliac plexus neurolysis for improving pain control in patients with pancreatic cancer.

Endosonographic Anatomy

Digestive wall: Whatever the digestive tract segment, USG frequency of 7-12 MHz discloses within the digestive wall a pattern of five concentric lines or layers:

1. First line is hyperechoic arising from the interface between the wall and intraluminal water (free/within the balloon).
2. The second/internal hypoechoic layer arises from the merging patterns of the mucosa and muscularis mucosa.
3. The third/medial hyperechoic layer is the submucosa.
4. Fourth/external hypoechoic layer is the muscularis propria.
5. Fifth/superficial hyperechoic layer arises from the interface between the muscularis and peridigestive connective tissue (esophagus and rectum) or serosa when it exists (stomach).

Lymph Nodes

Esophageal EUS yields images of posterior mediastinal nodes. Celiac, perigastric nodes, and nodes at hepatic and splenic hila are displayed through the stomach. Endoscopic ultrasonography may also show the perirectal nodes.

Several features have been used to describe their lymph nodes size which generally ranges from 3 to 10 mm in normal individuals. Descriptive characteristics include shape (rounded vs elongated), borders (hyperechoic vs hypoechoic) and echotexture (homogenous vs heterogenous). All LN when images should be described using these five characteristics.

Mediastinum

Transesophageal transverse sections of postmediastinum resemble those of CT, but the field covered is smaller, limited to periesophageal area. Air within the trachea and bronchi impedes the EUS study of medial and anterior mediastinum.

The mediastinal fat is clearly echogenic. Thus LN are clearly outline. In upper part of postmediastinum, the aorta and azygus vein are vascular landmarks. Thoracic duct is seen along its entire course as a rounded structure 2-3 mm in diameter, anterior to vertebral bodies. Lateral echogenic stripes arise from the mediastinal pleura and from air in the lungs.

Pancreas and Biliary Tract

The pancreas and hepatoduodenal ligament are studied during extraction of EE from the 3rd part of the duodenum. The aorta, mesenteric root, SMA, uncinate process, and aortocaval area are also displayed. A thickening of 5 mm of the 2nd hypoechoic layer in the 2nd part of duodenum marks the level of ampulla. The merging of the bile duct with the pancreatic duct is displayed behind and above this area. Bending enables one to see the CBD, pancreatic duct, pancreatic head, portal axis. While passing through the duodenal flexure (between and 1st and 2nd) EE shows the suprapancreatic part of bile duct, hepatic artery, cystic duct confluence portal trunk, and pancreatic neck. The body and tail of pancreas are examined through the stomach, using vascular landmarks like splenic artery.

Pelvis the rectal surroundings including the LN are studied through rectal wall. The prostate and seminal vesicles in the male patient, uterus and vagina in the female patient and the anterior border of the sacrum are readily seen. The bundles of the levator ani are more difficult to display due to obliquity. The study of the anal canal is possible during retraction of the probe, but the proximity of sphincter compromises the precise analysis of the difficult muscular layers.

Digestive Pathology

Digestive Carcinomas

Endoultrasonography is neither suitable for screening nor for achieving a diagnosis of the nature of tumors. Its purpose is the evaluation of tumor extension through the digestive wall and beyond, after an initial diagnosis by endoscopy and optically guided biopsies.

Stages of Tumoral Infiltration of Digestive Wall

- UT1—Invasion of mucosa and submucosa with integrity of medial hyperehoic layer
- UT2—Invasion of the muscularis propria with interruption of the medial hyperechoic layer, integrity of the superfecial hyperechoic layer
- UT3—Invasion of juxta-digestive fat; interruption of superficial hyperechoic layer
- UT4—Invasion of surrounding structures; disappearance of the hyperechoic fatty interface with adjacent organs.

  Thus EUS enables one to differentiate a superficial tumor (T_1) from an infiltrative tumor (T_2) or more

  EUS, however, has its own limitations

- The distinction between true invasion of adjacent structures and more adhesion may be inconclusive
- The hypoechoic peritumoral desmoplastic reaction may induce confusing images; so many also difficult technical conditions like obstructive stenosis impeding the progression of EE, oblique planes of section
- Superficial tumors developing within the mucosa are often nonvisualized. It is 'however' possible to grade such tumors as UT1 provided the operator is sure the optical tumoral zone has been effectively examined with USG.

Lymph Node Involvement

In general, it is thought that rounded shape, sharp demarcation, homogeneous hypoechoic features suggests malignancy, whereas elongated, heterogeneous, hyperechoic LN with indistinct borders are more likely to be benign/inflammatory. Using three criteria, i.e. rounded shape, clear border line, and hypo/isoechogenicity with primary tumor, has a positive predictive value of 95%. That it is possible to disclose such subtle abnormal measurements EUS has a higher sensitivity than CT, which is not able to disclose adenopathy without adenomegaly or to differentiate malignant LN from inflammatory.

However, EUS has its limitations
- Display of only two criteria is inconclusive
- Endoultrasonography fails to show intraganglionic microdeposit, very small LN + LN located at a distance from the transducer (like retroperitoneum). Difficult technical condition also use its sensitively (like marrow digestive stenosis).

Esophagus

Carcinoma: Contribution of EUS in evaluation of esophageal carcinoma is well-established. It is complementary to CT for assessing periesophageal invasion and well permits one to contraindicate surgery in some extensive tumors. It is of more interest where the therapeutic strategy, i.e. decision between surgery and palliative methods relies on staging. Endoultrasonography is also very sensitive in detecting enlarged LN. Numerous studies have shown a staging accuracy of 80–90% of tumor invasion compared to 40–70% for T1, T3 tumors by CT) and 85–95% for LN involvement. Endoultrasonography has a sensitivity of 95% in detecting recurrence after surgery. It also enables one to study the reduction in tumor volume after non surgical therapeutics.

Carcinoma of Stomach and Gastroesophageal Junction

The results of EUS are inferior to those obtained from esophageal carcinomas due to technical and anatomic difference. The clinical contribution of EUS to evaluation is also less evident than for esophageal carcinoma because most lesions, whatever their size and extension are treated by radical gastrectomy. However, it is invaluable in evaluation of carcinomas of gastroesophageal junction since it may disclose invasion of esophageal submucosa, which escapes esophagoscopy. Endoultrasonography is also used to follow up of esophageal and gastric lymphoma treated by chemotherapy or radiotherapy.

Endoultrasonography is also useful in evaluation of submucosal tumors (like leiomyoma, polyps, varices, lipomas, and ganglioneuromas, EUS readily distinguishes these from extrinsic compression/mucosal lesions. These lesions can be localized to their layer of origin and separated into cystic and solid.

Portal HT: Endoscopy remains the most important technique for detection of esophageal varices, being superior to EUS for their detection and grading and predicting those at risk for bleeding. However, with EUS also a large part of the portal venous system can be visualized. The azygus vein, splenic vein, and mesenteric portal veins are seen in normal subjects and the esophageal gastric varices, periesophageal, and gastric collateral veins in patients with portal HT. It can also visualize the small dilated vessels within gastric wall in patients with congestive gastropathy which is as such difficult to assess by endoscopy or barium studies. Endoultrasonography demonstrates not only enlarged perigastric veins and collaterals, but also varices within the gastric submucosa.

Scanning immediately after sclerotherapy of varices shows their disappearance with presentation of the deeper collaterals. It may be possible with EUS to predict those at greatest risk of bleeding.

Lower Gastrointestinal Tract

Rectal endosonography has a few limitations, i.e. narrow stenosis impede progression of the probe and with rigid probes, very high lesions are difficult to study. Endoultrasonography is now considered essential to therapeutic management of rectal carcinomas in most institutions. It is only in very large and extensive lesions that CT or MRI should be associated with EUS to assess resectability. Endoultrasonography is particularly useful in tumors of the lower one-third rectum since it enables surgeon to consider the preservation of the sphincter in T1N0 tumors, despite the classical 5 cm rule which would otherwise imply rectal amputation. Endoultrasonography is also efficacious in detection of local recurrence.

Endoultrasonography is also useful in evaluation of submucosal tumors, polyps, inflammatory bowel disease (IBD) and in patients with anal incontinance.

Biliopancreatic Pathology

Endoultrasonography is at present the single best modality for the early diagnosis and accurate local and regional staging of patients with pancreatic cancer. It may improve the prognosis of patients with pancreatic cancer. Guided fine needle aspiration cytology (FNAC) helps in procuring a tissue diagnosis while simultaneously obtaining additional tumor and nodal staging information, avoiding additional diagnostic testing and surgery and in providing prognostic information related in accurate TN staging. In additions EUS also proved cost effective by excluding patients with unresectable tumors from undergoing exploratory laparotomy. Recent data suggest that all patients thought to have operable disease based on CT imaging should undergo EUS and FNA prior to any surgical intervention. Endoultrasonography guided neurolysis is done for improving pain control in patients with carcinomas. Endoultrasonography is also useful in diagnosis and staging of patients with chronic pancreatitis and pseudocysts. Endoultrasonography coupled with endoscopic retrograde cholangiopancreatography (ERCP) may also become a combined interventional technique for the detection and removal of CBD stones. PHS with moderate probability of choledocholithiasis should be evaluated with EUS first if EUS shows stones, patient can be taken up for therapeutic ERCP. However, if no stones are seen on EUS, ERCP can be avoided and patients can go in for laparoscopic cholecystectomy, thereby decreasing the number of non-therapeutic ERCPs. The greatest role of EUS however, appears to be in the evaluation of CBD stone in patients with severe acute pancreatitis where ERCP is contraindicated. EUS interpretation common errors are of two types:

- Misinterpretation of normal structures
- Artifacts and technical problems because of insufficient scanning and using oblique transducer positioning. These errors can be minimized if the role of EUS is not overstated. It must be remembered that EUS does not replace histologic diagnosis. With few exceptions, it almost never is a primary imaging modality. Rather it should be used in conjunction with other diagnostic testing.

To summarize, EUS is a highly technical procedure requiring considerable experience and knowledge of human anatomy and its variations. Its use in the assessment of a variety of upper and lower GI diseases has been valuable. Measurement of structures by EUS is routinely accomplished although with uncertain accuracy, reproducibility and interobserver variation.

27

CHAPTER

Contrast Agents for Ultrasound

Administered contrast is not new to the field of ultrasound. Nonvascular applications are common in day to day practice like water can be introduced into the bowel lumen orally, to distinguish a fluid filled stomach from a left upper quadrant collection and rectally to distinguish a large bowel collection from a pelvic collection. Hydrocolosonography in which the colon is meticulously prepared and filled with water/saline can be used for evaluation of wall of colon with ready diagnosis of polyps and malignancies. Microbubbles produced by the injection of small quantities of agitated saline can be used to confirm the location of biopsy needles and catheters during interventional procedures. Intravascular contrast agents were first introduced more than two decades ago. The principal requirements for such agents are:

- Should be easily introducible into the vascular system.
- Should have low toxicity.
- Should be stable for the duration of diagnostic examination.
- Should modify one/more of the acoustic properties that determine the ultrasound imaging process.
- Should be capable of passing through the pulmonary, cardiac and capillary circulations. Although, it is conceivable that applications may be found for USG contrast agents that will justify their injection directly into arteries, the clinical context for contrast sonography requires that they be capable of administration intravenously.

MODE OF ACTION

Contrast agents might act by their presence in the vascular system, from where they are ultimately metabolized (blood pool agents) or by their selective uptake into a tissue after a vascular phase. Of the properties of tissue that influence the USG image, the most important are backscatter coefficient, attenuation and acoustic propagation velocity. Most agent seek to enhance the echo by increasing as much as possible the backscatter of the tissue that bears them, while increasing as little as possible their attenuation in the tissue.

The degree of signal enhancement generated a contrast agent depends on the density, compressibility, concentration, and size of the contrast particle, as well as the interrogating ultrasound frequency. Maximum impedance mismatch occurs at an air tissue interface, so that many ultrasound contrast agents are based on stabilized gas bubbles. The toxicity of the contrast agent is also an important consideration which is directly influenced by the agent's biochemical composition, particularly its osmolarity, viscosity, and particle size. Because of these considerations, only a few biochemical groups of compounds have been assessed in both animal models and clinical trials.

CLASSIFICATION OF ULTRASOUND CONTRAST AGENTS

- Free gas bubbles.
- Encapsulated gas bubbles.
- Colloidal suspensions.
- Lipid emulsions.
- Aqueous solutions.

Free Gas Bubbles

These are excellent scatterer of USG beam because of the large impedance mismatch between gas and the surrounding body tissues. The intensity of the reflected ultrasound signal is directly proportional to the sixth power of the bubble radius. Such gas bubbles may (i) pre-exist in solution, (ii) result from vigorous shaping during preparation, (iii) occur with a change in temperature of the solution (e.g. the vaporization of ether at body temperature, (iv) through cavitation at the catheter tip following a rapid, high volume injection, (v) through ultrasonic microcavitation.

The fundamental limitations of free gas bubbles are that they are relatively large (10–100 mm), so they are effectively filtered by the pulmonary capillary circulation and short-lived. Smaller bubbles capable of traversing the pulmonary bed (<8 mm) have high surface tension and internal pressures, leading to their dissolution, before the pulmonary bed is reached. For these reasons, free gas bubbles are only suitable for delineation of right sided heart structures and intracardiac shunts. However, opacification of left atrium and left ventricles has been reported following injection of sonicated bubbles in solution. Intra-arterial injections are possible, but may cause embolization of largest particles and are contrary to the noninvasive nature of USG examination.

Some of such agents include:
- SHU 454 (Echovist, Schering, and Berlin) is a powdered polysaccharide (galactose), that when mixed with a diluent forms a crystalloid microbubble suspension. The crystals have varied shapes and range in size from 1-10 mm (median 3-5 mm). Since it does not survive the passage through the lungs, its contrast effect is limited to imaging of venous system, right heart structures and intracavitory injections as in contrast enhanced TVS guided HSG.
- SHU 508A (Levovist, Schering AG, and Berlin) is a second generation contrast agent, that was derived from Echovist by addition of small bubbles of palmitic acid. It is a stable mixture consisting of 99.9% microcrystalline galactose microparticles and 0.1% palmitic acid. Upon dissolution and agitation in sterile water for injection, the galactose disintegrates into microparticles that provide an irregular surface for the adherence of microbubbles 3-4 mm in size stabilization of microbubbles takes place as they become coated with palmitic acid, which separates the gas to liquid interface and slows their dissolution. These microbubbles are highly echogenic and are sufficiently stable for transit through the pulmonary circuit. The estimated median particle size is 1.8 mm and the median bubble diameter approximately 2 mm, with the 97th percentile approximately 6 mm. Both preclinical and clinical studies with Levovist demonstrate its capacity to traverse the pulmonary bed in sufficient concentrations to enhance both color Doppler and in some instances, the B mode image itself.

It has been shown to increase the Doppler signal by up to 15-20 dB for 1-5 minutes, after an I/V injection and improves vascular studies by showing flow through regions with absent/weak Doppler signals.

Encapsulated Gas Bubbles

To tackle the natural instability of free gas bubbles, various attempts have been made to encapsulated gas within a shell so as to create a more stable particle. The early agents included gelatin encapsulated nitrogen microspheres (GENM). The echogenicity of this gas containing contrast agent is based on the presence of multiple solid gas interfaces with a large acoustic impedance mismatch. However, the large size of the particles (80 mm) precluded IV administration.

In the mid-80's, sonicated albumin microspheres (Albunex: molecular biosystems, San Diego, CA) were introduced as a nontoxic contrast medium, composed of air-filled human albumin microspheres produced by sonication, of 5% human serum albumin having a mean size of approximately 3.5 µ, ranging from 1 to 8 mm. The microbubbles are stable *ex-vivo*, with acoustic properties lasting 8-12 minutes, in an albumin solution. Albunex has been shown to pass successfully through the pulmonary capillary circulation of the lungs and can produce left ventricular cavity opacification. Additionally, it is stable enough following injection to produce consistent, dose related Doppler signal enhancement in large and small arteries within the abdomen of small animals. However, transpulmonary survival of the agent in humans in sufficient concentration to provide diagnostic enhancement of images or Doppler studies of small vessels has yet to be demonstrated. Imaging studies of small, experimental hepatic tumors demonstrate the dramatic impact I/V contrast injection can have on the detection of small vessels. The agent is available prepacked in ready to use 4 mL vials and particle concentration is high (4×10^8 spheres/mL).

Cardiac applications of albumen are most promising. Albumen crosses the pulmonary bed and opacifies the left atrial and ventricular cavities. Following intracoronary injections, perfused myocardium increases markedly in echogenicity, allowing quantification of myocardial perfusion.

Many potential cardiac applications can be proposed include delineation of endocardial borders, calculation of left ventricular ejection fraction, quantification of regurgitation and shunt lesions and enhancement of low intensity Doppler signals.

Albunex has been studied with abdominal imaging in small animals. It is not yet approved for human use.

Colloidal Suspensions

Consist of solid particles suspended in a liquid carrier. These agents are selectively taken up by the RE system and lead to increase in backscatter or attenuation of tissues. The agents included in this category are:
- Collagen/Gelatin spheres.
- IDE (Iodipamide ethylester particles).
- *Perfluorochemicals:* These are a class of compounds composed entirely of carbon and fluorine atoms. These are inert, and dense liquids with high gas solubility. In ultrasonic terms, the high density and compressibility of perfluorocarbons leads to a large tissue impedance mismatch and they therefore act as highly reflective ultrasound agents.

Perfluoroctyl bromide (PFOB) is a type of perfluorochemical in which the bromine atom is substituted for a fluorine atom, resulting in a compound that is radio-opaque and nearly twice as dense as water. It is emulsified in lecithin to produce a 100% weight/volume emulsion. The particles 0.1-0.2 mm in size are unable to leak out of normal capillaries, thus initially limiting the I/V space. Perfluorooctyl bromide hours is subsequently removed by the reticuloendothelial system and finally breathed out by the lungs and secreted in the bile. Echo-enhancement of the liver or spleen is noticeable about 6 hrs after administration. Toxicity of the compound is low, but not insignificant with side effects like pain in low back, fever, chills, reduced platelet counts, mild cholestasis and modification of blood lipid levels. The side effects of these compounds, what appearing to be relatively mild, may handicap their application is routine clinical practice.

Perfluorochemicals, particularly PFOB, have shown great promise as ultrasound and Doppler contrast agents. Proper applications include hepatic and renal ultrasound and CT, for detection of focal lesions, Doppler imaging for tumor blood flow, blood flow ultrasound imaging for organ perfusion and assessment of renal concentrating ability.

Advantages of PFOB include its long half-life, allowing thorough, imaging, gray scale changes in echogenicity proportional to blood flow both color and spectral doppler enhancing properties and potential to be used in conjunction with CT. The major limitations include possible side effects and the complex relation of preinjection sonographic appearance of parenchymal lesions to the dynamic role of PFOB, including perfusion imaging, RE deposition and macrophage imaging.

Lipid Emulsions

Because excess fat deposition in hepatocytes produces enhanced backscatter, lipid emulsions have been evaluated as ultrasound contrast agents; it was hypothesized that transient hepatic lipid accumulation would lead to increased echogenicity of normal liver parenchyma, compared to abnormal parenchyma. However, preliminary studies using lipid emulsions suggest that a perceptible difference in echogenicity between control and lipid containing liver has not been readily achieved, apparently because of their small particle size and relatively low concentration within the liver.

Aqueous Emulsions

It has been shown that a transient impedance mismatch is created between the vascular and nonvascular beds in the time immediately following an I/V injection of an agent with a significantly different acoustic impedance from normal body tissues. Materials like this include buffered sodium citrate, calcium gluconate, and calcium disodium edetic acid (EDTA).

OTHER NEWER AGENTS

- FSO69 (Mallinckrodt Inc) is a perfluoropropane filled albumin shell with a size distribution similar to that of albunex. The stability of bubbles in its population is the probable cause of the greater enhancement observed with this agent
- Echogen is an emulsion of dodecafluoropentane droplets that undergo a phase change in the blood, bilaterally boiling at body temperature. Recent reports suggest that this agent produces visible enhancement of renal parenchyma on conventional gray scale imaging
- DMP 115 is a perfluoropropane microbubble coated with a bilipid shell; it also shows improved stability and high enhancements at low doses
- The use of polymeric microballoons as new ultrasound contrast agents has recently been proposed. These microballoons are ultrathin firm resilient shells around air microbubbles with an outstanding resistance to pressure and survive pulmonary passage in all animal species studied till date. In IV injections, these agents produce enhancement of the liver parenchyma lasting for 1–2 hours. Thus, these can be considered promising as USG contrast agents for liver imaging.

CLINICAL APPLICATIONS

USG contrast media and tumor vessels: Ultrasonography contrast agents should increase the ability to detect smaller vessels by enhancing back scatter and in both tumor and normal vessels. By increasing the reflectively of blood, a contrast agent will enable better detection of blood flow in small deep vessels, than is possible with conventional Doppler techniques. Tumors detection and blood flow mapping using contrast agents have been reported in prostate, kidney, liver, and breast tumors.

Contrast media in renal ultrasonography: Contrast agents have a future role in the assessment of vesicoureteral reflux (VUR) in children (thus avoiding the problems of repeated examination, and avoiding ionizing radiation) and to detect renal artery stenosis.

ULTRASONOGRAPHY CONTRAST MEDIA AND VASCULATURE

- Ultrasonography contrast agents may prove to be of particular benefit in delineating cerebral circulation as they can improve the Doppler signal strength by up to 17 dB and thus compensate for the overlying bone attenuation
- Contrast studies may also be used to distinguish total occlusion of the carotid artery from a severe stenosis
- Veins can be examined with contrast agents resulting in better detection of venous thrombi and clots
- Ultrasonography contrast agents may also enhance the Doppler signal from a variety of vessels like retinal, ovarian and penile arteries.

CONTRAST ECHOCARDIOGRAPHY

- Has been employed for assessing both the anatomy and function of cardiac chambers and valves for assessing valvular diseases, intracardiac shunts and congenital heart diseases.
- Selective intracoronary/intra-aortic contrast agents may be used to demonstrate and quantify myocardial perfusion. In addition, direct coronary artery visualization may be important in determining the location and physiological significance of carotid artery stenosis.

USG contrast hysterosalpingography/Sonosalpingography: This is a technique which allows evaluation of fallopian tube patency without the risks of ionizing radiation and offering a high tolerance by the patient. In the last few years there has been great interest in evaluation of tubal patency by ultrasound. The first studies assessed patency on transabdominal sonography after injecting saline per vagina. When fluid was seen in the cul-de-sac, one and/or both tubes were concluded to be patent. On comparison with standard HSG, these studies quoted to be simpler and cost effective. More recently, transvaginal sonography (TVS) guided sonosalpingography has been reported to be a safe and accurate diagnostic and screening technique in the evaluation of tubal patency. Several authors have used transcervical instillation of Echovist in place of saline and reported it to be superior to saline as direct observation of flow into the fallopian tube is possible. Some authors also recommend the combined use of Echovist and color Doppler sonography to assess the same. Sonohysterography is reportedly to be useful in assessment of intraluminal disorders like polyps, submucosal fibroids, intrauterine synechial and uterine malformation. A thin flexible catheter is put through the cervix into the uterine, lumen with its tip near the fundus. Slow injection of 3-10 mL of sterile saline/contrast agent usually produces adequate distention of uterine lumen. The study should be done in the secretory phase of the cycle, when the endometrium is most echogenic.

Future directions: Till date, USG contrast agents are essentially experimental. However, several agents offer great promise for improved diagnostic accuracy, with each agent offering different applications tailored to its physical characteristics. Echovist is best studied for intracavitary use and venous imaging. Albunex is best suited for flow imaging with color Doppler, allowing improved detection of small deep vessels, distinguishing high grade stenosis from complete occlusion and identification of neovascularity.

28
CHAPTER

Normal Ultrasound Measurements

1. Liver — Craniocaudal scan
   Right midclavicular line — <13.0 cm (craniocaudal) to a maximum of 15.0 cm (depending on body habitus)

   Marginal angulation — <30° (left hepatic lobe laterally)
   <45° (right hepatic lobe, caudally)

   Midclavicular AP diameter of liver –8.1 ± 1.0 cm
   Midline longitudinal diameter of liver –8.3 ± 1.2 cm
   Midline AP diameter of the liver –5.7 ± 1.5 cm

2. Gallbladder — Wall thickness
   <0.4 cm (postprandial up to 0.7 cm)
   Maximal diameter
   <11.0 cm (longitudinal pre-prandial)
   <4.0 cm (transverse pre-prandial)

3. Biliary duct — Bile duct
   <0.6 cm (if gallbladder is present)
   <0.9 cm (status post-cholecystectomy)
   intrahepatic
   <0.4 cm

4. Hepatic veins — Luminal width
   <0.6 cm (distal to last confluence before the inferior vena cava)
   >0.6 cm = Right cardiac insufficiency

5. Spleen — Maximal size
   <11.0 cm (length)
   <7.0 cm (width)
   <4.0 cm (depth when measured between splenic hilum and surface)

6. Splenic vein — Luminal width
<1.0 cm
>1.2 cm = Portal hypertension or splenomegaly
7. Superior mesenteric artery — Luminal diameter <0.5
8. Aortomesenteric angle — <30°
9. Aortovertebral distance — <0.5 cm
10. Abdominal aorta — Luminal diameter
<2.5 cm (cranial portion)
<2.0 cm (caudal portion)
2.5–3.0 cm = ectasia
>3.0 cm = aneurysm
11. Pancreas — Size of head — AP −2.7 ± 0.7 cm
Craniocaudal −3.6 ± 1.2 cm
Size of body — AP −2.2 ± 0.7 cm
Craniocaudal −3.0 ± 0.6 cm
Size of tail — AP −2.4 ± 0.4 cm
Craniocaudal −2.9 ± 0.4 cm
Luminal diameter of duct — < 0.2 cm
12. Inferior vena cava — Luminal width
<2.0 cm (<2.5 cm in young athletes)
>2.5 cm (without expiration collapse = suspicious of right cardiac insufficiency)
13. Kidneys — Maximal size
10.0–12.0 cm (longitudinal)
4.0–6.0 cm (transverse)
Respiratory mobility
3.0–7.0 cm
Parenchymal width
1.3–2.5 cm
Parenchymal pyelon index
≥1.6:1 (under 30 years)
1.2:1–1.6:1 (31–60 years)
≥1.1:1 (above 60 years)
Depth
Oblique — 3.578 mean cm
Prone — 5.0 cm mean
Renal volume
0.49 × L × W × AP
14. Adrenal glands — Maximal size
<5.0 cm (length)
<1.0 cm (width of an Individual limb)
15. Lymph nodes — Maximal diameter
<1.0
16. Portal vein — Luminal width
<1.3 cm
>1.5 cm = portal hypertension
17. Prostate gland — Size
<5.0 cm (transverse)
<3.0 cm (craniocaudal)
<3.0 cm (anteroposterior, sagittal)
Volume <25 mL

18. Thyroid gland	—	Size 4.0–7.0 cm (craniocaudal) 1.0–3.0 cm (transverse) 1.0–2.0 cm (sagittal) Volume both lobes combined <20 mL (women) <25 mL (men)
19. Uterus	—	Maximal size 5.0–8.0 cm (longitudinal-nullipara) 1.5–3.0 cm width
20. Ovaries	—	Volume 5.5–10.0 cm^3 (each ovary premenopausal) 2.5–3.5 cm^3 (each ovary postmenopausal)
21. Cervical subcutaneous tissue		Width (in prenatal measurements) <3.0 mm (if more-nuchal edema or post-cervical edema)
22. Endometrium	—	Width (both layers) <15.0 mm (premenopausal) <8.0 mm (postmenopausal)
23. Urinary bladder		Wall thickness <0.4 cm (if bladder is full) <0.8 cm (after voiding) Postvoid residue <100 mL Volume <550 mL (women) <750 mL (men)
24. Volume calculation	—	$0.5 \times A \times B \times C$
25. Yolk sac	—	Diameter 3.0–7.0 mm
26. IUD-fundus distance	—	<20.0 mm (if increased-dislodged)
27. IUD-endometrium distance	—	<5.0 mm

TABLE 28.1: Measurement of extrahepatic bile ducts in healthy subjects, patients with gallstones, and postcholecystectomy patients by ultrasound.

	Mean ± SD	Range	95th Percentage
Normal subjects			
Porta hepatis	2.5 ± 1.1	1–7	4
Widest point	2.8 ± 1.2	1–7	4
Patients with gallstones			
Porta hepatis	3.8 ± 2.0	1–10	8
Widest point	4.8 ± 2.2	2–12	9
Patients after cholecystectomy			
Porta hepatis	5.2 ± 2.1	1–11	10
Widest point	6.2 ± 2.5	1–13	11

CHAPTER 28: Normal Ultrasound Measurements

TABLE 28.2: Sonographic measurements of the normal pediatric gallbladder and biliary tract.

Age range (year)	AP diameter		Coronal diameter (cm)		Length (cm)		Wall thickness (mm)		Common hepatic duct size (mm)		Right portal vein size (mm)	
	Mean	Range	Mean	Range	Mean	Range	Mean	Range	Mean	Range	Mean	Range
0–1	0.9	0.5–1.2	0.9	0.7–1.4	2.5	1.1–1.4	1.7	1.0–3.0	1.1	1.0–2.0	1.8	3.0–5.0
2–5	1.7	1.4–2.5	1.0	1.0–3.9	4.2	2.9–5.2	2.0	None	1.7	1.0–3.0	4.8	3.0–7.0
6–8	1.8	1.0–2.4	2.0	1.2–3.0	5.6	4.4–7.4	2.2	2.0–3.0	2.0	None	5.7	6.0–9.0
9–11	1.9	1.2–3.2	2.0	1.0–3.6	5.5	3.4–6.5	2.0	1.0–3.0	1.8	1.0–3.0	6.8	4.0–9.0
12–16	2.0	1.1–2.8	2.1	1.6–3.0	6.1	3.8–8.0	2.0	1.0–3.0	2.2	1.0–4.0	7.8	6.0–10.0

Normal GB wall thickness <2 mm
Normal mean PV diameter = 11 ± 2 mm

TABLE 28.3: Measurement of cerebral ventricular size in infants by ultrasound.

	The sonographic intracranial measurements and the mean values and 95% confidence limits for ratios are shown		
	n	Mean (mm)	SD
Frontal mantle thickness	71	26.5	4.9
Occipital mantle thickness	8	20.6	5.1
Ventricular diameter at caudate	72	25.0	5.6
Ventricular diameter at atria	70	37.9	6.0
Brain diameter at caudate	73	77.0	12.4
Brain diameter at atria	72	75.4	10.0

TABLE 28.4: Mean values and 95% confidence limits for ratios.

Ratio	n	Mean	95% confidence limits
Occipital frontal mantle	8	0.78	0.49–1.07
Ventricles brain at caudate	73	0.12	0.21–0.42
Ventricles brain at atria	73	0.51	0.40–0.60

Measurement of fetal cerebral ventricle size by ultrasound

TABLE 28.5: Dates from 196 normal fetuses.

Menstrual age (wk)	Lateral ventricular width (cm)	Ratio Hemispheric width (cm)	(LVW/HW) (% = 2 SD)
15	0.75	1.4	56(40–71)
16	0.86	1.5	57(45–69)
17	0.85	1.5	52(42–62)
18	0.83	1.8	46(40–52)
19	—	—	—
20	0.82	1.9	43(29–57)
21	0.76	2.2	35(27–43)
22	0.82	2.6	32(26–38)
23	0.83	2.5	33(24–42)
24	0.83	2.7	31(23–39)
25	1.1	3.0	34(26–42)
26	0.9	3.0	30(24–36)
27	0.9	3.0	28(23–34)
28	1.1	3.3	31(18–45)

Contd...

Contd...

Menstrual age (wk)	Lateral ventricular width (cm)	Ratio Hemispheric width (cm)	(LVW/HW) (% = 2 SD)
29	1.0	3.4	29(22–37)
30	1.0	3.4	30(26–34)
31	1.0	3.4	29(23–36)
32	1.1	3.6	31(26–36)
33	1.1	3.4	31(25–37)
34	1.1	3.8	28(23–33)
35	1.1	3.8	29(26–31)
36	1.1	3.9	28(23–34)
37	1.2	4.1	29(24–34)
Term	1.2	4.3	28(22–33)

Measurement of the normal bladder wall in children by ultrasound
The normal bladder wall thickness is given as

TABLE 28.6: Bladder wall thickness in millimeters (±SD) according to age and state of bladder.

	Empty	+Full	Full	Full ±
<1 month	2.62 ± 0.51	2.10 ± 0.31	1.92 ± 0.51	1.67 ± 0.57
1 month–1 year	2.61 ± 0.62	1.93 ± 0.27	1.65 ± 0.47	2
1–6 years	2.76 ± 0.73	2.06 ± 0.35	1.87 ± 0.37	1.44 ± 0.52
6–12 years	2.82 ± 0.46	2.17 ± 0.32	1.97 ± 0.42	1.43 ± 0.53
>12 years	2.83 ± 0.51	2.18 ± 0.32	1.89 ± 0.39	1.64 ± 0.74

The normal bladder wall has a mean thickness of 2.76 mm when the bladder is almost empty and 1.55 mm when it is distended. The upper limits are 3 and 5 mm for a full or empty bladder, respectively.

Measurement of the gestational sac by ultrasound for determination of fetal maturity
The measurements are given as.

TABLE 28.7: Gestational sac measurement.

Mean predicted gestational sac (mm)	Gestational age (wk)	Mean predicted gestational sac (mm)	Gestational age (wk)
10.0	5.0		
11.0	5.2	36.0	8.8
12.0	5.3	37.0	8.9
13.0	5.5	38.0	9.0
14.0	5.6	39.0	9.2
15.0	5.8	40.0	9.3
16.0	5.9	41.0	9.5
17.0	6.0	42.0	9.6
18.0	6.2	43.0	9.7
19.0	6.3	44.0	9.9
20.0	6.5	45.0	10.0
21.0	6.6	46.0	10.2
22.0	6.8	47.0	10.3
23.0	6.9	48.0	10.5
24.0	7.0	49.0	10.6
25.0	7.2	50.0	10.7
26.0	7.3	51.0	10.9
27.0	7.5	52.0	11.0

Contd...

Contd...

Mean predicted gestational sac (mm)	Gestational age (wk)	Mean predicted gestational sac (mm)	Gestational age (wk)
28.0	7.6	53.0	11.2
29.0	7.8	54.0	11.3
30.0	7.9	55.0	11.5
31.0	8.0	56.0	11.6
32.0	8.2	57.0	11.7
33.0	8.3	58.0	11.9
34.0	8.5	59.0	12.0
35.0	8.6	60.0	12.2

Equation: $\text{Gestational age (wk)} = \dfrac{\text{Gestational sac (mm)} + 25.43}{7.02}$

Measurement of biparietal diameter as an indicator of gestational age by ultrasound

TABLE 28.8: Composite biparietal diameter.

mm	Wk with variation	mm	Wk with variation
20	12.0	60	22.3–25.5
21	12.0	61	22.6–25.5
22	12.2–13.2	62	23.1–26.1
23	12.4–13.6	63	23.4–26.4
24	12.6–13.8	64	23.8–26.8
25	12.9–14.1	65	24.1–27.1
26	13.1–14.3	66	24.5–27.5
27	13.4–14.6	67	25.0–27.8
28	13.6–15.0	68	25.3–28.1
29	13.9–15.2	69	25.8–28.4
30	14.1–15.5	70	26.3–28.7
31	14.3–15.9	71	26.7–29.1
32	14.5–16.1	72	27.2–29.4
33	14.7–16.5	73	27.6–29.8
34	15.0–16.8	74	28.1–30.1
35	15.2–28.2	75	28.5–30.5
36	15.4–17.4	76	29.0–31.0
37	15.6–17.8	77	29.2–31.4
38	15.9–18.1	78	29.6–32.0
39	16.1–18.3	79	29.9–32.5
40	16.4–18.8	80	30.2–33.0
41	16.5–19.3	81	30.7–33.5
42	16.6–39.8	82	31.2–34.0
43	16.8–20.0	83	31.5–34.5
44	16.9–20.7	84	33.9–35.1
45	17.0–21.2	85	32.3–35.7
46	17.4–21.4	86	32.8–36.2
47	17.8–21.6	87	33.4–36.6
48	18.2–21.8	88	33.9–37.1
49	18.6–22.0	89	34.6–37.6

Contd...

Contd...

mm	Wk with variation	mm	Wk with variation
50	19.0–22.2	90	35.1–38.1
51	19.3–22.5	91	35.9–38.5
52	19.5–22.9	92	36.7–38.9
53	19.8–23.2	93	37.3–39.3
54	20.1–23.7	94	37.9–40.1
55	26.4–24.0	95	38.5–40.9
56	20.7–24.3	96	39.1–41.5
57	21.1–24.5	97	39.9–42.1
58	21.5–24.9	98	40.5–43.1
59	21.9–25.1		

Measurement of fetal head circumference as an indicator of gestational age by ultrasound

TABLE 28.9: Predicted menstrual age for head circumferences.

Head circumference (cm)	Menstrual age (wk)	Head circumference (cm)	Menstrual age (wk)
8.0	13.4	22.5	24.4
8.5	13.7	23.0	24.9
9.0	14.0	23.5	25.4
9.5	14.3	24.0	25.9
10.0	14.6	24.5	26.4
10.5	15.0	25.0	26.9
11.0	15.3	25.5	27.5
11.5	13.6	26.0	28.0
12.0	15.9	26.5	28.1
12.5	16.3	27.6	29.2
13.0	36.6	27.5	29.8
13.5	17.0	28.0	30.3
14.0	17.3	28.5	31.0
14.5	17.7	29.0	31.6
15.0	18.1	29.5	32.2
15.5	18.4	30.0	32.8
16.0	18.8	30.5	33.5
16.5	19.2	31.0	34.2
17.0	19.6	31.5	34.9
17.5	20.0	32.0	35.5
18.0	20.4	32.5	36.3
18.5	20.8	33.0	37.0
19.0	21.2	33.5	37.7
19.5	21.6	34.0	38.5
20.0	22.1	34.5	39.2
20.5	22.5	35.0	40.0
21.0	23.0	35.5	40.8
21.5	23.4	36.0	41.6
22.0	23.9		

Measurement of fetal abdominal circumference as an indicator of gestational age by ultrasound Measurement (Table 28.10)

TABLE 28.10: Predicted menstrual age for abdominal circumference values.

Abdominal circumference (cm)	Menstrual age (wk)	Abdominal circumference (cm)	Menstrual age (wk)
10.0	15.6	23.5	27.7
10.5	16.1	24.0	28.2
11.0	16.5	24.5	28.7
11.5	16.9	25.0	29.2
12.0	17.0	25.5	29.7
12.5	17.8	26.0	30.1
13.0	18.2	26.5	30.6
13.5	18.6	27.0	31.1
14.0	19.1	27.5	33.6
14.5	19.5	28.0	32.1
15.0	20.0	28.5	32.6
15.5	20.4	29.0	33.1
16.0	20.8	29.5	33.6
16.5	21.4	30.0	34.1
17.0	21.7	30.5	34.6
17.5	22.2	31.0	35.1
18.0	22.6	31.5	33.6
18.5	23.1	32.0	36.1
19.0	23.6	32.5	36.6
19.5	24.0	33.0	37.1
20.0	24.5	33.5	37.6
20.5	24.9	34.0	38.1
21.0	25.4	34.5	38.7
21.5	25.9	35.0	39.2
22.0	26.3	35.5	39.7
22.5	26.8	36.0	40.2
23.0	27.3	36.5	40.8

Measurement of fetal femur length as an indicator of gestational age by ultrasound

TABLE 28.11: Predicted menstrual age for femur lengths.

Femur length (mm)	Menstrual age (wk)	Femur length (mm)	Menstrual age (wk)
10	12.8	45	24.5
11	13.1	46	24.9
12	13.4	47	25.3
13	13.6	48	25.7
14	13.9	49	26.1
15	14.2	50	26.5
16	14.5	51	27.0
17	14.8	52	27.4
18	15.1	53	27.8
19	15.4	54	28.2
20	15.7	55	28.7
21	16.0	56	29.1
22	16.3	57	29.6
23	16.6	58	30.0
24	16.9	59	30.5
25	17.2	60	30.9
26	17.6	61	31.4

Contd...

Contd...

Femur length (mm)	Menstrual age (wk)	Femur length (mm)	Menstrual age (wk)
27	17.9	62	31.9
28	18.2	63	32.3
29	18.6	64	32.8
30	18.9	65	33.3
31	19.2	66	33.8
32	19.6	67	34.2
33	19.9	68	35.2
34	20.3	69	35.7
35	20.7	70	36.2
36	21.0	71	36.7
37	21.4	72	37.2
38	21.8	73	37.7
39	22.1	74	37.7
40	22.5	75	38.3
41	22.9	76	38.8
42	23.3	77	39.3
43	23.7	78	39.8
44	24.1	79	40.4

NORMAL VALUES IN PRENATAL ULTRASONOGRAPHY

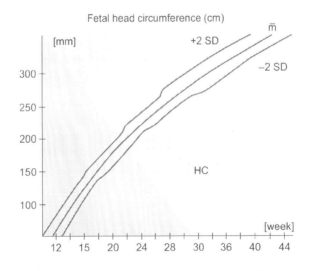

Weeks	Fetal head circumference (cm)		
	3rd	50th	97th
14	8.8	9.7	10.6
16	11.3	12.4	13.5
18	13.7	15.1	16.5
20	16.1	17.7	19.3
22	18.3	20.1	21.9
24	20.4	22.4	24.3
26	22.4	24.6	26.8
28	24.2	26.6	29.0

Contd...

Contd...

Weeks	Fetal head circumference (cm)		
	3rd	50th	97th
30	25.8	25.4	31.0
32	27.4	30.1	32.8
34	28.7	31.5	34.3
36	29.9	32.8	35.8
38	30.8	33.8	36.8
40	31.5	34.6	37.7

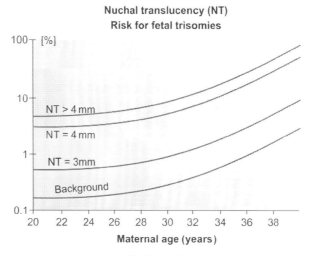

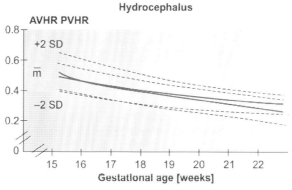

AVHR = Anterior ventricular hemisphere ratio
PVHR = Posterior ventricular hemisphere ratio
Ref.: Chudleigh P, Pearce JM: Obstetric Ultrasound. Churchill Livingstone; 1992

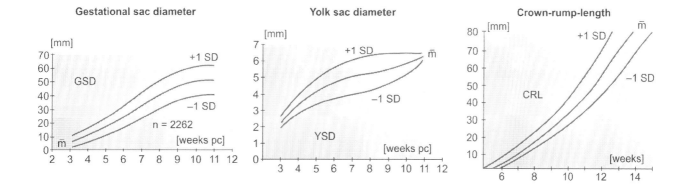

Contd...

Week	GSD	Week	GSD	Week	GSD
5.0	1.0	7.5	2.7	9.9	4.4
5.2	1.1	7.6	2.8	10.0	4.5
5.3	1.2	7.8	2.9	10.2	4.6
5.5	1.3	7.9	3.0	10.3	4.7
5.6	1.4	8.0	3.1	10.5	4.8
5.8	1.5	8.2	3.2	10.6	4.9
5.9	1.6	8.3	3.3	10.7	5.0
6.0	1.7	8.5	3.4	10.9	5.1
6.2	1.8	8.6	3.5	11.0	5.2
6.3	1.9	8.8	3.6	11.2	5.3
6.5	2.0	8.9	3.7	11.3	5.4
6.6	2.1	9.0	3.8	11.5	5.5
6.8	2.2	9.2	3.9	11.6	5.6
6.9	2.3	9.3	4.0	11.7	5.7
7.0	2.4	9.5	4.1	11.9	5.8
7.2	2.5	9.6	4.2	12.0	5.9
7.3	2.6	9.7	4.3	12.2	6.0

(mean values in (cm))

Week	CRL	Week	CRL	Week	CRL
		5 + 5	1.2	5 + 6	2.1
6	3.0	8	16.7	10	33.3
6 + 1	3.8	8 + 1	17.8	10 + 1	34.6
6 + 2	4.7	8 + 2	18.9	10 + 2	35.9
6 + 3	5.7	8 + 3	20.0	10 + 3	37.2
6 + 4	6.6	8 + 4	21.1	10 + 4	38.5
6 + 5	7.5	8 + 5	22.3	10 + 5	39.9
6 + 6	8.5	8 + 6	23.5	10 + 6	41.3
7	9.5	9	24.6	11	42.6
7 + 1	10.5	9 + 1	25.8	11 + 1	44.0
7 + 2	11.5	9 + 2	27.0	11 + 2	45.4
7 + 3	12.5	9 + 3	28.3	11 + 3	46.9
7 + 4	13.5	9 + 4	29.5	11 + 4	48.3
7 + 5	14.6	9 + 5	30.7	11 + 5	49.8
7 + 6	15.6	9 + 6	32.0	11 + 6	51.2

(mean values in (mm))

Body Height (cm)	m − 2SD	Liver (m)	m + 2 SD	m − 2SD	Spleen (m)	m + 2 SD	5%	Kidney 50%	95%
Neonates	3.47	5.53	7.59	2.90	4.07	5.24	3.40	4.16	4.92
<55	3.40	5.50	7.60	2.13	2.91	3.69	3.00	4.35	5.83
55–70	4.53	6.59	8.65	2.44	3.46	4.48	3.60	5.00	6.40
71–85	5.48	7.20	8.92	2.23	3.71	5.19	4.50	5.90	7.30
86–100	5.98	7.68	9.38	2.61	4.69	6.77	5.30	6.60	7.90
101–110	6.76	8.74	10.72	3.02	4.88	6.74	5.85	7.10	8.35

Contd...

Contd...

Body Height (cm)	m – 2SD	Liver (m)	m + 2 SD	m – 2SD	Spleen (m)	m + 2SD	5%	Kidney 50%	95%
111–120	6.56	8.71	10.83	3.38	5.26	7.14	6.35	7.65	8.95
121–130	7.38	9.40	11.42	3.37	5.31	6.87	6.90	7.20	9.50
131–140	8.63	9.99	11.35	4.10	5.96	7.82	7.40	8.70	10.00
141–150	8.48	10.42	12.36	4.61	5.81	7.01	7.90	9.25	10.60
>150	9.48	11.36	13.24	4.36	6.18	8.00	8.60	9.95	11.30

Age	m – 1SD	Girls (m)	m + 1SD	m – 1SD	Boys (m)	m + 1SD
Neonates	0.5	1.1	1.7	0.4	1.2	2.0
<1 year	0.6	1.6	2.6	0.6	1.2	1.8
<4 years	1.6	2.4	3.2	1.0	1.7	2.4
<8 years	1.9	3.4	4.9	1.9	3.2	4.5
<12 years	3.2	5.7	8.2	3.5	5.7	7.9
>12 years	4.8	8.0	11.2	4.5	7.9	11.3
Adults		<20			<25	

NORMAL VALUES IN PRENATAL ULTRASONOGRAPHY

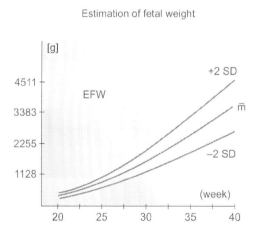

Estimation of fetal weight

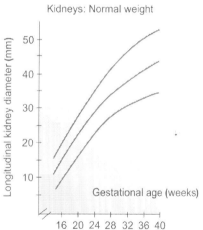

Kidneys: Normal weight

Log FW = 1.36 + 0.05AC + 0.18FL – 0.0037 (AC × FL)
FW = Fetal weight
AC = Abdominal circumference
FL = Femur length
Kidneys: Normal weight

Checklist Right Cardiac Insufficiency
- Dilatation of the inferior vena cava >2.0 cm (2.5 cm in trained athletes)
- Dilated hepatic vein >6.0 mm in the hepatic periphery
- Absent caval collapse with forced inspiration
- Possible pleural effusion, initially almost always on the right.

Checklist Aortic Aneurysm
- Normal lumen: suprarenal <2.5 cm
- Ectasia 2.5-3.0 cm
- Aneurysm >3 cm
- Risk of rupture increased by: progressing dilatation diameter >6 cm eccentric lumen saccular dilation (instead of fusiform dilation)

Checklist Portal hypertension
- Demonstration of portocaval collaterals at the porta hepatis
- Diameter of the portal vein at the porta hepatis >15 mm
- Dilatation of the splenic vein >1.2 cm
- Splenomegaly

- Demonstration of ascites
- Recanalized umbilical vein (Cruveilhier-Baumgarten syndrome)
- Esophageal varices (by endoscopy)

Normal measurements in abdominal ultrasonography in children

For liver and spleen, the median values (m) ± 2 SD in (cm) are related to body height and measured along the right and left median axillary line (not the MCL). The renal measurements (cm) are confidence intervals of the standard percentiles:

Normal Volumes of the Thyroid Gland (mL)

Both lobes combined, calculated according to the volume formula (0.5 × A × B × C).

Normal CSF Measurements in Neonates

SCW (sinucortical width)	≤3 mm
CCW (craniocerebral width)	≤4 mm
IHW (interhemispheric width)	≤6 mm
Width of lateral ventricles (frontal horn):	≤13 mm

Checklist of Criteria for Establishing a Cyst
- Spherical configuration
- Echo-free interior
- Smooth outline
- Distal acoustic enhancement
- Sharp defined distal wall
- Edge shadowing due to critical angle phenomenon

Checklist of Criteria for Establishing Hepatic Cirrhosis
- Absence of thin, hyperechoic capsular line
- Paucity of peripheral hepatic vessels
- Obtuse angulation of the hepatic veins >45°
- Accentuated echogenic wall of the portal vein
- Abrupt caliber changes of the branches of the portal vein
- Regenerating nodules with displacement of adjacent vessels
- Nodular liver contour (advanced stage only)
- Contracted liver (advanced stage only)
- Signs of portal hypertension

29
CHAPTER

Obstetric Ultrasound

The use of clinical ultrasound has revolutionized the practice of obstetrics. As of today, no biologically adverse effects of ultrasound are known and sonography has become the most versatile diagnostic modality used in obstetrics. The general consensus as stated by American Institute of Ultrasound in Medicine (AIUM) Bioeffects Committee is that "no confirmed biological effects on patients or instrument operators caused by exposure at intensities typical of present diagnostic ultrasound instruments have ever been reported." Current data indicate that the benefits to patients with the prudent use of diagnostic ultrasound outweigh the risks, if any, that may be present. A single routine screening ultrasound in a clinically normal pregnancy is usually recommended between 18 and 20 weeks of gestation and the scan time should be restricted to the minimum necessary to obtain adequate diagnostic information. As the Doppler ultrasound involves using much higher power intensities, its use should be further restricted for the assessment of the 'at-risk' fetus.

COMMON INDICATIONS FOR AN ULTRASOUND EXAMINATION

- Confirmation of the presence of intrauterine pregnancy and viability.
- Differentiation of intrauterine pregnancy from ectopic pregnancy.
- Estimation of gestational age.
- Detection of multiple gestational sacs.
- Evaluation of fetal growth, fetal weight, presentation, fetal anomalies, fetal death, suspected poly, or oligohydramnios.
- Evaluation of the placenta and complications related to it.
- Evaluation of vaginal bleeding of undetermined etiology.
- Evaluation for suspected molar pregnancy.
- As an adjunct to procedure like amniocentesis.
- For intrauterine contraceptive device (IUCD) localization.
- For suspected uterine abnormalities and pelvic masses.
- Biophysical profile after 28 weeks.
- Adjunct to special procedures such as fetoscopy, intrauterine transfusion, shunt placement, in vitro fertilization, embryo transfer, or chorionic villus sampling.
- Follow-up observation of identified fetal anomaly.

Equipment

The three types of transabdominal transducers used are:
1. *Sector transducers:* These are ideal for first trimester pregnancy as the access is limited.
2. *Linear array transducers:* These provide excellent axial and lateral resolution and a longer field of view and are best utilized in second and third trimester pregnancy. The larger surface area required for skin contact may however be problematic.
3. *Convex transducers:* These combine the advantages of both sector and linear transducers.

The appropriate frequencies for all the above transducers lie between 3 and 5 MHz. A moderately distended urinary bladder is essential for evaluating patients in the first trimester, those suspected of having placenta previa and those having cervical problems. The bladder should rise approximately 1 or 2 cm only above the uterine fundus.

Transvaginal transducers: Usually have a frequency of 6.5 MHz which provides better resolution. Avoidance of subcutaneous fat and scanning the patient with an empty bladder are its other advantages. In general the sonographic milestones of early pregnancy can be routinely delineated one week earlier with transvaginal sonography. It is also more sensitive in detection of ectopic pregnancy and for evaluating other complications of early pregnancy.

Guidelines for First-trimester Sonography

- Documentation of location of gestation sac. Embryo identified and crown rump length (CRL) measured.
- Presence or absence of fetal life recorded. Fetal cardiac motion seen around six weeks transabdominally and one week prior by transvaginal sonography (TVS) but if there is any doubt as to the viability repeat scan after 7–10 days.
- Document fetal number.
- Evaluation of uterus and adnexal structures.

Guidelines for Second and Third-trimester Sonography
- Document fetal life, number, and presentation.
- An estimate of the amount of amniotic fluid (increased, decreased, normal) should be reported.
- Record placental location and its relationship to internal os.
- Assess gestational age using biparietal diameter, head circumference, femur length or a combination of these fetal weight should also be assessed.
- Evaluate the uterus and adnexal structures.
- Fetal anatomy should be demonstrated cerebral ventricles, spine, stomach urinary bladder, umbilical cord insertion on the abdominal wall and kidneys Associated anomalies are demonstrated.

Evaluation of First-Trimester Pregnancy

The location and number of gestation sacs are noted. The presence of yolk sac and embryo with or without fetal heart beat/pulsations is established. The mean sac diameter, and the crown rump length (CRL) of the fetus are used for establishing the gestational age. The uterus and adnexal structures are also examined **(Figs. 29.1A and B)**.

The uterus enlarges in relation to the length of pregnancy. The gestation sac (GS) is first seen when the mean sac diameter (MSD) reaches 5 mm, corresponding to five menstrual weeks. With TVS the sac may be identified half week earlier when the MSD is 2 or 3 mm. The MSD equals the sum of the length, width, and height of the GS divided by three. The distance is measured between the inner walls of the sac and it is a highly accurate predictor of the gestational age as shown in **Table 29.1**. However once the embryo becomes visible, i.e., by 6.5 menstrual week the CRL is used.

The sac is seen as a well-defined ring having uniformly thick echogenic walls in the fundus or middle of the uterus. Initially it appears echofree and should be differentiated from other intrauterine fluid collections that may have similar appearance including bleeding, endometritis, endometrial cysts, cervical stenosis, and the pseudogestational sac of ectopic pregnancy.

A normal sac has round/oval shape. External compression due to overdistended bladder or bowel or fibroids in the uterine wall or myometrial contraction may distort the sac shape.

A sonolucent space may be seen around a portion of the sac between the sixth and eighth week of pregnancy as a normal variant and is thought to represent implantation bleeding in unobliterated uterine cavity.

The double decidual sac sign (DDSS)**(Fig. 29.2)** consisting of two concentric echogenic rings (joined at one portion) and surrounding at least a part of the gestational sac, is thought to represent the decidua parietalis and adjacent decidua capsularis. This sign is visible at 5 weeks menstrual age on transabdominal sonography (TAS) and helps to distinguish the two gestational sacs of intrauterine pregnancy from the pseudogestational sac seen in ectopic pregnancy in which only a single echogenic layer of decidua surrounds an intraendometrial fluid collection **(Fig. 29.3)**.

The earliest embryonic structures are not seen consistently until the mean sac diameter reaches 15 mm, i.e., around 6 weeks menstrual age. The first structure to be seen is a combination of the yolk sac and the developing amniotic sac. This double bleb is only briefly and therefore uncommonly seen in gestation sacs of 6–7 weeks maturity. The yolk sac grows slowly and is visible (earlier than the embryo) both on transabdominal sonography and transvaginal sonography by 6–7 weeks and 5 weeks respectively. Using

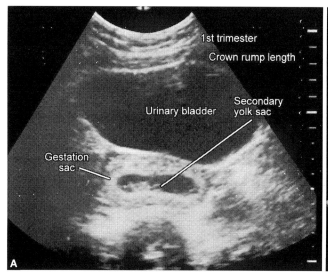
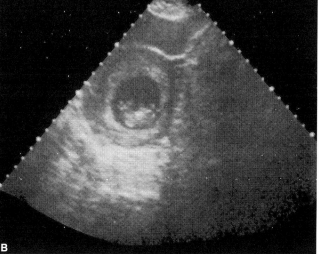

Figs. 29.1A and B: (A) Early pregnancy showing gestation sac, embryo and yolk sac. The measurement of crown rump length (CRL) is shown; (B) Normal gestational sac. Transverse scan of uterus shows a double ring gestational sac with a small embryo. CRL is measured with calipers, placenta is seen on the anterior aspect.

TABLE 29.1: Gestational sac measurement.

Gestational Age (Weeks) = $\dfrac{\text{Gestational Sac (mm)} + 25.43}{7.02}$

Gestational sac (mm)	Gestational age (weeks)	Gestational sac (mm)	Gestational age (weeks)
10.0	5.0	36.0	8.8
11.0	5.2	37.0	8.9
12.0	5.3	38.0	9.0
13.0	5.5	39.0	9.2
14.0	5.6	40.0	9.3
15.0	5.8	41.0	9.5
16.0	5.9	42.0	9.6
17.0	6.0	43.0	9.7
18.0	6.2	44.0	9.9
19.0	6.3	45.0	10.0
20.0	6.5	46.0	10.2
21.0	6.6	47.0	10.3
22.0	6.8	48.0	10.5
23.0	6.9	49.0	10.6
24.0	7.0	50.0	10.7
25.0	7.2	51.0	10.9
26.0	7.3	52.0	11.0
27.0	7.5	53.0	11.2
28.0	7.6	54.0	11.3
29.0	7.8	55.0	11.5
30.0	7.9	56.0	11.6
31.0	8.0	57.0	11.7
32.0	8.2	58.0	11.9
33.0	8.3	59.0	12.0
34.0	8.5	60.0	12.2
35.0	8.6		

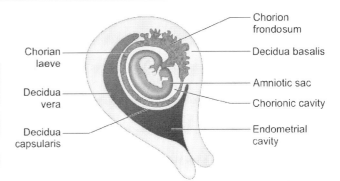

Fig. 29.2: Double decidual sign.

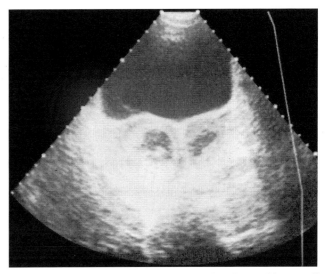

Fig. 29.3: Bicornuate uterus with a gestational sac with a small embryo seen inside, the right horn. Fluid collection is seen in the left horn without a double decidual sign—pseudogestational sac.

TAS yolk sac is seen when mean gestational sac diameter is approximately 10-15 mm and always visualized by an MSD of 20 mm and with TVS it should always be visualized by an MSD of 8 mm. When the sac reaches 15-18 mm diameter, i.e., approximately 6.5 weeks the embryo with a CRL of 5 mm can be seen. The fetal heart pulsations can be demonstrated as early 6½ weeks and 5½ weeks respectively by TAS and TVS **(Table 29.2)**. Embryonic cardiac activity identified routinely by TVS when CRL >5 mm. Transvaginal sonography can often demonstrate cardiac activity in embryos with a CRL of 2-4 mm. When the embryo achieves a CRL of 5 mm it should have visible cardiac pulsations if alive. At this age MSD is usually 15-18 mm. When an embryo reaches approximately 12 mm in CRL the head can be discriminated from the torso.

The embryo technically becomes the fetus by end of 10th menstrual week or beginning of the 11th menstrual week, at which time the CRL measures approximately 30-35 mm **(Table 29.3)**.

The crown-rump length is the longest length of the curved embryo (view should also show fetal heart) and care should be taken not to include the yolk sac in this measurement. Between 6.5 and 10 menstrual weeks CRL measurement is the most accurate method of pregnancy dating **(Table 29.4)**.

Complication of Early Pregnancy

Bleeding in the first trimester, with or without associated pain is a common problem in early pregnancy. Although such symptoms may be caused by a cervical erosion or polyp, they usually suggest a threatened abortion.
The possible causes include:
- *Threatened abortion (50%):* Intact intrauterine pregnancy corresponding to the patients date, with closed cervix.
- *Incomplete abortion:* Only a part of the products of conception remain within the uterus, the remainder having been expelled along with the vaginal bleeding. Sonographically the uterus appears enlarged. An empty, ill-defined gestational sac or a sac with internal echoes

TABLE 29.2: Sonographic milestones.

Sign or fetal structure	Menstrual age when detected	
	Transvaginal sonography (TVS)	Transabdominal sonography (TAS)
Gestational sac	4½ wk	5 wk
Double decidual sac sign (DDSS)	–	5 wk
Double bleb sign	–	6–7 wk
Yolk sac	5 wk	6–7 wk
Fetal heart beat	5½ wk	6½ wk
Head	8 wk	9 wk
Ventricles	8½ wk	11 wk

TABLE 29.3: Early diagnosis of non-viable pregnancy. Correlation of gestational sac diameter with detection of the yolk sac and embryo.

	Mean sac diameter	
	Transvaginal sonography (TVS)	Transabdominal sonography (TAS)
Yolk sac not detected	>8 mm	>20 mm
Embryo not detected	>16 mm	>25 mm

TABLE 29.4: Gestational age estimation by crown-rump length.

Crown rump length (CRL) (mm)	Gestational age Weeks	Crown rump length (CRL) (mm)	Gestational age Weeks
5	6.0	43	10.9
6	6.2	44	11.0
7	6.4	45	11.1
8	6.6	46	11.2
9	6.8	47	11.3
10	7.0	48	11.4
11	7.2	49	11.4
12	7.4	50	11.5
13	7.5	51	11.6
14	7.7	52	11.7
15	7.8	53	11.8
16	8.0	54	11.8
17	8.1	55	11.9
18	8.3	56	12.0
19	8.4	57	12.1
20	8.5	58	12.2
21	8.7	59	12.2
22	8.8	60	12.3
23	8.9	61	12.4
24	9.0	62	12.4
25	9.1	63	12.5
26	9.3	64	12.6
27	9.4	65	12.7
28	9.5	66	12.7
29	9.6	67	12.8
30	9.7	68	12.9
31	9.8	69	12.9
32	9.9	70	13.0
33	10.0	71	13.1
34	10.1	72	13.2
35	10.2	73	13.2
36	10.3	74	13.3
37	10.4	75	13.4
38	10.5	76	13.4
39	10.6	77	13.5
40	10.7	78	13.5
41	10.8	79	13.6
42	10.8	80	13.7

that are not clearly fetal is seen within the uterus. Sometimes no sac at all can be identified, but large clumps of echoes representing parts of fetus, placenta and blood are seen in the uterine cavity **(Fig. 29.4)**.

- *Complete spontaneous abortion:* All products of conception are expelled. Sonographically the uterus appears enlarged, the cervix is closed, no sac or fetus is identified, instead a line of central echoes representing blood and decidual reaction is seen.
- *Missed abortion:* The fetus dies but is retained within the uterus. It occurs most commonly between 6 and 14 weeks. Sonographically the uterus appears too small for the expected dates. In an early missed abortion the gestation sac containing a dead fetus (absent heart and/or limb motion) is seen. If detected later the fetus appears smaller than expected for the sac size or may appear formless and abnormal in shape. The placenta may become large and develop hydropic changes and resemble a hydatidiform mole **(Fig. 29.5)**.
- *Blighted ovum:* This is an embryonic pregnancy in which the gestational sac is present but empty. The main sonographic finding is a trophoblastic ring within the uterus which may look like a gestational sac, but unlike a gestational sac which has thick echogenic walls, it is more ill-defined and irregular in contour. Its walls are thin and measure less than 2 mm in thickness. The double decidual sac sign is absent and sac besides having a abnormal shape may be quite low in position or have a fluid-level within it. No fetal pole is seen within sac. If the mean sac diameter is 25 mm or more and no fetal pole is seen, or the MSD is 20 mm and no yolk sac is seen, a blighted ovum is considered to be present. Transvaginally, these structures should be seen when the sac diameter is 16 mm and 8 mm or more respectively **(Fig. 29.6)**. The normal sac grows at the rate of 1.1 mm per day and growth of less than 0.6 mm/day indicates abnormal development.

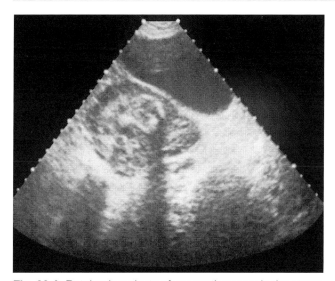

Fig. 29.4: Retained products of conception seen in the uterus in a case of incomplete abortion.

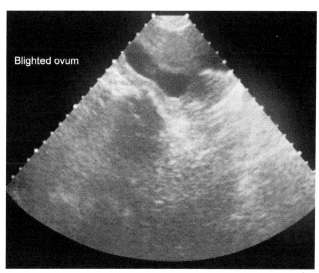

Fig. 29.6: Embryonic gestational sac—no yolk sac is seen in the gestational sac.

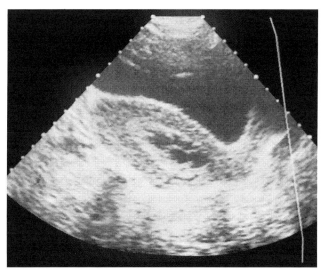

Fig. 29.5: Missed abortion—an irregular gestational ring with echoes inside it in normal sized uterus.

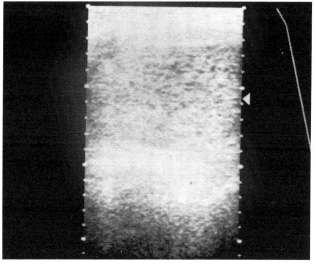

Fig. 29.7: Hydatidiform mole—sonographic snow storm appearance.

There may be a discrepancy between the size of the sac and the uterine size, with the sac being too large or too small for the uterus.

- *Inevitable abortion:* The gestational sac and fetus become detached from the implantation site and lie in the lower uterine segment or the dilated cervix. A sonolucent space may be preset around the sac where the sac has dissected away from the uterine wall. A fluid level may be present within the aborting sac.
- *Septic abortion:* Following a incomplete spontaneous, induced or surgical abortion, the retained product of conception may get infected. Sonographically the uterus is enlarged and there are increased endometrial echoes. Infection with gas producing organism or retained bony fragments may result in posterior acoustic shadowing from the endometrial echoes.
- *Hydatidiform mole:* The uterus is enlarged and contains echogenic cystic areas of varying sizes. The echoes and small cysts represent the vesicles and larger cystic areas represent areas of degeneration and hemorrhage **(Fig. 29.7)**.
- *Intrasac or perisac bleeds:* Bleeds in or around the sac are common. Bleeds are seen as (i) group of echoes within the amniotic sac adjacent to the fetus, (ii) between the amniotic and chorionic membrane, (iii) in a crescentic shape around the chorionic membrane, in the endometrial cavity, or (iv) behind the placenta (abruption) **(Fig. 29.8)**. Intra amniotic and chorioamniotic bleeds are not specifically harmful to the fetus.
- Ectopic pregnancy is pregnancy in any location, other than the body of the uterus. The most common site is

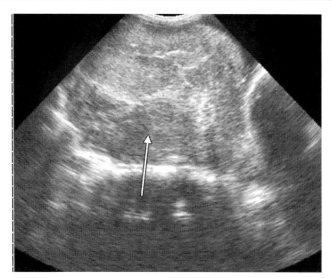

Fig. 29.8: A large retroplacental hematoma (white arrow) causing abruption of placenta.

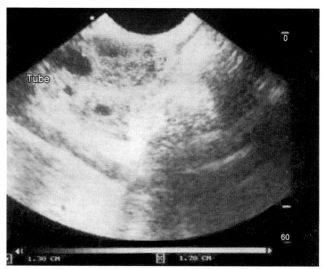

Fig. 29.9: Ectopic pregnancy—right ovary is seen separate from the right fallopian tube which contains a gestational sac. There is also free fluid in abdomen.

the ampullary/isthmic portion of fallopian tube (95-97%). Other sites include—uterine cornua/intramural portion of tube (2–5%), cervix, ovary, fimbrial end of tube/abdominal (very rare). Rupture usually occurs at or before the eight week of gestation.

Transvaginal scanning should always be done in addition to the transabdominal scanning as it greatly increases the diagnostic yield. As coexistent intra and extrauterine gestations are very rare, demonstration of an intrauterine pregnancy reasonably rules out the diagnosis of ectopic pregnancy. Transvaginal sonography can reliably detect the normal gestation sac of an intrauterine pregnancy as early as 4½ weeks from the last menstrual period. Also all other features of true intrauterine pregnancy like the double decidual sac sign, yolk sac identification and embryonic visualization is possible reliably at least one week earlier than TAS. In the absence of an intrauterine pregnancy the following sonographic features are strongly suggestive of an ectopic pregnancy:

- Uterine enlargement and endometrial thickening (decidual cast) and intraendometrial fluid collections (pseudogestational sac) occurs as a result of hormonal stimulation in many cases of ectopic pregnancy. The pseudogestational sac can be differentiated from the true gestational sac by double decidual sac sign and its central location within the uterus unlike the asymmetrical location of a true sac. Also no echogenic structure is present within the pseudogestational sac of ectopic pregnancy, except for low level echoes due to a blood clot sometimes.
- Adnexal findings:
    - With TVS a live embryo and a yolk sac may be seen in ectopic gestational sac in the adnexa, in many patients. These sacs are usually small and thick walled and may be confused with a hemorrhagic corpus luteal cyst, with which they may coexist **(Fig. 29.9)**.
    - When no identifiable embryo is seen in the gestational sac in the adnexa, the term adnexal ring is used. This is a cystic structure, surrounded by a thick echogenic ring, and can also be seen in some other conditions like pelvic inflammatory disease (PID), endometriosis and dermoid.
    - After rupture occurs, adnexal mass with a variable appearance is seen, depending on the organization of the surrounding hematoma. A rounded hypoechoic or complex predominantly echogenic mass is seen in the adnexa.
- Moderate to large amount of cul-de-sac and intraperitoneal fluid is highly suggestive of ruptured ectopic pregnancy. Initially the fluid is hypoechoic, later when the blood clots the cul-de-sac fluid becomes more echogenic than the adjacent myometrium and simulates a solid mass. This appearance is highly suggestive of hemoperitoneum.

Even an unruptured ectopic might be associated with small amount of loculated intraperitoneal fluid as a result of the oozing from the fimbrial end of the tube. The other differential diagnoses of small amount of cul-de-sac fluid include ruptured/hemorrhagic corpus luteal cyst or PID.

A normal pelvic sonogram however does not exclude an ectopic pregnancy. If the serum βHCG levels are more than 1800 IU/mL and there is no history of vaginal bleeding (i.e., no suggestion of a spontaneous abortion) and no evidence of identifiable intrauterine pregnancy (which should be definitely demonstrable at these high levels of βHCG), ectopic pregnancy is a strong possibility.

However, if the levels of βHCG are less than 1800 IU/mL possibility of an early normal pregnancy or spontaneous abortion cannot be ruled out. However, serial estimations of βHCG levels can include these possibilities:

- In a normal intrauterine pregnancy HCG levels double over a period of two days.

Ovarian Ectopic Pregnancy

Ovarian ectopic pregnancy appears similar to hemorrhagic corpus luteum.

Role of Doppler Sonography in Ectopic Pregnancy

It is particularly useful in patients with a nondescript adnexal mass, and/or small to moderate amount of pelvic fluid or no pelvic findings at all. Transvaginal color and pulsed Doppler are particularly useful in demonstrating previously unseen, small adnexal masses and further characterization of these masses. Adnexal masses seen in ectopic pregnancy have a surrounding ring of trophoblastic tissue which on color Doppler shows as an intense area of color flow (peritrophoblastic flow) and having a low resistance pattern of waveform (i.e., high diastolic flow) and on Duplex Doppler analysis.

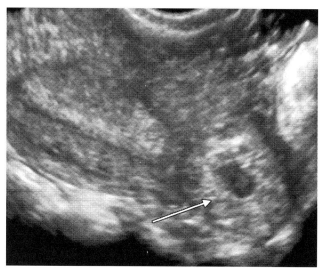

Fig. 29.10: An eccentrically placed GS (white arrow) in the region of fundus in a proven case of interstitial pregnancy in a transvaginal scan.

Second and Third Trimesters

- Fetal number, lie, presentation, and life should be documented.
- Assessment of gestational age is done using biparietal diameter, femur length, head circumference and abdominal circumference. Fetal weight can also be assessed.
- Amount of amniotic fluid and location of placenta is noted.
- The following fetal anatomy should be routinely demonstrated—cerebral ventricles, spine, stomach, urinary bladder, kidneys, and umbilical cord insertion on the anterior abdominal wall.
- The uterus and adnexa should also be evaluated.

- Patients with spontaneous abortion show declining levels of HCG.
- Patients with ectopic pregnancy show a subnormal increase in the levels of HCG.

Interstitial Pregnancy (Fig. 29.10)

Usually presents later (8 to 10 weeks) than the usual ectopic pregnancy with catastrophic bleeding. It is associated with a higher risk of shock and hemoperitoneum and subsequent higher maternal mortality due to delayed diagnosis and associated high vascularity of myometrium. Sonographically it may be misdiagnosed initially as normal intrauterine pregnancy, but its eccentric location and relative absence of surrounding myometrium, which is less than 5 mm in thickness, is highly suggestive but nonspecific indicator of interstitial pregnancy, and should alert the sonographer. Presence of an echogenic line between the gestation sac and endometrial cavity (interstitial line sign) is highly sensitive and specific sign. Differential diagnoses include pregnancy in a bicornuate uterus and fibroid uterus.

Cervical Pregnancy

The gestational sac is low in position with little or no myometrium surrounding its inferior aspect. These also present at a later date (8 to 10 weeks) with severe bleeding.

Abdominal Pregnancy

These develop outside the tube within the peritoneal cavity. It can be differentiated from intrauterine pregnancy by lack of surrounding uterine walls, the uterus is small and identified separate from the fetus, placenta, and amniotic fluid. Also, there is oligohydramnios and presence of intraperitoneal fluid.

The biparietal diameter can be measured from around 9 weeks onwards and is an accurate predictor of menstrual age before 20 weeks **(Table 29.5)**. Measurements are made on a standard transverse axial plane passing through the widest portion of the skull. The instrument should be set at medium gain so that the parietal bones measure approximately 3 mm in thickness. The intracranial landmark should include the falx cerebri anteriorly and posteriorly, the cavum septi pellucidi anteriorly in the midline, the thalamic nuclei (seen as blunted diamond-shaped structures on either side of the midline in the center of the brain) third ventricle between the thalmi and the choroid plexus in the atria of the lateral ventricles. The middle cerebral artery pulsation may be seen in the Sylvian fissure. The widest distance between the outer surfaces of the skull table nearest the transducer to the inner margin of the opposite skull gives the BPD **(Fig. 29.11)**.

However, the biparietal diameter (BPD) is a reliable parameter, only when the shape of the skull is normal, ovoid shape. Accuracy with this technique is ± 1 week prior to 20 weeks and ± 10 days until about 28 weeks. Beyond this point accuracy decrease to ± 2 to 4 weeks therefore, dating by BPD is undesirable after about 28 weeks. The cephalic index is used for assessing the fetal head shape. Cephalic

TABLE 29.5: Gestational age estimation by biparietal diameter.

BPD or BPDc* (mm)	Gestational age (weeks)	BPD or BPDc (mm)	Gestational age (weeks)
20	13.2	60	24.2
21	13.4	61	24.5
22	13.6	62	24.9
23	13.8	63	25.3
24	14.0	64	25.7
25	14.3	65	26.1
26	14.5	66	26.5
27	14.7	67	26.9
28	14.9	68	27.3
29	15.1	69	27.7
30	15.4	70	28.1
31	15.6	71	28.5
32	15.8	72	29.0
33	16.1	73	29.4
34	16.3	74	29.9
35	16.6	75	30.3
36	16.8	76	30.8
37	17.1	77	31.2
38	17.3	78	31.7
39	17.6	79	32.2
40	17.9	80	32.7
41	18.1	81	33.2
42	18.4	82	33.7
43	18.7	83	34.2
44	19.0	84	34.7
45	19.3	85	35.2
46	19.6	86	35.3
47	19.9	87	36.3
48	20.2	88	36.9
49	20.5	89	37.4
50	20.8	90	38.0
51	21.1	91	38.6
52	21.4	92	39.2
53	21.7	93	39.8
54	22.1	94	40.4
55	22.4	95	41.0
56	22.8	96	41.6
57	23.1	>97	42.0
58	23.5		
59	23.8		

*BPD, biparietal diameter; BPDc, corrected-BPD

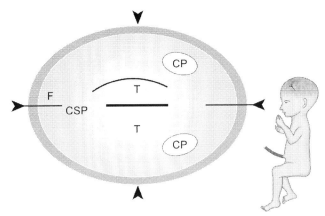

Fig. 29.11: Measurement of head circumference. (CP: choroid plexus; CSP: cervical spine; F: front; T: thalamus)

index is equal to the biparietal diameter (measured outer to outer) divided by occipital frontal diameter × 100. The normal range for this measurement is 78.4 ± 4.3.

- The occipitofrontal diameter is measured from the outer to the outer margin of the skull and is the longest distance from the front to the back of head. It is measured in the same plane as is used for measuring the BPD.

  Corrected BPD = Square root of (BPD × OFD/1.265)

  The rationale for corrected BPD is that it represents standard shaped head (one with an OFD/BPD ratio of 1.265) of the same cross-sectional area.

  Same tables used to determine gestational age from BPD are used for corrected BPD.

- Head circumference is a more accurate predictor of gestational age when the skull shape is abnormal. The same axial plane used to measure the BPD is used. Ideally it should be calculated by tracing the outer perimeter of the calvarium in centimeters using a trackball. The menstrual age can then be determined by using a standard reference **(Table 29.6)**. In most cases where the cephalic index is normal it can reliably be obtained using the following formula,

  Head circumference = $D_1 + D_2 \times 1.57$

  Where D_1 = short axis and D_2 = long axis of the fetal head, i.e., outer to outer BPD and OFD respectively (the same diameters as used to calculate the cephalic index).

- *The abdominal circumference:* This measurement is made from a transverse axial image of the upper abdomen of the fetus at the level of the liver. The image should be as round as possible and the image plane should be perpendicular to the long axis of the fetus. The various landmarks that should be seen in this plane include the stomach and a short section of the umbilical vein lying in the anterior portion of the abdomen, equidistant from the lateral walls of the abdomen. The spine and adrenal glands and aorta are seen in the posterior portion of the fetal abdomen **(Fig. 29.12)**.

  The abdominal circumference can be obtained by either tracing along the outer margin of the abdomen or by measuring two trunk diameters at right angle to each other (from the outer to outer abdominal wall) and using the formula AC = $D_1 + D_2 \times 1.57$.

- *Femur length:* The femur is the only long bone routinely used for predicting age because of its size and ease of measurement **(Table 29.7)**. Measurement is made

TABLE 29.6: Gestational age estimation by head circumference.

HC (mm)*	Gestational age Weeks	HC (mm)	Gestational age Weeks
80	13.4	225	24.5
85	13.7	230	25.0
90	14.0	235	25.5
95	14.3	240	26.1
100	14.7	245	26.6
105	15.0	250	27.1
110	15.3	255	27.7
115	15.6	260	28.3
120	16.0	265	28.9
125	16.3	270	29.4
130	16.6	275	30.0
135	17.0	280	30.7
140	17.3	285	31.3
145	17.7	290	31.9
150	18.1	295	32.6
155	18.4	300	33.3
160	18.8	305	33.9
165	19.2	310	34.6
170	19.6	315	35.3
175	20.0	320	36.1
180	20.4	325	36.8
185	20.3	330	37.6
190	21.3	335	38.3
195	21.7	340	39.1
200	22.2	345	39.9
205	22.6	350	40.7
210	23.1	355	41.6
215	23.6	360	42.4
220	24.0		

*HC, head circumference

TABLE 29.7: Gestational age estimation by femur length.

FL (mm)*	Gestational age (weeks)	FL (mm)	Gestational age (weeks)
10	13.7	45	24.5
11	13.9	46	24.9
12	14.2	47	25.3
13	14.4	48	25.7
14	14.6	49	26.2
15	14.9	50	26.6
16	15.1	51	27.0
17	15.4	52	27.5
18	15.6	53	28.0
19	15.9	54	28.4
20	16.2	55	28.9
21	16.4	56	29.4
22	16.7	57	29.9
23	17.0	58	30.4
24	17.3	59	36.9
25	17.6	60	31.4
26	17.9	61	31.9
27	18.2	62	32.5
28	18.5	63	33.0
29	18.8	64	33.6
30	19.1	65	34.1
31	19.4	66	34.7
32	19.7	67	35.3
33	20.1	68	35.9
34	20.4	69	36.5
35	20.7	70	37.1
36	21.1	71	37.7
37	21.4	72	38.3
38	21.8	73	39.0
39	22.2	74	39.6
40	22.5	75	40.3
41	22.9	76	40.9
42	23.3	77	41.6
43	23.7	≥ 78	42.0
44	24.1		

*FL, femur length

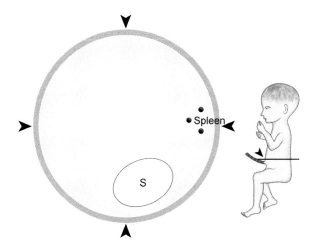

Fig. 29.12: Abdominal circumference.

along the long axis of the diaphysis, disregarding the curvature of the medial border and also the nonossified proximal and distal epiphyseal cartilages. Measurement is made along the straight lateral border and both ends appearing blunt, rather than pointed. Round echogenic cartilaginous femoral head and femoral condyles are seen at the ends. A portion of the femoral condyle may be ossified as the distal femoral epiphysis and this should never be included in the measurement **(Fig. 29.13)**.

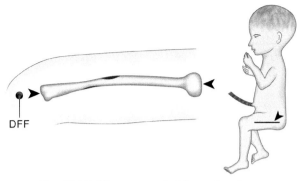

Fig. 29.13: Measurement of femur length.

- The presence or absence of certain epiphyseal ossification centers may play a role in increasing the accuracy of the above mentioned biometric age estimates. The distal femoral epiphysis is initially seen at 32 to 33 weeks, the proximal tibial epiphysis at 35 to 36 weeks and the proximal humeral epiphysis at 37 to 38 weeks.

Beyond the first trimester of pregnancy, age estimate should be based on the multiple parameter technique, because there is progressive increase in variability in predicting gestational age from any one fetal parameter as the pregnancy advances. The optimal combination of parameters is that based on head circumference and femur length.

Fetal Growth Abnormalities

Clinically large for date pregnancy has several causes including:
- Wrong dates—most common
- Polyhydramnios—excess of amniotic fluid; consequently the limbs stand out, separated by large echofree areas, devoid of any fetal structures. Between 20 and 30 weeks mild polyhydramnios is a normal variation.
  It may be associated with fetal anomalies, diabetes, multiple pregnancy, hydrops and intrauterine infections like toxoplasmosis and rubella.
- Multiple pregnancy.
- Uterine mass/ovarian cysts with pregnancy.
- Hydatidiform mole.
- Large for date fetus (i.e., whose weight is above the 90th percentile for gestational age) **(Table 29.8)** and macrosomia (i.e. fetus with birth weight above 4000 g) **(Table 29.9)**. Large fetuses have increased risk of perinatal mortality and morbidity because of obstetric complications. Various risk factors for large fetuses include—maternal obesity, diabetes, previous history of large fetus, prolonged pregnancy, multiparity, excess weight gain during pregnancy, and advanced maternal age.
- *Hydrops fetalis:* A large for date fetus may be the first indication of fetal hydrops with polyhydramnios. It is characterized by excess of total body water, causing soft tissue edema and fluid accumulation in body cavities.

TABLE 29.8: *In utero* fetal sonographic weight standards.

Menstrual week	Estimated fetal weight (g)				
	3rd	10th	50th	90th	97th
10	26	29	35	41	44
11	34	37	45	53	56
12	43	48	58	68	73
13	55	61	73	85	91
14	70	77	93	109	116
15	88	97	117	137	146
16	110	121	146	171	183
17	136	150	181	212	226
18	167	185	223	261	279
19	205	227	273	319	341
20	248	275	331	387	414
21	299	331	399	467	499
22	359	398	478	559	598
23	426	471	568	665	710
24	503	556	670	784	838
25	589	652	785	918	981
26	685	758	913	1068	1141
27	791	876	1055	1234	1319
28	908	1004	1210	1416	1513
29	1034	1145	1379	1613	1724
30	1169	1294	1559	1824	1949
31	1313	1453	1751	2049	2189
32	1465	1621	1953	2285	2441
33	1622	1794	2162	2530	2703
34	1783	1973	2377	2781	2971
35	1946	2154	2595	3036	3244
36	2110	2335	2813	3291	3516
37	2271	2513	3028	3543	3785
38	2427	2686	3236	3786	4045
39	2576	2851	3435	4019	4294
40	2714	3004	3619	4234	4524

Causes Include

- Rh incompatibility, now uncommon, also known as immune hydrops.
- Nonimmune hydrops causes of which include— underlying fetal cardiovascular anomalies (most common), placental tumors, viral diseases, and chromosomal anomalies.
  The presence of any two of the following features allows a diagnosis of hydrops:
  - Fetal edema/skin thickening of more than 5 mm. Evidence of scalp and skin edema is seen as a double outline around the fetal parts
  - Placental enlargement. Placenta is often markedly enlarged measuring more than 4 cm in thickness

TABLE 29.9: Predicting fetal weight by ultrasound.

Biparietal Diameters	Abdominal circumferences											
	15.5	16.0	16.5	17.0	17.5	18.0	18.5	19.0	19.5	20.0	20.5	21.0
3.1	224	234	244	255	267	279	291	304	318	332	346	362
3.2	231	241	251	263	274	286	299	312	326	340	355	371
3.3	237	248	259	270	282	294	307	321	335	349	365	381
3.4	244	255	266	278	290	302	316	329	344	359	374	391
3.5	251	262	274	285	298	311	324	338	353	368	384	401
3.6	259	270	281	294	306	319	333	347	362	378	394	411
3.7	266	278	290	302	315	328	342	357	372	388	404	422
3.8	274	286	298	310	324	337	352	366	382	398	415	432
3.9	282	294	306	319	333	347	361	376	392	409	426	444
4.0	290	303	315	328	342	356	371	386	403	419	437	455
4.1	299	311	324	338	352	366	381	397	413	430	448	467
4.2	308	320	333	347	361	376	392	408	424	442	460	479
4.3	317	330	343	357	371	387	402	419	436	453	472	491
4.4	326	339	353	367	332	397	413	430	447	465	484	504
4.5	335	349	363	377	393	408	425	442	459	478	497	517
4.6	345	359	373	388	404	420	436	454	472	490	510	530
4.7	355	369	384	399	415	431	448	466	484	503	523	544
4.8	366	380	395	410	426	443	460	478	497	517	537	558
4.9	376	391	406	422	438	455	473	491	510	530	551	572
5.0	387	402	418	434	451	468	486	505	524	544	565	587
5.1	399	414	430	446	463	481	499	518	538	559	580	602
5.2	410	426	442	459	476	494	513	532	552	573	595	618
5.3	422	438	455	472	489	508	527	547	567	589	611	634
5.4	435	451	468	485	503	522	541	561	582	604	627	650
5.5	447	464	481	499	517	536	556	577	598	620	643	667
5.6	461	477	495	513	532	551	571	592	614	636	660	684
5.7	474	491	509	527	547	566	587	608	630	653	677	701
5.8	488	505	524	542	562	532	603	625	647	670	695	719
5.9	52	520	539	558	578	598	649	642	664	688	713	733
6.0	57	535	554	573	594	615	636	659	682	706	731	757
6.1	532	550	570	590	610	632	654	677	700	725	750	777
6.2	547	566	586	606	627	649	672	695	719	744	770	797
6.3	563	583	603	624	645	667	690	714	738	764	790	817
6.4	580	600	620	641	663	686	709	733	758	784	811	838
6.5	597	617	638	659	682	705	728	753	778	805	832	860
6.6	614	635	656	678	701	724	748	773	799	826	853	882
6.7	632	653	675	697	720	744	769	794	820	848	876	905
6.8	651	672	694	717	740	765	790	816	842	870	898	923
6.9	670	691	714	737	761	786	811	838	865	893	922	952
7.0	689	711	734	758	782	807	833	860	888	916	945	975
7.1	709	732	755	779	804	830	856	883	912	941	971	1,002
7.2	730	763	777	801	827	853	880	907	935	963	990	1,927
7.3	751	775	799	824	850	876	904	932	961	991	1,022	1,054

Contd...

Contd...

Biparietal Diameters	Abdominal circumferences												
	15.5	16.0	16.5	17.0	17.5	18.0	18.5	19.0	19.5	20.0	20.5	21.0
7.4	773	797	822	847	874	901	928	957	987	1,017	1,040	1,081
7.5	796	820	845	871	898	925	954	983	1,013	1,044	1,076	1,102
7.6	819	844	870	896	923	951	980	1,009	1,040	1,072	1,104	1,137
7.7	843	868	894	921	949	977	1,007	1,037	1,068	1,100	1,133	1,167
7.8	868	894	920	947	975	1,004	1,034	1,065	1,096	1,129	1,162	1,197
7.9	893	919	946	974	1,003	1,032	1,062	1,094	1,126	1,159	1,193	1,228
8.0	919	946	973	1,002	1,031	1,061	1,091	1,123	1,156	1,189	1,224	1,259
8.1	946	973	1,001	1,030	1,060	1,090	1,121	1,153	1,187	1,221	1,256	1,292
8.2	974	1,001	1,030	1,059	1,089	1,120	1,152	1,185	1,218	1,253	1,288	1,325
8.3	1,002	1,030	1,059	1,089	1,120	1,151	1,183	1,217	1,251	1,286	1,322	1,359
8.4	1,032	1,060	1,090	1,120	1,151	1,183	1,216	1,249	1,284	1,320	1,356	1,394
8.5	1,062	1,091	1,121	1,151	1,183	1,216	1,249	1,283	1,318	1,355	1,392	1,430
8.6	1,093	1,122	1,153	1,184	1,216	1,249	1,283	1,318	1,354	1,390	1,428	1,467
8.7	1,125	1,155	1,186	1,218	1,250	1,284	1,318	1,353	1,390	1,427	1,465	1,505
8.8	1,157	1,188	1,220	1,252	1,285	1,319	1,354	1,390	1,427	1,465	1,504	1,543
8.9	1,191	1,222	1,254	1,287	1,321	1,356	1,391	1,428	1,465	1,503	1,543	1,553
9.0	1,226	1,258	1,290	1,324	1,358	1,393	1,429	1,456	1,504	1,543	1,533	1,624
9.1	1,262	1,294	1,327	1,361	1,396	1,432	1,468	1,506	1,544	1,584	1,624	1,656
9.2	1,299	1,332	1,365	1,400	1,435	1,471	1,508	1,546	1,586	1,626	1,667	1,700
9.3	1,337	1,370	1,404	1,439	1,475	1,512	1,550	1,588	1,628	1,663	1,710	1,753
9.4	1,376	1,410	1,444	1,480	1,516	1,554	1,592	1,631	1,671	1,712	1,755	1,793
9.5	1,416	1,450	1,486	1,522	1,559	1,597	1,635	1,675	1,716	1,758	1,800	1,844
9.6	1,457	1,492	1,528	1,565	1,602	1,641	1,680	1,720	1,762	1,804	1,847	1,892
9.7	1,500	1,535	1,572	1,609	1,547	1,686	1,726	1,767	1,809	1,852	1,895	1,940
9.8	1,544	1,580	1,617	1,654	1,693	1,733	1,773	1,815	1,857	1,900	1,945	1,990
9.9	1,589	1,625	1,663	1,701	1,740	1,781	1,822	1,864	1,907	1,951	1,996	2,042
10.0	1,635	1,672	1,710	1,749	1,789	1,830	1,871	1,914	1,958	2,002	2,048	2,094

SD = + 106.0 gm/kg of birth weight.

Abdominal circumferences												
21.5	22.0	22.5	23.0	23.5	24.0	24.5	25.0	25.5	26.0	26.5	27.0	27.5
378	395	412	431	450	470	491	513	536	559	584	610	638
388	405	423	441	461	481	502	525	548	572	597	624	651
397	415	433	452	472	493	514	537	560	535	611	688	666
408	425	444	463	483	504	526	549	573	598	624	652	680
418	436	455	475	495	517	539	562	587	612	638	666	695
429	447	466	486	507	529	552	575	600	626	653	681	710
440	458	478	498	519	542	565	589	614	640	667	696	725
451	470	490	510	532	554	578	602	628	654	682	711	741
462	482	502	523	545	568	592	616	642	669	697	727	757
474	494	514	536	558	581	606	631	657	684	713	743	773
486	506	527	549	572	595	620	645	672	700	729	759	790
498	519	540	562	585	609	634	660	688	716	745	776	807
511	532	554	576	600	624	649	676	703	732	762	793	825

Contd...

Contd...

					Abdominal circumferences							
21.5	22.0	22.5	23.0	23.5	24.0	24.5	25.0	25.5	26.0	26.5	27.0	27.5
524	545	567	590	614	639	665	692	719	749	779	810	843
538	559	581	605	629	654	680	708	736	765	796	828	861
551	573	596	620	644	670	696	724	753	783	814	846	880
565	588	611	635	660	686	713	741	770	801	832	865	899
580	602	626	650	676	702	730	758	788	819	851	884	919
594	617	641	666	692	719	747	776	806	837	870	903	938
610	633	657	683	709	736	765	794	824	856	889	923	959
625	649	674	699	726	754	783	812	843	876	909	944	980
641	665	690	717	744	772	801	831	863	895	929	964	1,001
657	682	708	734	762	790	820	851	883	916	950	986	1,023
674	699	725	752	780	809	839	870	903	936	971	1,007	1,045
691	717	743	771	799	828	859	891	924	958	993	1,030	1,068
709	735	762	789	818	848	379	911	945	979	1,015	1,052	1,091
727	753	780	809	838	869	900	933	966	1,001	1,038	1,075	1,114
745	772	800	829	858	889	921	954	989	1,024	1,061	1,099	1,139
764	792	820	849	879	911	943	977	1,011	1,047	1,085	1,123	1,163
784	811	840	870	900	932	965	999	1,035	1,071	1,109	1,148	1,189
804	832	861	891	922	955	988	1,023	1,058	1,095	1,134	1,173	1,214
824	853	882	913	945	977	1,011	1,046	1,083	1,120	1,159	1,199	1,241
845	874	904	935	967	1,001	1,035	1,071	1,107	1,145	1,185	1,226	1,268
867	896	927	958	991	1,025	1,059	1,096	1,133	1,171	1,211	1,253	1,295
889	919	950	982	1,015	1,049	1,084	1,121	1,159	1,198	1,238	1,280	1,323
911	942	973	1,006	1,039	1,074	1,110	1,147	1,185	1,225	1,266	1,308	1,352
935	965	997	1,030	1,065	1,100	1,136	1,174	1,213	1,253	1,294	1,337	1,381
958	990	1,022	1,056	1,090	1,126	1,163	1,201	1,241	1,281	1,323	1,367	1,411
983	1,015	1,048	1,082	1,117	1,153	1,190	1,229	1,269	1,310	1,353	1,397	1,442
1,008	1,040	1,074	1,108	1,144	1,181	1,219	1,258	1,298	1,340	1,383	1,427	1,473
1,033	1,066	1,100	1,135	1,171	1,209	1,247	1,287	1,328	1,370	1,414	1,459	1,505
1,060	1,093	1,128	1,163	1,200	1,238	1,277	1,317	1,358	1,401	1,445	1,491	1,538
1,087	1,121	1,156	1,192	1,229	1,267	1,307	1,348	1,390	1,433	1,478	1,524	1,571
1,114	1,149	1,184	1,221	1,259	1,297	1,338	1,379	1,421	1,465	1,511	1,557	1,605
1,143	1,178	1,214	1,251	1,289	1,328	1,369	1,411	1,454	1,499	1,544	1,592	1,640
1,172	1,207	1,244	1,281	1,326	1,360	1,401	1,444	1,487	1,533	1,579	1,627	1,676
1,202	1,238	1,275	1,313	1,352	1,393	1,434	1,477	1,522	1,567	1,614	1,663	1,712
1,232	1,269	1,306	1,345	1,385	1,426	1,468	1,512	1,557	1,603	1,650	1,699	1,749
1,264	1,301	1,339	1,378	1,418	1,460	1,503	1,547	1,592	1,639	1,687	1,737	1,787
1,296	1,333	1,372	1,412	1,453	1,495	1,538	1,583	1,629	1,676	1,725	1,775	1,826
1,329	1,367	1,406	1,446	1,488	1,531	1,575	1,620	1,666	1,711	1,763	1,814	1,866
1,363	1,401	1,441	1,482	1,524	1,567	1,612	1,657	1,704	1,753	1,803	1,854	1,906
1,397	1,436	1,477	1,518	1,561	1,605	1,650	1,696	1,744	1,793	1,843	1,895	1,948
1,433	1,473	1,513	1,555	1,599	1,643	1,689	1,735	1,784	1,833	1,884	1,936	1,990
1,469	1,510	1,551	1,594	1,637	1,682	1,728	1,776	1,825	1,875	1,926	1,979	2,033
1,507	1,548	1,589	1,633	1,677	1,722	1,769	1,817	1,866	1,917	1,969	2,022	2,077

Contd...

Contd...

	Abdominal circumferences												
21.5	22.0	22.5	23.0	23.5	24.0	24.5	25.0	25.5	26.0	26.5	27.0	27.5
1,545	1,586	1,629	1,673	1,717	1,764	1,811	1,859	1,909	1,960	2,013	2,067	2,122
1,584	1,626	1,669	1,714	1,759	1,806	1,854	1,903	1,953	2,005	2,058	2,113	2,169
1,625	1,667	1,711	1,756	1,802	1,849	1,897	1,947	1,998	2,050	2,104	2,159	2,216
1,666	1,709	1,753	1,799	1,845	1,893	1,942	1,992	2,044	2,097	2,151	2,207	2,264
1,708	1,752	1,797	1,843	1,890	1,938	1,938	2,039	2,091	2,144	2,199	2,255	2,313
1,752	1,796	1,841	1,888	1,936	1,984	2,035	2,086	2,139	2,193	2,248	2,305	2,363
1,796	1,841	1,887	1,934	1,982	2,032	2,083	2,135	2,188	2,242	2,298	2,356	2,414
1,842	1,887	1,934	1,982	2,030	2,080	2,132	2,184	2,238	2,293	2,350	2,407	2,467
1,889	1,935	1,982	2,030	2,080	2,130	2,182	2,235	2,289	2,345	2,402	2,460	2,520
1,937	1,984	2,031	2,080	2,130	2,131	2,233	2,287	2,342	2,398	2,456	2,515	2,575
1,986	2,033	2,082	2,131	2,181	2,233	2,286	2,340	2,396	2,452	2,510	2,570	2,631
2,037	2,085	2,133	2,183	2,234	2,286	2,340	2,395	2,451	2,508	2,567	2,627	2,688
2,089	2,137	2,186	2,237	2,288	2,341	2,395	2,450	2,507	2,565	2,624	2,684	2,746
2,142	2,191	2,241	2,292	2,344	2,397	2,452	2,507	2,564	2,623	2,682	2,743	2,806

Biparietal	Abdominal circumferences											
Diameters	28.0	28.5	29.0	29.5	30.0	30.5	31.0	31.5	32.0	32.5	33.0	33.5
3.1	666	696	726	759	793	828	865	903	943	985	1,029	1,075
3.2	680	710	742	774	809	844	882	921	961	1,004	1,048	1,094
3.3	695	725	757	790	825	861	899	938	979	1,022	1,067	1,114
3.4	710	740	773	806	841	878	916	956	998	1,041	1,087	1,134
3.5	725	756	789	823	858	896	934	975	1,017	1,061	1,107	1,154
3.6	740	772	805	840	876	913	953	993	1,036	1,080	1,127	1,175
3.7	756	788	822	857	893	931	971	1,012	1,056	1,101	1,147	1,196
3.8	772	805	839	874	911	950	990	1,032	1,076	1,121	1,168	1,218
3.9	789	822	856	892	930	969	1,009	1,032	1,096	1,142	1,190	1,240
4.0	806	839	874	911	949	988	1,029	1,072	1,117	1,163	1,212	1,262
4.1	828	857	892	929	968	1,008	1,049	1,093	1,138	1,185	1,234	1,285
4.2	841	875	911	948	987	1,028	1,070	1,114	1,159	1,207	1,256	1,308
4.3	859	893	930	968	1,007	1,048	1,091	1,135	1,181	1,229	1,279	1,331
4.4	877	912	949	987	1,027	1,069	1,112	1,157	1,204	1,252	1,303	1,353
4.5	896	932	969	1,008	1,048	1,090	1,134	1,179	1,226	1,275	1,326	1,380
4.6	915	951	989	1,028	1,069	1,112	1,156	1,202	1,249	1,299	1,351	1,404
4.7	934	971	1,010	1,049	1,091	1,134	1,178	1,225	1,273	1,323	1,375	1,430
4.8	954	992	1,031	1,071	1,113	1,156	1,201	1,248	1,297	1,348	1,401	1,455
4.9	975	1,013	1,052	1,093	1,135	1,179	1,225	1,272	1,322	1,373	1,426	1,482
5.0	996	1,034	1,074	1,115	1,158	1,203	1,249	1,297	1,347	1,399	1,452	1,508
5.1	1,017	1,056	1,096	1,138	1,181	1,226	1,273	1,322	1,372	1,425	1,479	1,535
5.2	1,039	1,078	1,119	1,161	1,205	1,251	1,298	1,347	1,398	1,451	1,506	1,563
5.3	1,061	1,101	1,142	1,185	1,229	1,276	1,323	1,373	1,425	1,478	1,533	1,591
5.4	1,084	1,124	1,166	1,209	1,254	1,301	1,349	1,399	1,452	1,506	1,562	1,620
5.5	1,107	1,148	1,190	1,234	1,279	1,327	1,376	1,426	1,479	1,534	1,590	1,649
5.6	1,131	1,172	1,215	1,259	1,305	1,353	1,402	1,454	1,507	1,562	1,619	1,678
5.7	1,155	1,197	1,240	1,285	1,332	1,380	1,430	1,482	1,535	1,591	1,649	1,709
5.8	1,180	1,222	1,266	1,311	1,358	1,407	1,458	1,510	1,564	1,621	1,679	1,739

Contd...

Contd...

Biparietal Diameters	Abdominal circumferences											
	28.0	28.5	29.0	29.5	30.0	30.5	31.0	31.5	32.0	32.5	33.0	33.5
5.9	1,205	1,248	1,292	1,338	1,386	1,435	1,486	1,539	1,594	1,651	1,710	1,770
6.0	1,231	1,274	1,319	1,366	1,414	1,464	1,515	1,569	1,624	1,682	1,741	1,802
6.1	1,257	1,301	1,346	1,393	1,442	1,493	1,545	1,599	1,655	1,713	1,773	1,835
6.2	1,284	1,328	1,374	1,422	1,471	1,522	1,575	1,630	1,686	1,745	1,805	1,868
6.3	1,311	1,356	1,403	1,451	1,501	1,552	1,606	1,661	1,718	1,777	1,838	1,901
6.4	1,339	1,385	1,432	1,481	1,531	1,583	1,637	1,693	1,751	1,810	1,872	1,935
6.5	1,368	1,414	1,462	1,511	1,562	1,615	1,669	1,725	1,784	1,844	1,906	1,970
6.6	1,397	1,444	1,492	1,542	1,594	1,647	1,702	1,759	1,817	1,878	1,941	2,006
6.7	1,427	1,474	1,523	1,574	1,626	1,679	1,735	1,792	1,852	1,913	1,976	2,042
6.8	1,458	1,505	1,555	1,606	1,658	1,713	1,769	1,827	1,887	1,949	2,012	2,078
6.9	1,489	1,537	1,587	1,639	1,692	1,747	1,803	1,862	1,922	1,985	2,049	2,116
7.0	1,521	1,570	1,620	1,672	1,726	1,781	1,839	1,898	1,959	2,022	2,087	2,154
7.1	1,553	1,603	1,654	1,706	1,761	1,817	1,875	1,934	1,996	2,059	2,125	2,193
7.2	1,586	1,636	1,688	1,741	1,796	1,853	1,911	1,971	2,044	2,098	2,164	2,232
7.3	1,620	1,671	1,723	1,777	1,832	1,890	1,948	2,009	2,072	2,137	2,203	2,272
7.4	1,655	1,706	1,759	1,813	1,869	1,927	1,987	2,048	2,111	2,176	2,244	2,313
7.5	1,690	1,742	1,795	1,850	1,907	1,965	2,025	2,087	2,151	2,217	2,265	2,354
7.6	1,727	1,779	1,833	1,888	1,945	2,004	2,065	2,127	2,192	2,258	2,326	2,397
7.7	1,764	1,816	1,871	1,927	1,985	2,044	2,105	2,168	2,233	2,300	2,369	2,440
7.8	1,801	1,855	1,910	1,966	2,025	2,085	2,146	2,210	2,275	2,343	2,412	2,484
7.9	1,840	1,894	1,949	2,006	2,065	2,126	2,188	2,252	2,318	2,386	2,456	2,528
8.0	1,879	1,934	1,990	2,048	2,107	2,168	2,231	2,296	2,362	2,431	2,501	2,574
8.1	1,919	1,975	2,031	2,089	2,149	2,211	2,275	2,340	2,407	2,476	2,547	2,620
8.2	1,960	2,016	2,073	2,132	2,193	2,255	2,319	2,385	2,462	2,522	2,594	2,667
8.3	2,002	2,059	2,116	2,176	2,237	2,300	2,364	2,431	2,499	2,569	2,641	2,715
8.4	2,045	2,102	2,160	2,220	2,282	2,345	2,410	2,477	2,546	2,617	2,689	2,764
8.5	2,089	2,146	2,205	2,266	2,328	2,392	2,457	2,525	2,594	2,665	2,739	2,814
8.6	2,134	2,192	2,251	2,312	2,375	2,439	2,505	2,573	2,643	2,715	2,789	2,864
8.7	2,179	2,238	2,298	2,359	2,423	2,488	2,554	2,623	2,693	2,765	2,840	2,916
8.8	2,226	2,285	2,346	2,408	2,472	2,537	2,604	2,673	2,744	2,817	2,892	2,968
8.9	2,274	2,333	2,394	2,457	2,521	2,587	2,655	2,725	2,796	2,869	2,944	3,021
9.0	2,322	2,382	2,444	2,507	2,572	2,639	2,707	2,777	2,849	2,923	2,998	3,076
9.1	2,372	2,433	2,495	2,559	2,624	2,691	2,760	2,830	2,903	2,977	3,053	3,131
9.2	2,423	2,484	2,547	2,611	2,677	2,744	2,814	2,885	2,958	3,032	3,109	3,187
9.3	2,475	2,536	2,599	2,664	2,731	2,799	2,869	2,940	3,014	3,089	3,166	3,245
9.4	2,527	2,590	2,653	2,719	2,786	2,854	2,925	2,997	3,070	3,146	3,224	3,303
9.5	2,582	2,644	2,709	2,774	2,842	2,911	2,982	3,054	3,129	3,205	3,283	3,362
9.6	2,637	2,700	2,765	2,831	2,899	2,969	3,040	3,113	3,188	3,264	3,343	3,423
9.7	2,693	2,757	2,822	2,889	2,958	3,028	3,099	3,173	3,248	3,325	3,404	3,484
9.8	2,751	2,815	2,881	2,978	3,017	3,088	3,160	3,234	3,309	3,387	3,466	3,547
9.9	2,810	2,874	2,941	3,009	3,078	3,149	3,222	3,296	3,372	3,450	3,529	3,611
10.0	2,870	2,935	3,002	3,070	3,140	3,211	3,285	3,359	3,436	3,514	3,594	3,676

Contd...

Contd...

						Abdominal circumferences						
34.0	34.5	35.0	35.5	36.0	36.5	37.0	37.5	38.0	38.5	39.0	39.5	40.0
1,123	1,173	1,225	1,279	1,336	1,396	1,458	1,523	1,591	1,661	1,735	1,812	1,893
1,143	1,193	1,246	1,301	1,358	1,418	1,481	1,546	1,615	1,686	1,761	1,838	1,920
1,163	1,214	1,267	1,323	1,381	1,441	1,504	1,570	1,639	1,711	1,786	1,865	1,946
1,183	1,235	1,289	1,345	1,403	1,464	1,528	1,595	1,664	1,737	1,812	1,891	1,973
1,204	1,256	1,311	1,367	1,426	1,488	1,552	1,619	1,689	1,762	1,839	1,918	2,001
1,226	1,278	1,333	1,390	1,450	1,512	1,577	1,645	1,715	1,789	1,865	1,945	2,029
1,247	1,300	1,356	1,413	1,474	1,536	1,602	1,670	1,741	1,815	1,893	1,973	2,057
1,269	1,323	1,379	1,437	1,498	1,561	1,627	1,696	1,768	1,842	1,920	2,001	2,086
1,292	1,346	1,402	1,461	1,523	1,586	1,653	1,722	1,794	1,870	1,948	2,030	2,115
1,315	1,369	1,426	1,486	1,548	1,612	1,679	1,749	1,822	1,898	1,977	2,059	2,145
1,338	1,393	1,451	1,511	1,573	1,638	1,706	1,776	1,849	1,926	2,005	2,088	2,174
1,361	1,417	1,475	1,536	1,599	1,664	1,733	1,804	1,878	1,954	2,035	2,118	2,205
1,385	1,442	1,500	1,562	1,625	1,691	1,760	1,832	1,906	1,984	2,064	2,148	2,236
1,410	1,467	1,526	1,588	1,652	1,718	1,788	1,860	1,935	2,013	2,094	2,179	2,267
1,435	1,492	1,552	1,614	1,679	1,746	1,816	1,889	1,964	2,043	2,125	2,210	2,298
1,460	1,518	1,579	1,641	1,706	1,774	1,845	1,918	1,994	2,073	2,156	2,241	2,330
1,486	1,545	1,605	1,669	1,734	1,803	1,874	1,948	2,024	2,104	2,187	2,273	2,363
1,512	1,571	1,633	1,697	1,763	1,832	1,904	1,978	2,055	2,136	2,219	2,306	2,396
1,539	1,599	1,661	1,725	1,792	1,861	1,924	2,009	2,086	2,167	2,251	2,339	2,429
1,566	1,626	1,689	1,754	1,821	1,891	1,964	2,040	2,118	2,200	2,284	2,372	2,463
1,594	1,655	1,718	1,783	1,851	1,922	1,995	2,071	2,150	2,232	2,317	2,406	2,498
1,622	1,683	1,747	1,813	1,882	1,953	2,027	2,103	2,183	2,266	2,351	2,440	2,532
1,651	1,713	1,777	1,843	1,913	1,984	2,059	2,136	2,216	2,299	2,386	2,475	2,568
1,680	1,742	1,807	1,874	1,944	2,016	2,091	2,169	2,250	2,333	2,420	2,510	2,604
1,710	1,773	1,838	1,906	1,976	2,049	2,124	2,203	2,284	2,368	2,456	2,546	2,640
1,740	1,803	1,869	1,938	1,008	2,082	2,158	2,237	2,319	2,403	2,491	2,582	2,677
1,770	1,835	1,901	1,970	2,041	2,115	2,192	2,272	2,354	2,439	2,528	2,619	2,714
1,802	1,866	1,934	2,003	2,075	2,150	2,227	2,307	2,390	2,475	2,564	2,657	2,752
1,834	1,899	1,966	2,037	2,109	2,184	2,262	2,342	2,426	2,512	2,602	2,694	2,790
1,866	1,932	2,000	2,071	2,144	2,219	2,298	2,379	2,463	2,550	2,640	2,733	2,829
1,899	1,965	2,034	2,105	2,179	2,255	2,334	2,416	2,500	2,588	2,678	2,772	2,869
1,932	1,999	2,069	2,140	2,215	2,291	2,371	2,453	2,538	2,626	2,717	2,811	2,909
1,967	2,034	2,104	2,176	2,251	2,328	2,408	2,491	2,577	2,665	2,757	2,851	2,949
2,001	2,069	2,140	2,213	2,288	2,366	2,446	2,530	2,616	2,705	2,797	2,892	2,991
2,037	2,105	2,176	2,250	2,326	2,404	2,485	2,569	2,656	2,745	2,838	2,933	3,032
2,073	2,142	2,213	2,287	2,364	2,43	2,524	2,609	2,696	2,786	2,879	2,975	3,075
2,109	2,179	2,251	2,326	2,403	2,482	2,564	2,649	2,737	2,827	2,921	3,018	3,117
2,147	2,217	2,290	2,365	2,442	2,522	2,605	2,690	2,778	2,869	2,964	3,061	3,161
2,184	2,255	2,329	2,404	2,482	2,563	2,646	2,732	2,821	2,912	3,007	3,104	3,205
2,223	2,295	2,368	2,444	2,523	2,604	2,688	2,774	2,863	2,955	3,050	3,149	3,250
2,262	2,334	2,409	2,485	2,564	2,646	2,730	2,817	2,907	2,999	3,095	3,193	3,295
2,302	2,375	2,450	2,527	2,607	2,689	2,773	2,861	2,951	3,044	3,140	3,239	3,341
2,343	2,416	2,491	2,569	2,649	2,732	2,817	2,905	2,996	3,089	3,186	3,285	3,388
2,384	2,458	2,534	2,612	2,693	2,776	2,862	2,950	3,041	3,135	3,232	3,332	3,435

Contd...

Contd...

						Abdominal circumferences							
34.0	34.5	35.0	35.5	36.0	36.5	37.0	37.5	38.0	38.5	39.0	39.5	40.0
2,426	2,501	2,577	2,656	2,737	2,821	2,907	2,996	3,088	3,182	3,279	3,380	3,483
2,469	2,544	2,621	2,700	2,782	2,866	2,953	3,042	3,134	3,229	3,327	3,428	3,531
2,513	2,588	2,666	2,746	2,828	2,912	3,000	3,090	3,182	3,277	3,376	3,477	3,581
2,557	2,633	2,711	2,792	2,874	2,959	3,047	3,137	3,230	3,326	3,425	3,526	3,631
2,603	2,679	2,757	2,838	2,921	3,007	3,095	3,186	3,279	3,376	3,475	3,576	3,681
2,649	2,725	2,804	2,886	2,969	3,056	3,144	3,235	3,329	3,426	3,525	3,627	3,733
2,695	2,773	2,852	2,934	3,018	3,105	3,194	3,286	3,380	3,477	3,577	3,679	3,785
2,743	2,821	2,901	2,983	3,068	3,155	3,244	3,336	3,431	3,529	3,629	3,732	3,838
2,791	2,870	2,950	3,033	3,118	3,206	3,296	3,388	3,483	3,581	3,682	3,785	3,891
2,841	2,920	3,001	3,084	3,169	3,257	3,348	3,441	3,536	3,634	3,735	3,839	3,945
2,891	2,970	3,052	3,135	3,221	3,310	3,401	3,494	3,590	3,688	3,790	3,894	4,000
2,942	3,022	3,104	3,188	3,274	3,363	3,454	3,548	3,644	3,743	3,845	3,949	4,056
2,994	3,074	3,157	3,241	3,328	3,417	3,509	3,603	3,700	3,799	3,901	4,005	4,113
3,047	3,128	3,210	3,295	3,383	3,472	3,565	3,659	3,756	3,855	3,958	4,063	4,170
3,101	3,182	3,265	3,351	3,438	3,528	3,621	3,716	3,813	3,913	4,015	4,120	4,228
3,155	3,237	3,321	3,407	3,495	3,585	3,678	3,773	3,871	3,971	4,074	4,179	4,287
3,211	3,293	3,377	3,464	3,552	3,643	3,736	3,832	3,930	4,030	4,133	4,239	4,347
3,268	3,350	3,435	3,522	3,611	3,702	3,795	3,891	3,989	4,090	4,193	4,299	4,408
3,326	3,409	3,494	3,581	3,670	3,761	3,855	3,951	4,050	4,151	4,254	4,361	4,469
3,384	3,468	3,553	3,641	3,738	3,822	3,916	4,013	4,111	4,213	4,316	4,423	4,532
3,444	3,528	3,614	3,701	3,791	3,884	3,978	4,075	4,174	4,275	4,379	4,486	4,595
3,505	3,589	3,675	3,763	3,854	3,946	4,041	4,138	4,237	4,339	4,443	4,550	4,659
3,567	3,651	3,738	3,826	3,917	4,010	4,105	4,202	4,302	4,404	4,508	4,615	4,724
3,630	3,715	3,802	3,890	3,981	4,074	4,170	4,267	4,367	4,469	4,573	4,680	4,790
3,694	3,779	3,866	3,956	4,047	4,140	4,236	4,333	4,433	4,536	4,640	4,747	4,857
3,759	3,845	3,932	4,022	4,113	4,207	4,303	4,400	4,501	4,603	4,708	4,815	4,924

and has an abnormal, homogeneous, and echogenic texture
- Polyhydramnios.
- Ascites—fluid is seen around the bowel or liver and outlining the greater omentum, which is seen as a membrane.
- Pleural effusion—fluid outlines the lung and diaphragm.
- Pericardial effusion—fluid surrounds the heart.

Clinically Small for Date Pregnancy

Causes include:
- Wrong dates
- Oligohydramnios due to
  - Premature rupture of membrane
  - Intrauterine growth retardation
  - Fetal renal anomalies.

Intrauterine Growth Retardation (IUGR)

It is defined as a fetal growth disorder, where the weight of the fetus is less than the 10th percentile for the gestational age **(Table 29.8)**. Such fetuses are also known as small for age, and constitute a mixed population of growth retarded and constitutionally small babies. Such fetuses have a high perinatal mortality and morbidity.

Types of Intrauterine Growth Retardation

- *Symmetric:* There is uniform reduction in size and weight of all organs. Affected fetuses show a higher incidence of chromosomal anomalies, congenital malformations, intrauterine diseases, chronic exposure to nicotine, and certain drugs. It begins in the second trimester.
- *Asymmetric:* The trunk of fetus is affected earlier and more severely than the head and weight more than length. The major factor is uteroplacental insufficiency

due to maternal hypertension, renal disease, diabetes mellitus, and idiopathic causes. It occurs in the third trimester and is more common, accounting for 70–80% of all cases.

There are many sonographic parameters used for the antenatal diagnosis of IUGR, some of which are very specific and sensitive. The best criterion is the HC/AC ratio and even this parameter has a positive predictive value of only 62%, which means that 38% of the fetuses diagnosed as having abnormally high HC/AC ratio will not be growth retarded. Hydrocephalus can also result in a high HC/AC ratio. A low HC/AC ratio may be associated with microcephaly and microsomia **(Fig. 29.14)**.

Other even less sensitive and specific criteria include: Decreased amniotic fluid volume, low effective fetal weight, slow rate of BPD growth, small BPD and advanced placental grade, small BPD, low total intrauterine volume, elevated FL/AC (normal is between 22 and 26), advanced placental grade. FL/BPD ratio may also be used, normal being 0.79 ± 0.06.

Even though no single criterion permits confident diagnosis of IUGR, a combination of the following three parameters helps in establishing the diagnosis with greater certainty.
- Estimated fetal weight
- Amniotic fluid volume
- Maternal blood pressure status (normal versus hypertensive) **(Table 29.10)**.

Doppler Ultrasound Analysis

Both the fetoplacental and uteroplacental circulation may be studied with Doppler ultrasound. As pregnancy advances, the blood flow through the placenta increases due to decrease in placental vascular resistance. In IUGR there is an increase in the placental resistance and a reduction

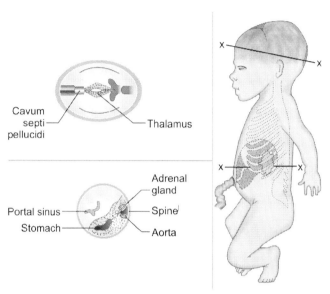

Fig. 29.14: Measurement of head and abdominal circumference.

TABLE 29.10: Critical values* for estimated fetal weight (in grams) for diagnosing or excluding growth retardation.

	Status of maternal blood pressure and amniotic fluid volume*					
	Nl BP	Nl BP	Nl BP	Htn	Htn	Htn
GA	Nl/Poly	M-M Oligo	Sev Oligo	Nl/Poly	M-M Oligo	Sev Oligo
26	516–660	646–826	743–950	610–780	763–976	878–1123
27	597–761	745–949	855–1090	704–898	878–1119	1009–1285
28	693–877	859–1087	982–1244	813–1030	1008–1276	1153–1460
29	803–1008	988–1239	1124–1410	937–1176	1152–1446	1312–1646
30	931–1155	1132–1405	1281–1589	1078–1337	1311–1627	1483–1840
31	1075–1317	1293–1584	1452–1779	1234–1512	1484–1819	1667–2042
32	1235–1493	1468–1774	1635–1976	1405–1698	1670–2018	1860–2248
33	1411–1682	1656–1973	1830–2180	1590–1895	1865–2223	2061–2456
34	1600–1880	1853–2177	2031–2386	1785–2098	2067–2429	2266–2662
35	1798–2083	2055–2382	2236–2590	1987–2302	2272–2633	2471–2863
36	1997–2285	2257–2583	2437–2789	2189–2504	2474–2830	2671–3056
37	2192–2479	2452–2774	2631–2976	2383–2696	2666–3016	2861–3236
38	2371–2658	2631–2949	2807–3147	2563–2872	2843–3186	3034–3400
39	2526–2812	2785–3101	2961–3296	2717–3025	2996–3335	3185–3545
40	2645–2933	2906–3223	3083–3419	2838–3147	3118–3458	3307–3668
41	2717–3013	2985–3310	3166–3511	2915–3232	3202–3551	3396–3766
42	2736–3045	3016–3356	3205–3567	2942–3274	3243–3609	3447–3836

*For each pair, estimated weight less than the lower value allows confident diagnosis of IUGR (positive predictive value, 74%). Estimated weight greater than the upper value virtually exclude IUGR (negative predictive value, 97%). Estimated weight between the two values is indeterminate for IUGR (likelihood of IUGR, 13%).
GA, gestational age; Nl BP, normal blood pressure; Htn, hypertension; Nl, normal fluid; Poly, polyhydramnios; M-M, mild to moderate; Oligo, oligohydramnios; Sev, severe

in blood flow which manifests as decreased or absent end diastolic flow. Both uterine and umbilical arteries have been evaluated for their systolic/diastolic ratio, resistive, and pulsatility indices to quantify these changes, and increase in all these indices is seen in IUGR.

However, none of these criteria are better than the conventional criteria at predicting IUGR. Doppler may however play a role in determining the prognosis of a fetus with IUGR, as a reversed diastolic flow in the umbilical artery carries a grave prognosis and absent diastolic flow or an elevated s/d ratio is associated with increased likelihood of intrapartum fetal distress and perinatal mortality **(Fig. 29.15)**.

The optimal approach (using regression analysis) to diagnose IUGR includes three parameters:
1. Estimated fetal weight.
2. Amniotic fluid volume.
3. Maternal blood pressure category (Normotensive versus hypertensive).

The above three key parameters can be combined into a composite IUGR score.

Intrauterine growth retardation (IUGR) Score Maternal blood pressure score + amniotic fluid volume score + fetal weight +39.2.

Maternal blood pressure score
  0 = Normotensive patient
  8.8 = Hypertensive patient.
Amniotic fluid volume score
  0 = Normal or increased fluid
  9.1 = Mild to moderate oligohydramnios
  14.8 = Severe oligohydramnios.

Fetal weight score = No. of standard deviations the estimated fetal weight falls from mean for the gestational age multiplied by 13.1.

Finally, constant value of 39.2 is added to give IUGR score from 0 to 100.

IUGR score above 60 = 74% likelihood of IUGR.
IUGR score below 50 = 3% likelihood of IUGR.
Between 50 and 60 = Indeterminate for IUGR

A single cut off score of 60 can be used in Pre 20 week's sonogram.

IUGR score above 60 = 36% likelihood of IUGR.
IUGR score below 60 = 3% likelihood of IUGR.

Once IUGR is diagnosed careful fetal assessment and careful monitoring for the remainder of the pregnancy is mandatory. Sonographic features to be followed include amniotic fluid volume, biophysical profile score, estimated fetal weight percentile and umbilical artery Doppler.

Biophysical Scoring

Many pregnancies are at risk for fetal distress or fetal death:
- Maternal risk factor which include:
  - Chronic hypertension
  - Pre-eclampsia
  - Diabetes mellitus
  - Narcotics addiction.
- Fetal anomalies
- Placental insufficiency or abruption
- Previous history of stillbirth and fetal distress.

Such high risk patients and patients complaining of decreased fetal movements need special monitoring for early detection of fetal distress. The biophysical profile provides information regarding the fetal health and influence the obstetric management. Manning and his colleagues used five fetal biophysical variables to predict perinatal outcome. They used a scoring system in which each biophysical activity was scored as zero when abnormal or two when normal. This scoring system is illustrated in the **Table 29.11**. Another scoring system which was proposed by Vintzelios and coworkers included placental grading as one of the biophysical variables **(Table 29.12)**. In both system the fetal evaluation starts with the performance of

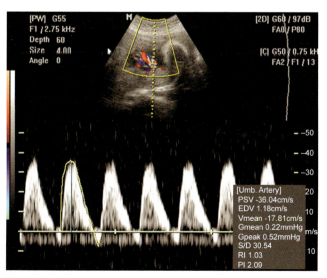

Fig. 29.15: Presence of reversed diastolic flow and absence of the forward diastolic flow in an intrauterine growth retardation fetus.

TABLE 29.11: Biophysical profile scoring according of Manning and coworkers.

Parameters	Score of 2	Score of 0
Breathing	30 s or more of breathing noted in 30 min period	Less than 30 s period or no breathing in 30 min
Movement	3 or more gross body/limb movements in 30 min period	Less than 3 gross body/limb movements in 30 min
Tone	At least 1 episode of flexion or extension with return to normal position in a 30 min period	Failure to observe any flexion or extension in a 30 min period
Fluid	One pocket of amniotic fluid measuring 2 cm in both vertical and horizontal planes	Failure to identify fluid pocket measuring 2 cm in any plane
Nonstress test	Negative or reactive test	Less than 2 accelerations of at least 15 bpm

Total Possible Score 10

TABLE 29.12: Criteria for scoring biophysical variables according to Vintzelios.

Parameter	Score of 2	Score of 1	Score of 0
Nonstress test	5 or more FHR accelerations of at least 15 bpm in amplitude and at least 15 s duration associated with fetal movement in a 20 min period (NST 2)	2–4 accelerations of at least 15 bpm and at least 15 seconds duration associated with fetal movements in a 20 min period (NST 1)	1 or 0 accelerations in a 20 min period (NST 0)
Fetal movements	At least 3 gross (trunk and limbs) episodes of fetal movements within 30 min. Simultaneous limb and trunk movements are counted as a single movement (FM 2)	1 or 2 fetal movements within 30 min (FM 1)	Absence of fetal movements within 30 min (FM 0)
Fetal breathing movements	At least one episodes of fetal breathing of at least 60 s duration within a 30 min observation period (FBM 2)	At least one episode of fetal breathing lasting 30–60 s within 30 min (FBM 1)	Absence of fetal breathing, or breathing lasting less than 30 s within 30 min (FBM 0)
Fetal tone	At least one episode of extension of extremities with return to position of flexion and also one episode of extension of spine with return to position of flexion (FT 2)	At least one episode of extension of extremities with return to position of flexion or one episode of extension of spine with return to point of flexion (FT 1)	Extremities in extension. Fetal movements not followed by return to flexion. Open hand (FT 0)
Amniotic fluid volume	Fluid evident throughout the uterine cavity. A pocket that measures 2 cm or more in vertical diameter (AF 2)	A pocket that measures less than 2 cm but more than 1 cm in vertical diameter (AF 1)	Crowding of fetal small parts. Largest pocket less than 1 cm in vertical diameter (AF 0)
Placental grading	Placental grade 0, 1, or 2 (PL 2)	Placenta posterior; difficult to evaluate (PL 1)	Placental grade 3 (PL 0)

FHR, fetal heart rate; NST, nonstress test; FM, fetal movement; FBM, fetal breathing movement; FT; fetal tone; AF amniotic fluid; PL, placental grade

the nonstress test (NST) followed by real time evaluation of the other fetal biophysical components. The examination is ended when each of the parameters meets normal criteria or 30 minutes of real time ultrasonography have elapsed. In both scoring systems fetal biophysical scores of eight or more are associated with good perinatal outcome.

- Fetal breathing is visible in all normal fetuses from 26 weeks on, but is intermittent. It can be identified by observing the movement of the diaphragm as reflected in stomach and liver movement. One should observe prolonged period of fetal breathing lasting 30 seconds or more to assign a normal biophysical profile score of 2.
- *Fetal movements:* The most important component of biophysical profile. At least three gross body or limb movements (i.e., twisting or hitching) during the 30 minutes period give a normal BPS of 2. Simultaneous limb and trunk movements are counted as a single movement.
- *Fetal tone:* Fetal flexion and extension movements are monitored. There should be at least one episode of flexion and extension of fetal limbs or body followed by return to normal position. If the fetal hand and fingers open and close, or there are hitching movements or arching of the spine with return to normal position the BPS is 2.
- *Amniotic fluid volume:* At least one pocket of amniotic fluid free of fetal parts, umbilical cord measuring 2 cm in both the horizontal and vertical planes gives a BPS of 2. Amniotic fluid index gives a better estimation of the actual amniotic fluid volume. The abdomen/uterus is divided in 4 quadrants and sum of the maximum vertical diameter of the amniotic fluid pockets in each of the 4 quadrants is equal to the amniotic fluid index (AFI). The normal range is 5–29.
- *Nonstress test:* The normal fetal heart rate is approximately 120–160 bpm. Brief period of bradycardia lasting less than 30 seconds followed by return to normal heart rate is considered normal. For NST the fetal heart is monitored for 20 minutes. A reactive (or negative) NST is 2 or more acceleration (15 bpm above the baseline) in a 20-minutes period. If the first 20 minutes is non reactive, the NST is continued for an additional 20 minutes using artificial stimulation. If the results of the NST are negative (reactive) the BPS is 2.
- *Placental grading:* Placental grade of 0, 1, or 2 equals a BPS of 2. A placental grade of 3 is assigned 0 for BPS.

Pitfalls of Biophysical Profile

- A false-positive BPS result occurs if a normal fetus is observed during a sleep or rest cycle.
- Fetal movements and tone is difficult to assess even normally in the third trimester; with oligohydramnios and with premature rupture of membranes.
- Calculation of AFI makes it less likely that oligohydramnios will be overlooked even by inexperienced observer.

Sonographic Appearances of Fetal Death

Fetal demise is most common in the first trimester. Immediately following death, absent fetal heart motion is the only sonographic sign of fetal demise. Within a couple of days other findings develop:

- Subcutaneous edema this appears as a double outline surrounding the fetus with a sonolucent center.

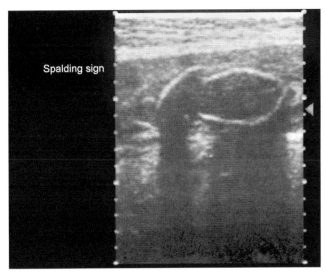

Fig. 29.16: Spalding' sign—overriding of fetal skull bones are seen.

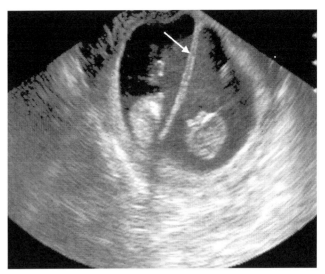

Fig. 29.18: A thin uterine septum (white arrow) in a case of twin pregnancy in a septate uterus.

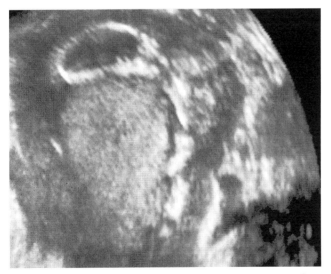

Fig. 29.17: A compressed macerated fetus with loss of definition of internal structures.

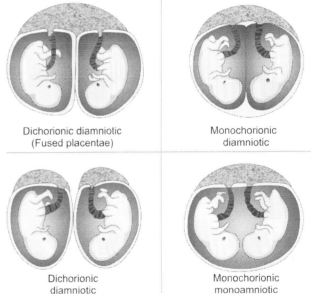

Fig. 29.19. Multiple gestations.

- Unnatural/unusual fetal position like a position of extreme flexion or extension or fetus curled into a tight ball shape.
- Spalding's sign overlapping of skull bones. Often the fetal head becomes grossly distorted **(Fig. 29.16)**.
- Loss of definition of structures in the fetal trunk. Anatomical structures cannot be made out and echoes start to appear in the fetal brain **(Fig. 29.17)**.
- Robert's sign: Air develops in the fetal abdomen and may obscure the fetal anatomy. Shadowing is seen posterior to strong echoes.
- Maceration causes echoes to develop in the amniotic fluid.

Ultrasound Evaluation in Multiple Gestations

It is important to establish whether there is a multiple pregnancy in a uterus that appears large for date. All multiple gestations have substantially higher risks of fetal morbidity and mortality than singleton pregnancies do. The risks become greater progressively as the number of fetuses increases and if there is associated uterine anomaly **(Fig. 29.18)**. Among twin pregnancies, the twins that share a single placenta (monochorionic) are at higher risks than those having two separate placenta (dichorionic). A still greater danger exists if the monochorionic twins also share a single amniotic cavity (monoamniotic monochorionic twins (MA/MC) **(Fig. 29.19)**.

Sonography not only allows early detection of multiple pregnancy, it can accurately determine the number of placentas and amniotic sacs and also identify the various pathologic condition that may complicate a multiple pregnancy.

Sonographic Determination of Amnionicity and Chorionicity

In the First Trimester, before 10 Weeks

It is established by counting the number of gestational sacs, and the number of embryonic heartbeats.

Transvaginal sonography (TVS) can identify the gestational sac/chorionic cavity as early as 4.5–5.5 weeks menstrual age as an echogenic ring within the thickened decidua (intradecidual sign). The double decidual sac sign helps identification of the sac beyond 5.5 menstrual weeks. Presence of two gestational sacs implies a dichorionic pregnancy and single gestational sac implies monochorionic pregnancy. In case of the latter presence of one or two separate amniotic sacs within the chorionic cavity is searched. The amnion is very thin and filamentous and very difficult to visualize if TAS is used. Transvaginal sonography (TVS) is often more successful. At approximately 5.5 menstrual weeks the amniotic cavity is first visualized as a 2 mm bleb adjacent to the yolk sac. It then becomes difficult to visualize until the CRL is 8–12 mm, at which point it is seen as a thin delicate membrane surrounding each embryo suggesting MC/DA twins.

By approximately 10 weeks gestation the amniotic have grown enough to contact each other resulting in the sonographic appearance of a single, thin membrane separating the two fetuses.

After the first trimester the determination of amnionicity and chorionicity is more difficult. The presence of two placentas is indicative of a dichorionic, diamniotic twin pregnancy. However, the problem arises when (i) The two placentas of a DC/DA pregnancy fuse to appear as a single placental mass, as is seen in 50% of DC/DA twins, (ii) rarely two placentas may be present in monochorionic twins due to a large succenturiate lobe of placenta. In such circumstances, the following features help to establish the chorionicity and amnionicity:

- Identification of two umbilical cords originating from two placentas differentiates between DC/DA and a monochorionic pregnancy with a succenturiate lobe.
- Fetal sex determination—If one fetus is male and the other is a female, dizygotic twin pregnancy and thus DC/DA pregnancy is established.
- Identification of a membrane separating the fetuses indicates that the pregnancy is not a MC/MA twin pregnancy **(Fig. 29.20)**.
- Presence of a chorionic peak or twin peak sign. The chorionic peak is defined as a projection of tissue of similar appearance and echogenicity to the placenta, extending into the intertwin membrane and tapering to a point within this membrane. The presence of a chorionic peak is diagnostic of DC/DA twin pregnancy, its nonvisualization however does not suggest otherwise.
- If the above criteria are indeterminate/absent assess the thickness of the separating membrane. The membrane in DC/DA pregnancy appears thicker and more

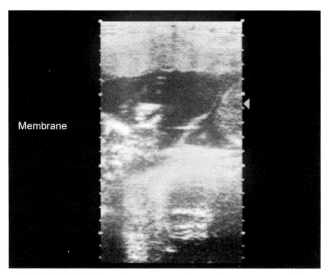

Fig. 29.20: A thin echogenic membrane is seen separating the two amniotic sacs in a case of twin pregnancy.

echogenic than that seen in MC/DA pregnancy as it is composed of two layers of chorion and two layers of amnion. However, as the pregnancy advances this membrane thins progressively and thus membrane thickness is an accurate predictor of chorionicity only prior to 22 weeks gestation. The membrane in MC/DA pregnancy is composed of only two layers of amnion and is thin and wispy. Problem may arise when it appears artifactually thicker owing to specular reflection when it is exactly orthogonal to the sonographic beam.

- In the absence of a visible intertwin membrane, two causes are likely (a) if the two umbilical cords can be followed to a common tangle, the diagnosis is a MC/MA twin pregnancy, (b) the membrane may be difficult to visualize in a MC/DA twin pregnancy in a condition known as the stuck twin syndrome in which the intertwin membrane is closely applied to the smaller twin. The stuck twin has severe oligohydramnios and is persistently positioned close to a portion of the uterine wall. The other twin has gross polyhydramnios and rolling the patient to her side is not accompanied with gravity dependent downward shift of the fetus because of the presence of a restricting membrane. A segment of this membrane may be visualized between a limb and the torso or the head and shoulder at least transiently as the fetus attempts to stretch or move.

Chorionicity and amnionicity of higher order multifetal pregnancies can be inferred by applying the same principles as those used for twin.

Sonographic Diagnoses of Complications of Multifetal Pregnancies

- *First trimester pregnancy loss:* There is an increased risk for spontaneous loss of one or more embryos early in pregnancy. Abnormal sonographic findings including gestational sac discrepancy, fibroid or a subchorionic

hemorrhage were associated with increased risk of fetal loss.
- *Prematurity:* The intrauterine growth pattern for twins is similar to that of singletons until 30–34, after which growth of the twins slows probably because uteroplacental insufficiency sets in earlier than in singleton pregnancy. Thus, the mean duration of gestation for twins is approximately 37 weeks. Part of the problem of preterm labor is also because of cervical incompetence, which is more common in multifetal pregnancies. Thus sonographic assessment of the cervix is important and helps to identify the patients that may need a cerclage.
- *Intrauterine growth retardation/discordant growth:* Monitoring for fetal wellbeing is best accomplished by use of the biophysical profile. It has been suggested that twice-weekly biophysical testing should be performed, beyond the state of viability, in any twin pregnancy showing growth discordance or abnormal Doppler velocimetry or oligohydramnios or triplets (or higher order multifetal pregnancies). In fact, some recommend that all twin pregnancies beyond 26 weeks should undergo a twice weekly biophysical assessment.

  Discordant growth, as defined as an intrapair birth weight discrepancy of 15–20% is associated with a 2.5 times higher perinatal mortality. The various indicators of discordant intertwin birth weight are:
  - Intrapair abdominal circumference difference of 20 mm or more.
  - A difference in umbilical artery Doppler systolic/diastolic ratio of 15% or more.
  - Difference in 2nd trimester biparietal diameter of 5 mm or more.
  - Difference in head circumference of 5% or more.
- *Problems of monochorionicity:* These occur due to vascular anastomoses in the shared placenta of monochorionic twins. In DC/DA pregnancies the placenta may fuse, but there is no vascular anastomoses.
  - *Twin transfusion syndrome:* The classic findings are that of a hypovolemic, anemic donor, usually small, hypotensive and having oligohydramnios and a fluid overloaded, edematous, hypertensive, polycythemic recipient having polyhydramnios. The donor twin usually suffers from IUGR and since the disparity in amniotic fluid volume is progressive stuck twin syndrome often results. There may be a disparity in the size or number of vessels within the umbilical cord. Also umbilical artery systolic/diastolic ratio difference of more than 0.4 is noted. In some patient with twin transfusion syndrome, a superficial communicating vessel with an arterial waveform may be demonstrated at the placental insertion of the intertwin membrane, using color flow Doppler ultrasound.
  - *Twin embolization syndrome:* In demise of the cotwin in DC/DA pregnancy the surviving twin is not at significant risk. If the cotwin demise occurs in the second trimester, as the surviving twin grows, the water content and most of the soft tissue of the dead fetus may be reabsorbed resulting in a small, flattened fetus surrounded by minimal or no amniotic fluid referred to as fetus papyraceus.

    In a monochorionic twins demise of the cotwin may result in renal, hepatic, and cerebral damage in the surviving twin. This occurs either due to embolization of clot and debris across the placental vascular anastomoses to the surviving twin or more probably due to transplacental exsanguination of the survivor.
  - *Acardiac parabiotic twin:* This is a rare occurrence where flow direction in the umbilical arteries and vein of the recipient fetus is reversed resulting in limited development of the upper half of the body of the acardiac twin. A multiloculated dorsal cystic hygroma is usually present and the acardiac twin usually has severe oligohydramnios. The acardiac twin usually dies in utero or at the time of delivery. The normal twin also has perinatal mortality rate of 50% because of high cardiac output and polyhydramnios.
  - Congenital anomalies are more common in monozygotic twins as compared with dizygotic twins, which have the same risk for anomalies as singleton.
    - Malformation occurring in late pregnancy due to limited intrauterine space includes torticollis, talipes and hip dislocation.
    - Anomalies related to twin transfusion syndrome (TTS), TER and acardiac parabiotic twinning.
    - Early defects of morphogenesis include conjoined twins, neural tube defects, holoprosencephaly, VACTERAL association, congenital heart disease, cloacal exstrophy, sirenomelia, and gonadal dysgenesis.
- Problems specific to monoamniotic twinning (MC/MA)
  - Conjoined twins there is partial fusion of the twins and sharing of body parts. The most common form is fusion of the anterior thorax and/or abdomen. Conjoined twins should be suspected if the twins maintain a constant and often usual relative position and more together and if the neck and head are constantly hyperextended.
  - Cord entanglement and cord knotting are potential complications in nonconjoined MA/MC twins.

    In patients with cord entanglement, frequent fetal monitoring with amniocentesis at 32 weeks and delivery as soon as long maturity is demonstrated is recommended.

Fetal Anomalies

Ultrasound plays a central role not only in the primary diagnoses of fetal structural anomalies, but also in the guidance of amniocentesis needles and chorionic villous sampling catheters by which genetic material is made available for prenatal analysis of genetic disorders.

CNS anomalies are amongst the most common birth defects. Fetal anomalies are often associated with certain risk factors and should specifically be looked for in the presence of these. The various risk factors include:
- Maternal drug intake.
- Maternal infections/diseases like diabetes.
- Maternal age of 35 or more.
- Family history of an affected sibling, parent or cousin.
- Absent or slow fetal mobility.
- *Polyhydramnios:* Certain fetal anomalies are associated with interference with the intake and absorption of amniotic fluid leading to polyhydramnios and include the following:
  - Gut anomalies with impaired gut motility or obstruction
    - Omphalocele
    - Gastroschisis
    - Diaphragmatic hernia
    - Esophageal atresia and tracheoesophageal fistula
    - Small bowel atresia.
  - Swallowing problems
    - Cleft palate
    - Tracheo-esophageal fistula
    - Small lower jaw (micrognathia)
  - Central nervous system anomalies (if the swallowing center is impaired)
    - Anencephaly
    - Hydrocephalus
    - Encephalocele
  - Neck problems
    Goiter
    - Cystic hygroma
    - Cervical teratoma
  - Short limbed dwarfism with small chest (presumably compressing the esophagus)
    - Thanatophoric dwarfism
    - Achondrogenesis
    - Osteogenesis imperfecta
  - Lung problems (with esophageal compression)
    - Cystic adenomatoid malformation
    - Isolated pleural effusion
  - Nonimmune or immune hydrops
  - Renal problem with too much urine production or renal enlargement compressing gut as with PUJ obstruction.
- Oligohydramnios: Too little urine output causes less or no amniotic fluid at all **(Fig. 29.21)**.
  - Renal anomalies
    - Renal agenesis
    - Infantile polycystic kidney
    - Bilateral dysplastic kidney
    - Posterior uretheral valves

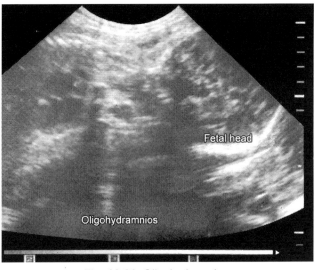

Fig. 29.21: Oligohydramnios.

  - Prune belly syndrome
  - Megacystis microcolon syndrome
  - Others
    - Amniotic band syndrome (limb/body wall malformation)
    - Some spina bifida
    - Some cranial problems
- Very severe IUGR occurring before 28 weeks has a strong chance of being related to a chromosomal anomaly.
- Increased maternal alpha fetoprotein
  - Open neural crest defects
    - Spina bifida variant
    - Encephalocele
    - Anencephaly
    - Inencephaly
  - Abdominal wall defects
    - Omphalocele
    - Gastroschisis
    - Limb/body wall syndrome (amniotic bands)
  - Tumor lesions
    - Cystic hygroma
    - Sacrococcygeal teratoma
  - Renal problems (rarely)
    - Renal agenesis
    - Posterior uretheral valve
    - Hydronephrosis
    - Finnish nephropathy

Other conditions than can cause elevated AFP include
- Pregnancy that is more advanced than expected
- Twins
- A dead fetus
- Placental problem like triploidy
- A lesion in the mothers' liver that is producing AFP. The maternal serum AFP evaluates AFP produced by both mother and fetus. AFP produced by the fetus can be assessed in the amniotic fluid obtained by amniocentesis. Acetyl cho linesterase found in the amniotic fluid is increased only with anomalies.

- Decreased Maternal Serum AFP
  - Down syndrome /trisomy 21.
  - Most fetal anomalies however are unexpectedly discovered during a sonographic study. To distinguish normal from pathologic a detailed knowledge of normal fetal anatomy is essential.

Relevant Fetal Anatomy

Central Nervous System (CNS)

Fetal head

- With TVS it is possible to distinguish the fetal head and torso from 7 weeks gestation and as early as 9 weeks by TAS. By the end of first trimester the two lateral ventricles filled with brightly echogenic choroid plexuses and surrounded by a thin cerebral mantle are apparent. The thalamus, third ventricle, midbrain, brainstem and cerebellar hemispheres are also fully formed and remain unchanged except progressively enlargement throughout the pregnancy.
- Cross-sectional anatomy of the fetal head should be defined at varying levels starting at the level of the lateral ventricles and moving inferiorly **(Figs. 29.22A to D)**. Structures that should be routinely identified are the thalamus, the lateral ventricles, the third ventricle, the cavum septum pellucidum, the sylvian fissures, the cerebellar hemispheres and the vermis of the cerebellum and the cisterna magna.
- A vast majority of the anomalies of both head and spine can be excluded if the following three structures appear well within the normal range-cavum septum pellucidi, the ventricular atrium and the cisterna magna.
- At 12–13 weeks the lateral ventricles appear ovoid in shape and are largely filled with choroid plexus. A demarcation between lateral ventricles and the surrounding hypoechoic cerebral mantle can be appreciated from specular reflection arising from the walls of lateral ventricles. By 18 weeks there is marked thickening of the cerebral cortex and the ventricles appear less prominent. Also the occipital and temporal horns develop and the lateral ventricles assume their normal shape.

  From 13 to 40 weeks the size of the atria remains largely unchanged and the transverse ventricular diameter at the level of atria is approx 8–10 mm throughout the rest of pregnancy. The choroid plexus fills most of the atrium and the gap between the choroid plexus and the wall of lateral ventricles should not be more than 3 mm.
- The cisterna magna is a cystic space between the occipital bone and the cerebellum and should not be more than 10 mm in diameter as measured on an inferiorly angled axial view. The correct plane includes the cavum septum pellucidi, cerebral peduncles, cerebral hemispheres and the cisterna magna. This transcerebellar view is also used for calculating the transcerebellar diameter which in millimeters corresponds to the gestational age throughout the first 25 weeks of pregnancy.

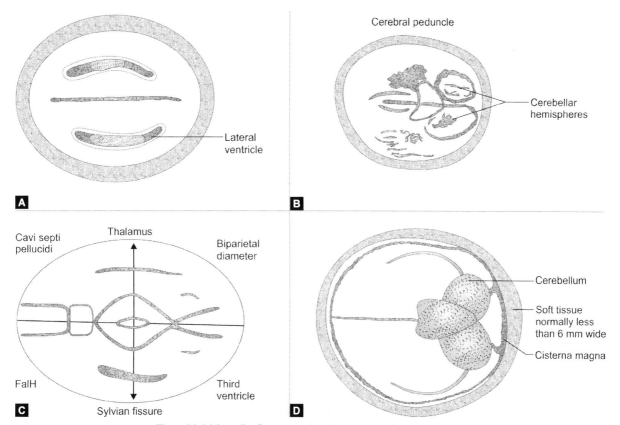

Figs. 29.22A to D: Cross-sectional anatomy of the fetal head.

- *Fetal head:* The nuchal skin fold thickness is typically measured between 15 and 21 weeks. Menstrual age in the transcerebellar plane in fetuses suspected to have Down syndrome as redundant nuchal skin folds are present in 80% of newborns with Down syndrome. Nuchal skin fold thickness is measured from the outer skull table to the outer skin surface and should be less than 6 mm in normal fetuses.

Fetal Spine

The spine can be delineated as early as 7–8 weeks by TVS and is seen as 2 parallel echogenic lines from 12 weeks on with TAS. The fetal vertebral is composed of three ossification centers, the anterior, which forms the vertebral body (centrum) and two posterior centers which form the posterior neural arch. The centers are ossified first in the lower thoracic and upper lumbar regions, followed by progressive ossification in both the cephalic and caudal directions. Ossification in the posterior centers begins in the cervical region and progresses sequentially downwards, and may not be seen in the sacral spine even until 25 weeks.

Full assessment of the spine requires imaging in three planes: the oblique coronal (through the anterior center and one posterior center), the coronal (through both posterior centers which became visible by 12 weeks) and the transverse plane taken throughout the spine and showing all the three ossification centers. A profile sagittal view showing the skin posterior to the spine helps to pick up subtle meningoceles.

The normal spine has a gentle curve forwards in the thoracic area and a posterior bend in the sacral area on the longitudinal view. The fetal spine widens slightly in the cervical and lumbar regions and tapers in the sacral region.

The spinal cord may be seen within the spinal canal and can be traced to the level of L_1. It is more echogenic than the other contents of the spinal canal.

Orbit

The standard axial view for the BPD is taken. The transducer is turned to right angle axis. The axis is continually changed till the plane where the orbits appear largest and the intraorbital distance is maximal. Measurements of the orbit represent another method of estimating gestational age.

Face

Views of the maxilla and lips are essential to include cleft palate. The gap between the upper lip and maxilla beneath the nose is seen on a plane through the orbits angled downwards to include the maxilla **(Fig. 29.23)**.

Profile

The transducer is placed at right angles to the views that show the maxilla, should not include the orbits and includes the chin.

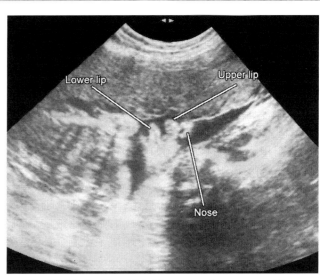

Fig. 29.23: Profile of fetal face showing nose and lips.

Nose

When taking views of the maxilla, a view through the nose is taken to ensure two nostrils. One nostril suggests holoprosencephaly.

Neck

The cervical spine area of the neck is visualized to include small cystic hygromas and to check for small encephaloceles.

Genitourinary System

The prenatal sonographic assessment of the genitourinary system includes visualization of the fetal kidneys and bladder and an assessment of the volume of amniotic fluid.

The appearance of the normal kidneys varies through pregnancy, the pelvicalyceal system becoming relatively more prominent with increasing gestational age. The kidneys can be reliably identified sonographically at 14–16 weeks as hypoechoic areas on either side of the lower thoracic lumbar spine. Longitudinally the kidneys exhibit an elliptical shape and in transverse section they have a circular appearance. The normal kidneys span the length of 4½ vertebral bodies and have a lobulated outline. The hypoechoic fetal renal pyramids orient in anterior and posterior rows. The menstrual age in weeks approximates the normal renal length in millimeter and is twice the AP diameter in millimeters. A small degree of dilatation of the central sinus echoes is permissible as a normal variant. The dilatation is accepted as normal if it is less than 5 mm in the AP direction and probably normal if it is between 5 and 10 mm. The fetal bladder is seen in the pelvis, anteriorly in the midline and has barely perceptible walls. It empties and fills over the course of about an hour and is rarely completely empty. The nondilated urethra is difficult to detect in females, and in males it is imaged when the penis is flaccid. It appears as an echogenic line in an erect penis.

By 16–18 weeks the fetal kidneys are major producers of the amniotic fluid, the volume of which is an important prognostic determinant. Thus, although a normal amniotic fluid volume may be seen early in the second trimester in the absent renal function, later in the pregnancy there will be inevitable oligohydramnios, which inturn makes detailed sonographic assessment of the fetus and fetal urinary tract more difficult.

Polyhydramnios is categorized as mild, moderate, and severe if the amniotic fluid pocket measures 8, 10, and 12 cm in the AP dimensions respectively.

Oligohydramnios: The lowest limit of normal is defined as one pocket of fluid 1 cm or less in its broadest diameter.

Genitalia

The penis and scrotum can be made out from 16–20 weeks onwards **(Fig. 29.24)**. The testicles normally descend into the scrotum at 28 weeks providing a 100% distinction between the labia and scrotum. Females are recognized by the labia with linear echoes from the vagina in between.

Fetal Abdomen

The umbilical cord insertion into the ventral abdominal wall should be routinely examined. As the fetal intestines grow faster than the fetal abdomen, they tend to herniate out of the abdominal cavity into the base of the umbilical cord. This physiologic cord herniation is seen as a bulge in the proximal cord near the fetal abdomen between 9 and 12 menstrual weeks. Thus unless the bulge is large and clearly pathologic the diagnosis of ventral abdominal wall defects should be deferred until at least 14 menstrual weeks. The liver, gallbladder, and spleen are seen as distinct structures in every normal fetus by the mid second trimester. The liver occupies a large part of the fetal abdomen and has the same homogenous appearance as an adult liver. On transverse view, the cause of umbilical vein in the falciform ligament is an important landmark. The gallbladder appears an oblong, anechoic structure to the right of the portal/umbilical vein within the liver contour. The spleen is visible on the side of the abdomen opposite to the liver. Fetal pancreas is usually not visualized because of paucity of retroperitoneal fat. The kidneys are identified in almost all fetuses by 17–22 weeks in the flanks. The fetal adrenal glands are readily visualized in the third trimester of pregnancy. They have a relatively thick hypoechoic outer zone and an echogenic inner zone, representing the adrenal cortex and medulla respectively.

Gastrointestinal System

The stomach appears as an anechoic crescent shaped structure in the left hemidiaphragm in nearly all fetuses after 18 weeks. If the stomach is not visualized the patient should be examined again in 30 minutes to 1 hour. Occasionally a pseudomass is seen in the stomach in the second trimester, due to swallowed cells and debris. Small bowel loops filled with meconium are echogenic and can appear mass like (fetal abdominal pseudomass) in the second trimester. They lie centrally and show peristalsis and are more difficult to visualize compared with the colon. Later in gestation as the fetus swallows amniotic fluid they appear as anechoic tubular fluid filled loops with individual segments not more than 6 mm in diameter and 15 mm in length. The normal colon appears as an aperistaltic hypoechoic tubular structure around the perimeter of the abdominal cavity and is seen in all fetuses at 28 weeks. It is hypoechoic with low level internal echoes due to the intraluminal meconium and has well-defined walls. The normal colonic diameter increases linearly during gestation and is 20 mm or more at term.

Fetal Thorax

The fetal chest: By middle of second trimester fetal thorax is identified as dome-shaped cavity framed by echogenic ribs on coronal section. The chest shape, size, and symmetry, cardiac size, and morphology and pulmonary echotexture are evaluated by taking coronal, sagittal and transverse axial views of the chest. Chest circumference measurements are obtained in the transverse plane at the level of the four-chamber view of the heart. The thoracic/abdominal circumference, i.e., TC:AC ratio is more than 0.80 in all normal pregnancies beyond 20 weeks. Small pericardial effusions may be seen in normal fetuses; however pleural fluid is abnormal at any gestational age. The fetal lungs appear as two paracardiac structures of moderate and uniform echogenicity. Early in gestation the primary parenchyma appears similar to or slightly less echogenic than the liver and as gestation progresses there is a trend towards increased pulmonary echogenicity relative to the liver. The diaphragm appears as a sonolucent curved band separating the lungs and the liver.

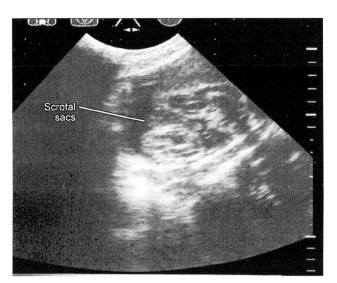

Fig. 29.24: Normal male genitalia showing penis and scrotum.

Fetal Heart

The four chamber view of the fetal heart should be routinely obtained in all fetuses older than 16 weeks. This basic view is excellent for defining the comparative size of the cardiac chambers. The apical four-chamber view allows good visualization of the atrioventricular valves while the subcostal view will demonstrate the aorta and pulmonary arteries. Long axis views obtained through both the left and right ventricles allows assessment of their respective outflow tracts, while the aortic arch is best imaged in the longitudinal axis of the fetus. A short axis view allows for detailed assessment of the great vessels and can rule out a transposition.

The fetal heart lies transversely in the chest toward the left side and occupies about one-third of the thorax. For determining the situs the left and right sides of the body is established. The left atrium lies closer to the vertebral column and the right ventricle is closer to the anterior chest wall.

M-mode and Doppler echocardiography can evaluate not only the cardiac chambers and great vessels, dysarrhythmias and stenotic and regurgitant valvular lesions can be diagnosed and quantified.

Musculoskeletal System

The upper arm and thigh which contain single bones generate only a single linear echo, whereas the distal limbs generate two parallel linear echoes. Bones are seen as echogenic lines with acoustic shadowing. Soft tissue can be seen around the bones and some structures. Epiphysis can be seen as cartilaginous structure such as the femoral head are visible. The distal femoral epiphysis and the proximal tibial epiphysis are used to aid dating.

If the femur is short by more than two standard deviations all long bones—the tibia, fibula, radius, ulna, and humerus should be measured. Bowing, absence or unduly short or large limbs indicate fetal anomalies. Grossly short (less than the fifth percentile), barely visible long bones are associated with polyhydramnios. To diagnose specific lethal defects the following should be visualized.
- The chest/abdomen ratio.
- The amount of soft tissue around the limbs.
- The amount of ossification of the spine, and
- The shape of the head.

If the bones appear poorly ossified angulations and fractures in the long bones should be looked for.

Hands

The hands should be mildly flexed with all fingers and thumbs aligned **(Fig. 29.25)**. They should flex and extend frequently. The number of fetal digits (Fingers and toes) can be counted from 16 weeks onwards. Extra-digits are seen in certain syndromes like Meckel's syndrome and Ellis-van Creveld syndrome or a digit may be missing (e.g., Holt Oram syndrome). A small fifth-finger (clinodactyly) is seen with

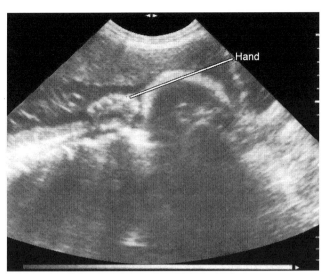

Fig. 29.25: Fetal hand.

Down syndrome. To find the hands scanning is started at the trunk. The humerus is identified, followed by the radius and ulna, and once the knuckles are found the transducer is angled slightly so that the fingers and thumb are seen simultaneously and their alignment is noted. If the fourth finger is overlapped by the third or fifth finger, there may be an associated chromosomal anomaly. Unusual thumb positions may be due to a chromosomal anomaly or a particular type of dwarfism (i.e., Hitchhiker thumb in diastrophic dwarfism).

Feet

The feet are found by tracing the hips to the femur to the fibula and tibia. The toes are inspected for number, alignment and position. The angle between the foot and leg is noted and it should not be too small or too large. Acute angulation of the foot is a feature of clubfoot and rocker bottom feet, both are common with chromosomal anomalies.

Major Fetal Anomalies

Most fetal anomalies are discovered unexpectedly during a sonographic study. The various abnormal sonographic findings can be grouped under the following:
- Cyst in the abdomen
- Cyst in the chest
- Cyst in the head
- Head and brain malformations
- Limb shortening
- Mass arising from the head or neck
- Mass arising from the trunk abdominal wall defects
- Stomach not seen
- Fetal ascites
- Skin thickening
- Bilateral large echogenic kidneys
- Absent or small kidneys
- Chromosomal abnormalities
- Fetal hydrops.

Cyst in the Abdomen

The two normal cystic structures seen in the abdomen are the stomach and the bladder. Other abnormal cystic processes are either renal, or from gastrointestinal tract, intraperitoneal or pelvic.

Renal Cystic Processes

These are paraspinal in location.
- *Infantile polycystic renal disease (Potter type I):* Is inherited as an autosomal recessive disorder. The kidneys are symmetrically enlarged and appear echogenic. Severe cases associated with absence of bladder and oligohydramnios may be diagnosed by 16 weeks gestation.
- *Multicystic dysplastic kidneys (Potter type II)* **(Fig. 29.26)**: There is a wide spectrum of sonographic appearances. Involvement may be bilateral, unilateral, or segmental and both kidneys may be large (Potter type IIA) or small (Type IIB). The kidneys may appear echogenic due to numerous small parenchymal cysts, and fibrous tissue. When cysts are large the condition is called a multicystic kidney rather than dysplasia. Large cysts of varying sizes that do not communicate with each other are seen. In up to 40% of cases with unilateral dysplastic kidney the contralateral kidney may show malrotation, PUJ obstruction, hypoplasia and horse-shoe kidney. Other associated anomalies may be seen in the CNS (anencephaly, hydrocephalus, and spina bifida), chest (diaphragmatic hernia) and abdomen (duodenal stenosis and imperforate anus).
- *Adult polycystic disease:* May be seen in utero and is autosomal dominant.
- Renal obstruction/hydronephrosis resulting is cysts that connect with each other and the pelvis, kidney parenchyma is seen around them. Diagnosis of hydronephrosis is made when the AP diameter of renal pelvis is more than 10 mm or the pelvis/kidney ratio is more than 50%.
  - *Unilateral obstruction:* Amniotic fluid volume is usually normal.
    - *PUJ obstruction:* Most common cause of neonatal hydronephrosis. A dilated pelvicalyceal system is seen on the affected side. Severe cases may show a large fluid, filled structure with a thin surrounding rim of parenchyma distending the abdomen and compressing the thorax. The ureter is not seen as it is not dilated **(Figs. 29.27A and B)**.
    Amniotic fluid volume is normal if the condition is unilateral. In 10–30% cases both kidneys may be involved and such conditions are associated with oligohydramnios. Polyhydramnios may also occur as a result of associated gastrointestinal

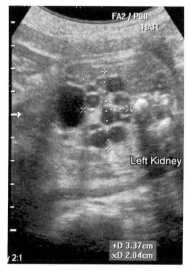

Fig. 29.26: A multicystic dysplastic kidney in the fetal abdomen.

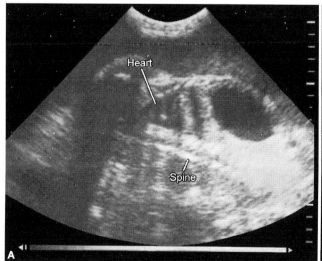 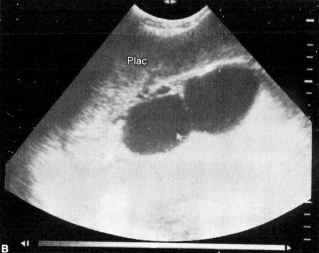

Figs. 29.27A and B: PUJ obstruction.

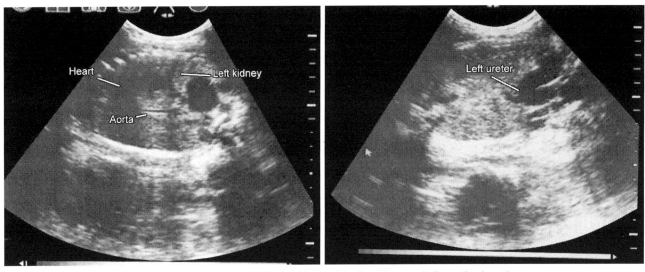

Fig. 29.28: Dilated pelvis of left kidney with dilated ureter in its entire length.

atresia or because of impaired concentrating ability of the affected kidney.

The contralateral kidney may show anomalies and in up to 20% cases extraurinary anomalies may be seen.

- *Ureterovesical junction obstruction due to ureterocele:* A tortuous dilated ureter can be traced from the renal pelvis to the bladder and a small spherical membrane—the wall of the ureterocele can be seen in the bladder. The ureterocele may be draining only the upper half of the kidney and the lower half of the kidney may not be hydronephrotic if it is a double collecting system. The dilated ureter should be differentiated from fluid filled bowel loops and normal hypertrophied psoas.
- *Reflux:* The ureter is dilated and the pelvis is usually small. The size of the renal pelvis and the ureter varies during the study **(Fig. 29.28)**. The condition may be bilateral.
- *Bilateral obstruction:* If severe there will be associated oligohydramnios.
  - *Bilateral ureteropelvic junction obstruction:* Usually asymmetrical. The renal pelvis is large in comparison with the calyces.
  - Posterior uretheral valves affect male fetuses, membranous valves in the posterior urethra cause obstruction to the urinary flow. The bladder wall is thickened (> 2 mm) and there is a persistent dilatation of the fetal bladder. In nearly 50% cases the dilated posterior urethra may be seen as an extension from the bladder base **(Fig. 29.29)**. Secondary hydronephrosis with dilatation of the ureter and pelvicalyceal system is seen in nearly half the cases **(Fig. 29.30)**. In 10 percent cases spontaneous bladder decompression with formation of urinary ascites or perirenal urinoma may occur.

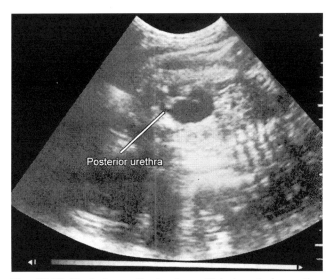

Fig. 29.29: Posterior urethral valve—dilated posterior urethra and dilated urinary bladder is seen in this 34 weeks gestation age fetus.

Poor prognostic signs include—oligohydramnios, absent caliectasis, extensive urinary ascites (leading to stenting and elevation of diaphragm and secondary primary pulmonary hypoplasia) and dystrophic abdominal calcification at the site of previous bladder perforation.

- *Idiopathic megaureter:* Ureters are dilated and there may be is some dilatation of the renal pelvis. Distal portion of the ureter do not function properly and this condition may be confused with reflux.

Gastrointestinal Cystic Processes

- *Duodenal atresia:* The large sonolucent spaces (dilated stomach and duodenum) are seen in the upper abdomen and constitute the double bubble sign.

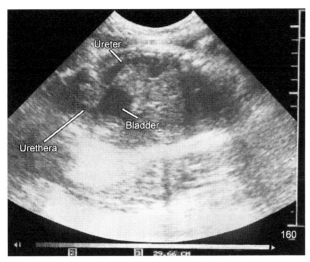

Fig. 29.30: Posterior urethral —a longitudinal scan showing dilated posterior urethra, urinary bladder, ureter and left kidney.

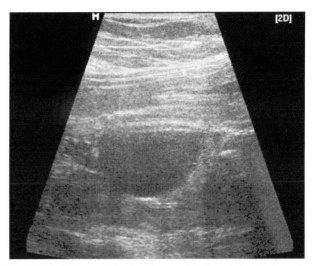

Fig. 29.31: A foregut duplication cyst in the abdominal cavity.

There is a strong association with Down syndrome and cardiac anomalies. Polyhydramnios is present after 24 weeks. Other causes of sonographic double bubble are duodenal web, Ladd's band and annular pancreas.

- *Intestinal atresia:* Multiple fluid filled bowel loops can be visualized proximal to the level of obstruction and stomach is dilated. Polyhydramnios, evidence of malrotation and odd position of the stomach is seen. Other differential diagnoses include midgut volvulus, meconium ileus, meconium plug syndrome and Hirschsprung's disease.

Intraperitoneal Cystic Processes

- *Meconium cyst:* A peritonitis results from bowel perforation with spillage of bowel contents (meconium) in the peritoneal cavity resulting in ring-like calcification in the peritoneum. Associate finding include ascites, bowel dilatation, polyhydramnios and cystic peritoneal masses.
- Mesenteric cyst and duplication are extremely rare **(Fig. 29.31)**. There is no associated polyhydramnios **(Fig. 29.32)**.
- Choledochal cyst is seen adjacent to the liver. A dilated bile duct may be seen entering it **(Fig. 29.33)**.
- Ovarian cyst seen in female fetuses as a round, cystic echofree lesion lying in the anterior part of abdomen close to the liver rather than in the pelvis. Internal echoes may be seen in the cyst representing blood.

Pelvic Cystic Processes

- Bladder
  - Prune belly syndrome is a combination of a hypotonic abdominal wall, large hypotonic bladder with dilated ureters and cryptorchidism.

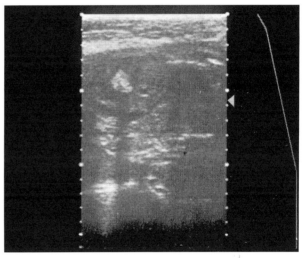

Fig. 29.32: Fetal teratoma—large echogenic mass with a central area of calcification seen in the fetal abdomen.

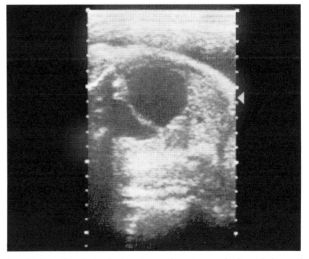

Fig. 29.33: Choledochal cyst—a large anechoic sub-hepatic cyst was seen which was confirmed on surgery to be a choledochal cyst.

- Megacystic microcolon syndrome seen almost always in a female fetus. There is normal or excessive amount of amniotic fluid. Bladder is overdistended with or without dilatation of ureter and pelvicalyceal systems. The bowel is small, malformed, and obstructed but is not seen as such.
- *Rectum and colon:* Normal meconium filled large bowel can appear cystic in the third trimester. The rectum may be mistaken for a cyst.
- *Hydrometrocolpos:* In a female fetus an obstructed vagina may appear as a cystic structure arising from the pelvis posterior and slightly inferior to the bladder.

Cysts in the Chest

- Pleural effusion
  - *Unilateral:* The most common cause is congenital chylothorax secondary to the disruption of the thoracic duct. Sonographically appears as an anechoic collection conforming to the shape of thoracic cavity. Mediastinal shift, diaphragmatic inversion, compression of superior vena cava and impaired venous return to the heart leading to polyhydramnios is associated with large pleural effusions.
  - *Bilateral:* Usually seen with diaphragmatic hernias or fetal hydrops.
- *Cystic adenomatoid malformation:* In the type I and II forms of the entity there are multiple cysts with echogenic areas in between filling the entire/part of the chest with displacement of the heart. Polyhydramnios and nonimmune hydrops are often present. Type III form has multiple microcysts that appear as echogenic areas in the lung.
- *Diaphragmatic hernias:* Left sided hernia is more common. Both types are very difficult to diagnose and a definitive diagnosis can only be made if bowel loops are seen in the thorax behind the heart. Other findings include stomach not seen in the abdomen, but in chest next to the displaced heart, small abdominal circumference and polyhydramnios. Incidence of other congenital anomalies like omphalocele and myelomeningocele are particularly high. The differential diagnoses include cystic adenomatoid malformations, bronchogenic and enteric cysts, pulmonary sequestration and cystic teratoma.
- *Bronchogenic and neuroenteric cysts:* Seen as single cyst in the lung in the upper part with associated vertebral anomalies. Other predominantly cysts varies include pericardial cysts and lymphangiomas.

Cysts in the Head

Hydrocephalus (Fig. 29.34)

Most cystic lesions in the head represent dilatation of two or more ventricles. At any stage of pregnancy beyond 12 weeks the width of lateral ventricle at the level of the atrium should not be more than 10 mm and the choroid plexus should fill most of the atrium. The choroid plexuses are gravity dependent and in a normal ventricle they are angled at less than 25° from ventricle. In hydrocephalus the choroid plexus angle is 75° or more (**Figs. 29.35 A and B**).

Selective dilatation of the lateral ventricles is unusual and suggests hydranencephaly and holoprosencephaly.

- Aqueduct stenosis (**Fig. 29.36**) sonographic feature include
  - Symmetrical dilatation of both lateral ventricles with intact interhemispheric fissure
  - Dilated third ventricle
  - Dilated aqueduct may be seen as a small tube extending towards the tentorium.

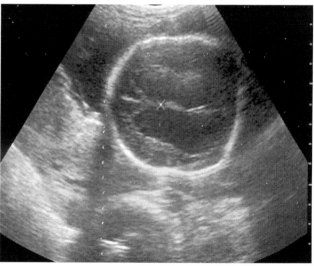

Fig. 29.34: Symmetric dilatation of the lateral ventricle s/o hydrocephalus.

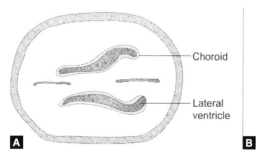
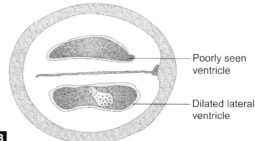

Figs. 29.35A and B: Hydrocephalus.

- Arnold Chiari malformation usually associated with spina bifida. The spinal cord ends at a lower level than L₂ due to tethering, so a portion of the cerebellum lies below the skull and is compressed as it is pulled through cisterna magna. The sonographic features include:
  - Dilatation of the lateral ventricles usually asymmetrical and severe **(Fig. 29.37)**.
  - Partial absence of the septum pellucidum.
  - Dilatation of the third ventricle and aqueduct.
  - Obliteration of the cisterna magna (Banana sign) **(Fig. 29.38)**. The cerebellum has a banana shape instead of the usual bilateral apple shape. Cerebellum may not be seen if it is in the upper cervical region.
  - Lemon sign **(Figs. 29.39 and 29.40)**. The combination of this sign and ventricular dilatation is virtually pathognomonic for spina bifida. The anterior portion of the skull is narrow and has a lemon shape. Spinal defects are usually small and resolution of the lemon sign invariably occurs by 34 weeks.
- *Hydranencephaly:* The head is filled with CSF, contained in a cavity lined with leptomeninges. The sonographic

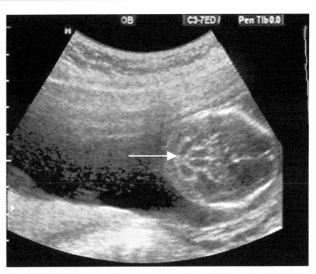

Fig. 29.38: Banana shaped cerebellum (white arrow) due to small sized posterior fossa in Arnold Chiari malformation.

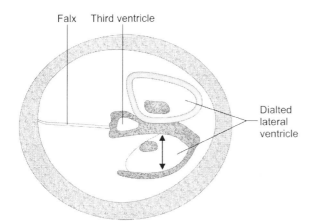

Fig. 29.36: Aqueduct stenosis.

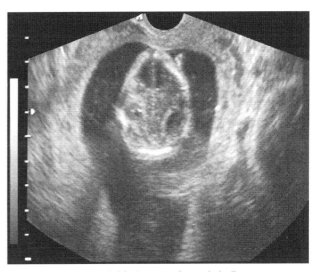

Fig. 29.39: Lemon shaped skull.

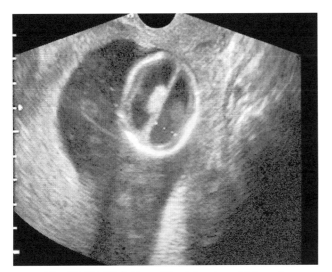

Fig. 29.37: Dilatation of the lateral ventricles s/o hydrocephalus.

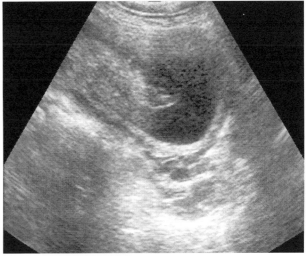

Fig. 29.40: Lumbosacral meningomyelocele accompanied with lemon sign in the skull as shown in Fig. 29.39.

appearances of the brainstem protruding into this fluid-filled cavity are fairly characteristic. The cerebral hemispheres and the falx cerebri are totally or almost absent. The cerebral peduncles, brainstem, thalamus and cerebellum are preserved. Differential diagnosis include severe hydrocephalus (but a thin rim of compressed cortical tissue is seen) and alobar holoprosencephaly (but fusion of thalamus and facial abnormalities are not seen in hydranencephaly).

Microcephaly and polyhydramnios is seen in all cases.

- *Holoprosencephaly:* 50% cases are associated with trisomy 13. Fetus has associated facial, CNS and extra-CNS abnormalities. The condition results from failure of cleavage of the forebrain and depending on the degree of cleavage three types are recognized:
    – *Alobar holoprosencephaly:* Most severe form is associated with a monoventricular cavity, fusion of the thalami and absent corpus callosum, falx cerebri, optic tracts and olfactory bulbs.
    – *Semilobar holoprosencephaly:* The two cerebral hemispheres are partially separated posteriorly but there is still a single ventricular cavity and partial fusion of the thalami.
    – *Lobar variety:* The interhemispheric fissure is well developed and there is some separation of the thalamus. Prenatal diagnosis of this condition is usually not possible. Posterior fossa is normal in all types.
- Dandy-Walker Cyst **(Figs. 29.41 and 29.42)**
    – Cystic enlargement of the fourth ventricle
    – Dilatation of the third ventricle and aqueduct
    – Dilatation of the lateral ventricles to a variable degree. Cerebellar lobes are small, abnormal in shape and split apart
    – Agenesis of cerebellar vermis
    – Associated anomalies include agenesis of corpus callosum, encephaloceles, polycystic kidneys, and cardiovascular defects.
- *Vein of Galen aneurysm:* A midline, cystic tubular structure showing turbulent venous/arterial flow on Doppler examination is seen extending posteriorly

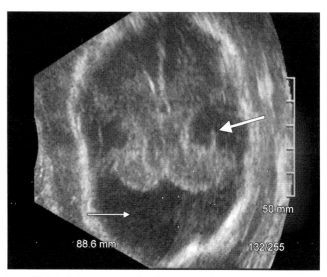

Fig. 29.41: A large posterior fossa cyst (thin white arrow) with proximal hydrocephalus as evident by dilated temporal horns (thick white arrow) of the lateral ventricles in Dandy Walker syndrome.

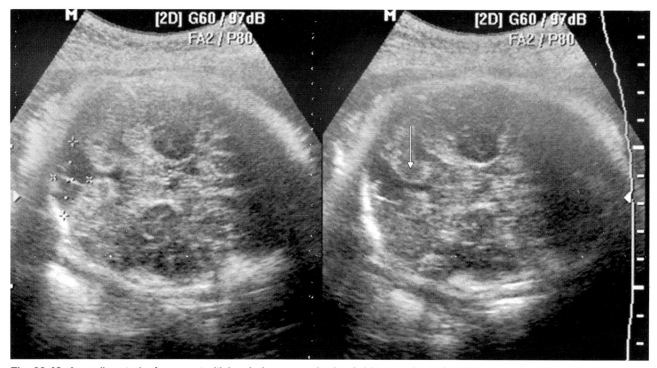

Fig. 29.42: A small posterior fossa cyst with key-hole communication (white arrow) with fourth ventricle s/o Dandy Walker variant.

from above the thalami to a vein called the straight sinus superior to the cerebellum. Heart and the venous supplying the brain may be enlarged. Fetal ascites may be seen, due to high output of congestive cardiac failure.
- Arachnoid cyst is a cystic lesion in the brainstem of any shape and in any location, not communicating with the ventricles.
- Agenesis of corpus callosum
  The sonographic features include:
  – Increased separation of the lateral ventricles with a parallel course of both ventricular walls
  – Disproportionate enlargement of the occipital horns and atria
  – Upward displacement of the third ventricle
  – Abnormal gyral pattern along falx, where the sulci radiating towards the third ventricle may be seen as a vary appearance of the midline in axial sections
  – Possible cystic enlargement of the third ventricle.

Agenesis of corpus callosum may be an isolated anomaly, when the prognosis is good may be associated with holoprosencephaly, the Dandy-Walker malformation, microcephaly, macrocephaly, median cleft lip syndrome and CVS, GIT and GUT anomalies.
- Intracranial tumors are rare.
- Intracranial teratoma seen as cystic and echogenic areas distributed randomly throughout a greatly enlarged head.
- Choroid plexus papilloma-seen as a bright echogenic mass adjacent to the choroid within the lateral ventricle with hydrocephalus.

Head and Brain Malformations

- Anencephaly **(Fig. 29.43)** is the most common anomaly of the CNS. Associated anomalies include spinal defects in nearly 50%, midline, facial defects and polyhydramnios, sonographically there is a symmetrical absence of the cranial vault and cerebral hemispheres above large and prominent orbits. Only the structures at the base of the brain are present and seen as a ribbon of tissue at the cranial end of the trunk.
  Exencephaly and acrania are variants of anencephaly where some or all the cortical brain tissue is present respectively.
- *Microcephaly:* A head circumference that is less than three standard deviations below the mean is suggestive. Serial sonograms show decreased head growth and low head to trunk ratio. Ventriculomegaly with a small head is diagnostic of microcephaly. Ventricles dilate due to cerebral atrophy. Periventricular calcification may be seen if the cause of microcephaly is cytomegalic inclusion disease. In microcephaly due to toxoplasmosis there is patchy calcification within the brain.
  In the absence of ventriculomegaly the head size has to fall below the 5th percentile before the diagnosis of microcephaly can be made because there are many normal variant small heads.

Limb Shortening

Limb shortening may be disproportionate, involving either the proximal or the distal bones.
- Thanatophoric dwarfism
  – Grossly shortened bowed limbs
  – Tiny chest with normal shaped abdomen, giving a bell shape to the trunk
  – Severe polyhydramnios resulting from compression of esophagus
  – Flattened vertebral bodies
  – Redundant soft tissue-normal quantity of soft tissues around a short limb
  – Head is large and a bulge may be seen off the top of the head contributing to a deformity known as a clover leaf skull or Kleebattschadel deformity due to the fusion of some of the skull sutures.
  – Short and stubby fingers and feet.
- *Achondrogenesis:* Findings are similar to those in thanatophoric dwarfism except that the spine is very poorly ossified and the cloverleaf deformity is absent.
- Osteogenesis imperfecta two types are seen
  – Lethal recessive form:
    - Multiple fractures, bowing and irregular contours of the limb bones
    - Poorly ossified skull, so the brain is seen too well and can be compressed by the transducer (also seen in hypophosphatasia)
    - The chest is small
    - Spine is poorly ossified
    - Polyhydramnios is present.
  – Mild dominant form
    - Limbs are normal in length and mildly shortened
    - Limb bones may show a few fracture with marked angulation.

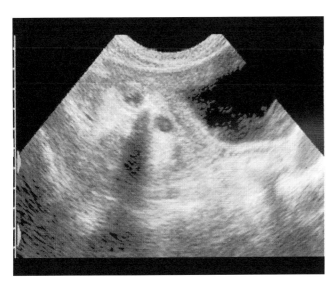

Fig. 29.43: Frog's eye appearance in a case of anencephaly.

- Achondroplasia
  - Heterozygous form is common, limbs do not became short until after 24 weeks. Rhizomelic shortening, i.e., proximal limbs are more shortened than the distal limbs is seen. The head is large and ventricles may be mildly dilated.
  - Homozygous form is fatal and limbs are very short. Family history of both parents being achondroplastic dwarfs differentiates it from thanatophoric dwarfism.
- *Phocomelia:* Long bones are missing and the hands and foot come off the shoulder or hip.
- *Limb/body wall defect syndrome:* It is a lethal multisystem disease thought to be due to amniotic bands. The components are as follows:
  - Liver and small bowel are seen outside the abdominal wall
  - Myelomeningocele, sometimes with hydrocephalus
  - Absence of one or more limbs
  - Gross kyphoscoliosis, sometimes with loss of sacrum (caudal regression)
  - Oligohydramnios.

Short femur length—if the femur length is less than 0.91 of the expected femur length for the gestational age, nuchal fold thickness is 6 mm or more, and serum AFP is low and maternal age is high then Down syndrome should be suspected. A more obscure sign is a short middle phalanx of the little finger. Duodenal atresia and endocardial cushion defects of the heart both have a strong association with Down syndrome.

Masses Arising from the Head or Neck

- *Encephalocele (Fig. 29.44):* A bony calvarial defect which allows herniation of the meninges alone (cranial meningocele) or both brain and meninges (encephalocele) occurs in the occipital midline (75%), or frontal midline or parietal regions. Sonographically detected as fluid or solid-filled structure protruding from the calvarium, an encephalocele is easy to demonstrate, the bony defect is usually difficult to demonstrate. Microcephaly and hydrocephalus are associated findings.

  When associated with polydactyly and polycystic kidney the condition is known as Meckel-Guber syndrome which is lethal.

- *Cystic hygroma (Fig. 29.45):* Multiseptate cystic structure are seen located in the occipitocervical region of the fetus. Large lesions demonstrate a thick midline septum corresponding to the nuchal ligament. This condition occurs due to failure of normal communication between the fetal lymphatic system and jugular vein. In the milder form a small cystic area is seen in the posterolateral or posterior aspect of the neck. The condition may progress to a generalized lymphoedema and nonimmune hydrops. Bilateral pleural effusions, ascites, pericardial effusions and polyhydramnios and severe skin thickening with multiple septae within the thickened skin may be present.

  Chromosomal analysis may show a high incidence of Turner's syndrome or Down syndrome.

- *Goiter:* A smooth bordered, homogeneous solid mass is seen on the anterior aspect of the neck due to the enlarged thyroid. Head is extended and as swallowing is impeded by the neck mass polyhydramnios results.

- *Teratoma of the neck:* Appear as a solid mass of heterogeneous echotexture in the anterior neck region.

Masses Arising from the Trunk

- *Omphalocele (Fig. 29.46):* There is a midline defect in the anterior abdominal wall, through which the abdominal contents, usually some portion of the gut,

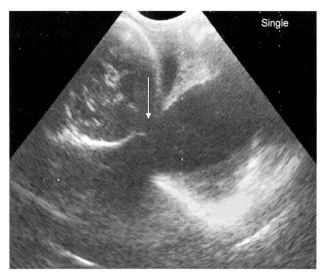

Fig. 29.44: A large encephalocele arising from the defect in skull (white arrow).

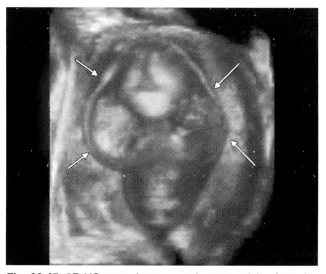

Fig. 29.45: 3D US scan shows a cystic mass arising from the cervical region in a case of cystic hygroma (white arrows).

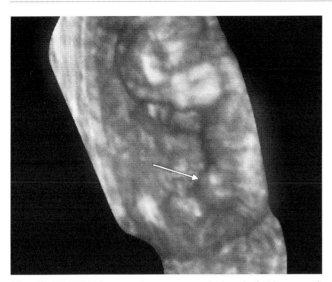

Fig. 29.46: 3D US scan shows an omphalocele (white arrow) as a midline umbilical mass.

stomach and liver herniate out into the base of the umbilical cord. The herniated organ is covered with a membrane of intact peritoneum. Omphalocele may be a component of the Pentology of Cantrell. Ectopia cordis-heart lying outside the chest, and interrupted diaphragm are other components. Other anomalies like cardiac problem and cystic hygroma are seen half the time. Chromosomal anomalies may be seen with omphalocele that contain only gut.

Sonographic criteria for diagnosis of omphalocele
- Central anterior abdominal wall defect containing bowel/solid viscera
- Mass encompassed by umbilical cord
- Limiting membrane covering the defect.

- *Gastroschisis:* It is less common than omphalocele. Here a full thickness defect of the abdominal wall is located to the right of the umbilical cord which has normal insertion. The defect is generally small and usually only the bowel loops, herniate through it and float freely in the amniotic fluid as there is no peritoneal sac around them. Although, complications like bowel obstruction, or peritonitis or ischemia may be seen, other concurrent abnormalities are rarely seen in gastroschisis.

Sonographic criteria for diagnosis of gastroschisis
- Full-thickness abdominal wall defect
- Paraumbilical location of the defect; generally right sided
- Small (i.e., 2 to 4 cm) defect
- No limiting membrane
- Free floating loops of bowel in the amniotic fluid.

- *Pentalogy of Cantrell:* This represents an association of omphalocele and an ectopic heart.

Sonographic criteria for diagnosis of pentalogy of Cantrell
- Midline anterior wall defect usually involving the upper abdomen
- Ectopic heart
- Pericardial or pleural effusions
- Craniofacial anomalies
- Ascites
- Two-vessel cord.

- *Limb-body wall complex:* This is a complex malformation caused by failure of the ventral body wall to close. The maldevelopment of the cranial, caudal and lateral body fold results in a short or absent umbilical cord with evisceration of abdominal organs that are attached to placenta.

Sonographic criteria for limb-body wall complex
- Large ventral wall defect of the abdomen and thorax (often left sided)
- Craniofacial anomalies
- Marked scoliosis and/or spinal dysraphism
- Limb defects
- Short or absent umbilical cord
- Amniotic bands.

- *Bladder and cloacal exstrophy:* They are midline defects of the infraumbilical anterior abdominal wall. In bladder exstrophy there is failure of muscle development of the anterior abdominal wall with inappropriate eversion of the bladder mucosa. In cloacal dystrophy there is maldevelopment of cloacal membrane **(Table 29.13)**.

Sonographic findings in cloacal exstrophy
- Large infraumbilical anterior wall defect with irregular anterior wall mass.
- Absent bladder
- Malformation of genitalia
- ± neural tube defect.

- Teratomas most commonly seen posterior to the sacrum where they are called sacrococcygeal teratoma. Other locations include head and neck region.
Majority is solid or mixed cystic and solid with calcification. Only 15% are entirely cystic and they need to be differentiated from myelomeningocele. They have an intrapelvic component which may extend superiorly, posterior to the bladder and cause obstruction of the bladder and kidneys. Hydrops, placentomegaly and oligohydramnios are poor prognostic findings **(Fig. 29.47)**.

- *Spina bifida/myelomeningocele:* These are most common in the lumbosacral region and almost all are posterior to the spine, they may rarely be anterior. More than 90% are meningomyeloceles, the remainder being meningoceles. Sonographic findings can be grouped under: (i) dysraphic spinal defect (ii) soft tissue findings (myelomeningocele with disruption of overlying integument) and (iii) cranial findings.

- *Dysraphic spinal defect* **(Fig. 29.48)**: Sonographic diagnosis may be difficult and the spine should be imaged in all three planes-coronal, sagittal, and transverse. The spectrum of abnormalities ranges from complete spinal disorganization, isolated abnormalities at different levels and subtle splaying of the posterior neural arches, as seen on the coronal

TABLE 29.13: Typical features of anterior abdominal wall defects.

	Gastroschisis	Omphalocele	Limb body wall complex	Cloacal exstrophy
Location	Right paraumbilical	Midline cord	Lateral	Infraumbilical
Size defect	Small (2–4 cm)	Variable (2–10 cm)	Large	Variable
Membrane	–	+	+ (contiguous with placenta)	variable
Liver involvement	–	Common	+	+
Ascites	–	Common	–	+
Bowel thickening	+	– (unless ruptured membrane)	–	+
Bowel complications	Common	–	–	–
Cardiac anomalies	Rare (ASD, PDA)	Common (complex)	Common	10-15%
Other anomalies	Rare	Common	Always (Scoliosis) cranial defects limb defects)	Always (genitourinary, spinal)
Chromosome abnormalities	–	Common	–	Always

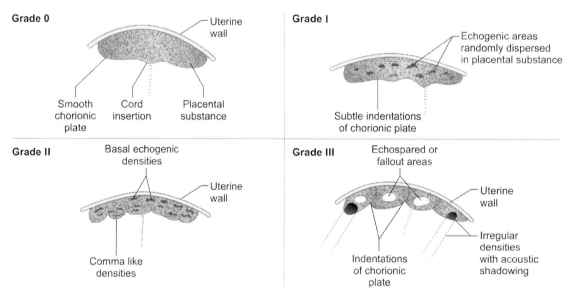

Fig. 29.47: Placental grading.

views. On the transverse view the two posterior elements appear widely separated and a U or V shape is formed. The sagittal view shows an absence of the posterior element at the level of the defect with a pouch seen posterior to spine. The spine may be angulated at the level of the defect.
- *Soft tissue findings:* Myelomeningoceles appear as fluid filled sacs containing echogenic lines representing nerves. The sac may rupture or be compressed against the adjacent structures.
- *Cranial findings:* May be more apparent than spinal defect itself. These findings are usually due to Arnold-Chiari malformations which is almost always present.

These findings include
- Hydrocephalus—seen in more than 75% fetuses with spina bifida. One-third of the cases of hydrocephalus have spina bifida
- Lemon sign

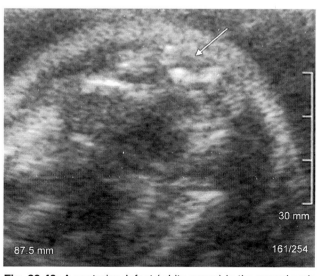

Fig. 29.48: A posterior defect (white arrow) in the neural arch in a case of occult spina bifida.

- Banana sign
- Decreased head measurements. BPD is small even when hydrocephalus is present, in fetuses less than 24 weeks. Tethering of the spinal cord is common. Diastematomyelia with widening of the lumbar spine and a central bony spur may also show tethering of the cord. An echogenic lipoma may also be associated with cord tethering. In hemivertebrae, the spine appears to be out of alignment and confusion with diastematomyelia is possible.

Absent Stomach

Stomach may be difficult to visualize even in normal fetuses, associated polyhydramnios however, helps is differentiating from a normal variant. Absent stomach is associated with the following:
- Cleft palate is difficult to diagnose. A gap is seen in the lip or in the maxilla or in both. An abnormal nostril may be seen in profile. Polyhydramnios is usually present. Cleft palate is frequently associated with hypotelorism and holoprosencephaly.
- *Tracheoesophageal atresia:* The esophagus may be absent (atresia), but more commonly it connects with the trachea which in turn connects with the stomach. It is difficult to diagnose because a small stomach is seen usually because of the connection between the trachea and stomach. If no connection exists (10%) stomach is not seen and there is polyhydramnios. Cardiac, chromosomal, GIT, and GUT malformations occur in 50% cases.
- *Diaphragmatic hernia:* In left sided hernias the stomach lies in the chest. It is usually not visualized in right sided hernias.

Fetal Ascites (Fig. 29.49)

The bowel is outlined by free fluid in a dependent position. Pseudoascites occurs when the fetus is prone and paraspinous muscles look like fluid on either side of the spine or a thin translucent band is seen around the anterior and lateral aspect of the fetal abdomen due to the hypoechoic abdominal wall muscles.

Isolated fetal ascites is most often seen with GIT or GUT anomaly with oligohydramnios. Most often ascites is associated with other features of hydrops.

Skin Thickening

Skin thickening is seen with the following conditions:
- Macrosomia
- Hydrops
- Fetal death.

Bilateral Echogenic Large Kidneys

- Polycystic kidneys—infantile and adult type
- Bilateral multicystic dysplastic kidney.

Absent or Small Kidneys or Abnormally Located Kidneys

- Renal agenesis if bilateral there is no amniotic fluid production after 15–18 weeks. Adrenals assume a flattened discoid shape and tend to be located lower and more lateral than normal and since in utero they have an echogenic center they may be mistaken for the kidneys.
- Ectopic kidneys usually lie in the pelvis and more prone to dysplastic changes.
- Horse-shoe kidneys lie at a lower level in front of the spine in the midline.

Fetal Chromosomal Abnormalities

Most fetuses with chromosomal abnormalities have external or internal defect which can be detected by detailed ultrasound examination. Hence, ultrasound is a powerful tool for detection of these abnormalities prenatally and in prompting for further obstetric and genetic counseling and fetal karyotyping.

The sonographic features of five main chromosomal disorders are detectable by prenatal ultrasound.
- Sonographic features of trisomy 21 Down's syndrome
    - Cystic hygroma
    - Nuchal thickening
    - Nonimmune hydrops
    - Hydrothorax.

    Craniofacial malformations
    - Round low ears
    - Protruding tongue

    CNS abnormalities
    - Mild ventriculomegaly

    CVS abnormalities
    - ASD, VSD, PDA, ASVA

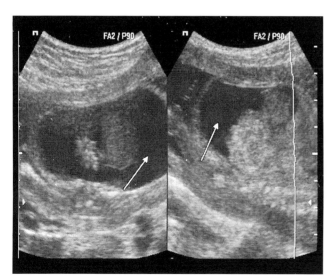

Fig. 29.49: Gross fetal ascites (white arrows) with floating bowel loops and liver.

Gastrointestinal tract malformation
- Duodenal atresia
- Esophageal atresia
- Anorectal atresia
- Omphalocele
- Echogenic bowel.

Genitourinary tract abnormalities
- Undescended testis
- Mild hydronephrosis.

Skeletal malformations
- Widening of iliac wings
- Clinodactyly
- Short upper and lower extremities
- Increased space between first and second toes.

- Sonographic features of trisomy 18 detected antenatally
  - Intrauterine growth retardation
  - Polyhydramnios or oligohydramnios
  - Single umbilical artery (>80%)
  - Cystic hygroma
  - Nuchal edema
  - Nonimmune hydrops

Craniofacial abnormalities
- Dolicocephaly (Strawberry-shaped head)
- Microcephaly
- Low set ears or 'pixie' ears
- Micrognathia
- Cleft lip or palate (10–20%)

Central nervous system abnormalities
- Choroid plexus cysts
- Absent corpus callosum
- Enlarged cisterna magna
- Hydrocephalus
- Myelomeningocele (10–20%).

Cardiovascular abnormalities
- ASD, VSD, PDA, double outlet ventricle.

Gastrointestinal tract anomalies
- Esophageal atresia/tracheoesophageal fistula
- Omphalocele
- Diaphragmatic hernia
- Anorectal atresia

Genitourinary abnormalities
- Horse-shoe kidney
- Hydronephrosis

Skeletal malformations
- Short extremities
- Radial aplasia
- Rocker bottom feet
- Overlapping fingers, flexed hand
- Generalized arthrogryposis
- Shortened first toe.

- Sonographic features of trisomy 13
  - Single umbilical artery

Craniofacial abnormalities
- Microcephaly
- Cyclopia
- Anophthalmia
- Microphthalmia
- Cleft lip and palate
- Low-set, deformed ears
- Capillary hemangiomas.

Central nervous system abnormalities
- Holoprosencephaly
- Agenesis of the corpus callosum

Cardiovascular malformations
- VSD, ASD, PDD.

Gastrointestinal tract malformation
- Omphalocele, umbilical hernia

Genitourinary anomalies
- Cystorenal dysplasia
- Hydronephrosis
- Duplicated kidney

Skeletal malformation
- Polydactyly (70%)
- Rocker-bottom feet.

- Sonographic features of triploidy
  - Early onset (second trimester) IUGR
  - Third trimester polyhydramnios

Central nervous system anomalies
- Holoprosencephaly
- Agenesis of corpus callosum
- Mild ventriculomegaly
- Meningomyelocele

Cardiovascular malformations
- VSD, ASD, dextrocardia

Craniofacial malformations
- Micrognathia
- Sloping forehead
- Cleft lip/palate

Skeletal abnormalities
- Overlapping digits
- Postaxial polydactyly
- Syndactyly

Renal malformations
- Renal cortical cysts
- Hydronephrosis
- Horse-shoe kidney

Abdominal wall defects
- Omphalocele.

- Sonographic features of Turner's syndrome
  - Cystic hygromas
  - Nonimmune hydrops

Craniofacial malformations
- Abnormal ears
- Small mandible

Cardiovascular malformations
- Coarctation of aorta

Skeletal malformations
- Cubitus valgus
- Short stature

Genitourinary tract malformations
- Horse-shoe kidneys
- Double renal pelvis.

Sonographic biometry for detection of cytogenetic abnormalities
- *Nuchal skin fold thickness:* It is measured between 15 and 21 weeks of menstrual age. Transverse axial image directed in suboccipital-bregmatic plane is used. Internal landmarks are cavum septi pellucidi, cerebral peduncles, cerebellar hemispheres and cisterna magna. It is measured from outer skull table to outer skin surface. Values of greater than or equal to 6 mm are considered abnormal.
- *Nuchal translucency:* It is the sonolucent area in the nuchal region typically observed between 10 and 14 weeks. Measurement of nuchal translucency should be performed with the fetus in the sagittal plane. The maximal area of translucency is measured between occipital bone and subcutaneous interface. Measurement of 3 mm or more is considered abnormal; however, at younger gestational ages even 2 mm is abnormal. Increased nuchal translucency (NT) is associated with various chromosomal abnormalities including trisomy 21, 18, and 13.
- *Femur length:* It is an indirect measure of stature so fetuses with Down syndrome have shorter femur than with fetuses with normal chromosomes. Any fetus with a BPD/FL ratio above 1.5 standard deviations for menstrual age is considered as having a positive screening test or if the observed-to-expected femur length ratio is below 2 standard deviation is indicative of disproportionate shortening of femur.
- *Humeral length:* It is also shorter than expected in trisomy 21.

Approach to the Patient with an Ultrasound Identified Fetal Abnormality

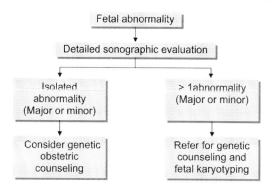

Isolated abnormalities with increased probability of fetal chromosomal anomaly
- Borderline ventriculomegaly
- Posterior fossa abnormality
- Nuchal fold
- Cystic hygroma
- Nuchal translucency
- AV septal defect
- Omphalocele
- Duodenal atresia
- Echogenic bowel
- Genitourinary abnormalities
- Nonimmune hydrops (NIH).

Fetal Hydrops

Fetal hydrops is defined as abnormal accumulation of serous fluid in at least two body cavities or tissues.

Classification
- Immune hydrops
- Nonimmune hydrops.

Nonimmune hydrops (NIH) is characterized by the absence of a detectable circulating antibody against red blood cells (RBC) in the mother.

Sonographic features of hydrops
- Ascites
- Pleural effusions
- Subcutaneous edema
- Placental edema (placental thickness >5 cm)
- Arterial or venous Doppler abnormalities
- Alteration of fetal "wellbeing".

Causes of hydrops
Immune hydrops: It occurs when sensitized mother has antibodies to fetal red blood cells.

Hydrops develops when the fetal hemoglobin (Hb) deficit is <7 g/dL probably due to decreased oncotic pressure.

Nonimmune hydrops
Causes can be classified as:
- Fetal
- Maternal
- Placental.

Fetal

Cardiovascular anomalies
- Structural anomalies like left or right heart hypoplasia, single ventricle, closure of foramen ovale, severe AV regurgitation, Ebstein anomaly, biventricular outflow tract obstruction
- Cardiac tumors
- Myocarditis/cardiomyopathy
- Brady/Tachyarrhythmias
- High-output failure—placental chorioangioma, large fetal angioma, sacrococcygeal teratoma, vein of Galen aneurysm twin/twin transfusion, acardiac liver.

Neck/Thoracic Anomalies
- Cystic hygroma
- Chylothorax/hydrothorax
- Congenital cystic adenomatoid malformation
- Diaphragmatic hernia
- Pulmonary sequestration
- Thoracic tumors.

Gastrointestinal Anomalies

- Hepatic—cirrhosis, hepatitis, and tumors
- Bowel—atresia, volvulus, meconium, and peritonitis.

Urinary Tract Anomalies

- Congenital nephrotic syndrome
- Urinary tract obstruction
- Polycystic kidney.

Chromosomal

- Trisomy 21, 18, and 13, triploidy and 45, X.

Anemia

- α thalassemia (homozygous)
- G6PD deficiency
- Fetomaternal hemorrhage
- Twin/twin transfusion (donor).

Infection

- Cytomegalovirus (CMV)
- Parvovirus
- Toxoplasmosis
- Syphilis
- Coxsackie
- Rubella.

Genetic Disorders

- Metabolic—Gaucher's disease, GM1 gangliosidosis, mucopolysaccharidosis

Skeletal Dysplasia

- Achondrogenesis, osteogenesis, thanatophoric dysplasia
- Asphyxiating thoracic dystrophy.

Idiopathic (15–20%)

Maternal
- Severe diabetes mellitus
- Severe anemia
- Severe hypoproteinemia.

Placental
- Chorioangioma
- Venous thrombosis
- Cord torsion, knot or tumor.
  Evaluation of Hydrops by Ultrasound—Methodical Approach

Fetus
- Biometry
- Full anatomical study
- Careful search for associated structural anomalies
- Distribution and size of fluid collections
  – Ascites
  – Pleural effusion
  – Pericardial effusions.
- Distribution and thickness of skin edema
- Fetal echocardiography
- Normal bladder (usually excludes urinary ascites).

Placenta
- Thickness
- Texture
- Exclusion of AVM

Amniotic fluid: Semiquantitative assessment.

Functional assessment
- Biophysical studies
- Doppler blood flow studies
- Functional cardiac assessment.

A comprehensive approach should be taken to the investigation of hydrops, both for management and for future counseling.

Sonographic Evaluation of the Placenta

Anatomy

The placenta appears as a relatively echogenic discoid mass of tissue and can be distinguished from the surrounding chorion and the underlying myometrium from 10 to 12 weeks of gestation onwards. A network of vascular channels at the placental myometrial function seen as a subjacent hypoechoic area is a normal variant and may be mistaken for abruption to placenta. Real-time visualization will document pulsations in this region. The volume of normal placenta increase through gestation, however, it is cumbersome to measure the placental volume. Instead the thickness of mid placenta, measured perpendicular to the plane of placenta is obtained in millimeters and roughly equals the menstrual age in weeks. Thus the normal placental thickness is upto 4 cm.

With advancing pregnancy calcium deposition occur normally in the placenta along the basal plate and along the septa separating placental lobes. They appear as bright intraplacental echoes with or without acoustic shadowing. Placental grading (0 to III) is done based on the appearance of calcification in the placenta **(Fig. 29.47)**.

Grade 0   Homogeneous placental substance with no visible calcification and a smooth chorionic plate on the fetal surface of the placenta

Grade I   Scattered bright echoes in the placental substance with subtle indentations of the chorionic plate

Grade II Increased basal echogenicities and comma like echogenicities extending into the placental substance from indentation of the chorionic plate

Grade III Extensive basal echogenicities and curvilinear echogenicities extending from the chorionic plate up to the basal plate with echospared or fall-out areas in the placental substance. Irregular densities with acoustic shadowing are also seen within the placental substance.

Echopenic areas in the placenta in a subchorionic location are a normal finding if represent subchorionic fibrin deposition.

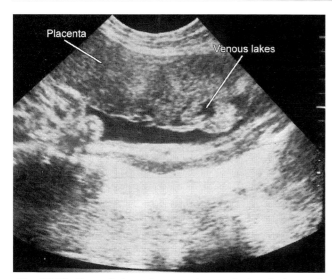

Fig. 29.50: Normal placenta seen along anterior uterine wall showing venous lakes.

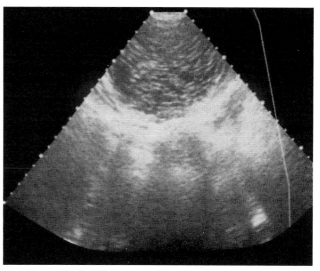

Fig. 29.51: Hydatidiform mole (complete). The entire uterus is filled with a heterogeneous mass with multiple anechoic cystic areas in a female with five month amenorrhea.

Intraplacental anechoic/hypoechoic lesions are frequently visualized in normal placentae and may represent venous lakes perivillous fibrin deposition, intervillous thromboses and septal cysts. Slow flow is often seen in all the above lesions at real time sonography, but color Doppler often fails to demonstrate the flow (Fig. 29.50).

Small placental infarcts are common and have no clinical significance. However, large infarcts involving more than 10% of the placenta are associated with IUGR, fetal hypoxia and fetal demise.

Infarcts appear as triangular shaped lesions based on the maternal surface of the placenta and are only visualized when complicated by hemorrhage and contain fluid, blood or fibrin.

Placental Tumors

Nontrophoblastic

- Primary placental tumors include the rare teratoma and the chorioangioma.
  The later appears as a well-demarcated, complex mass within the placenta. Most chorioangiomas are small and of no clinical significance. Teratomas also appear as large complex masses.
- Metastatic lesions from melanoma, Ca breast and carcinoma of lung.
- Metastases from fetal neuroblastoma and leukemia.

Trophoblastic Tumors

- Hydatidiform mole is not a neoplastic condition itself but is premalignant is some patients. The normal placenta is completely replaced by an intrauterine, solid echogenic mass with numerous anechoic spaces of varying sizes. Massive bilateral ovarian enlargement with multiple theca lutein cysts may also be associated. Presence of a fetus with true mole is extremely rare

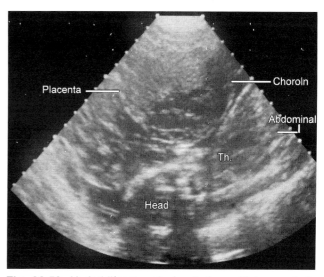

Fig. 29.52: Hydatidiform mole (partial)—multiple anechoic spaces in the region of placenta. Fetal parts are seen adjacent to it.

and usually occurs in case of multiple ovulations with molar transformation of one binovular twin placenta (Fig. 29.51).

- *Partial mole (triploidy):* Sonographically a large placenta which contains multiple, diffuse anechoic areas and a retarded or dysmorphic fetus is seen (Fig. 29.52).
  A few patients may develop an invasive mole characterized by extensive myometrial and parametrial invasion. A small number of patients develop choriocarcinoma with distant metastases and extensive local ulcerations.

Variation in Shape of Placenta

- *Succenturiate lobes:* These are single/multiple accessory lobes of the placenta connected to the main placenta by

fetal blood vessels crossing through the membranes. Their presence could be associated with complications like their retention following delivery, implantation of the accessory lobe over the cervical os and bleeding from the connecting vessels.
- Extrachorial placenta **(Fig. 29.53)**
  - *Circummarginate:* The fetal membranes form a flat ring at the site of attachment to the chorionic plate.
  - *Circumvallate:* Here there is a fold in the membranes at the site of attachment.
  - *Placenta membranacea:* A rare condition in which the entire surface of the amniotic sac is covered with villi due to failure of regression in early pregnancy.
  - *Annular placenta:* Is also rare and probably a variant of the placenta membranacea.

Placenta Creta

In this condition the placenta adheres to (placenta accreta vera), invades (placenta increta) or completely penetrates (placenta percreta) the myometrium because of partial or complete absence of decidua basalis. This usually occurs at the site of uterine scars due to previous cesariean section or other etiology. Nearly one-third of the cases are associated with placenta previa.

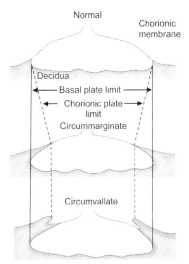

Fig. 29.53: Extrachorial placenta.

Placental Previa (Fig. 29.54)

The placenta is normally situated in the upper uterine segment, and its lower edge may extend into the lower uterine segment.
- *Low lying placenta:* When the lower edge of placenta is within 2 cm from the internal os.

Marginal Previa

- *Marginal placenta:* Previa extends up to the margin of internal os without covering it.
- *Partial placenta previa:* The lower edge of the placenta completely covers the closed internal os.
- Complete placenta previa **(Fig. 29.55)** Could be symmetric (central) or asymmetric. In symmetric the placenta is centered over the internal os and in asymmetric a large part of the placenta is implanted on one side of the cervical os. In both types the internal os is completely covered by the placenta, even when it is fully dilated.

A moderately full bladder is required for the exact localization of the placenta. False positive diagnosis results from:
- Overdistended bladder causing artefactual lengthening (>3.5–4 cm) of the cervical canal.
- Myometrial contractions may simulate placental tissue in an abnormally low location. A repeat scan 30–60 minutes later resolves this problem.
- Due to differential growth of the lower uterine segment a low position detected in early pregnancy may become normal in the third trimester due to so-called placental migration.

Placental Abruption

It is defined as the premature separation of a normally implanted placenta. Sonographic findings depend on the size, site, and age of hematoma.
- *Retroplacental hematomas:* Separate the basal plate of the placenta from the myometrium **(Fig. 29.56)** and are clinically significant if they involve 30–40% of the maternal surface of the placenta. A fresh hematoma is difficult to diagnosis as it is echogenic and isoechoic with the overlying placenta. With time

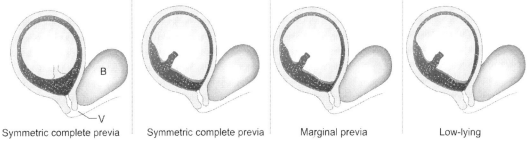

Fig. 29.54: Different types of placenta previa.

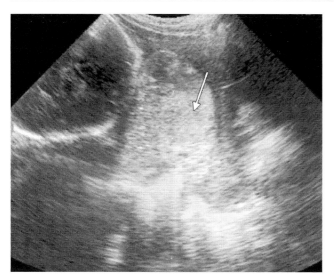

Fig. 29.55: Longitudinal US scan shows central placenta previa (white arrow) lying in between the head and the internal os.

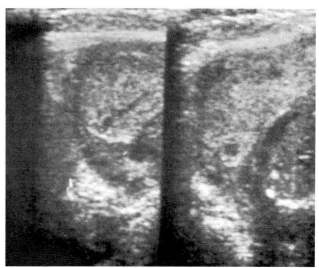

Fig. 29.58: Resolving retroplacental clot—focal isoechoic thickening of the placenta caused by a resolving retroplacental clot.

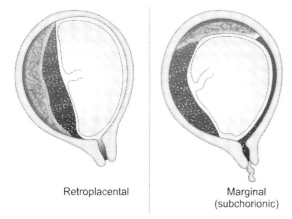

Fig. 29.56: Retroplacental hematomas.

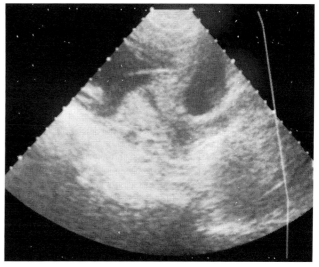

Fig. 29.59: Echolucent area seen in the region of the cervix at the margin of placenta lifting the membranes with internal echoes in it, representing subchorionic hemorrhage.

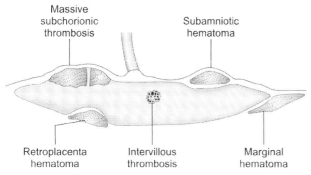

Fig. 29.57: Marginal hematoma.

it eventually becomes heterogeneous and finally anechoic in 1–2 weeks. Differential diagnoses include-a myometrial contraction, a fibroid and the normally seen subplacental venous network.

- *Marginal hematoma:* Includes the subchorionic and the subamniotic bleeds. These are seen at the periphery of the placenta and commonly elevate the edge of the placenta. In some cases they may appear remote from the placenta. Hematoma volumes of less than 60 mL tend to have a favorable outcome (**Figs. 29.57 to 29.59**).
- *Preplacental hematomas:* Also known as massive subchorial thrombosis or Breu's mole are rarer and appear as a mass extending from the anterior placental surface bulging into the amniotic cavity. They are difficult to differentiate from subamniotic hemorrhage, which are also seen on the anterior surface of the placenta.
- *Intraplacental hematomas:* Seen as focal masses of varying echogenicities within the placenta and are related to infarcts and or massive retroplacental hematoma dissecting into the placenta.

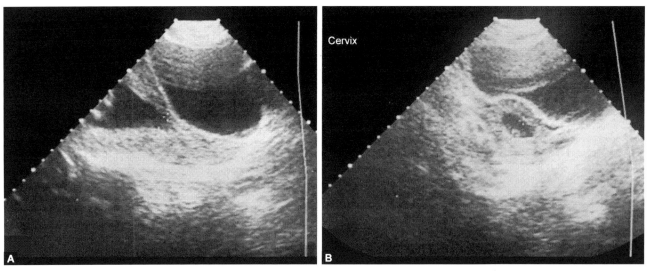

Figs. 29.60A and B: Cervical incompetence—(A) longitudinal; and (B) Transverse scans at the level of internal os. Ultrasound show opened internal os.

- *Intra-amniotic:* May be focal or diffuse and seen as internal echoes in the amniotic fluid.

Umbilical Cord

Normal umbilical cord has three vessels—two equal sized arteries and one larger vein all surrounded by Wharton's jelly. Ten to twenty percent of cases with single umbilical artery are associated with one or more additional malformations including trisomy 18, trisomy 13, urinary tract anomalies CNS and CVS anomalies, omphalocele, sirenomelia and the VATER association.

The normal umbilical cord measure 1–2 cm in diameter, enlargement may be a normal variant or due to edema or hematoma.

Tumors of the umbilical cord are rare and include the echogenic hemangioma and teratoma. Umbilical cysts may also occur.

The umbilical cord usually inserts eccentrically on the fetal surface of the placenta.

Marginal insertion (Battledore placenta): May be seen occasionally and has no clinical significance. The cord may insert on the membranes at a variable distance from the placenta (velamentous insertion). The unprotected intramembranous vessels may bleed in the antepartum period and also during labor and delivery. Vasa previa is the condition where these vessels overly the internal os and color flow Doppler is useful in this situation.

Cervix

Evaluation of the cervix is valuable, both to identify factors such as a large cervical fibroid which may influence the mode of delivery and also for assessment of cervical. Incompetence, changes in length, finding of cervix, and dilatation of the conical canal are important sonographic

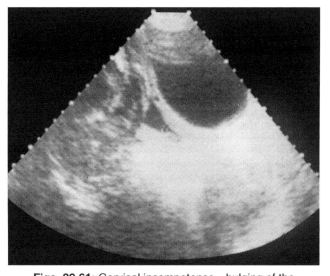

Figs. 29.61: Cervical incompetence—bulging of the membranes with amniotic fluid is seen at the internal os.

findings **(Figs. 29.60 and 29.61)**. Serial measurements allow distinction between nonprogressive shortening of the cervix and true progressive cases of incompetence. It is also possible to check the placement of cerclage and monitor the success or failure of this technique.

There are three approaches to scanning the cervix.

SCANNING TECHNIQUE

- Transabdominal using a 3.5 MHz sector or convex transducer, scanning is done in the midlines of the lower abdomen through a moderately distended urinary bladder.
- Transperineal (translabial) approach-using a 3.5 MHz probe, covered with a plastic scanning is performed with an empty bladder, patient lies supine and hips abducted,

the transducer is placed between the labia minora at the vaginal introitus. The ultrasonic beam is oriented in a sagittal plane along the direction of the vagina. The vagina is seen in a vertical plane between the bladder and the rectum and the cervix is oriented horizontally at a right angle with the vagina.
- *Transvaginal approach:* Endovaginal probes with a wide scanning angle (>90%) allow visualization of the entire cervix provided the probe is inserted only 3.4 cm into the vagina.

Normal Cervix

The endocervical canal appears an echogenic line representing the mucosal interface and mucous plug, surrounded by a hypoechoic zone attributed to endocervical glands. The lower uterine segment and cervix normally have a Y shaped configuration. By the transabdominal approach 30 mm is taken as the lower limit of normal cervical length and less than 8 mm is taken as the normal cervical canal width. With the transvaginal approach 25 mm is taken as the cut off cervical length and anteroposterior diameter of the internal os of >5 mm before 30 weeks of gestation is regarded significant dilatation.

Besides shortening of the cervix and dilatation of the cervical canal, funneling of the internal os (i.e., early herniation of the membranes into the internal cervical os with an intact external os) is an important and in fact an early sign of incompetent cervix. Protrusion of membranes for a distance of >6 mm is significant.

30

CHAPTER

Interventional Radiology

Interventional radiology deals with diagnostic and therapeutic management of pathologic lesions by the radiologist. This management may be palliative, supplementary to other therapy or definitive.

Improvement in imaging technology, especially the 3-dimensional imaging techniques has opened new possibilities of approaching a lesion. Availability of better catheters, guide wires, biopsy sampling instruments and needles, have also contributed to make these techniques simpler, and hence, the radiologists are venturing into newer areas, making interventional radiology a separate, new and adventurous branch of radiology, with a lot of clinical overlap.

Vascular interventional techniques have a longer history than the nonvascular ones. This chapter only intends to provide an introductory overview of these procedures.
Prerequisites of interventional procedures:
- *Informed consent:* Most of the interventional procedures are alternatives to other methods used previously, before interventions became possible. Therefore, consent of the patient as well as that of the referring clinician is not only desirable but mandatory before any intervention is undertaken.
- Assurance and adequate sedation.
- Local anesthesia as required.
- *Complete asepsis:* Complete asepsis of standards equipment, premises and personnel is a must. A separate ultrasound machine/probe or fluoroscopic unit could be reserved for interventional procedures wherever possible. Suitable sterile covers for ultrasound probes and computed tomography (CT) table or fluorotables could be alternatively used.
- Check on and correction if required of bleeding disorders, e.g., prothrombin time.
- Antibiotic/steroid cover wherever required.

Imaging modalities used for guidance in interventional procedures must provide three dimensional information. Fluoroscopic guidance especially with plain fluoroscopy or C-arm; ultrasound guidance or CT scanning are the modalities used for this purpose. Magnetic resonance has rarely been used although its role is being explored at present as a guiding tool for interventional procedures.

Ultrasound provides dynamic information and can visualize the lesion as well as the needle in real-time. It is, perhaps, the most versatile guiding modalities used in hepatobiliary and other abdominal and pelvic interventions. It is also used in thorax, cranium and skeletal lesions wherever an acoustic window is available.

Fluoroscopy is mostly used for vascular interventions, although it can be successfully used for thoracic and bony lesions as well. Although time consuming, CT is ideal modality for management of deep seated and small lesions in abdominal, intrathoracic lesions and for skeletal lesions.

Interventional techniques are broadly classified into nonvascular and vascular procedures.

Nonvascular procedures
- Biopsy techniques
- Drainage techniques for various collections
- Percutaneous or endoscopic stent placement
- Lesion ablation.

Vascular procedures
- Embolization techniques
- Vascular dilatation with or without stenting
- Vascular therapy
    - Chemotherapeutic agents
    - Dilators/constrictors
    - Intravascular thrombolysis
    - Intravascular extractions
    - IVC filters.

NONVASCULAR PROCEDURES

Biopsy Techniques

Various equipments like biopsy track guides used with ultrasound equipment, **(Figs. 30.1A and B)** surface grids tailor-made for CT or mammographic guidance and head frames used for stereotactic guidance under CT/MRI imaging are available to facilitate needle placement in the lesion for obtaining tissue samples for histologic evaluations. However, most experienced radiologists prefer a free hand technique under dynamic imaging control of sonography. Fine needle aspiration (FNA) yields smaller cellular sample and may give false-negative results while

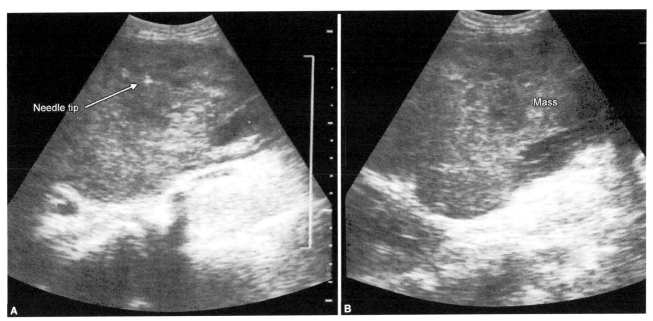

Figs. 30.1A and B: Heterogeneous mass with needle tip in mass for biopsy under ultrasound guidance transverse (A) and longitudinal (B) scan of liver shows.

core biopsy needles although more risky are more efficient in providing the requisite tissue samples. Whenever there is presence of coagulopathies like prolonged prothrombin time and fear of traversing vessels or important organs, FNA is preferred over cutting or boring needles.

At times, the biopsy needle track needs to be embolized after obtaining the tissue sample, e.g., in presence of bleeding tendency or biopsy leakage. In such cases, a coaxial needle is used in which the inner needle obtains the sample while the outer sheath is used to embolize the leak with material like gel foam. Needle placement under CT guidance is more time consuming as repeated scans are required to check the position of the needle tip. However, it is indispensable for transthoracic or of intrapulmonary/mediastinal lesions, small deep-seated abdominal pelvic lesions and even some spinal/skeletal lesions. For fluoroscopic guidance, at times the lesion needs to be rendered radio-opaque by contrast, e.g., by IVU in renal biopsies, ERCP, angiography/renography.

At times, transjugular approach can also be tried in cases with severely deranged coagulation and gross ascites with small lines where percutaneous biopsy is difficult and hazardous.

Drainage Techniques (Fig. 30.2)

Drainage procedures are now accepted and widely used not only as palliative procedures or adjuncts to surgery but as the treatment of choice in various situations.

They are suitable for large collections not responding to medical treatment or where there is fear of impending complications, e.g., large liver abscesses with or without biliary pseudocysts and pancreatic abscesses, large splenic abscesses/perisplenic collections, subphrenic collections,

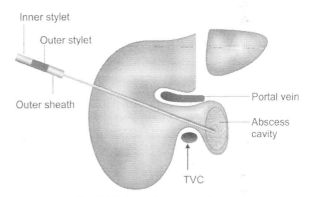

Fig. 30.2: The abscess drainage.

encysted pleural collections, postoperative intra-abdominal collections, bilomas, urinoma, hematometra, pelvic abscesses, and psoas abscesses, etc.

The draining catheter needs to be self retaining, i.e., Foley's, Malecot's or pigtail catheter of appropriate caliber having adequate number or size of draining holes (in case of pigtail catheters which are most frequently used). At times, larger holes are punched on the catheter which is re-sterilized before insertion.

Percutaneous Insertion Techniques

The draining bag used can be an ordinary passive collection bag or bag employing active suction, e.g., concertina suction bag or aseptic syringe. These suction bags providing active drainage are more effective in keeping the cavities collapsed while enhancing healing.

The drainage time may vary from 5 days to even 5 months or even longer in cases where the cavity refills due to a communication. Maintenance of asepsis is of paramount importance during that period. Percutaneous feeding gastrostomy/enterostomy employs the same technique used to place a self retaining catheter in distended stomach under local anesthesia and anchoring it to the skin. It also provides a very useful portal for feeding neurologically ill or debilitated patients.

Similarly percutaneous nephrostomy is a useful technique for decompression of hydronephrotic kidney due to supravesical obstruction. Nephrostomy may further be followed by stricture dilatation, stenting, biopsy, and stone removal, etc. as required in a particular case.

Percutaneous/Endoscopic Stent Placement

Technically, percutaneous stenting is an extension of the percutaneous drainage technique where instead of a draining catheter, a stent is threaded over the guidewire through the dilated tract.

Percutaneous stenting is used extensively in hepatobiliary obstruction as well as in ureteric obstructions.

Endoscopic stent placement is used in lower common bile duct (CBD) obstruction and in esophageal and rectosigmoid strictures. The technique is useful for both benign and malignant strictures.

Hepatobiliary drainage techniques (with or without stenting) are as follows:
- External drainage
- Internal drainage
- Internal-external drainage.

Chief indications for biliary drainage in space occupying lesion (SOL) are:
- Palliation in cases of unresectable growth
- Therapeutic in benign strictures
- Infective obstructive jaundice.

In the percutaneous technique, a guidewire is advanced into the biliary system through the percutaneous transhepatic cholangiographic (PTC) needle and manipulated into the common bile duct with the help of high-torque catheters. The external drainage catheters are mainly for short-term; used whenever the obstruction cannot be passed with the guidewire. Internal drainage catheters are usually self retaining and designed for long-term drainage. Internal drainage is performed by placing stents either percutaneously or endoscopically. Multiple stents may at times be required for multiple levels of obstruction. Usually obstruction at or above porta hepatis is managed percutaneously while below porta endoscopy is preferred. Cholangitis, sepsis, loss of bile salts and electrolytes, biliary peritonitis, pancreatitis, pneumothorax, bilothorax, hemorrhage and hemobilia are the common complications of biliary intervention procedures.

Lesion Ablation

Technique of lesion ablation involves placing a suitable needle at the center of the lesion and causing local tissue death by instilling fluids like alcohol, hypertonic saline or hot contrast material or by coagulating the lesion by heat or laser diathermy.

Unilocular hydatid cysts are effectively treated by alcohol/saline injection. Similarly symptomatic simple cysts of liver and kidney can be ablated by this technique.

Hepatic malignancies like hepatocellular carcinoma shows progressive size reduction on serial intralesional alcohol injections. Similarly, hepatic metastases especially those from colorectal malignancies when less than 4 in number can be effectively treated by laser ablation when the primary is completely resectable.

In cases of induced pregnancies where multiple gestation sacs are common, selective ablation of sacs is accomplished by intrasac or even intracardiac instillation of potassium chloride (KCl) solution.

VASCULAR PROCEDURES

Embolization

A vascular interventionist must be an expert in angiographic technique as these procedures require great skill and experiences. The process of emboliation attempts to cut of completely or partially, the blood supply to a specific region or organ in the body.

The effects of embolation depend on the end organ and the type of embolizing material used. For example, organs like liver with dual blood supply can sustain embolization of hepatic artery while embolization of a renal artery results in definite ablation of the part or whole of the kidney supplied as it has no alternative blood supply.

Total asepsis, adequate sedation and post-procedure analgesia are necessary parts of the procedure.

The catheter tip is placed as selectively as possible to avoid ischemia to adjacent tissues.

Reflux of emboli from catheterized artery must be avoided at all costs as it can result in considerable morbidity and even mortality. Delivery of particulate material must be stopped once the flow is severely reduced.

Ideal embolizing material should be non-toxic, thrombogenic, easy to inject, radio-opaque, rapid, and permanent in effect, sterile, and readily available.

Materials for Embolization

- Absorbable materials
  - Analogous blood clot
  - Oxidized cellulose (Oxycel)
  - Gel foam.
- Nonabsorbable materials
  - Particulate analogous fat/muscle
    Ivalon (Polyvinyl alcohol sponge)
    Silastic spherules
    Silastic and steel spheres
    Acrylic spheres
  - Injectible fluid embolic agents

isobutyl 2-cyano acrylate (IBCA)
Modified IBCA
Tissue glue
Silicon rubber
- Sclerosants
Ethanol
Hypertonic saline
Boiling contrast medium
- Nonparticulate agents
Steel coils
Modified coils
Detachable balloons
- Endovascular electrocoagulation diathermy

Common applications of embolization procedures are as follows:

- *Arteriovenous malformations:* The aim is to use permanent embolic material as distally within the nidus by super selective catheterization of all feeding vessels one by one. Towards the end of the procedure when the blood flow decreases, there is risk of reflux of particulate embolic material into adjacent circulation. This should at all costs be avoided.
- *Arteriovenous fistula:* For example caroticocavernous fistula. Usually a balloon of appropriate size is placed at the fistulous communication. The procedure has minimal risk and shows excellent therapeutic results.
- *Pulmonary AV fistula:* are closed by using coils or balloons; particulate embolic material if used can cross and go into coronary or cerebral circulation with disastrous results.
- *Splenic artery embolization:* Proximal splenic embolization is performed to decrease vascularity or to occlude a splenic artery aneurysm or an acutely bleeding vessel. Distal splenic artery embolization is performed as an alternative to splenectomy. This procedure has many complications like splenic abscess formation, rupture, necrosis of gastric wall, pancreatitis, etc.
- *Management of acute gastrointestinal (GI) bleeding:* Embolization is helpful in upper GI hemorrhage as lots of collaterals exist. In lower GI bleeding, the complications outweigh the uses of embolization and collateral circulation is very poor. Microcatheters are used for super selective arterial canalization and embolization.
- *Management of hemoptysis:* Massive life-threatening hemoptysis due to tuberculosis, bronchiectasis or malignant disease can be effectively managed only by embolization of the responsible bronchial artery.
- Preoperative embolization to decrease tumor vascularity is required in highly vascular tumors like nasopharyngeal angio-fibroma, glomus jugulare, renal cell carcinoma, hepatic tumors etc.
- Internal pudendal artery embolization in cases of priapism is preferred over medical management which is ineffective and over surgical management which is more often detrimental to future physiological functioning.
- *Venous embolization:* Embolization of testicular veins by balloons or coils is a standard treatment for varicoceles. Obliteration of adrenal veins is also at times performed in cases of Cushing syndrome secondary to adrenal tumors.

Complications of Embolization

General: General complications of embolization procedures are same as those due to the angiographic procedures or due to contrast reaction.

Specific: Immediate postembolization complications may vary from mild to severe in clinical importance; pain, and nausea are relatively common while embolization of adjacent normal structures, adherence of catheter tip to vessel wall by liquid adhesives and reaction to embolic agents are uncommon but severe reactions.

Delayed reactions include pain, fever, infection, septicemia, tissue infarction and necrosis, extension of the thrombus beyond intended area and acute renal failure secondary to tissue necrosis and dehydration.

Any of the above severe reactions may potentially result in iatrogenic mortality.

Vascular Therapy

Chemoembolization

High concentrations of a chemotherapeutic agent can be superselectively delivered to one organ by this technique. The agent may be mixed with iodized oils and particulate embolic material. The technique is used for certain musculoskeletal, genitourinary, and gastrointestinal neoplasia.

Constrictor/Dilator Therapy

Constrictors like vasopressin or dilators like papaverine, nitroglycerine, etc. are used during angiography to improve the quality of vascular opacification. Vasopressin in the dose of 0.1 to 0.4 IU/Kg body weight is used to control active GI bleeding. Dilators may be used as adjuncts to angioplasties in management of stenotic vascular lesions.

Intra-arterial Thrombolysis

Agents like streptokinase, urokinase, prourokinase and plasminogen activator cause local thrombolysis when delivered selectively at the site of thrombus by catheters. Urokinase is being used in treatment of coronary artery thrombolysis, embolic stroke, and pulmonary embolism with encouraging results. In peripheral arteries and in cases of central venous thrombolysis, the therapy has been recognized as standard. Certain cases of loculated pleural effusion and peritonitis instillation of thrombolytic agents locally help in disruption of dense adhesions and septations.

Transluminal Angioplasty

Transluminal angioplasty is widely used as an alternative to surgical angioplasty in different parts of the body. Initially PTA was used in atherosclerotic narrowing of passage but now variety of other lesions like congenital defects fibromuscular dysplasia, arteritis and other lesions causing vessel narrowing are also being managed by this technique. The basic technique in PTA is to place the balloon catheter in the region of vascular stenosis, dilating the balloon under fluoroscopic control resulting in distention of the stenotic segment, and thereby improving blood flow. The narrowed segment is crossed with the guidewire and contrast injected to delineate the exact length and position of the lesion which are marked with radio-opaque markers. The exchange wire is replaced over the diagnostic catheter and balloon catheter is then introduced over it and manipulated into the stenosis. Careful inflation to predetermine volumes of the balloon must be done under fluoroscopic guidance.

The balloon inflation is maintained for one to two minutes. A check angiogram is done to evaluate the effect of dilatation and to look for complications, if any. If required repeated balloon dilatations are done at later dates to achieve better results. Main complications of PTA include groin hematomas, distal embolic complications, elevation of intimal flaps, false aneurysm, and arterial rupture. Transluminal angioplasty of renal arteries is a standard procedure for management of renovascular hypertension. Stenotic lesions resulting from various causes like atherosclerosis, fibromuscular dysplasia and aortoarteritis are managed by PTA. In experienced hands, the results of renal angioplasty compare favourably with surgical results. In lower extremities, management of arterial stenosis which may be isolated or multiple is successfully done by PTA. In fact, PTA is performed in almost any vessel which if dilated will improve the end organ perfusion.

Alternatives to PTA or adjuncts to PTA have come to stay in interventional vascular radiology due to various reasons.

- Arterial blockage which do not allow the guidewire in which case a passage needs to be created by using various newer methods like application of heat (lasers, radiofrequency probes), mechanical energy (atherectomy catheters, atherolytic wires), or thrombolytic agents.
- Restenosis is generally managed by reducing atheromatous bulk using lasers and also by providing supportive framework with intravascular stents. One or more new developments in the interventional vascular work is the introduction of angioscopes, which are miniaturized flexible fiberoptic bundles that can be introduced percutaneously to visualize the arterial lumen.

The impact of interventional techniques has been very profound in clinical medicine. The intervention is practically applied to every branch of medicine. The greatest benefits of interventional radiology include reduction of mortality, hospitalization costs, and in selected areas is considered as the primary modality of choice in the clinical management of the patient. The discriminating application of interventional radiology can bring benefits in completely avoiding surgery or postponement of major procedures.

31
CHAPTER

Color Doppler

INTRODUCTION

Doppler effect is observed in every day life due to relative motion of sound waves between sound source and observer. But Doppler principle and effect was originally formulated by Austrian Mathematician and Scientist, Johann Christian Doppler in 1942. It was Satomura who first used this to measure blood flow in the heart in 1956. Since then, the clinical uses of blood flow imaging have expanded and refined to present day medical applications of Doppler.

Ultrasound imaging is especially useful in showing cardiovascular anatomy and detecting the flowing blood through many points within the vascular system. Various approaches for identification of the moving structures include relative pulse echo imaging, motion mode (M mode) display of reflected ultrasound pulse, and the Doppler's shift method.

Doppler systems emit a short burst of ultrasound waves which is then reflected off the moving blood and return to the transducer at a different frequency dependent on the speed and direction of moving blood. The change in sound frequency caused by moving blood can be displayed as a color image, spectral waveform pattern or as an audible signal.

Doppler Effect

When there is relative motion between a source and a receiver of ultrasound, the frequency of the received ultrasound differs from that emitted by the source.

If the source and receiver are moving away from each other, the frequency measured by the observer will be lower than the frequency measured by stationary observer. Conversely, if they are moving towards each other, the frequency will be higher. This difference between the frequency of sound emitted and received is known as a frequency shift.

The shift in frequency (f_D) is given by
$$f_D = 2f_o v/c$$
f_o = True frequency
c = Speed of sound
v = Velocity of source

If an object is moving towards the source, shift in frequency is positive while if object is moving away from source, the Doppler shift (f_D) is negative, that is the frequency of detected ultrasound is lower than that emitted by the source.

The above discussion has assumed that ultrasound beam is parallel to the motion of an object. If the source and observer are not moving directly towards or opposite to each other, but an angle θ, then the equation becomes,
$$f_D = \frac{v\cos\theta}{c}$$

This technique is used to study motion, primarily that of circulatory system. This is based on scattering of ultrasound beam by red blood cell (RBC) known as Rayleigh Tyndall scattering. Since RBCs are not continuous they act as rough surface and are the particulate components of blood that interact with the ultrasound.

The Doppler frequency f_D is defined as the difference between received and transmitted frequency and is given by:
$$f_D = f_r - f_o = \frac{2f_o n \cos\theta}{c}$$

f_r is receiver frequency and f_o is transmitted frequency; θ is called Doppler angle.

As a general guideline, the Doppler angle should be between 30 and 60 degrees whenever possible.

Determining the volumetric flow of blood in the units of cubic centimeter per second requires an estimation of the area of vessel as well as Doppler angle. Volumetric flow Q is the product of average velocity v and cross section area of A of vessel
$$Q = vA$$

Instrumentation

Basic Doppler systems used in Doppler sonography is
- Continuous wave Doppler
- Single-gated pulsed wave Doppler
- Multi-gated pulsed wave Doppler
- Duplex Doppler
- Color flow imaging
- Power Doppler imaging.

Continuous Wave Doppler (CW Doppler)

The most basic Doppler system through which first Doppler blood velocity measurements were performed is a continuous wave Doppler system.

Such a system requires a separate transmitter and receiver, i.e., two piezoelectric transducers mounted in same enclosure.

Basic CW Doppler units are simple to use as they usually have only a few controls, like the transmitting power to vary the amplitude of signal from the transmitter to transducer thus changing the sensitivity to weak echoes whereas some simple units omit this control as well keeping the transmitting level constant.

A basic CW Doppler instrument allows detection of magnitude of Doppler frequency, but it provides no information of whether flow is towards or away from the transducer that is whether Doppler shift is positive or negative.

Since the frequencies used in medical ultrasound and velocity encountered in the human body combines to produce Doppler frequency shift in audible range, it is customary to send the Doppler signal directly to loudspeakers and significant diagnostic information can be obtained from the audio output.

Another way of processing the Doppler signal is to digitize it in an analogue to digital converter (ADC) and then use, Fast Fourier Transform (FFT) to extract the spectral information.

Continuous wave instruments are good for superficial vessel such as carotid. They are also very sensitive to weak signal such as might be found in digital artery of a finger. CW system has no limit on the maximum velocity measures and can therefore measure any velocity correctly. Other advantage includes the high accuracy of Doppler shift estimate with the narrow frequency band width that is used.

However, this system suffers from few major constraints. Since the information is received from an entire ultrasound beam, it is impossible to determine the depth of specific blood vessel and also it does not provides information whether flow is towards or away from the transducer (that is whether Doppler shift is positive or negative) and thus the direction of the flow cannot be determined.

Pulsed Wave Doppler (PW Doppler)

Pulsed wave Doppler unit use the echo ranging principle to provide quantitative depth information of the Doppler signals from different depths, thus allowing detection of moving interface and scatter only from within a well-defined sample volume. This sample volume can be positioned any where along the axis of the ultrasound beam. Depth selection is achieved with the use of electronic gating.

In PW Doppler, scattered and reflected echo signal are detected by same transducer. The transducer is excited with a short duration burst and then no sound sent for brief period of time that is transducer is silent for a period of time to listen for echoes before another burst of ultrasound is generated. This differs from continuous wave Doppler where one transducer is continuously excited.

Detected signal is amplified by receiver and applied to demodulator. The received signal is electronically gated for processing so that only those echoes detected in a narrow time interval after pulse, corresponding to a specific depth contribute to the Doppler signal and all other echoes are rejected by the electronics. Gate parameter such as position (axial location of the sample volume or depth) and duration are controlled by operator and can be adjusted.

The received echo must be evaluated to determine if the reflector is moving. This is accompanied by comparing the phase of the echo with a reference signal for which phase is synchronized with the transmitter pulse. Two waves are described as being in phase if their maximum, minimum and zero point occur concurrently. The echo from stationary reflector has the same phase as the reference signal where as the echoes from moving structure undergoes a phase shift via the Doppler Effect.

The system is repeatedly pulsed. The pulse repetition frequency (PRF) is the frequency at which sound pulses are transmitted. One sample per period is acquired until enough data for an accurate estimation of Doppler shift have been collected, (typically 64–128 samples). The technique is known as range gating.

Limitation of Doppler Systems

The use of CW and PW Doppler ultrasound raises a number of problems and ambiguities all of which influence the performance of Color Flow Images (CFI) system as well.

Even when only one vessel is studied and only one frequency is emitted, a range of Doppler frequencies will be received. This phenomenon is known as spectral broadening. It is due to either to flow profile variation within the vessel or to transit time effect. The latter is a fundamental uncertainty inherent in Doppler measurement.

An echo must have returned to the receiver before the next pulse is transmitted, if the depth of origin is to be unambiguously determined. The maximum depth accessible is therefore limited by the propagation or velocity and the interpulse duration of the system (i.e., 1/PRF).

Further more, there is a limit to the maximum velocity measurable. This is due to digitization applied. If the Doppler signal changes too rapidly then it is impossible to reconstruct the correct Doppler shift frequency. This is known as aliasing.

To avoid aliasing the PRF must be at least 2 times the frequency of Doppler signal to construct the signal successfully. When PRF equals $2 \times f_D$, it is known as Nyquist limit. If the frequency of Doppler shift is above Nyquist limit then aliasing occur.

To measure reflector moving with high velocity and producing large Doppler shift a high PRF is necessary. But a high PRF limits the depth that can be sampled because a certain time is required to collect the echoes arising from that depth before the next pulse is sent out. So while the maximum velocity measurable, v_{max} increases with increasing PRF, the maximum depth measurable, d_{max} decreases.

The maximum depth and velocity are inversely related. As sample volume depth increases the maximum detectable Doppler signal frequencies increases and hence the maximum reflector velocity that can be detected decreases.

The trade off between maximum velocity and depth measurement constitute an important compromise inherent in PW Doppler system.

An additional problem affecting all Doppler scanner is the angular dependence when converting the Doppler shift from a frequency (in Hz) to a velocity in (m/s).

MULTIGATED PW DOPPLER SYSTEMS

A single-gated PW Doppler system limits the information to one particular location or depth along the scan line. In order to obtain data from several depths simultaneously a so called multigated (MG) PW Doppler system must be employed. Multigated PW systems typically contain 64–128 gates with a minimum axial length of 1mm for each sample volume.

Basically after demodulation the received signal is directed to a number of parallel processing channels. Each has a slightly different range gate setting. This allows number of adjacent sample volumes to be positioned across a vessel. The problem of locating a vessel is greatly reduced.

Since the assessment of the blood flow velocity is performed simultaneously in each sample volume, the velocity distribution along the vessel cross section can be determined as a function of time. The velocity profile will be influenced by the presence of for example plaques or stenosis and can be therefore a useful diagnostic tool.

Duplex Doppler Systems

In spite of the advantage afforded by MG Doppler system, orientation and locating the desired vessel remain a problem. One way to overcome this is to combine 2D B-mode scan with flow information from Pulsed wave Doppler data. The first such combined system was referred to as Duplex Doppler scanner. This is because without some visual guidance to the vessel of interest, PW Doppler would be of little use.

In Duplex system, a PW Doppler beam is visualized across the B-mode image with a sample volume position indicated by a cursor. This permits vessels to be easily selected for further evaluation.

An advantage of a Duplex system is that the angle of incidence can be estimated from the B-mode. Thus Doppler frequency shift can be transferred to flow velocity estimates. One should always have a beam flow angle from 30 to 60 degree. In spite of the name "Duplex" the B-mode and Doppler scanning do not occur simultaneously. It takes significantly longer to acquire Doppler data than B-mode data, and early Duplex scanner often "freez" the B-mode completely when obtaining flow information.

The loss of real-time imaging was a major drawback. More recently Duplex system employed mechanical changes that might lower the frame rate but will not freeze the image.

The Doppler method has a number of applications in clinical medicine, including detection of fetal heart beat, detection of air embolism, blood pressure monitoring, detection and characterization of blood flow and localization of blood vessel occlusion.

To understand all the clinical applications of Doppler to imaging, it is necessary to understand basic principles of the dynamics of blood circulation (normal physiology of blood circulation) and the hemodynamics of occlusive disease.

Blood Flow Dynamics

Flow between two points in certain direction occurs only when there is difference in energy level (pressure gradient) between these two points.

Circulatory system generally consists of a high pressure, high energy, arterial reservoir and a venous pool of low pressure and energy. These reservoirs are connected by a system of distributing vessels (smaller arteries) and by the resistance vessels of the microcirculation, which consists of arterioles, capillaries and venules. During flow, energy (pressure and energy levels) is continuously lost from arterial to the venous ends due to internal friction/viscosity. The volume and pressure in arteries should be within limits for smooth function and this is achieved by maintaining a balance between the amount of blood that enters and leaves the arterial reservoir. The amount that enters the arteries depends on the cardiac output. The amount that leaves depends on the arterial pressure and on the total peripheral resistance which is controlled in turn by the amount of vasoconstriction in the microcirculation.

Under normal circumstances, flow to all the body organs and tissues is adjusted according to tissues particular need at a given time.

Arterial System

Laminar Flow

In most vessels, blood moves in concentric layers and hence, the flow is said to be laminar. The flow velocity profile in the initial portion of the segment is very flat (entrance effect, plug flow), further along the distal segment the flow gradually reaches its steady-state parabolic velocity profile.

The relation between flow volume per unit time q, viscosity η, length of vascular segment l, vessel radius r and pressure difference (P_2-P_1) at proximal and distal end of tube is described by Hagen and Poiseuille's law as expressed in equation as:

$$P_2 - P_1 = \frac{8l\eta q}{r^4}$$

Because the length of the vessels and the viscosity of blood do not change much in the cardiovascular system, alteration in blood flow occur mainly as a result of changes in the radius of the vessels and in the difference in the pressure energy level available for flow. Hence, the Poiseuille's equation can be written as:

$$R = \frac{P_2 - P_1}{q}$$

Hence, by measuring pressure difference and blood flow (q), the resistance can thus be calculated.

In small vessels, there is significant resistance to flow. The major part of the total resistance of vascular system originates from the arterioles—the part of arterial vascular tree with the largest capacity for vasomotor regulation.

Pulsatile Flow

The pulsatile variation in blood volume and energy occurring with each cardiac cycle are manifested as a pressure wave that can be detected throughout the arterial system. Pulsatile changes in pressure are associated with corresponding acceleration of blood flow with systole and deceleration in diastole.

The arteries become progressively stiffer from the aorta towards the periphery. Therefore, the speed of propagation of the wave increases as it moves peripherally (as it increases with stiffness of arterial walls). Therefore, the pulse and systolic pressure in the aorta and proximal arteries are relatively lower than in peripheral vessels.

Disturbed Flow and Turbulence

Various degree of deviation from normal laminar flow occurs in the circulation under both normal and abnormal conditions. Various factors responsible for these deviations are—the flow velocity (changes throughout the cardiac cycle), alteration in the lines of flow (vessel changes dimension with each pulse), types of flow (distorted at curves, bifurcations).

Turbulent flow can be recognized in color Doppler study by a mixture of different color pixels next to one another representing flow in different directions.

The existence of turbulent flow depend on the vessel diameter d (2r), the average flow velocity v, across the lumen, the density of the fluid and viscosity of the fluid.

Turbulence develops more readily in large vessels under conditions of high flow and can be detected clinically by the findings of bruits or thrills. Distortion of laminar flow velocity profile can be assessed using ultrasound flow detectors, and such assessments can be applied for diagnostic purpose, e.g., in arteries with severe stenosis, pronounced turbulence is a diagnostic feature observed in poststenotic zone.

Hemodynamics at Stenosis

A basic understanding of flow dynamic is essential for the correct interpretation of most phenomena encountered in Doppler studies of arterial system. Prestenotic, intrastenotic and poststenotic changes in absolute and relative flow velocities and flow pattern are the variables that lead to a correct diagnosis and permit a quantitative assessment of pathologic finding regardless of Doppler technology used.

The detection and determination of the severity of vascular stenosis with Doppler ultrasound is based on recording the relative velocity increase or Doppler frequency shift that is produced by the stenosis.

The degree of stenosis can be determined from velocity measurements only by measuring both intrastenotic flow velocity and the flow velocity at a more distal site in a segment having normal lumen size, well away from stenotic jet or turbulence. Alternatively, the degree of proximal stenoses of internal carotid artery can be estimated from empirically derived ratios of the maximum systolic velocities at the prestenotic and intrastenotic levels.

There are two basic methods in Duplex sonography for determining the severity of a stenoses on the basis of flow velocity.

As a basic rule, the maximum flow velocity in a given vascular segment should be measured. The use of maximum systolic velocities permits the most accurate assessment of the degree of stenoses. If the time averaged velocities are used, the severity of the lesion will be underestimated due to entrance effects and changes in the flow velocity profile during pulse cycle.

It is also absolutely mandatory to perform a Doppler angle correction when flow velocities are calculated from Doppler frequency shift.

Intrastenotic and Poststenotic Flow Changes

Distal to stenosis, the maximum flow velocity continues to be elevated (Poststenotic jet) at least in certain zone of the vascular cross section with exit effects playing significant roles. This may cause marked turbulence to develop in the poststenotic segments in addition to zones of flow separation and flow reversal along the vessel walls.

Turbulence and flow reversal are easily recognized in color duplex imaging using Doppler frequency analysis. Turbulent flow produces broadening of the Doppler spectrum that may completely fill in the systolic window beneath the spectrum envelope and simultaneous occurrence of positive and negative Doppler frequency shifts.

VENOUS HEMODYNAMICS

In large veins such as the vena cava, flow and pressure changes during the cardiac cycle. Such oscillation in pressure and flow at times is transmitted to more peripheral vessels.

There are three positive pressure waves. These reflect corresponding changes in pressure in atria. Wave 'a' is caused by atrial contraction and relaxation. The upstroke of 'c' wave is related to the increase in pressure when the atrioventricular values are closed and bulge during isovolumetric ventricular contraction. The subsequent down stroke results from the fall in pressure caused by pulling the atrioventricular valve rings towards the apex of heart during ventricular contraction. The upstroke of 'v' wave results from a passive rise in atrial pressure during ventricular systole when the atrioventricular valve are closed and atria fill with blood from the peripheral veins. The 'v' wave downstroke is caused by fall in pressure that occurs where the blood leaves the atria rapidly and fills the ventricles soon after the opening of atrioventricular valve early in ventricular diastole.

In abnormal condition such as congestive heart failure or tricuspid insufficiency venous pressure is increased and this leads to the transmission of phasic changes in pressure and flow to the peripheral vein of the upper and lower limb.

Venous Effect of Respiration

Respiration has profound effect as venous pressure and flow. During inspiration, the volume in the veins of thorax increases and the pressure decreases in response to reduced intrathoracic pressure. Expiration leads to the opposite effect, with decreased venous volume and increased pressure. The venous response to respiration is reversed in the abdomen where the pressure increases during inspiration because of the descent of diaphragm and decreases during expiration as the diaphragm ascends. Increased abdominal pressure during inspiration decreases pressure gradient between peripheral veins in the lower extremities and the abdomen thus reducing flow in the peripheral vessels while opposite effect is seen during expiration.

In the veins of the upper limbs, the changes in flow with respiration are opposite to those in the lower extremities because of reduced intrathoracic pressure during inspiration.

Venous Obstruction

Venous obstruction can be acute or chronic. In the case of severe chronic obstruction, edema may occur.

Acute obstruction, usually associated with thrombosis may lead to potentially fatal pulmonary embolism. Color Doppler and duplex scanning may be used for the diagnosis.

The presence or absence of obstruction is also gauzed by increasing flow towards the site of examination by squeezing the limb distally or by activating the distal muscle group and thus increasing venous flow towards the flow detecting probe. This is called augmentation and absence of increased flow/augmentation suggests obstruction between the probe location and the site from which the enhancement of venous flow was attempted.

When veins are competent, flow in peripheral veins, is towards the heart. When there are incompetent veins proximally, there may be retrograde filling in the peripheral veins such as those in ankle region. This feature is evaluated better with Valsalva maneuver as mild incompetence is also unmasked on greatly increased abdominal pressure.

Display of Doppler Information

The blood flow information (direction as well as magnitude of flow) obtained through Doppler can be displayed variably for example as color (Color flow imaging), spectral pattern (Duplex Doppler) or an audible signal.

Color Flow Imaging

This imaging is one of most important development in ultrasound imaging. This imaging method superimposes a blood flow image on a standard gray scale, ultrasound image, permitting instantaneous visual assessment of blood flow. The estimated velocity of each sample volume is mapped in a color representing the direction of flow as well as its magnitude (via the color and hue).

Typically shades of red and blue are used for flow towards and away respectively, from the transducer. The variance of velocity estimate, i.e., spectral broadening of the Doppler signal can be included as a third color often green. The blood flow information provided by CFI is qualitative and not quantitative.

Principles of Color Flow Imaging

Color Doppler instruments are different from gray scale instrument because they use the Doppler shift information besides information of distance from echo to the transducer and strength of echo. Therefore the information from a color Doppler image is:
- The site of the echo or depth of the signal
- The strength or amplitude of ultrasound signal
- The Doppler frequency shift present
- The magnitude of the Doppler frequency shift which is proportionate to the blood flow velocity and the Doppler angle
- The direction of the Doppler shift

It is customary to show flow in one direction in blue and flow in the other direction in red. However, the operator can select other color schemes if desired. The way to show color has two different ways:
1. Different colors are used to represent different frequency levels (e.g., blue, green, yellow, white with increasing frequency).
2. *Changing shades method:* Here same color is used but the color gets lighter as frequency increases (e.g., dark red, light red pink and white).

Clinical Advantages of Color Flow Imaging

Perhaps the greatest advantage of color flow imaging is technical efficiency. When moving blood is encountered, the vessel lights up even if the vessel is too small to be resolved on the gray scale image. Because vessels stand out in vivid color, they may be located and follow much more easily than with gray scale instruments. Further more basic judgement about blood flow can be made easy with color flow imaging. One can quickly determine the presence or absence of flow, the direction of flow and the presence of local flow disturbances and therefore sonographer can quickly examine long vascular segments such as vascular bypass graft, with relative ease.

Another advantage of color flow imaging simplifies differentiation between vascular and nonvascular structure, which is particularly useful in the abdomen, e.g., porta hepatis anatomy.

Flow assessment in entire lumen, a major advantage of color flow imaging is the depiction of blood flow throughout a large segment of a vessel, rather than solely at the Doppler sample volume. Because flow features are visible over a large area, localized flow abnormalities are readily apparent and are less likely to be overlooked than with gray scale Duplex methods. The sonographer becomes immediately aware of the location of any flow abnormalities which speeds up the examination and permit rapid assessment of long segment of vessels for obstruction and other pathology.

As compared with gray scale ultrasound, color flow imaging makes it easier to define the residual lumen in stenotic vessels permitting more precise visual measurement of arterial stenoses.

The ability of color flow imaging to detect low velocity flow in a tiny residual lumen may facilitate the differentiation between occlusion of an artery and near occlusion with a trickle of residual flow.

Limitation of Color Flow Imaging

Flow information is qualitative because:
- Flow image is based on the average Doppler shift within the vessel, rather than the peak Doppler shift and therefore is not helpful for actually grading the stenosis.
- It is not corrected for Doppler angle.
- Only a few frequency levels are shown.

Power Doppler Flow Imaging

Power or intensity of Doppler signal is measured and mapped and thus ignores the velocity of Doppler signal detected from each location.

The amplitude and this intensity or a power of back scattered signal depends on the number of RBCs present within the sample volume, the size of vessel and the attenuation of intervening tissue. Since the Doppler frequency shift information is not utilized, power Doppler images is nondirectional and does not suffer from aliasing. The advantages of this modality over color flow imaging are therefore:
- Power Doppler imaging is more sensitive in detecting blood flow. Hence, anything that represents noise is blue and anything that represents flow is another color (usually gold).
- Power Doppler imaging is not affected by aliasing. Even the aliased portion of signal has the power and can be displayed as flow.
- Power Doppler is significantly less angle dependent.
- Power Doppler display improves in functional lumen definition.
- Since the advent of ultrasound contrast agents, Power Doppler imaging is less subject to blooming than the standard color Doppler imaging. Blooming is the spread of color outside of the blood vessel that occurs when amplification of Doppler signal is too great.

The two major limitations of power Doppler imaging are:
1. Frame rate is slow, which render this imaging method useless for rapidly moving vessels, rapidly moving patients (especially children) and areas subject to respiratory or cardiac motion.
2. Power Doppler imaging does not provide flow direction information and therefore cannot assess effects such as pulsatility and flow reversal.

Because the color flow images are qualitative, Doppler spectrum analysis must be used to derive detailed quantitative flow data. The spectral pattern provides a real-time display of the detected range of frequencies with time on horizontal axis and Doppler shift frequency on the vertical axis.

In addition to such qualitative uses of Doppler technique, spectral analysis of the signals allows more detailed quantitation. The outline of the maximum Doppler shift frequency corresponds to the time variation of the maximum flow velocity within the vessel. The pulsatility of this waveform is related to the vascular impedance downstream to the point of measurement. In addition, the range of frequency present in the Doppler spectrum yields information about distribution of velocities across the vessel lumen. This provides evidence of the flow conditions, whether there is a plug or parabolic flow profile, whether there are flow disturbances or turbulence related to vessel wall abnormality.

Clinical Applications of Doppler Imaging

A Doppler examination can be undertaken to simply confirm the presence or absence of flow or determine direction of blood flow, for example in patients with cirrhosis, reversed flow in the portal vein may accompany severe portal hypertension. The presence of flow in portal vein or renal vessels can be most helpful in excluding occlusion, while flow signals from solid mass can indicate neovascularization associated with malignancy.

The Doppler characteristic which can be quantified using a variety of parameters, enable a description of a signal that is fairly specific to a particular vessel or even vessel site. Alteration of the normal pattern occurs in various disease conditions causing local, regional or generalized hemodynamic changes evident on Doppler examination.

RETROPERITONEAL VESSELS

Aorta

The abdominal aorta is a compliant tube that supplies blood to the digestive organs, the kidneys, the adrenals, the gonads, the abdominal, paraspinal musculature the pelvis, and lower limbs. It contributes significantly to the continuous forward flow of blood during diastole by acting as a reservoir of fluid during systole when it has a very pulsatile, inflow.

The main aortic branches that are frequently seen on ultrasound are the coeliac artery, the superior mesenteric artery, and the paired renal arteries. At the L4 level, it bifurcates into paired common iliac arteries, which further bifurcates into external and internal iliac arteries.

Good acoustic window for scanning the abdominal aorta include:
- The midline in the upper abdomen
- The left flank.

The entire aorta should be visualized in transverse and longitudinal planes and its maximum anteroposterior and transverse diameter measured accurately. At sonography aorta is shown as a hypoechoic tubular structure with echogenic walls. It is usually located just to the left of the midline. The abdominal aorta tapers from its cranial to caudal and usually measures less than 2.3 cm in diameter for men and 1.9 cm for women. The normal flow pattern in the aorta is classified as plug flow, a situation in which most of the blood is moving at the same velocity showing a clear window below the systolic time velocity pulse **(Figs. 31.1A and B)**. During the remainder of diastole there is some low velocity antegrade flow. In iliac arteries, flow is typically of the high resistance type with a sharp increase in antegrade velocity during systole followed by a rapid decrease in velocity and culminating in a brief period of reversed flow. In fact, this flow that is found below the renal vessels results in the renal arterial flow being maintained during diastole. Relatively continuous flow in the renal artery may be of importance in renal function.

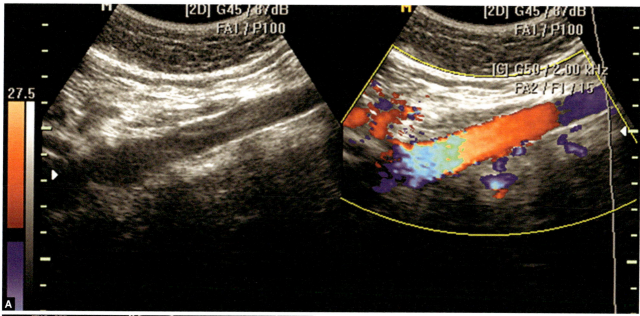

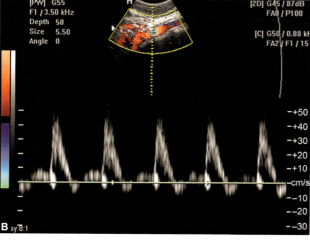

Figs. 31.1A and B: B-mode and color Doppler image (A) and spectral Doppler from aorta (B).

Aortic Pathology

The abdominal aorta and its main branches are affected by atheroma, aneurysm formation, connective tissue disorders, rupture, thrombosis, infections and displacement by and invasion from disease in adjacent structures.

Atheromatous Disease

Atheroma or arteriosclerosis is a vascular wall disorder characterized by the presence of lipid deposits in the intima causing luminal stenosis of the aorta, iliac arteries and the other aortic branch arteries. Stenotic or occlusive disease most often occurs in the infrarenal portion of the aorta. Atheroma may also be associated with mural weakening and aneurysm formation.

Ultrasound can demonstrate thickening and calcification of the aortic intima. Patency of the aorta and its branch vessels can be confirmed with color Doppler analysis and where aliasing occurs, a Doppler spectral tracing helps to determine whether a true stenosis is present or not and determine the grade of stenosis into five categories (i) Normal (ii) 1-19% diameter reduction (iii) 20-49% diameter reduction (iv) 50-99% diameter reduction (v) Total occlusion.

Stenosis of 50-99% diameter reduction is considered hemodynamically significant. Reverse velocity is absent in these stenosis, the systolic peak is increased by 100% or more and spectral broadening is usually prominent. Occluded arteries have no detectable flow and velocity is markedly decreased in the segments proximal to occlusion.

Thus, duplex scanning can localize and classify peripheral arterial stenosis. It is helpful to the angiographer to tailor the angiography technique to fit the needs of patient. Angiography is the definitive test for symptomatic aortic iliac disease. The invasive nature and relative high cost of angiography makes it unsuitable for screening purpose or routine follow-up.

In addition, duplex scanning provides a baseline for assessing the early and long-term results of PTA. Duplex scanning can detect restenosis of segments dilated by angioplasty or bypass graft stenosis.

The ability of duplex scanning to distinguish high grade stenosis from occlusion, to detect hemodynamically significant disease and to localize disease accurately is unique among noninvasive tests.

Aortic Aneurysms

Abdominal aortic aneurysm is a common disease with potentially catastrophic complications like rupture with a high mortality of 50-90%, while elective surgical resection has an excellent prognosis and low mortality (2-4%). Most patients are asymptomatic and not diagnosed until detected on imaging.

A true aneurysm of abdominal aorta is a localized dilatation of wall greater than 3 cm in diameter containing all these layers of the vessel while false aneurysm (pseudoaneurysm) is essentially a perforation of the aorta with subsequent hematoma formation limited by adventitial or surrounding vascular. Growth of aneurysm is approximately at 4 mm per year and the risk of rupture increase over 5 cm.

Sonography and color Doppler are ideal for screening and follow-up of uncomplicated aneurysms. It also helps in recognizing complications of abdominal aortic aneurysm like rupture, thrombosis, dissection, distal embolism, and invasion of adjacent structures. Most common complications are branch artery occlusions or stenosis due to atheroma rather than with aneurysm, most commonly involving inferior mesenteric artery and renal artery. Rupture of an aneurysm appears as a pulsating hematoma or a hypoechoic collection in the periaortic region.

A dissecting aortic aneurysm is easily recognized on sonography with the classical appearance being a thin membrane fluttering in the lumen at different phases of cardiac cycle. Color Doppler shows blood flow in both channels, although flow rates frequently differ between the channels. Color Doppler also distinguishes a true dissection from a pseudodissection which is caused by liquefaction of aneurysm thrombus by absence of fluttering of the intravascular membrane, no flow in one lumen and a thick membrane in pseudolesion.

Abdominal aortic pseudoaneurysm formation involves an arterial injury, local hemorrhage and tamponade by surrounding tissues. It is an organized perivascular hematoma that has a lumen in continuity with the vascular lumen.

On gray scale sonography, pseudoaneurysms appear as anechoic saccular collections in proximity to arteries. These collections are more easily perceived by color flow mapping. The final diagnosis with Duplex Doppler sonography requires identification of the typical flow pattern within the neck of the pseudoaneurysm. It shows turbulent or arterial-like flow (swirling or whirl wind flow) within the pseudo-aneurysm lumen and systolic and diastolic continuous flow and the classic 'to and fro' spectral wave pattern, in the communicating channel.

The operative procedure for a patient with abdominal aortic aneurysms is a graft. This is appreciated sonographically by a rather sharp definition of parallel echogenic walls in the aorta. Duplex Doppler imaging may be used as the first line investigation to monitor patients following endovascular aneurysm repair.

Mesenteric Doppler

The arteries primarily responsible for mesenteric circulation include the SMA, IMA and branches of coeliac artery (common hepatic artery and gastroduodenal artery) which provide anastomotic links in case of occlusive disease. Chronic mesenteric ischemia results due to athero-sclerotic involvement of at least two of the three major vessels supplying the bowel. Mesenteric duplex scanning represents a noninvasive technique for anatomic and physiologic assessment of visceral vessels. It provides a rapid accurate method for the evaluation of patency of major splanchnic vessel. This aids in the selection of patients for arteriography and allow rational selection of alternative diagnostic studies.

Splanchnic Aneurysms

Splanchnic aneurysms may be mistaken for simple abscesses. It is prudent to evaluate with Doppler all collections prior to drainage. Real-time identification of pulsation in the aneurysm is helpful in characterising the vascular nature of mass. Pulsation may be absent or be diminished as a result of perianeurysmal fibrosis, where Doppler ultrasound will make a precise diagnosis.

Renal Arteries

Renal arteries are examined by color and duplex Doppler to evaluate cases of secondary hypertension to rule out renal artery stenosis. Other vascular lesions like aneurysm and A-V malformations are also detected and evaluated with the help of Doppler.

Doppler techniques have been applied to the renal artery with 83% sensitivity and 97% specificity in diagnosing stenosis greater than 60%.

The main renal arteries from the origin to the renal hilum may be interrogated with Duplex ultrasound or alternatively intrarenal spectral Doppler waveform may be evaluated to diagnose significant stenosis.

Renal artery aneurysms may be suspected due to pulsations in the hypoechoic lesion and confirmed when arterial flow is identified in them using Doppler ultrasound.

Renal arteriovenous malformations may form as a result of trauma, surgery, renal biopsy or neoplasms. It appears as a cluster of tortuous arteries and veins or more commonly a cystic structure (aneurysmal artery or vein) with arterial and venous pulsations. A dilated renal vein or inferior vena cava above the level of renal vein suggests the presence of this lesion.

Inferior Vena Cava

Anatomy

The inferior vena cava is a large vein that returns blood from the lower limbs, pelvis and abdomen to the right atrium. It is formed by the confluence of bilateral common iliac veins on the anterior surface of the L_5 vertebral body. Passing through the diaphragm, it enters the right atrium. Its main tributaries are the hepatic veins and the renal veins.

The inferior vena cava (IVC) lumen is anechoic although with slow flowing blood it becomes more echogenic and may show swirling and the classical tracing has a saw tooth pattern due to both cardiac and respiratory pulsations **(Fig. 31.2)**.

The most commonly encountered intraluminal pathology of the IVC is thrombosis which usually spreads from another vein in the pelvis, lower limbs, liver or kidney. It is seen as an intraluminal filling defect that

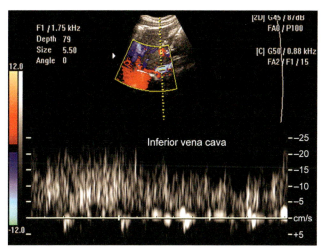

Fig. 31.2: Normal Doppler tracing of the inferior vena cava.

usually expands the diameter of the vessel. If a thrombus is hypoechoic or isoechoic with the liver, color Doppler is very helpful in making the diagnosis. Spectral Doppler analysis produces no signal from uncomplicated thrombus. Arterial type tracing may be seen within tumor thrombi.

A rare primary tumor leiomyosarcoma is seen as a soft tissue mass which distends the IVC and may contain scattered foci of cystic necrosis with detection of tumor neovascularity, arteriovenous shunting or low impedance high diastolic flow with Doppler ultrasound.

Inferior Vena Cava Branches and Tributaries

Renal veins are usually interrogated for renal vein thrombosis usually associated with acute glomerulonephritis, lupus, amyloidosis, sepsis, trauma dehydration and renal transplants. On sonography, one may see dilatation of vein proximal to the occlusion. The kidney enlarges and there is decreased echogenicity secondary to edema in the kidney. Doppler study shows no renal vein flow and a high resistive arterial flow pattern.

Hepatic Veins

Hepatic vein Doppler spectral tracings are usually triphasic and pulsatile reflecting transmitted cardiac pulsations **(Fig. 31.3)**. This pattern is abolished in cases of cirrhosis and portal hypertension, and it is exaggerated in right heart failure.

Ovarian Veins

Ovarian vein thrombosis usually occurs postpartum and is associated with endometritis and surgery. Sonography frequently shows massive enlargement of all part of the ovarian vein often with an echogenic thrombus within it.

Cerebrovascular

Doppler ultrasound is the principal investigation for patients with possible carotid disease both for screening

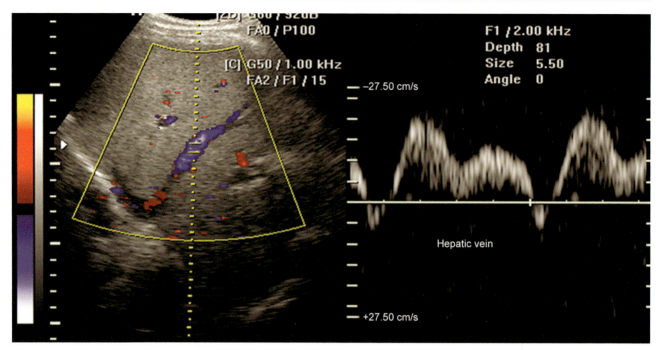

Fig. 31.3: Normal Doppler tracing of the hepatic veins.

and evaluation of atherosclerotic disease, resultant stenosis and the consequent hemodynamic effects.

Carotid Doppler examination in patients with severe stenosis with symptomatic ischemia is beneficial as they can be offered end-atherectomy. Following end-atherectomy, follow-up with carotid ultrasound is mandatory. Insufficient cerebral vascular supply due to subclavian steal syndrome and also cases of posterior fossa ischemia can be evaluated.

Patients who are to undergo surgery for peripheral or coronary artery disease, aneurysms or other vascular disease are also at risk and hence are candidates for carotid Doppler sonography.

Generally 7–10 MHz frequency transducer is used and transverse scanning from sternoclavicular region up in the neck is first done, followed by longitudinal scanning in color mode to outline the lumen of both carotid arteries. Turbulent flow is normally visualized in the carotid bulb region. Spectral Doppler is required to assess and quantify the abnormal flow. The severity of disease or stenosis in the arteries can be quantified either by velocity measurements in the area of narrowing or by direct visualization and measurement of the stenosis.

It is important to identify external carotid artery separate from the internal carotid artery, especially in the presence of disease, as significant disease alters the waveform characteristics, thus blurring the distinction between external carotid and internal carotid flow. Reversal of flow in the ophthalmic artery is diagnostic of significant carotid artery occlusion.

Common carotid and internal carotid artery usually show laminar flow pattern on color image. The external carotid artery can be differentiated from internal carotid

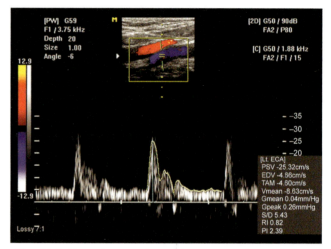

Fig. 31.4: Normal spectral trace from external carotid artery with a short reverse flow as in peripheral arteries.

artery by its medial location in neck; cervical branches; high pulsatility flow with little flow in diastole and the prominent dicrotic notch **(Fig. 31.4)**. In contrast, internal carotid arterial flow is less pulsatile flow with high diastolic flow and localized widening at its origin (carotid bulb) **(Fig. 31.5)**. Waveform of CCA resembles that of ICA.

Of the various indices used for measurements of blood flow, the most important are the peak systolic velocity, end diastolic velocity and the ratio of peak systolic velocities of the internal and the common carotid arteries. Internal carotid artery to common carotid artery (at a point 2–4 cm distal to bifurcation) peak systolic velocity ratio compensates for changes in cardiac output or arrhythmias.

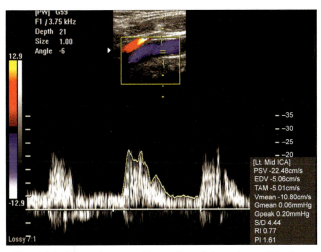

Fig. 31.5: Normal spectral trace from internal carotid artery with higher end-diastolic flow.

Direct stenotic measurements can be done either by the diameter reduction or area reduction method. For the purpose of measurement in the transverse image color and power Doppler are helpful. Very severe degree of stenosis (greater than ninety percent) with very narrow lumen, results in weak signals and low velocities because of small blood flow through the residual lumen. Hence, it is imperative to adjust the equipment settings to detect very low intensity and low velocity signals.

Gray scale scanning in longitudinal plane is useful for measurement of the intimal-media complex thickness for detection of early atherosclerotic disease. Plaques if present are assessed for their extent, location, characteristics and subsequent risk of a stroke. Softer and more delicate lipid-rich plaques (echopoor type 1 and 2) are more likely to fracture and dislodge than firm, more fibrotic (echo-reflective type 3 and 4) plaques.

The newer advances in ultrasound technology allow rendering of 3D reconstruction of acquired images have helped in improving the conspicuity and better delineation of the extent of pathology. This can be used to advantage for showing complex tortuosity of carotid arteries and their branches.

Contrast enhanced imaging of carotid arteries can be done for evaluating patients with difficult anatomy. Further, contrast agents improved conspicuity of luminal interface; improve visualization and characterization of plaque and analysis of the residual lumen.

Carotid occlusion: While even the critical carotid stenosis is surgically correctable, carotid occlusion is not. Hence, careful distinction should be made between the two by utilizing color Doppler or power Doppler and when required by the use of echo-enhancer agents.

Carotid dissection: This entity can also be assessed on ultrasound. There may be complete occlusion of vessels or a smoothly tapering stenosis with or without hematoma or thrombosis of false lumen that might be easily recognizable. On Doppler ultrasound double lumen with variable flow pattern in two channels may be seen.

Pulsatile neck masses can be due to prominent carotid bulb, ectatic neck arteries, lymph-adenopathy adjacent to carotid sheath, carotid artery aneurysm or carotid body tumors. These causes can be easily differentiated on Doppler ultrasound.

The vertebral arteries: The clinical significance of the stenotic disease in the vertebral arteries as compared with the carotid arteries is significant less, because basilar artery and posterior circulation is supplied by two vertebral arteries and are connected to circle of Willis allowing compensatory flow unless both of them are narrowed.

The direction of flow in the vertebral arteries should be noted to identify the phenomenon of the subclavian steal. This phenomenon can be unmasked in the latent cases by asking patient to do some muscular work by arm or inducing the reactive hyperemia. The direction of the blood flow in the vertebral arteries can be determined easily on Doppler.

Transcranial Doppler Ultrasound (TCD)

Pulsed transcranial color Doppler was first described in 1982 for adults. Now real-time Doppler not only provides useful physiological, pathological, and pharmacological information but also allows intraoperative and postoperative monitoring of endarteritis patients.

The three main access portals for transcranial Doppler examination are transtemporal, suboccipital, and transorbital window. The low frequency (2 MHz) is used with maximum possible sensitivity settings and maximum possible power for adult except in transorbital window to avoid excessive insonation and damage to lens.

For neonates, lowest possible power output is to be maintained regardless of the window to be used. Additionally the transfontanelle approach increases the indications of Doppler in the infants.

Applications of transcranial Doppler ultrasound (TCD) are:
- Identification of stenosed arteries and resultant collateral pathways
- Investigation of vasospasm secondary to subarachnoid hemorrhage (SAH)
- Brain death
- Assessment of the cerebral venous system
- Peroperatively during carotid surgery and neurointensive care
- Detection of emboli
- Estimation of the cerebral perfusion reserve
- Detection of intracranial aneurysms and large feeders to arteriovenous malformation (AVM).

Color Doppler gives better waveform and velocity information while Pulsed Doppler is better for monitoring cerebral perfusion reserve and emboli counting.

Liver

Sonography is considered to be the most effective primary investigation of choice in elucidation of liver pathology. Color Doppler sonography is a superb, noninvasive alternative to hepatic arteriography and splenoportography. Addition of duplex Doppler gives complete information in cases of portal hypertension (PHT), hepatic venoocclusive diseases, differentiation of various hepatic masses and cases of hepatic transplantation.

Technique

A low frequency (3 MHz) is chosen for examination of deep vessels and for detection of high velocities and a high frequency (5–7.5 MHz) transducer is used for the examination of superficial vessels, studies of children or detection of low blood flow velocities. The hepatic artery and portal veins are best interrogated by Doppler ultrasound of the porta hepatis using oblique intercostal scans. Color flow imaging allows rapid differentiation of bile duct from hepatic artery in cases of abnormal anatomy. The hepatic artery shows a high diastolic flow due to the low resistance of the hepatic vascular bed. Normal portal venous flow is hepatopetal and is usually monophasic with some fluctuation due to respiration and cardiac activity. The splenic vein and superior mesenteric vein are also examined for their caliber and flow pattern. The portal vein and splanchnic circulation has physiological changes due to respiratory, exertional, postural and postprandial variations **(Fig. 31.6)**. The hepatic veins and the inferior vena cava are also examined thoroughly in cases of Budd-Chiari syndrome for any localized increase or obliteration in caliber and/or flow velocity **(Fig. 31.7)**. The hepatic veins characteristically have a triphasic waveform which reflects right atrial and inferior vena cava pressures.

PORTAL HYPERTENSION (PHT)

Sonographic Findings in Portal Hypertension

Ascites, splenomegaly, and abnormal portal venous flow indicate development of PHT. Upper limit of normal portal vein diameter measured in basal conditions, i.e., quiet respiration, supine and fasting state is 13 mm. Varying

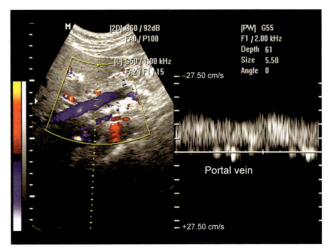

Fig. 31.6: Normal Doppler trace from portal vein.

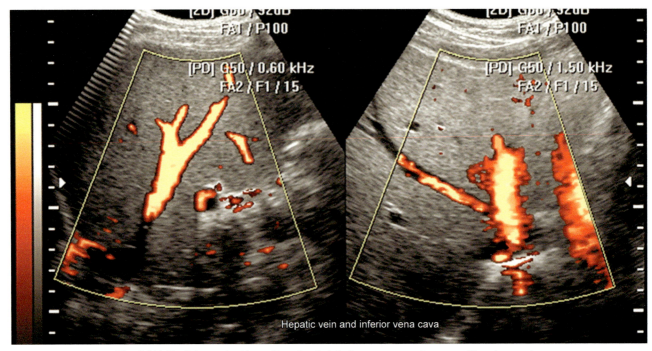

Fig. 31.7: Draining patent hepatic veins in inferior vena cava in power Doppler mode.

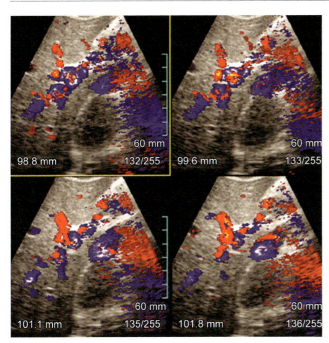

Fig. 31.8: Multiple color Doppler images in a case of portal cavernoma.

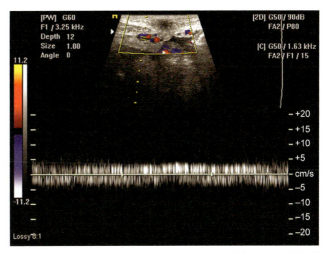

Fig. 31.9: Multiple anterior abdominal wall (paraumbilical) collaterals in portal hypertension secondary to cirrhosis of liver.

degrees of dilatation of splenic and superior mesenteric veins also occur in PHT. A significant caliber increase is noted during inspiration in normal patients. Whereas, loss of this variation is seen in early cases of PHT. Opening up of vessels (collaterals) between high pressure portal venous system and low pressure systemic circulation is usually seen with portal hypertension.

Doppler provides qualitative, semiquantitative, and quantitative assessment of the splanchnic vessels. The presence, direction, and characteristics of blood flow are the qualitative data. Semiquantitative measurements include vascular impedance which is calculated by means of pulsatility and resistance indices. Quantitative data includes calculation of the maximum and mean flow velocity and of the flow volume in larger diameter veins.

Hepatomegaly/shrunken liver with altered liver architecture, presence or absence of portal vein thrombosis, cavernous transformation of the portal vein are useful in establishing the etiology of PHT **(Fig. 31.8)**.

The specific diagnosis of portal hypertension must include search for collateral beds. Real-time USG and Doppler can explore the paraumbilical veins, splenorenal, esophageal, peripancreatic, and pericholecystic collaterals **(Fig. 31.9)**.

The impedance changes in the splanchnic vessels have been studied in the three main arterial beds—the superior mesenteric, splenic and hepatic. It reveals reduction of mesenteric arterial resistance leading to a hyperdynamic splanchnic circulation. Intra-parenchymal branches of the splenic artery and hepatic arterial impedance indexes are increased in patients with liver cirrhosis.

Quantitative measurements of the portal flow can provide information not only related to the diagnosis of portal hypertension but also in the evaluation of hemorrhage risk and the efficacy of pharmacological therapy and surgical portosystemic anastomosis.

Doppler has proved useful in preoperative evaluation of patients as well as postoperative follow-up. After splenorenal, lienorenal shunt or TIPS placement duplex Doppler is accepted as a reliable technique in the long-term surveillance for complications of stent dysfunction.

Budd-Chiari Syndrome (BCS)

Budd-Chiari syndrome includes hepatic venoocclusive disease at the level of the small centrilobular veins, major hepatic veins or IVC and presents with features of ascites, abdominal pain, hepatomegaly, and jaundice.

Angiography has been the mainstay of diagnosis in patients with Budd-Chiari syndrome, both before and after surgery but it is invasive. Doppler imaging is an appealing non-invasive technique in patients with Budd-Chiari syndrome and it can be used to assess the presence, direction and characteristics of flow within the hepatic veins and the IVC.

The flat wave profile was found in all the intrahepatic vessels resembling the hepatic veins and this has been defined as a major criterion for the diagnosis of Budd-Chiari syndrome with Doppler US.

COLOR DOPPLER IN HEPATIC LESIONS

Benign pathological processes occur frequently in the liver and need to be differentiated from malignant tumors. Color Doppler and Duplex sonography are also very useful in characterization of solid liver lesions.

Demonstration of blood flow in a hypoechoic rim of a focal liver lesion in patients without clinical suspicion of HCC or metastases suggest the diagnosis of FNH.

Hemangiomas generally have too low Doppler frequency shift to be detected by Doppler systems and thus demonstrate little or no detectable flow. Intratumoral venous flow on pulse Doppler signal is very suggestive of benignancy.

The occurrence of detour venous pattern has been reported in metastases. The simultaneous occurrence of both intra and peritumoral arterial flow in the same lesion strongly suggests malignancy. A basket pattern of peritumoral flow and a 'vessel-in-tumor' pattern are regarded as being very specific for hepatocellular carcinomas. Patients with lesions measuring less than 3 cm with detectable Doppler signals are likely to have HCC.

Power Doppler sonography is thought to be three to five times more sensitive than color Doppler sonography. The advantages of power Doppler sonography are that it detects lower velocity flows than color Doppler sonography, it decreases the noise background, it does not produce aliasing and it is independent of angle.

Contrast enhanced color Doppler sonography in liver tumors improves the detection of low velocity blood flow because they increase the signal-to-noise ratio, allowing a more complete display of the vascular pattern of the tumor in both color and pulsed Doppler Sonography.

Gallbladder Carcinoma

Gallbladder carcinoma is a common hepatobiliary tumor. When seen as a solid mass occupying the whole gallbladder, differentiation of gallbladder carcinoma from tumefactive biliary sludge is essential. Conventional gray scale US provide very little, if any, useful information for differentiation. The addition of color Doppler sonography offers a definite advantage for this purpose. Blood flow signals are seen in majority of cases of gallbladder carcinoma. In the tumefactive biliary sludge group, color Doppler sonography is devoid of any blood signals.

LIVER TRANSPLANTATION

Diagnostic ultrasound augmented with Duplex and color Doppler plays an important role in both preoperative (recipient and donor) and postoperative evaluation of the patient undergoing hepatic transplantation.

Prior to hepatic transplantation, significant hepatic parenchymal and vascular abnormalities must be identified to aid the surgeon in planning the operation. Ultrasound, aided by Doppler, is used to document the anatomy, and patency of the inferior vena cava, hepatic veins, and portal vein. If transplantation is being performed for treatment of hepatic malignancy, ultrasound may aid in defining the extent of the tumor and determining the presence of vascular invasion or biliary obstruction. A preoperative baseline measurement of splenic size is important to detect the portal vein stenosis or occlusion, recurrent liver disease or rejection in the postoperative period.

Spleen

Portal hypertension is the commonest indication for splenic Doppler examination. Besides portal vein varying degrees of dilatation of splenic and superior mesenteric veins also occurs in portal hypertension. Splenomegaly and caliber of splenic vein over 12 mm with lack of respiratory variations in caliber and presence of hepatofugal flow, is directly correlated with hepatic encephalopathy.

At level of lower splenic pole, splenorenal collaterals appear as tortuous vessels with a high velocity Doppler signal and a broad spectrum of frequencies due to turbulence.

Splenic Infarction

Severe infarct related complications might develop in the course of disease that can be detected by follow-up US and Doppler scanning which require splenectomy.

Patients demonstrating arterial signals within the infarction revealed superinfection of the splenic infarcts. The presence of arterial signals and increasing subcapsular hemorrhage are signs suggestive of spontaneous splenic rupture. Hence, with clear sonographic signs of life-threatening splenic rupture, splenectomy should be undertaken.

Intrasplenic Pseudoaneurysms

Intrasplenic pseudoaneurysms are formed by active bleeding from injured intrasplenic arterial branches and carry a risk, thereby necessitating a meticulous search for these lesions in all cases of blunt splenic trauma.

Intrasplenic pseudoaneurysms appear on gray scale sonography as nonspecific anechoic lesions. Their aneurysmal nature can be revealed by the demonstration of arterial flow on color Doppler sonography. Turbulent arterial flow within the lesion suggests a diagnosis of pseudoaneurysms. Some lesions develop late thus conservative management of blunt splenic trauma should include periodic follow-up with color Doppler sonography, even if admission scans are negative.

Pancreas

In the preoperative evaluation of pancreatic tumors patients showing signs of peripancreatic vessel involvement are considered to be unresectable and helps avoid unnecessary surgery. Color Doppler sonography has been found to be more sensitive than angiography in depicting vascular involvement of carcinoma. Hence, a preoperative assessment in suspected pancreatic carcinoma patients with initial color Doppler sonography helps in improved patient management. A vessel if normal or show abutment favored resectability whereas encasement or occlusions of vessel favor non-resectability.

Pancreatic Transplantation

As in other organ transplants, arterial and venous integrity is critical in pancreatic transplantation. Color and Duplex

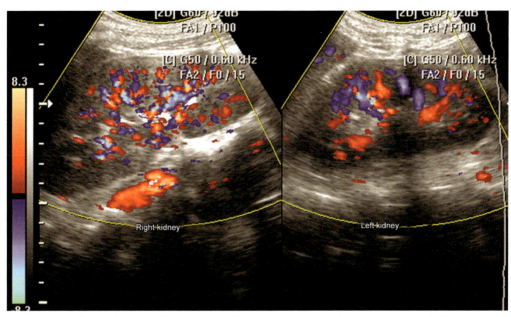

Fig. 31.10: Color Doppler flow in bilateral kidneys (right kidney is enlarged with increased vascularity due to pyelonephritis).

Doppler are commonly used to monitor blood flow postoperatively to the pancreas. Common complications of pancreatic transplantation are vascular thrombosis, intra-abdominal infections, rejection, anastomotic leaks, and pancreatitis. Sonography with Doppler is the procedure of choice in detecting fluid collections and identifying pancreatitis, vascular thrombosis and rejection to some extent.

URINARY SYSTEM

Gray scale ultrasound has greatly increased the morphologic detail that could be displayed within the kidney. Further, the addition of pulsed Doppler allowed arterial and venous perfusion to be assessed both qualitatively and quantitatively. Recent addition to color flow and power Doppler imaging now allow superb demonstration of the entire renovascular tree from the main renal arteries to their fine terminal branches **(Fig. 31.10)**.

The origin and proximal portion of the main renal arteries are best examined with the patient supine using a 3 MHz transducer and a transverse midline approach. Patients should ideally fast for at least 8 hours prior to examination. In larger patients, decubitus positioning is helpful and renal parenchymal vessels are best examined from a lateral intercostal approach.

The normal waveform of the main renal artery demonstrates a low impedance pattern with continuous forward diastolic flow reflecting the low resistance of the native kidney. Peak systolic velocity is usually less than 100 cm/sec. The resistive index (RI) should be less than 0.7.

The segmental renal branches which lie within the renal hilum as well as the more distal interlobar and arcuate vessels within the renal cortex are readily identified on color or pulse Doppler examination.

Pulsed Doppler interrogation of the intrarenal vessel reveals a low resistance waveform with a decreasing peak systolic velocities as the vessels are traced distally. Increase in downstream resistance result in a relative reduction in diastolic flow compared with systolic with intrarenal RI of 0.7.

Children and neonates will have RI (0.7-1.0) of higher value and decreases with age and stablises in the adult range by age 4-5 years.

Doppler signals from parenchyma or main renal veins demonstrates continuous flow in the opposite direction that of arterial flow with respiratory and cardiac variation.

Pyelocaliectasis identified by sonography is certainly not synonymous with true pelvicalyceal obstruction. Differentiation of true renal obstruction from non-obstructive dilatation cannot be resolved by gray scale sonography and often requires the use of invasive procedures and tests. However, intrarenal Doppler has a great value in identifying true renal obstruction, noninvasively.

Kidney with a dilated collecting system and a RI value of 0.70 or more is suggestive of obstruction, while RI value less than 0.70 is suggestive of nonobstructive dilatation. Complete obstruction may be associated with normal RI immediately after the onset of obstruction. But after 2 hours of obstruction, elevation of renal vascular resistance and hence RI occurs. In acute obstruction, Doppler study enables detection of marked elevation in renal arterial resistance by 6 hours of clinical obstruction at a time when conventional US often reveals little or no pyelocaliectasis.

As Doppler analysis **(Fig. 31.11)** provides physiologic rather than anatomic information, cases of partial or mild unilateral obstruction can also be picked up. In such cases a resistive index ratio (RIR), which is defined as the RI of the dilated kidney divided by RI of the contralateral nonobstructive kidney of 1.1 or greater is suggestive of obstruction.

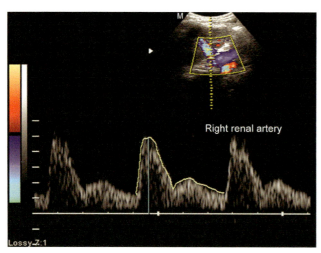

Fig. 31.11: Normal low impedance flow pattern in renal artery.

Color Doppler of vesicoureteric junction for ureteric jets within the bladder may also be useful in diagnosing ureteric obstruction. If a ureteric jet is not seen after 15 minutes of continuous observation, the ureter is considered obstructed.

The conditions associated with renal microangiopathy (e.g., Hemolytic uremic syndrome) have decreased arterial renal parenchymal blood flow causing resultant oliguria or anuria frequently requiring dialysis. Duplex Doppler demonstrates a renal parenchymal arterial waveform characterized by absent, reversed or markedly reduced diastolic flow and elevated intrarenal RI ≥ 0.9 during the oliguric phase. The reappearance of normal diastolic blood flow and drop of RI normal (0.65–0.70) accurately predicts recovery of renal function and urine output allowing dialysis to be terminated.

Renal Masses

Pulse and color Doppler examination can be useful for further evaluation of solid renal masses. Color Doppler imaging show most renal cell carcinomas to be hypervascular showing numerous arteriovenous shunts. High peak systolic frequency shifts demonstrated on pulse Doppler in renal cell carcinoma (RCC) help differentiate them from other vascular lesions in the kidney. Renal cell carcinoma also have a propensity to invade renal veins and inferior vena cava which can also be assessed on Doppler examination.

Acute Renal Vein Thrombosis (RVT)

It occurs most frequently as a result of dehydration, vascular congestion, hypercoagulopathies, malignancy or trauma. Sepsis, birth trauma, maternal diabetes or maternal hypertension in neonates and children are the other important causes. Prevention of renal failure by early institution of the diagnosis requires an accurate diagnosis.

Duplex Doppler sonography of the kidney with the study of the main renal vein is often used in the noninvasive evaluation of this condition. Typical findings include the presence of thrombosis and the absence of a Doppler signal in the renal vein besides the gray scale findings of enlarged and hypoechoic kidney.

Renal Artery Stenosis

Renovascular hypertension is the most common surgically curable cause of hypertension for which various causes have been implicated. Therefore, an imaging modality providing physiologic data and/or anatomic detail would be a more ideal screening technique.

Recently captopril scintigraphy has been demonstrated to have a very high sensitivity (91%) and specificity (93%) for diagnosis of renovascular hypertension but only provides physiologic study and no anatomic detail. Pulse Doppler waveform has the ability to suggest physiological information whereas real-time ultrasonography provides anatomic detail often identifying the stenotic lesion.

There are two basic approaches to the Doppler US diagnosis of renal artery stenosis (RAS). The first depends on the ability of both real-time and Doppler US to identify a focal area of increased peak systolic velocity (PSV) at the anatomic site of stenosis and the second involves demonstrating a decrease in the rate of systolic acceleration distal to a stenosis.

PSV > 100 cm/sec and or RAR > 3.5 (ratio of peak systolic renal artery velocity to peak systolic aortic velocity) have sensitivities of 79–91% and specificities of 73–92% for hemodynamically significant RAS (>50–60% diameter reduction).

Hemodynamically significant arterial stenosis cause changes in velocity waveforms that can be detected with Duplex sonography in distal contiguous arteries. Such changes in peripheral arteries are called tardus and parvus. Tardus refers to delayed or prolonged early acceleration and parvus to the diminished amplitude of the systolic peak shown by prolonged acceleration time (AT) and diminished acceleration index (AI).

Renal Transplant

Renal transplantation is the most commonly performed abdominal organ transplant worldwide. The sonographic evaluation of the transplanted kidney combines imaging and Doppler because transplant dysfunction arises from both vascular and nonvascular causes (**Fig. 31.12**).

Transplant dysfunction may result from vascular complication such as vessel stenosis or occlusion or parenchymal changes secondary to rejection, tubular necrosis, or drug toxicity. Vascular complications are usually arterial and venous stenosis and thrombosis and intrarenal or extrarenal arteriovenous fistula (AVF) and pseudoaneurysm. If detected early, many are amenable to graft sparing by surgical or radiologic intervention.

Renal Artery Stenosis/Thrombosis

Arterial stenosis usually occurs within the first 3 years after transplantation and easily evaluated on Doppler examination. Color Doppler sonography is likely to detect segmental infarcts in relation to renal artery thrombosis. Renal vein thrombosis can also be assessed on duplex Doppler by absence of renal venous flow and reversed plateau of diastolic arterial flow.

Intrarenal AVF and pseudoaneurysms are almost exclusively the result of trauma induced during percutaneous needle biopsy. The duplex Doppler findings of both AVF and pseudoaneurysms exhibit high velocity low impedance arterial waveform associated with arterialized venous tracings and highly turbulent pulsatile flow in their central lumen with classic to and fro flow at their neck in AVF and pseudoaneurysm respectively.

Important causes of altered renal blood flow resulting in transplant dysfunction are ATN, acute and chronic rejection and drug toxicity. Duplex and color Doppler ultrasound remain valuable tools for assessing response to therapy and for evaluating the allograft for other vascular abnormalities such as acute venous and arterial thrombosis, arterial stenosis or arteriovenous fistulas.

Urinary obstruction is an infrequent but serious complication of renal transplantation. Obstruction is a common cause of an elevated RI > 0.75 in a transplanted kidney with pyelocaliectasis.

Scrotum

Color Doppler imaging added on to high-resolution ultrasonography of scrotum has widened the diagnostic spectrum. Spectral waveforms of testicular flow typically show prominent diastolic component (**Fig. 31.13**). Normal low flow in the testis is readily seen on Doppler study and it is also possible to diagnose hypo or hypervascular states in various disease processes. It is usually used to diagnose varicocele (in erect position) and to differentiate infection from torsion in an acute scrotum.

TESTICULAR TORSION

Testicular torsion is a result of excessive mobility of testis. Ultrasonography findings vary depending on the time elapsed between the onset of episode and the time of examination and can be confused with epididymo-orchitis. Addition of color Doppler solves the diagnostic dilemma. Diminished or absent flow to the testis with decreased or increased peritesticular flow is seen in torsion while increased intratesticular vascularity is seen in infection.

Undescended testis when confused with a lymph node can be differentiated on color Doppler. Enlarged node is hypervascular as compared to virtually avascular undescended testis.

Varicocele is the most common correctable cause of male infertility. Ultrasonography and color Doppler play an important role in the diagnosis; particularly in subclinical cases. The veins of the pampiniform plexus are considered dilated if they exceed 2 mm in diameter. The veins often

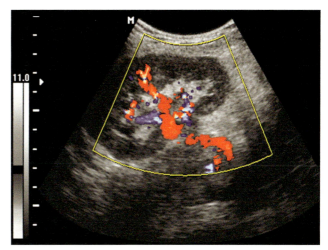

Fig. 31.12: A color Doppler image in a case of transplanted kidney with maintained vascular supply.

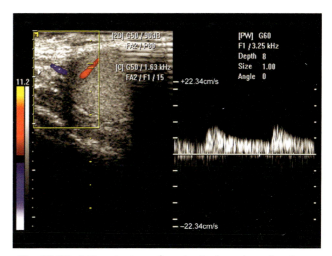

Fig. 31.13: A Doppler trace from testicular artery showing a low impedance flow with high diastolic flow.

dilate to 3 mm and more when the examination is performed in standing posture and during valsalva (**Fig. 31.14**).

Most neoplasms of testis are malignant and there is a wide spectrum of ultrasonographic features ranging from hypoechoic, isoechoic, hyperechoic, and even complex echoic. Color Doppler sonography may reveal flow in the periphery of the mass lesion.

Evaluation of Erectile Dysfunction

Impotence is defined as an inability to achieve rigidity. Vasculogenic impotence is the most common cause of organic impotence or erectile dysfunction (ED). Vascular ED can occur due to obstruction in penile inflow tract, termed as arterial ED and the inability to trap the incoming blood at sufficient pressure in the cavernosa, termed as veno-occlusive ED.

Pharmacopenile duplex ultrasonography (PPDU) is fast becoming the first line investigation to define vascular

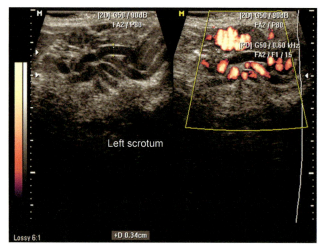

Fig. 31.14: Multiple varicoceles on gray scale and power Doppler image.

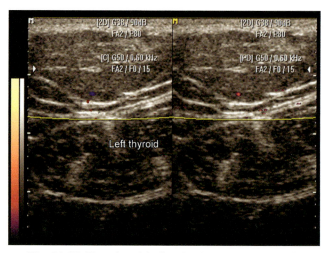

Fig. 31.15: Type I nodule (benign lipomatosis of skin).

ED and to differentiate between arterial insufficiency and incompetent veno-occlusive mechanism.

The sonographic evaluation begins with scanning of the flaccid penis in transverse plane to measure the diameter of the cavernosal arteries. Postpapaverine evaluation of the erectile function involves measurement of angle corrected flow velocities in cavernosal arteries at 5 minutes after the injection and repeated after short intervals till peak rigidity. Postpapaverine normal spectral waveform of cavernosal artery normally exhibits five reproducible phases. Various parameters and other accepted normal values include maximum recorded peak systolic velocity (PSV) of 30 cm/second or more, minimum end diastolic velocity (EDV) of 5 cm/second or less (zero or reversed diastolic flow included as normal), acceleration time (AT) of 0.11 second or less, and resistive index (RI) of 0.85 or more. Abnormal PSV and AT are suggestive of arterial cause while abnormal EDV and RI indicates venous leakage.

DOPPLER OF SMALL PARTS

Musculoskeletal System

Ultrasound is often the first step in the assessment of musculoskeletal soft tissue masses. Sonography is usually not able to distinguish benign from malignant mass lesions.

Color and pulsed wave Doppler data are more helpful in categorizing a lesion as benign or malignant compared to gray scale sonography alone. Absence of flow is a characteristic feature of the benign lesion. Presence of flow however, can be found in both benign and malignant lesions. Arrangement and not number of vessels in the lesion is useful. A regular arrangement with a linear course is usually suggestive of a benign mass. Randomly distributed vessels with abrupt variation in size as well as spot flow signals are seen in malignant lesions. On spectral evaluation, peak systolic velocity is the single most reliable parameter for discriminating benign and malignant lesions. A threshold of 50 cm/s is the best criterion.

Skin and Subcutaneous Tissues

Color Doppler sonography increases the specificity of sonography by providing real-time evaluation of the vascularity, which is an important clue in distinguishing benign from the malignant lesions.

The sonographic examination should be carried by a high resolution (10–20 MHz) linear transducer. Power Doppler can be used to increase vessel conspicuity and demonstrate vessel continuity. The nodules are classified as:
- *Type I:* Avascular
- *Type II:* Hypovascular with a single vascular pole in the hilum
- *Type III:* Hypervascular with multiple peripheral poles, and
- *Type IV:* Hypervascular with internal vessels.

Majority of the malignant nodules show both peripheral (Type III) and intralesional vascularity (Type IV), where as hypovascularity is seen mainly in the benign lesion **(Fig. 31.15)**.

VASCULAR LESIONS

Hemangioma

Hemangiomas are among one of the most common soft tissue masses in infants. On color Doppler flow imaging (CDFI), hemangiomas show presence of large number of intralesional vessels **(Fig. 31.16)**. Presence of more than five vessels per square centimeter has been seen. On spectral imaging, a high frequency shift measuring more than 2 kHz is seen.

Arteriovenous malformations may also show similar features on CDFI and pulse Doppler imaging; additionally Doppler evaluation may show arterialization of the waveform **(Fig. 31.17)**.

and resistive index. In malignant neoplasm peak systolic velocity is increased and a PI value of >1.4 and RI value of >0.8 have been suggested as clinically useful cut off points.

Thyroid and Parathyroid Glands

Ultrasound has been successfully used as an adjunct to nuclear scintigraphy in evaluating the thyroid gland. Development of color Doppler flow imaging has permitted the assessment of blood supply in addition to morphology.

High frequency transducers (7-12 MHz) are used for thyroid and parathyroid imaging. The patient is examined in supine position with neck extended. Doppler parameters are optimized for low flow sensitivity in the case of suspected parathyroid adenoma. Mean diameter of the thyroid arteries is 1-2 mm, the veins may be up to 8 mm in diameter. Peak systolic velocities are 20-40 cm/sec in major thyroid arteries and 15-30 cm/sec in intraparenchymal arteries.

Graves' disease: Graves' disease is characterized by generalised enlargement of the thyroid gland with biochemical hyperfunction. Color Doppler is useful in evaluation of this disease. Markedly increased vascularity is seen on CDFI and power Doppler imaging. This appearance has been referred to as "Thyroid inferno". Spectral Doppler shows increased peak systolic velocity, which may exceed 70 cm/sec. None of the other thyroid diseases show such high velocities. Doppler examination can also be used to monitor the response to therapy in these patients. Following treatment significant decrease in vascularity and the velocities of thyroid vessels is seen.

Thyroid nodules: With presently available high definition color Doppler systems, some degree of vascularity is demonstrated in all nodules. Two types of vascular distribution may be seen:
- Nodule with peripheral vascularity
- Nodule with internal vessels, which may or may not be associated with peripheral vessels.

Large majority of hyperplastic, adenomatous, and goiterous nodules show peripheral distribution of the blood vessels **(Fig. 31.18)**, while majority of the thyroid malignancies show internal vessels with or without peripheral vascularity.

Parathyroid Adenoma

Primary hyperparathyroidism is caused by an adenoma in 80-90% of the cases. Typical sonographic appearance of parathyroid adenoma on gray scale imaging is a hypoechoic ovoid or lobulated mass posterior or lateral to the thyroid gland. Parathyroid adenomas are hypervascular. Color Doppler flow imaging increases the sensitivity and specificity of sonographic examination, in localizing an adenoma.

Salivary Glands

Differentiation of benign from malignant salivary gland tumor may be difficult with gray scale sonography alone. Increased

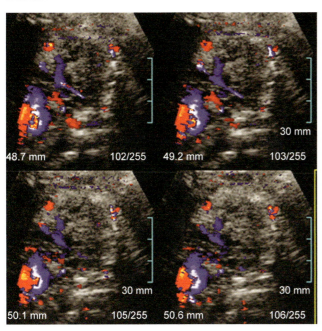

Fig. 31.16: Multiple color Doppler images in a case of hemangioma.

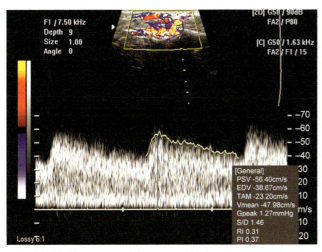

Fig. 31.17: Very low resistance and high velocity arterial flow in a case of arteriovenous malformation.

Breast

Application of Doppler studies in differentiation of benign and malignant lesions is based on the presumption that the malignant lesions are likely to be more vascular.

For the sonographic and Doppler examination of the breast 7.5 MHz linear transducer is usually required and gain settings are adjusted so that the clutter noise disappears. The tumor vessels are visualized with the help of CDFI and power Doppler imaging and the vessels with the largest diameters are interrogated with pulsed Doppler for spectral analysis.

Various Doppler parameters have been evaluated for their use in differentiating between benign and malignant lesions. These include peak systolic velocity, pulsatility index,

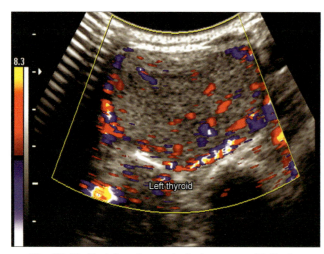

Fig. 31.18: Peripheral vascularity in a case of follicular adenoma of thyroid.

vascularity in salivary gland tumors can be recognized on color Doppler flow imaging (CDFI), a characteristic peripheral pattern for pleomorphic salivary gland adenoma has been described. The lesion may show fine centripetal branches. Warthin's tumor shows evenly scattered flow throughout the tumor. The peak systolic velocity is always less than 60 cm/sec in these tumors. The peak systolic velocity in malignant tumors is more than 60 cm/sec.

Vascular malformation in the salivary gland have similar feature as in other superficial organ. Multiple tortuous vascular channels with color flow are seen.

ORBIT

With color Doppler imaging, it is now possible to obtain information on the perfusion of the orbital structures in real-time.

The color Doppler examination can be performed with 7.5 MHz linear transducer. Arteries show evidence of pulsatile flow on color images and spectral tracing. While the veins show continuous or minimally pulsatile flow.

Normal Orbital Vessels

Central retinal artery (CRA) and central retinal vein (CRV), ciliary vessels, ophthalmic artery and vortex veins are visualized and interrogated.

Ocular Tumors

Color Doppler is being increasingly used to enhance the efficacy of gray scale USG to diagnose and differentiate intraocular mass lesions.

Choroidal melanomas show abnormal Doppler signals within the lesions. The flow spectrum pattern in these lesions is a medium to high systolic Doppler shift with high diastolic flow velocity. In choroidal hemangiomas, a high maximum systolic Doppler shift is seen along with high diastolic shifts. Evidence of increased flow is also seen in uveal metastases and retinoblastoma. Some intraocular lesions like age related macular degeneration, with subretinal hemorrhage and dense vitreous hemorrhage may simulate the appearance of tumor on B-mode imaging. Color Doppler flow imaging can help in differentiating these lesions by demonstrating lack of abnormal blood flow within these lesions.

In cavernous hemangiomas flow may be seen on decreased gain settings. Orbital varices have a characteristic pattern on Doppler imaging. They show dynamic changes throughout inspiration and expiration. On pulsed Doppler evaluation, the flow is continuous and nonpulsatile during both phases. This is characteristic of venous flow seen in this lesion.

A caroticocavernous sinus fistula (CCSF) is an abnormal communication between a branch of the carotid artery and the cavernous sinus. Color Doppler flow imaging clearly demonstrates the dilated arterialized superior ophthalmic vein with high velocity blood flow towards the transducer.

Retinal vessel abnormalities like occlusion of central retinal artery show absence or marked reduction in flow can be seen on CDFI.

Peripheral Vascular System

Easy accessibility of the limb arteries to sonography enables it to play a decisive role in the evaluation of disease involving peripheral arteries. Gray scale imaging has a limited role, it can detect presence of an atherosclerotic plaque, aneurysm and juxta vascular masses which may appear to be of arterial origin on clinical evaluation. Duplex scanning plays an important role by assessing the hemodynamic changes in a vessel after obtaining the spectral waveform. Thus, obstructive arterial lesions can be quantified, arterial stenosis can be differentiated from occlusion and the nature of perivascular masses can be determined. The addition of CDFI has transformed peripheral arterial imaging from a time consuming tedious task to an efficient practical examination. It has also improved the diagnostic accuracy of the examination. A rapid survey by CDFI can identify the zone of abnormal flow in a diseased vessel which can be evaluated by pulse Doppler. Color Doppler flow imaging enables accurate gate placement in the area of maximum flow disturbance. Power mode imaging or Doppler angio displays the peak amplitude of the flowing blood. The color obtained is uniform, aliasing is not a problem, as with pulsed and CDFI mode and slow flow is better detected, a disadvantage is the lack of information about the flow direction.

Doppler waveforms of lower limb arteries show a triphasic flow pattern in all the arteries **(Fig. 31.19)**. This triphasic wave form is characteristic of arteries supplying muscular bed, which has high peripheral resistance. During exercise or transient ischemia, there is loss of triphasic pattern. A monophasic pattern is characterized by persistent antegrade diastolic flow. Peak systolic velocities of arteries

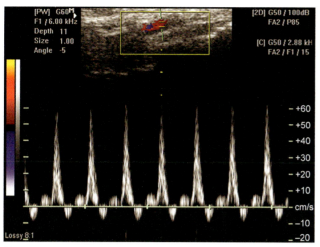

Fig. 31.19: Typical triphasic pattern of flow in the peripheral artery.

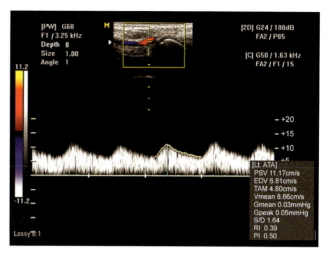

Fig. 31.20: Tardus parvus waveform in a case of Buerger's disease.

vary with location. It is approximately 100 cm/sec at the level of common femoral artery and 40–50 cm/sec in the leg arteries.

Technique

Lower Limb

Arterial occlusive disease is the main indication of the lower limb arterial Doppler study. Atherosclerosis is the major cause and as it also involves proximal vessels, evaluation of aortoiliac arteries should be integral part of Doppler study of lower limb arterial occlusive disease.

With the advent of CDFI, the aorta and iliac arteries can be visualized easily. With a 2.5–3.5 MHz transducer, the aorta, its bifurcation and common and external iliac branches are examined till the groin. Evaluation of vessels at and below the groin require high frequency transducers and involves assessment of common femoral artery, proximal segment of the profunda femoris, superficial femoral artery, popliteal artery, anterior tibial artery, posterior tibial artery, the peroneal artery, and the dorsalis pedis artery.

Any site of increased flow disturbance is noted. Entire length of each vessel must be scanned to avoid missing sites of localized stenosis. It is important to confirm the findings by taking the spectral tracing in the region of abnormality seen on CDFI.

Upper Limb

Arterial Doppler study of the upper limb involves evaluation of the subclavian artery, axillary artery, brachial artery and its bifurcation into radial, ulnar, and interosseous artery. Doppler flow pattern of the upper limb arteries is similar to that seen in the lower limb arteries.

Diagnosis on Doppler Imaging

The normal triphasic waveform is altered in presence of arterial stenosis or occlusion. Analysis of the velocity pattern provides the most useful information regarding the hemodynamic significance of atherosclerotic lesion. Color Doppler flow imaging enables rapid identification of site of flow abnormality, which is then interrogated by pulsed Doppler to obtain the spectral waveforms. Waveforms are also obtained proximal and distal to stenosis. Ratio of peak systolic velocity in the stenosed segment to that in proximal segment is calculated to determine hemodynamically significant stenosis.

Proximal to the stenosis the waveform is usually normal. The findings in the stenotic region depend upon the severity of lesion and help in the determining the degree of stenosis. In mild to moderate stenosis, the early diastolic reversal decreases and finally disappears. With increasing severity, increase in the diastolic flow is seen followed ultimately by the diastolic velocity approaching the systolic velocity. This increasing diastolic velocity is probably due to decreased peripheral resistance caused by dilatation of arterioles in the muscular bed in response to release of metabolites caused by local ischemia. Opening up of many small collateral pathways also contribute to decrease in peripheral resistance. Peak systolic velocity is less affected by vasodilatation. Therefore, this parameter is used to quantify the degree of stenosis. Artery distal to a high grade stenosis or occlusion shows a slow rise, low amplitude (Tardus-Parvus) waveform **(Fig. 31.20)**.

Color Doppler flow imaging and Duplex Doppler ultrasound are the techniques of choice for the postoperative monitoring of the bypass graft patency and to detect focal stenosis or any other cause of graft dysfunction.

Aneurysms

Peripheral arterial aneurysms (most commonly in popliteal artery) are usually due to weakening of the vessel walls because of arteriosclerosis.

A bulge or focal enlargement of 20% of the expected vessel diameter is consistent with diagnosis of aneurysm.

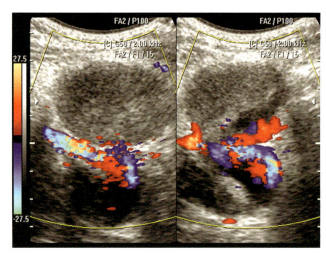

Fig. 31.21: Ying-yang sign in a case of pseudoaneurysm of superficial femoral artery in thigh.

Ultrasound can visualize the presence of intraluminal thrombus. With color Doppler patent lumen can be visualized and complete thrombosis can be diagnosed with more certainty.

Pseudoaneurysm (contained rupture of the arterial wall) can be differentiated from true aneurysm by demonstration of a cystic mass seen in relation to parent vessel. Communicating channel may be visualized on gray scale sonography. Characteristic finding on CDFI are swirling of color ('ying-yang' sign) within the cystic mass **(Fig. 31.21)**. The communicating channel or 'neck' of the pseudoaneurysm is seen well on CDFI. Duplex sonography shows typical "to and fro" flow in the communicating channel.

Arteriovenous Fistula

Communications between artery and veins result in arteriovenous fistula which may be congenital or acquired (dialysis shunt or traumatic).

The fistulous communication is more easily seen with CDFI than with the duplex scanning. On Duplex scanning the affected vein shows turbulence and arterialized waveform. Arterial waveform proximal to the communication will show increase in the diastolic flow due to reduced resistance in the vein. Distal artery will show a normal waveform.

Role of Color Doppler in Gynecology and Obstetrics

Color and power Doppler has important implications in the field of infertility and gynecological cancers.

Infertile females may show evidence of high resistance flow in the uterine arteries and even the presence of reverse diastolic flow. Power Doppler may fail to reveal vascularity reaching up to the endometrial lining at the most fertile period of the cycle. Color and power Doppler is very useful in demonstrating the highly echogenic and vascular stroma of polycystic ovaries. color Doppler flow imaging and power doppler imaging (PDI) also help to select right period of menstrual cycle for intrauterine semination in cases of infertility.

Blood clot and endometrial polyps can be easily differentiated on the basis of presence of detectable vascularity in the latter. Endometrial malignancies are associated with relative higher vascularity of low resistance than benign conditions. Ovarian malignancies can be characterized as malignant lesions based on the presence of septal blood flow of low resistance and haphazard neovascularization both at the periphery and center. Ectopic pregnancy in the adnexa can be characteristically recognized by the presence of ring of fire appearance on CDFI or PDI.

In obstetrics, CDFI has a complementary role in evaluating intrauterine growth retardation and at-risk babies. At risk babies may reveal presence of diastolic notch in the uterine arteries after 26 weeks, higher RI values in umbilical arteries or diastolic flow reversal, absence or reversal of diastolic flow in the middle cerebral arteries.

CHAPTER 32

Basics of Echo

The modalities of echo used clinically are:
- Image echo
  - Two-dimensional echo (2D echo)
  - Motion-mode echo (M-mode echo)
- Doppler echo
  - Continuous wave (CW) Doppler
  - Pulsed wave (PW) Doppler.

Different echo modalities are not mutually exclusive but complement each other and are often used together.

All of them follow the same principle of ultrasound but differ with respect to the manner in which reflected sound waves are received and displayed.

TWO-DIMENSIONAL (2D) ECHO

- Ultrasound reflected from a tissue interface distorts the piezoelectric crystal and generates an electric signal. The electric signal produces a dot (spot) on the display screen
- The location of the dot indicates the distance of the structure from the transducer. The brightness of the dot indicates the strength of the returning signal
- To create a 2D image, the ultrasound beam has to be swept across the area of interest. Ultrasound is transmitted along several (90–120) scan lines over a wide (45°–90°) arc and many (20–30) times per second
- The superimposition of simultaneously reflected dots, builds up a red-time image on the display screen. Production of images in quick succession creates an anatomical cross-section of structures. Any image frame can be frozen, studied on the screen or printed out on thermal paper or X-ray film
- 2D echo is useful to evaluate the anatomy of the heart and the relationship between different structures **(Figs. 32.1A and B)**
- Intracardiac masses and extracardiac pericardial abnormalities can be noted. The motion of the walls of ventricles and cusps of valves is visualized
- Thickness of ventricular walls and dimensions of chambers can be measured and stroke volume, ejection fraction, and cardiac output can be calculated
- 2D image is also used to place the "cursor line" for M-mode echo and to position the "sample volume" for Doppler echo.

MOTION-MODE (M-MODE) ECHO

- In the M-mode tracing, ultrasound is transmitted and received along only one scan line.
- This line is obtained by applying a cursor line to the 2D image and aligning it perpendicular to the structure being studied. The transducer is angulated till the cursor line is exactly perpendicular to the image
- M-mode is displayed as a continuous tracing with two axes. The vertical axis represents distance between the moving structure and the transducer. The horizontal axis represents time
- Since only one scan line is imaged, M-mode echo provides greater sensitivity than 2D echo for studying the motion of moving structures
- Motion and thickness of ventricular walls, changing size of cardiac chambers and opening and closure of valves is better displayed on M-mode **(Figs. 32.2A and B)**
- Simultaneous ECG recording facilitates accurate timing of cardiac events. Similarly, the flow pattern on color flow mapping can be timed in relation to the cardiac cycle.

PRINCIPLES OF DOPPLER

- The Doppler acoustic effect is present and used by us in everyday life, although we don't realise it. Imagine an automobile sounding the horn and moving towards you, going past you and then away from you

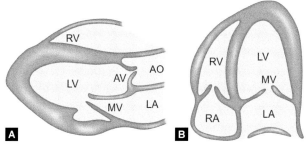

Figs. 32.1A and B: Two-dimensional echo (2D Echo): (A) Parasternal long-axis (PLAX) view; (B) Apical four-chamber (AP4CH) view. (AV: aortic valve; AO: Aorta; LA: left atrium; LV: left ventricle; MV: mitral valve; RV: right ventricle).

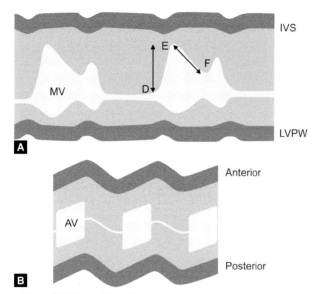

Figs. 32.2A and B: Motion-mode echo (M-mode echo): (A) Mitral valve (MV) level; (B) Aortic valve (AV) level.

- The pitch of the horn sound is higher when it approaches you (higher frequency) than when it goes away from you (lower frequency)
- The change of frequency (Doppler shift) depends upon the speed of the automobile and the original frequency of the horn sound
- This means that the nature of sound chiefly depends upon the relative motion of the listener and the source of sound
- Ultrasound reflected back from a tissue interface gives information about the depth and echo-reflectivity of the tissue being studied. On the other hand, Doppler utilizes ultrasound reflected back by moving red blood cells (RBCs)
- The Doppler principle is used to derive the velocity of blood flow. Flow velocity is derived from the change of frequency that occurs between transmitted (original) and reflected (observed) ultrasound signal
- The shift of frequency (Doppler shift) is proportional to ratio of velocity of blood to speed of sound and to the original frequency
- It is calculated from the following formula:

$$F_D = \frac{V}{C} \times F_O$$

F_D: Doppler shift $\quad$ F_o: Original frequency
V : Velocity of blood $\quad$ C : Speed of sound
Therefore, velocity of blood flow is:

$$V = \frac{F_D \times C}{F_o}$$

A further refinement of this formula is:

$$V = \frac{F_D \times C}{2F_o \cos\theta}$$

- The original frequency (F_o) is multiplied by 2 since Doppler shift occurs twice during forward transmission as well as during backward reflection
- Cosine theta ($\cos\theta$) is applied as a correction for the angle between the ultrasound beam and blood flow. The angle between the beam and flow should be less than 20° to ensure accurate measurement
- $\cos\theta$ is 1 if the beam is parallel to direction of blood flow and maximum velocity is observed. $\cos\theta$ is 0 if the beam is perpendicular to direction of blood flow and no velocity is detected
- It is noteworthy that for Doppler echo, maximum velocity information is obtained with the ultrasound beam aligned parallel to the direction of blood flow being studied
- This is in sharp contrast to conventional echo, where best image quality is obtained with the ultrasound beam aligned perpendicular to the structure being studied
- Since the original frequency value ($2 F_o$) is in the denominator of the velocity equation, it is important to remember that maximum velocity information is obtained using a low frequency transducer (2.5 MHz probe)
- There is a direct relationship between the peak flow velocity through a stenotic valve and the pressure gradient across it
- Understandably when the valve orifice is small, blood flow has to accelerate in order to eject the same stroke volume. This increase in velocity is measured by Doppler
- The pressure gradient across the valve can be calculated using the simplified Bernaulli equation:

$$\Delta P = 4 V^2$$

P : pressure gradient (in mm Hg)
V : peak flow velocity (in m/sec)

- This equation is frequently used during Doppler evaluation of stenotic valves, regurgitant lesions and intracardiac shunts
- The velocity information provided by Doppler echo complements the anatomical information provided by M-mode and 2D Echo
- Analysis of the returning Doppler signal not only provides information about flow velocity but also about flow direction
- By convention, velocities towards the transducer are displayed above the baseline (positive deflection) and velocities away from the transducer are displayed below the baseline (negative deflection) **(Fig. 32.3)**

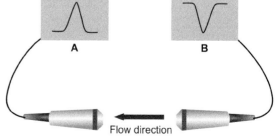

Fig. 32.3: Direction of blood flow and polarity of deflection: (A) Towards the transducer, positive deflection; (B) Away from transducer, negative deflection.

- The returning Doppler signal is a spectral trace of velocity display on a time axis. The area under curve (AUC) of the spectral trace is known as the flow velocity integral (FVI) of that velocity display
- The value of FVI is determined by peak flow velocity and ejection time. It can be calculated by the software of most echo machines
- Careful analysis of the spectral trace of velocity also gives densitometric information. Density relates to the number of RBCs moving at a given velocity
- When blood flow is smooth or laminar, most RBCs are travelling at the same velocity, since they accelerate and decelerate simultaneously
- The spectral trace then has a thin outline with very few RBCs travelling at other velocities **(Figs. 32.4A and C)**. This is known as low variance of velocities
- When blood flow is turbulent as across stenotic valves, there is a wide distribution of RBCs velocities and the Doppler signal appears "filled in" **(Fig. 32.4B)**. This is known as high variance of velocities, "spectral broadening" or "increased band width"
- It is to be borne in mind that turbulence and spectral broadening are often associated with but not synonymous with a high velocity signal
- The intensity of the Doppler signal is represented on the grey-scale as increasing shades of grey
- Maximum number of RBCs travelling at a particular velocity cast a dark shade on the spectral trace. Few RBCs travelling at a higher velocity cast a light shade
- This is best seen on the Doppler signal from a stenotic valve. The spectral display is most dense near the baseline reflecting most RBCs moving at a low velocity close to the valve **(Fig. 32.5A)**
- Few RBCs accelerating through the stenotic valve are at a high velocity **(Fig. 32.5B)**
- The Doppler echo modes used clinically are continuous wave (CW) Doppler and pulsed wave (PW) Doppler
- In CW Doppler, two piezoelectric crystals are used, one to transmit continuously and the other to receive continuously, without any time gap
- It can measure high velocities but does not discriminate between several velocity components. Therefore, CD Doppler cannot precisely locate the signal which may originate from anywhere along the length or breadth of the ultrasound beam

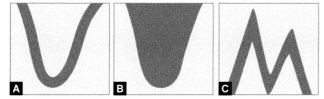

Figs. 32.4A to C: Various patterns of blood flow on Doppler: (A) Laminar flow across a normal aortic valve; (B) Turbulent flow across stenotic aortic valve; (C) Normal flow pattern across the mitral valve.

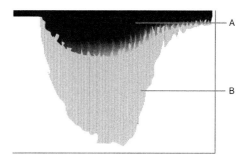

Fig. 32.5: Continuous wave Doppler signal from a stenotic aortic valve showing turbulent flow: (A) Most RBCs moving at low velocity, (B) Few RBCs moving at high velocity.

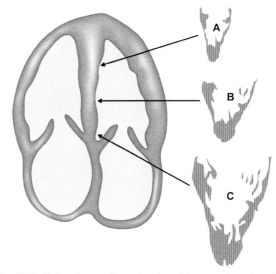

Fig. 32.6: Pulsed wave Doppler signal from various levels of the left ventricle: (A) LV apex; (B) Mid LV; (C) Subaortic.

- In PW Doppler, a single piezoelectric crystal is used to first emit a burst of ultrasound and then receive it after a preset time period. This time is required to switch-over into the receiver mode
- To localize the velocity, a 'sample volume' indicated by a small box or circle, is placed over the 2D image at the region of interest. The 'sample volume' can be moved in depth along the path of PW beam indicated as a broken line, until a maximum velocity signal is obtained **(Fig. 32.6)**
- PW Doppler can precisely localize the site of origin of a velocity signal, unlike CW Doppler
- Because of the time delay in receiving the reflected ultrasound signal, PW Doppler cannot accurately detect high velocities exceeding 2 m/sec.
- However, PW Doppler provides a spectral tracing of better quality than does CW Doppler **(Fig. 32.7)**
- The single crystal of PW Doppler can emit a fresh pulse only after the previous pulse has returned. The time interval between pulse repetition is therefore the sum of the time taken by the transmitted single to reach the target and the time taken by the returning signal to reach the transducer

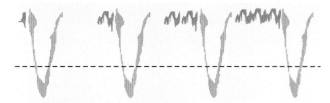

Fig. 32.7: Pulsed wave Doppler signal from a regurgitant aortic valve showing laminar flow.

- The rate at which pulses are emitted is known as the pulse repetition frequency (PRF). Obviously, greater the depth of interrogation, more is the time interval between pulse repetition and lower is the PRF
- Pulse repetition frequency (PRF) should be greater than twice the velocity being measured. The PRF decreases as the depth of interrogation increases
- The maximum value of Doppler frequency shift that can be accurately measured with a given repetition frequency (PRF) is called the Nyquist limit
- The inability of PW Doppler to defect high-frequency Doppler shifts is known as aliasing. Aliasing occurs when the Nyquist limited is exceeded
- Aliasing is an artificial reversal of velocity and distortion of the reflected signal. The phenomenon of aliasing is also called "wrap around"
- Aliasing can be tackled overcome by one of these modifications:
  - high pulse repetition frequency
  - multigate acquisition technique
  - reducing the depth of interrogation
  - shifting the baseline of spectral display.

CONTINUOUS WAVE DOPPLER

- Continuous wave (CW) Doppler transmits and receives ultrasound continuously. It can measure high velocities without any upper limit and is not hindered by the phenomenon of aliasing
- However, CW Doppler cannot precisely localize the returning signal which may originate anywhere along the length or width of the ultrasound beam **(Fig. 32.8)**
- This Doppler modality is used for rapid scanning of the heart in search of high velocity signals and abnormal flow patterns
- Since the Doppler frequency shift is in the audible range, the audio signal is used to angulate and rotate the transducer in order to obtain the best visual display
- Continuous wave Doppler display forms the basis for placement of "sample volume" to obtain PW Doppler spectral tracing
- Continuous wave Doppler is used for grading the severity of valvular stenosis and assessing the degree of valvular regurgitation
- An intracardiac left-to-right shunt such as a ventricular septal defect can be quantified

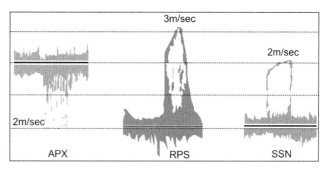

Fig. 32.8: Continuous wave (CW) Doppler signal of a stenotic aortic valve from multiple views. Maximum velocity 3 m/sec (APX: apical 5 chamber view; RPS: right parasternal view; SSN: suprasternal notch).

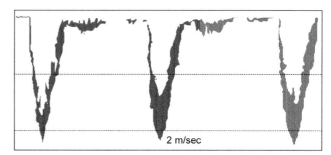

Fig. 32.9: Pulsed wave (PW) Doppler signal of a stenotic aortic valve from single view. Maximum velocity is 2 m/sec.

- By using CW Doppler signal of the tricuspid valve, pulmonary artery pressure can be calculated.

PULSED WAVE DOPPLER

- Pulsed wave (PW) Doppler transmits ultrasound in pulses and waits to receive the returning ultrasound after each pulse
- Because of the time delay in receiving the reflected signal which limits the sampling rate, it cannot detect high velocities
- At velocities over 2 m/sec., there occurs a reversal of flow known as the phenomenon of aliasing
- However, PW Doppler provides a better spectral tracing than CW Doppler, which is used for calculations **(Fig. 32.9)**
- Pulsed wave Doppler modality is used to localize velocity signals and abnormal flow patterns picked up by CW Doppler and color flow mapping, respectively
- The mitral valve inflow signal is used for the assessment of left ventricular diastolic dysfunction
- The aortic valve outflow signal is used for the calculation of stroke volume and cardiac output.

CLINICAL APPLICATIONS OF ECHO

2D Echo

- Anatomy of heart and structural relationships
- Intracardiac masses and pericardial diseases

- Motion of ventricular walls and valvular leaflets
- Wall thickness, chamber volume, and ejection fraction
- Calculation of stroke volume and cardiac output
- Architecture of valve leaflets and size of orifice
- Positioning for M-mode image and Doppler echo.

M-mode Echo

- Cavity size, wall thickness, and muscle mass
- Excursion of ventricular walls and valve cusps
- Timing of cardiac events with synchronous ECG
- Timing of flow pattern with color flow mapping.

Continuous Wave Doppler

- Grading the severity of valvular stenosis
- Assessing degree of valvular regurgitation
- Quantifying the pulmonary artery pressure
- Scanning the heart for high velocity signal.

Pulsed Wave Doppler

- Assessment of left ventricular diastolic function
- Calculation of stroke volume and cardiac output
- Estimation of orifice area of stenotic aortic valve
- Localization of flow pattern seen on CF mapping
- Localization of signal picked up on CW Doppler
- Application of spectral tracing for calculations.

PRINCIPLES OF COLOR DOPPLER

- Color Doppler echocardiography is an automated version of the pulsed-wave Doppler. It is also known as real-time Doppler imaging
- Color Doppler provides a visual display of blood flow within the heart, in the form of a color flow map
- The color flow map is rightly called a "noninvasive angiogram" since it simultaneously displays both anatomical as well as functional information
- After a burst of ultrasound is reflected back along a single scan-line, as in pulsed-wave Doppler, it is analyzed by the autocorrelator of the echo-machine
- The autocorrelator compares the frequency of the returning signal with the original frequency. It then assigns a color-code to the frequency difference, using an algorithm
- Analysis of several sample volumes down each scan-line and of several such scan-lines using multigate Doppler, creates a color-encoded map of the area being interrogated
- The color flow map encodes information about direction as well as velocity of blood flow. When this map is superimposed on the image sector of interest, appropriate interpretation is made
- The colors assigned to blood flow towards the transducer are shades of red white colors assigned to flow away from the transducer are hues of blue **(Fig. 32.10)**

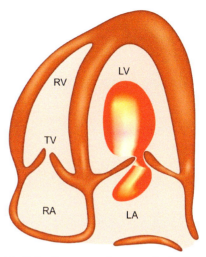

Fig. 32.10: Color flow map of a normal mitral valve from A4CH view showing a red-colored jet.

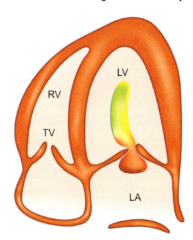

Fig. 32.11: Color flow map of a stenotic mitral valve from A4CH view showing a mosaic pattern.

- This is in accordance with the BART convention:
  Blue Away Red Towards
- As the velocity of blood flow increases, the shade or hue assigned to the flow gets progressively brighter. Therefore, low velocities appear dull and dark while high velocities appear bright and light
- When blood flow at high velocity becomes turbulent, it superimposes color variance into the color flow map. This is seen as a mosaic pattern with shades of aquamarine, green and yellow **(Fig. 32.11)**
- This reversal of color-code, as it "wraps around" and outlines the high velocity, is the color counterpart of aliasing observed on pulsed-wave Doppler
- The differences between a color-flow map and a spectral trace obtained from pulsed-wave Doppler are summarized in **Table 32.1**.

TECHNIQUES OF COLOR DOPPLER

- The technique of color Doppler is similar to that of conventional echo and pulsed-wave Doppler. The

TABLE 32.1: Differences between spectral trace and color-flow map.

	Spectral trace	Color flow-map
Display	Scan-line	Flow-map
Depiction	Direction	Color
Velocity	Velocity	Hue/shade
Turbulence	Aliasing	Variance

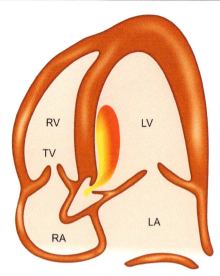

Fig. 32.13: Color flow map of a regurgitant aortic valve from AP5CH view showing a mosaic pattern jet. (TV: tricuspid valve)

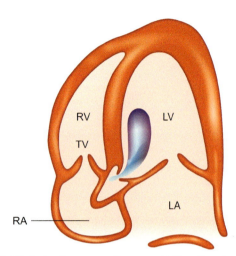

Fig. 32.12: Color flow map of a normal LV outflow tract from AP5CH view showing a blue-colored jet.

transducer is placed in the usual parasternal or apical window as done for standard echo imaging
- Once an anatomical image is obtained, the color is turned on. Color flow maps are automatically displayed and superimposed on the standard echo image **(Fig. 32.12)**.
- When the color map has been visualized, the transducer is slightly angulated. This is done to optimize the visual display. The final image is often a trade-off between an optimal anatomical image and a good color flow map
- The grey-scale tissue-gain setting must be just enough to provide structural reference. Setting the tissue-gain too low blurs the anatomical image. Setting the tissue-gain too high induces grey-scale artefact or "background noise" and distorts the color display **(Fig. 32.13)**
- The velocity-filter and color-gain settings must be optimal. Setting the filter high and gain low may miss color flow maps of low velocities. Setting the filter low and gain high may introduce color artefacts from normal structures and obscure genuine color flow maps.

ADVANTAGES OF COLOR DOPPLER

- The major advantage of color Doppler echo is the rapidity with which normal and abnormal flow patterns can be visualized and interpreted
- The spatial orientation of color flow mapping is easier to comprehend for those not experienced in Doppler. Conventional wave Doppler tracings have to be understood, before interpretation

- Color Doppler improves the accuracy of sampling with pulsed-wave and continuous-wave Doppler by helping to align the Doppler beam with the color jet. This facilitates localization of valve regurgitation and intracardiac shunts
- The phenomenon of aliasing, a disadvantage in pulsed-wave Doppler, is advantageous during color flow mapping. Introduction of color variance in the flow map is easily recognized as a mosaic pattern.

LIMITATIONS OF COLOR DOPPLER

- Like all other echo modalities, color Doppler may be limited by non-availability of a satisfactory echo window or by malalignment of the ultrasound beam with blood flow direction
- As with pulsed-wave Doppler, color Doppler is sensitive to pulsed repetition frequency (PRF) of the transducer and the depth of the cardiac structure being interrogated
- Color Doppler may inadvertently miss low velocities if the flow signal is weak. This occurs especially if the velocity filter setting is high and the color gain setting is low
- Color Doppler may spuriously pick up artefacts from heart muscle and valve tissue which falsely get assigned a color. This occurs especially if the velocity filter setting is low and the color gain setting is high **(Fig. 32.14)**
- Complex cardiac lesions may produce a multitude of blood flows in a small area, in both systole and diastole. The result is a confusional riot of color, hindering rather than helping an accurate diagnosis.

APPLICATIONS OF COLOR DOPPLER

Stenotic Lesions

- Color Doppler can identify, localize, and quantitate stenotic lesions of the cardiac valves. It visually displays

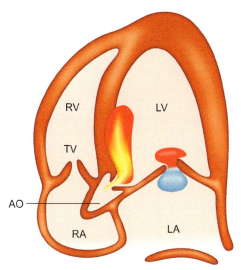

Fig. 32.14: Color flow map of the left ventricle from AP5CH view showing artefacts from the IV septum and mitral leaflets.

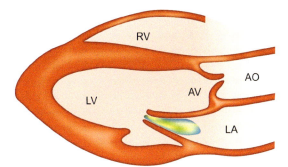

Fig. 32.16: Color flow map of a regurgitant mitral valve from PLAX view showing a jet in the left atrium.

- It would be ideal to measure the stenotic orifice from the color Doppler view. However, this is practically difficult since anatomical measurement requires perpendicular beam orientation while the Doppler signal requires a parallel beam orientation.

Regurgitant Lesions

- Color Doppler can diagnose and estimate the severity of regurgitant lesions of the valves. It displays the regurgitant jet as a flow-map distinct from the normal flow pattern
- A regurgitant valve produces a color-flow map in the receiving chamber. For instance, mitral regurgitation results in a left atrial flow map while aortic regurgitation causes a flow map in the left ventricular outflow tract **(Fig. 32.16)**
- A jet interrogated along its length produces a large flow area while scanning the same jet across reveals a smaller area. By using multiple views and windows for interrogation, the size and geometry of a pathological jet can be accurately estimated
- It is necessary to angulate the transducer, in order to scan across the length and width of the chamber being studied. This will improve the detection of eccentric regurgitant lesions
- Valvular regurgitation can be quantified by assessing the depth upto which color flow can be picked up. Mild regurgitation is confined to the valve plane while severe regurgitation can be mapped upto the distal portion of the receiving chamber
- Measuring the absolute jet area and calculating the ratio of jet area to atrial size is also used to assess the degree of ventriculo-atrial regurgitation
- A ratio of less than 25% indicates mild, 25–50% suggests moderate and more than 50% represents severe valvular regurgitation.

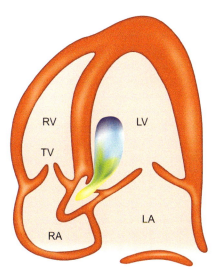

Fig. 32.15: Color flow map of a stenotic aortic valve from AP5CH view showing change in color to a mosaic pattern.

the stenotic area and the resultant jet as distinct from normal flow
- Stenosis of a valve produces a "candle-flame" shaped jet at the site of narrowing. The jet color assumes a mosaic pattern of aquamarine, green and yellow signifying increased velocity and turbulent flow **(Fig. 32.15)**
- The color Doppler signal has to be parallel to the direction of blood flow or else the degree of stenosis gets underestimated. Angulation of the transducer to improve the Doppler signal, inadvertently skews and distorts the anatomical image
- When there is calcification of the valve leaflets or annulus, the color flow display drops out of the image in the calcified area. Turning up the gain to image the calcified area causes blooming of both the anatomic image as well as the Doppler signal

Intracardiac Shunts

- An atrial septal defect produces a mosaic color flow map crossing from the left atrium to the right atrium. Because of low velocity, the color map is sometimes missed **(Fig. 32.17)**

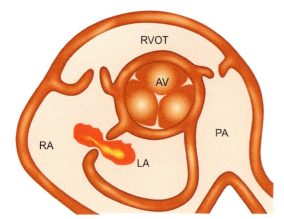

Fig. 32.17: Color flow map of an atrial septal defect from PSAX view showing a jet crossing from the left to right atrium.

- A ventricular septal defect produces a mosaic color flow map extending from the left ventricle to the right ventricle across the septum. The width of the map approximates the size of the septal defect
- A patent ductus arteriosus produces a retrograde mosaic color flow map extending from the descending aorta to the pulmonary artery.

CORONARY ARTERY DISEASE

Since coronary artery disease (CAD) is the leading form of heart disease in middle and old ages, it is therefore not surprising that CAD is the commonest clinical diagnosis in those on whom echo is performed.

INDICATIONS FOR ECHO IN CORONARY ARTERY DISEASE

- Detection and assessment of myocardial ischemia
- Prediction of infarction-related artery
- Assessment of left ventricular function
- Detection of right ventricular infarction
- Detection of complications of acute infarction
  - Acute mitral regurgitation
  - Acute ventricular septal defect
  - Ventricular aneurysm
  - Pericardial effusion
  - Mural thrombus
- Direct visualization of proximal coronary arteries
  - Proximal coronary stenosis
  - Coronary artery aneurysm
  - Coronary artery fistula
  - Anomalous origin of artery
- Diagnosis of cardiac conditions simulating CAD
  - Aortic stenosis (AS)
  - MV prolapse (MVP)
  - Hypertrophic CMP (HOCM)
- Stress echocardiography
  - If TMT is not possible, uninterpretable or equivocal.
- To localize the site and quantify extent of ischemia
- To assess myocardial stunning or hibernation.

MYOCARDIAL ISCHEMIA

- *Lack of systolic wall thickening:* reduced or absent. Systolic thickening of the ischemic myocardial segment during systole is either reduced in extent or altogether absent
- *Abnormal systolic wall motion:* hypokinesia, akinesia or dyskinesia. Inward motion of the ischemic myocardial segment during systole is partially reduced, entirely absent or paradoxically outwards
- These changes are transient if ischemia is reversed by giving rest or nitrate medication. Acute myocardial infarction causes similar abnormalities which are reversible by thrombolytic therapy or primary angioplasty
- Abnormal wall motion can be classified as in **Table 32.2**, with each pattern of wall motion assigned a score
- From the wall motion score, the wall motion index can be calculated as follows:

$$\text{Wall motion index} = \frac{\text{sum of scores of all segments}}{\text{number of segments studied}}$$

A wall motion index that exceeds 1.5 is abnormal.

MYOCARDIAL INFARCTION

- *Abnormal systolic wall thickening:* reduced or absent. Systolic thickening of the infarcted myocardial segment during systole is either reduced in extent or altogether absent
- There may be systolic thinning to less than 6 mm or by more than 30% compared to adjacent myocardium. This occurs if the infarct is old. The normal septal thickness is 6–12 mm
- The thinned infarcted myocardial segment is more echoreflective than the adjacent myocardium, due to postinfarction fibrosis and scarring
- *Abnormal systolic wall motion:* hypokinesia, akinesia or dyskinesia. Inward motion of the infarcted myocardial segment during systole is reduced, absent or paradoxically outwards respectively **(Fig. 32.18)**
- Dyskinetic segments and aneurysmal areas are more often due to old myocardial infarction than due to ischemia, because of prior myocardial scarring

TABLE 32.2: Left ventricle systolic wall motion score.

Score	Motion	Description
1.	Normal motion	Full inward motion
2.	Hypokinesia	Reduced (<50%) inward motion
3.	Akinesia	No inward motion
4.	Dyskinesia	Outward movement
5.	Aneurysmal	Outpouching of wall

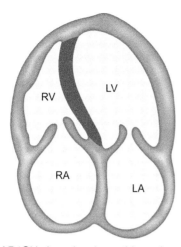

Fig. 32.18: AP4CH view showing a thin and scarred septum that moves paradoxically outwards in systole.

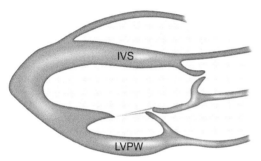

Fig. 32.19: Motion of IVS and LVPW as seen on PLAX view. (IVS, interventricular septum; LVPW, left ventricular posterior wall)

TABLE 32.3: Motion of IVS and LVPW.

Contractility	Amplitude (mm)	
	IVS	LVPW
Reduced	<3	<9
Normal	3–8	9–14
Exaggerated	>8	>14

IVS, interventricular septum; LVPW, left ventricular posterior wall

- Wall motion abnormalities due to infarction are not reversible by medication (nitrate) or intervention (thrombolysis or PTCA) **(Fig. 32.19)**
- The normal myocardial segment opposite the wall that shows reduced motion, exhibits compensatory hyperkinesia and exaggerated motion
- Besides myocardial infraction, reduced wall motion is also observed in cardiomyopathy and pericardial constriction. Exaggerated wall motion is due to compensatory hyperkinesia or in case of volume overload and hyperdynamic circulation. Motion of the IV septum may be paradoxical (away from LV cavity during systole) in certain situations
- Wall motion of the IV septum and LV posterior wall can be categorized as normal, reduced, and exaggerated as shown in **Table 32.3**
- Wall motion of the IV septums and LV posterior wall is abnormal in the following situations:

Posterior Wall (LVPW) Motion

Reduced	Left ventricular posterior wall infarction
	Dilated cardiomyopathy
	Constrictive pericarditis
Exaggerated	Left ventricular volume overload
	Right ventricular volume overload
	Mitral valve paraprosthetic leak
	Septal wall infarction

Ventricular Septal (IVS) Motion

Reduced	Septal wall infarction
	Hypertrophic myopathy
	Dilated cardiomyopathy
Exaggerated	Left ventricular volume overload
	Hyperdynamic state
	Posterior wall infarction
Paradoxical	Right ventricular volume overload
	Constrictive pericarditis
	Left bundle branch block

- The areas of the left ventricle which can be seen from various echo views are:
  - Interventricular septum **(Fig. 32.20)**
  - Left ventricular apex **(Fig. 32.21)**
  - Anterior wall **(Fig. 32.22)**
  - Lateral wall **(Fig. 32.23)**
  - Inferior wall **(Fig. 32.24)**.
- On 2D imaging, the left ventricle can be divided into several segments. This is useful to identify the location of ischemia or infarction and to quantify its extent
- Each wall can be further divided into basal (proximal), middle and apical (distal) segments. Multiple views are used to study wall motion
- From the location of regional wall motion abnormalities, it is possible to predict the coronary artery involved in the ischemic event **(Fig. 32.25)**.

LEFT VENTRICULAR DYSFUNCTION

- Presence of coronary artery disease ever without prior myocardial infarction can cause LV diastolic dysfunction (impaired myocardial relaxation)
- A single large myocardial infarction or repeated small infarcts leads to scarring of myocardium resulting in thin segments which do not thicken during systole and show reduced motion
- This is often associated with LV systolic dysfunction. Thinning of myocardium with reduced systolic motion is also observed in dilated cardiomyopathy.
- Triple vessel coronary artery disease may lead to impairment of LV systolic dysfunction even in the absence of prior myocardial infarction **(Fig. 32.26)**

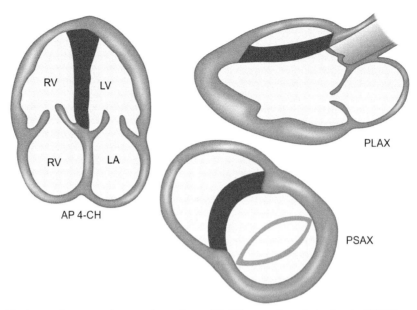

Fig. 32.20: The ventricular septum seen from various views. (PLAX: parasternal short axis; PSAX; parasternal long axis).

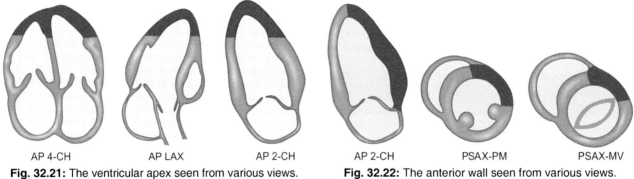

Fig. 32.21: The ventricular apex seen from various views.

Fig. 32.22: The anterior wall seen from various views.

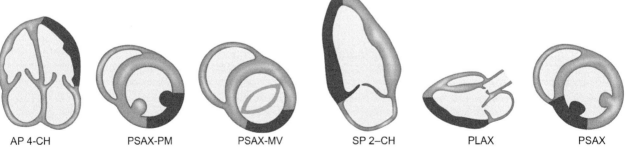

Fig. 32.23: The lateral wall seen from various views.

Fig. 32.24: The inferior wall seen from various views.

- This condition is referred to as ischemic cardiomyopathy (ICMP). ICMP superficially resembles a dilated cardiomyopathy (DCMP) with the following subtle differences:
    - In ICMP, atleast one portion of the LV moves normally while global hypokinesia is seen in DCMP
    - Dyskinetic areas and aneurysms are a feature of ICMP and are not observed in DCMP
    - In ICMP but not DCMP, wall motion abnormalities conform to specific coronary arterial territories.
    - The right ventricle is usually spared in ICMP and it is often involved in DCMP.

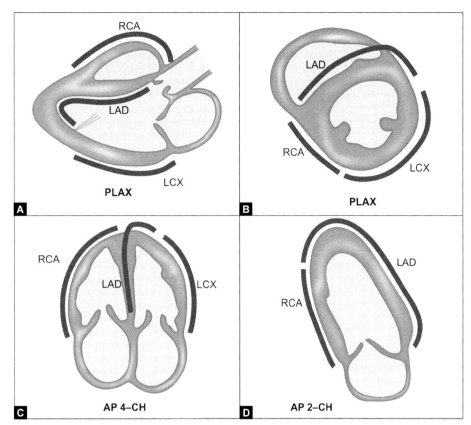

Figs. 32.25A to D: The coronary arterial supply to different areas of the heart: (A) PLAX view; (B) PSAX view; (C) AP4CH view; (D) AP2CH view (LAD: Left anterior descending; LCX: Left circumflex artery; RCA: Right coronary artery).

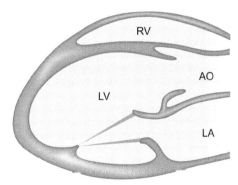

Fig. 32.26: PLAX view showing enlargement of the left ventricle in a patient of ischemic CMP.

- Following temporary coronary occlusion, impairment of myocardial contractile function may remain, even after restoration of blood supply without infarction
- This condition is termed as myocardial stunning and the myocardial tissue remains viable to regain normal function after 1–2 weeks
- Similarly, recurrent episodes of acute ischemia may result in temporary myocardial dysfunction which is termed as myocardial hibernation
- Myocardium that is stunned or hibernating does not have enough energy to contract but is still viable and able to repair wear and tear

- A stunned or hibernating myocardium causes LV systolic or diastolic dysfunction which is potentially reversible by a revascularization procedure
- Cardiogenic shock after acute myocardial infarction may be due to pump failure following extensive muscle damage. In this condition, echo shows severe impairment of LV systolic function
- Alternatively, it may be due to LV free wall rupture, hemopericardium and cardiac tamponade
- In acute mitral regurgitation or acute ventricular septal defect after myocardial infarction, LV systolic function remains active.

RIGHT VENTRICULAR DYSFUNCTION

- Whenever echocardiography is performed for assessment of coronary artery disease, the focus is on the left ventricle
- Nevertheless, evaluation of the right ventricle is important, particularly in patients of inferior wall infarction
- In them, prognosis is worse if there is right ventricular infarction and RV dysfunction
- The hemodynamic response of the right ventricle to myocardial infarction is different from that of the left ventricle

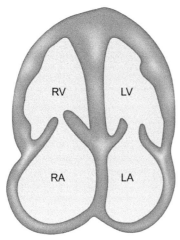

Fig. 32.27: AP4CH view showing dilatation of right ventricle and right atrium due to right ventricular infarction.

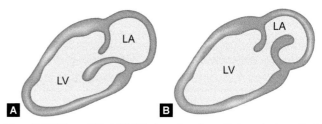

Figs. 32.28A and B: AP2CH view showing a flail posterior mitral leaflet with exaggerated motion towards: (A) Left ventricle in diastole; (B) Left atrium in systole.

- When there is RV infarction, cardiogenic shock is common and it requires a different therapeutic approach than does LV infarction (saline infusion and not diuresis)
- Right ventricular infarction is suspected clinically by the coexistence of hypotension (low BP) with elevated venous pressure (high JVP)
- RV infarction is associated with a dilated (> 23 mm) and hypokinetic right ventricle. There is paradoxical motion of the IV septum. The right atrium is dilated **(Fig. 32.27)**
- Due to RV failure, the inferior vena cava (IVC) is dilated more than 2 cm and fails to constrict by atleast 50 percent during the phase of inspiration
- Evaluation of RV function is also useful in assessing the prognosis of patients with ventricular septal defect (acute VSD) following myocardial infarction
- RV dysfunction is a predictor of cardiogenic shock and mortality in these patients.

ACUTE MITRAL REGURGITATION

- Acute MR in a setting of acute myocardial infarction occurs either due to papillary muscle rupture or because of papillary muscle dysfunction.
- Rupture of a papillary muscle causes a flail mitral valve leaflet. Since rupture of the posteromedial papillary muscle is more common than that of the anterolateral muscle, often it is the posterior mitral leaflet (PML) that is flail
- It generally follows inferior wall infarction due to occlusion of the posterior descending branch of the right coronary artery
- On 2D Echo, the flail leaflet exhibits an exaggerated whip-like motion (like a sail flapping in the wind). Its tip moves past the coaptation point into the left atrium and fails to coapt with the AML **(Figs. 32.28A and B)**
- Superficially, it resembles the floppy leaflet of mitral valve prolapse (see Valvular Diseases)
- Papillary muscle dysfunction is due to ischemic restriction of papillary function or akinesia of the inferobasal wall that does not shorten in systole
- As a result, the posterior MV leaflet fails to reach the plane of the MV annulus and the coaptation point of the AML with PML in systole, is located distally in the left ventricle
- On continuous wave (CW) Doppler or color flow mapping, the MR flow velocity or color jet is eccentric and directed towards the posterior left atrial wall
- The jet area may be much less than what the actual amount of MR would indicate hence there is a risk of underestimation of MR severity
- Unlike in the MR of valvular disease, in acute MR there is no dilatation of the left atrium and ventricle or abnormal architecture of the MV leaflets
- In acute MR due to acute MI, LV systolic function remains preserved unlike in pump failure due to extensive MI, where there is severe impairment of LV function.

VENTRICULAR SEPTAL DEFECT

- Ventricular septal defect (acquired VSD) in a setting of acute myocardial infarction occurs due to a breach in continuity of the interventricular septum
- It often occurs near the cardiac apex and is more common after damage to the inferior wall with right ventricular infarction
- The discontinuity of the IV septum can be seen as an echo drop-out on 2D echo in several views
- The perforation expands in systole and often there is an aneurysmal bulge of the septum close to the LV apex
- The VSD jet can be seen on color flow mapping and by tracking the pulsed wave (PW) Doppler sample volume along the right side of the septum **(Fig. 32.29)**
- Significant left-to-right shunting of blood across the VSD can cause RV volume overload. As in acute MR, the LV systolic function is preserved in acute VSD.

LEFT VENTRICULAR ANEURYSM

- An aneurysm is a large bulge-like deformity with a wide neck, located at or near the apex of the left ventricle. It is more common after damage to the anterior wall than after inferior wall infarction

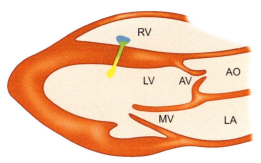

Fig. 32.29: PLAX view showing a color flow map across a ventricular septal defect.

TABLE 32.4: Differences between LV aneurysm and pseudo-aneurysm.

	LV aneurysm	Pseudo-aneurysm
Shape	Wide neck	Narrow neck
Location	Apex of LV	Posterior wall
Motion	Dyskinetic	Expansile
Wall	Myocardium	Pericardium
Rupture	Unlikely	Liable
Thrombus	Laminar	Fills cavity

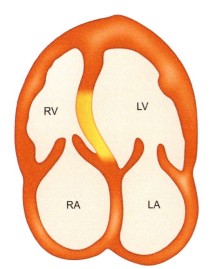

Fig. 32.30: AP4CH view showing an aneurysmal bulge of the basal IV septum.

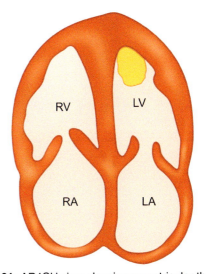

Fig. 32.31: AP4CH view showing a ventricular thrombus protruding into the LV cavity.

- The aneurysm exhibits dyskinesia of motion or outward systolic expansion and a persistent diastolic deformity (**Fig. 32.30**)
- The wall of the aneurysm is made of myocardium and is more echogenic than adjacent areas because of fibrous scar tissue. It does not rupture but is often associated with a pedunculated or laminated ventricular thrombus
- A false aneurysm (pseudo-aneurysm) follows a breach in the left ventricular free wall, when the resulting hemopericardium clots and seals off the hole by pericardial adhesions
- The neck of the pseudo-aneurysm that communicates with the left ventricle is narrower than the diameter of the aneurysm. Therefore, it appears as a globular extracardiac pouch, external to the LV cavity
- A false aneurysm is located on the posterolateral LV wall and is more common after inferior wall than after anterior wall infarction. Being thin-walled, it expands in systole
- The wall of the aneurysm is made of pericardium and it is less echogenic than adjacent areas. It is friable, liable to rupture and is often filled with a thrombus due to clotted hemopericardium

- The differences between a true and false LV aneurysm are enumerated in **Table 32.4**.

VENTRICULAR MURAL THROMBUS

- A ventricular thrombus may form on a dyskinetic, infarcted and scarred myocardial segment or within a left ventricular aneurysm
- It appears as a rounded pedunculated mass protruding into the LV cavity (**Fig. 32.31**) or as a flat laminated mural thrombus contiguous with the ventricular wall
- A mobile mural thrombus may be a source of peripheral embolization (see Intracardiac Masses).

ACUTE PERICARDIAL EFFUSION

- A small amount of pericardial effusion may accumulate due to pericardial reaction after infarction
- A rupture of the left ventricular free wall may lead to hemopericardium. This may cause cardiac tamponade which is usually fatal
- Sometimes the hemopericardium clots, seals off the hole by adhesions and forms a pseudoaneurysm.

- An autoimmune pericarditis with a small amount of effusion may follow acute myocardial infarction. This is known as the Dressler's syndrome.

CORONARY ARTERIAL ANOMALIES

- Echocardiography is not the best investigative modality to visualize the coronary arteries themself. Coronary angiography is the best investigation for this purpose
- Sometimes, direct visualization of the coronary arteries may reveal the following abnormalities:
  - Coronary stenosis at origin seen as focal reduction in lumen or increase in reflectivity of the proximal 1.0–1.5 cm of the artery.
- Coronary artery aneurysm seen as a circular echo-free space Kawasaki syndrome
- Coronary artery fistula seen as parallel echoes with a wide lumen separating them
- Anomalous origin of artery seen as a dilated right coronary artery with the left coronary artery arising from pulmonary artery. This condition is known as ALCAPA (anomalous left coronary artery arising from pulmonary artery).

SIMULATING CONDITIONS

- The commonest form of coronary artery disease (CAD) is narrowing of the vessel lumen by atherosclerotic plaque(s). The most frequent symptom of CAD is chest pain (angina pectoris) due to myocardial ischemia
- This anginal pain needs to be differentiated from other causes of chest pain such as esophageal disorders and musculoskeletal diseases
- Occasionally, the chest pain is caused by cardiac conditions that simulate CAD in their clinical presentation. These conditions can be readily diagnosed by echocardiography and they include:
  - Aortic valve stenosis (AS)
  - Mitral valve prolapse (MVP)
  - Hypertrophic CMP (HOCM)

  These have been discussed elsewhere in this book.

STRESS ECHOCARDIOGRAPHY

Principle

Stress echocardiography is a noninvasive technique to demonstrate abnormalities of regional wall motion and myocardial thick which are not present when an echo is performed at rest. In other words, it picks up the effects of ischemia which are inducible or provocable by stress.

Technique

The stress is delivered by one of the following methods:
- Physical exercise on a treadmill or bicycle as used for stress ECG testing
- Pharmacological stress with dobutamine, an inotropic sympathomimetic agent which increases the heart rate and blood pressure and therefore the myocardial oxygen demand
- Vasodilators like adenosine and dipyridamole may be used to dilate normal coronary arteries and in the process divert blood away from the stenotic artery and cause ischemia
- Electrical cardiac pacing may be employed to increase the heart rate and to simulate exercise.

Indications

- As an alternative to the stress ECG test. The situations in which stress ECHO is superior to the Stress ECG test are:
  - Inability to exercise on a treadmill or bicycle (due to prior stroke, arthritis, obesity or fraility)
  - Resting ECG abnormality (LBBB, LVH, digoxin)
  - Equivocal or inconclusive stress ECG testing.

  The sensitivity and specificity of stress echocardiography for detection of coronary disease (80% and 90% respectively), is higher than that of stress ECG (65% and 75%).

  It is quite similar to that of radionuclide myocardial perfusion imaging (stress thallium). Wall motion abnormalities appear earlier than either chest pain or ST segment depression.

- To localize the site and quantify extent of ischemia.

  As mentioned earlier, the left ventricle can be divided into several segments to study wall motion abnormalities. From the pattern of abnormal motion, not only can ischemia be quantified but the occluded artery can also be predicted.

  This is helpful in the following situations:
  - To select patients for early coronary angiography and revascularization e.g., a large wall motion abnormality in the LAD territory.
  - To stratify the risk of a future coronary event after acute myocardial infarction
  - To assess the functional significance of a known stenotic lesion while planning a revascularization procedure (angioplasty or by-pass surgery).

- To assess viability of the myocardium.

  Myocardium that is stunned or hibernating causes LV systolic or diastolic dysfunction which is reversible by revascularization. If hibernation is present but revasculariz, mortality is higher than if there was no viability at all.

  This fact underscores the importance of detecting hibernating myocardium. Stress echo is similar in sensitivity to position emission tomography (PET) in detecting myocardial viability.

Positive Test

The stress echo is considered to be positive if one or more of these findings are observed:
- Worsening of previous wall motion abnormality
- Appearance of a new wall motion abnormality

- Inability of myocardial thickness to increase
- Failure to rise or a fall in the ejection fraction
- Appearance or worsening of mitral regurgitation.

Negative Test

The stress echo may be falsely negative in the following situations:
- Small ischemic area with good collateralization
- Single vessel disease without prior infarction
- Difficult echo window, or operator inexperience
- Postexercise time-lag before echo.

Limitations

- The limitations of stress echo as a diagnostic modality for CAD are:
  - High degree of operator dependency in technique.
  - Difficult acoustic windows in the presence of obesity or pulmonary emphysema
  - Artefacts caused by hyperventilation during the immediate post-exercise period
  - Difficulty in delineation of the endocardial lining causing error in volumetric measurement
  - Presence of septal dyskinesia due to the presence of left bundle branch block.

SYSTEMIC ARTERIAL HYPERTENSION

Since systemic arterial hypertension is a fairly common clinical condition, echo is often performed in hypertensive subjects.

INDICATIONS FOR ECHO

- Detection of left ventricular hypertrophy (LVH) (see Echo Features below)
- Assessment of LV systolic and diastolic function (see Ventricular Dysfunction)
- Detection of coexisting coronary artery disease (see Coronary Artery Disease)
- Detection of mitral and aortic valve degeneration (see Valvular Diseases)
- Detection of aortic dilatation and coarctation (see Aortic Diseases).

LEFT VENTRICULAR HYPERTROPHY

Echo Features of Left Ventricular Hypertrophy

- Thickening of the interventricular septum (IVS) and left ventricular posterior wall (LVPW)
- The normal thickness of the IVS and LVPW in diastole is 6–12 mm. Thickness exceeding 12 mm indicates presence of left ventricular hypertrophy (LVH) (**Fig. 32.32**).

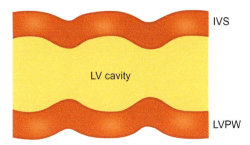

Fig. 32.32: M-mode scan of the left ventricle showing marked thickening of the IV septum and LV posterior wall with a small LV cavity.

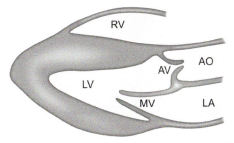

Fig. 32.33: PLAX view showing obliteration of the left ventricle cavity due to thickening of the septum and posterior wall.

- Normally the ratio of IVS : LVPW thickness is 1:1. Hypertrophy of the IVS to a greater extent than that of the LVPW indicates asymmetrical septal hypertrophy (ASH).
- If there is ASH in hypertension, the IVS : LVPW ratio is usually in the range of 1.3–1.5.
- Small left ventricular cavity less than 36 mm in diameter during diastole. Thickening of the IVS and LVPW leads to obliteration of the LV cavity in systole
- The normal left ventricular end-diastolic dimension (LVEDD) is 36 to 52 mm (**Fig. 32.33**)
- Since the LV systolic function is usually good, the amplitude of wall motion is normal
- Thick papillary muscles with prominent trabeculae carnae are seen parallel to the LV posterior wall.
- There is an increase in the left ventricular mass. The LV mass (in grams) is calculated by the equation:
$$1.05\,[(IVS + LVPW + LVEDD)^3 - LVEDD^3] - 14$$
LV mass =
IVS: Diastolic thickness of the IV septum
LVPW: Diastolic thickness of posterior wall
LVEDD: End-diastolic dimension of ventricle.
- LV mass can also be calculated by subtracting LV endocardial volume (LVV endo) from the LV epicardial volume (LVV epi) and multiplying it by the density of the muscle which is 1.05 g/cm^3 (mass = volume × density) (**Fig. 32.34**).
LV mass = [LVVepi – LVV endo] × 1.05
- In the presence of LV hypertrophy, the LV mass exceeds 136 grams in men and 112 grams in women per meter square body surface area (m^2 BSA)

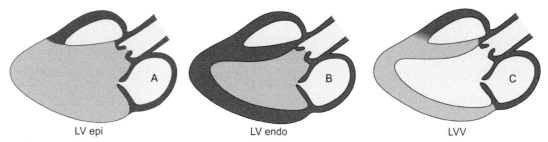

Fig. 32.34: Calculation of left ventricular mass from LV volume: LV epicardial volume (A) minus LV endocardial volume (B) is equal to LV volume (C).

- In LV hypertrophy due to hypertension, the increase in wall thickness occurs at the expense of reduction in cavity size. This is known as concentric LVH
- In concentric LVH, the relative wall thickness (RWT) ratio, which is LVPW thickness divided by LV radius in diastole, exceeds 0.45.

DIFFERENTIAL DIAGNOSIS OF LEFT VENTRICULAR HYPERTROPHY

- The echo picture of LVH due to hypertension is simulated by LVH due to other conditions causing LV pressure overload namely aortic valve stenosis and coarctation of aorta
- The asymmetrical septal hypertrophy (ASH) in hypertension may resemble ASH observed in case of hypertrophic cardiomyopathy (HOCM)
- However, the IVS: LVPW ratio in hypertension is generally in the range of 1.3–1.5 while it exceeds 1.5 in HOCM
- Myocardial thickening with LV diastolic dysfunction is also observed in restrictive cardiomyopathy (RCMP) and myocardial infiltrative diseases
- These can be differentiated from the effects of systemic hypertension by the lack of coexisting coronary arterial, valvular and aortic abnormalities
- Systemic hypertension, aortic stenosis and coarctation of aorta cause LV pressure overload. Mitral and aortic regurgitation, chronic anemia and chronic renal failure cause LV volume overload
- In conditions causing LV volume overload, there is predominant LV dilatation with a mild degree of LVH. In these conditions there is eccentric LVH which is inadequate for the degree of LV dilatation
- The relative wall thickness (RWT) ratio, which is LVPW thickness divided by LV radius in diastole, is less than 0.45
- In eccentric LV hypertrophy the degree of LVH, as determined only from wall thickness, may be underestimated. However, the left ventricular muscle mass is increased
- Therefore, LV muscle mass is a better indicator of LV hypertrophy than LV wall thickness
- Increase in LV mass precedes increase in blood pressure. LV diastolic dysfunction precedes LV systolic dysfunction
- In the advanced stages of hypertensive heart disease, there is LV dilatation, global hypokinesia and LV systolic dysfunction. The echo picture then resembles that of dilated cardiomyopathy (DCMP).

CLINICAL SIGNIFICANCE OF LEFT VENTRICULAR HYPERTROPHY

- Presence of LVH is the most common abnormality on echo in a hypertensive patient. Systemic hypertension is also the most important cause of LVH
- Left ventricular hypertrophy is an independent predictor of cardiovascular morbidity and 10-year mortality as a risk factor for myocardial infarction, heart failure, ventricular arrhythmias, and sudden cardiac death. The predictive value of LVH in hypertension is as strong as that of multi-vessel coronary artery disease
- Left ventricular hypertrophy may be indicated on the ECG by presence of tall QRS complexes. The voltage criteria of S in V_1 or V_2 plus R in V_5 or V_6 greater than 35 mm (Sokolow criteria) is often used. There may be an associated "strain pattern" with ST segment depression and T wave inversion in the lateral leads
- Echocardiography is 5–10 times more sensitive than an ECG in the detection of LVH. Precordial findings in LVH are visible aortic ejection mummur and a loud aortic component (A_2) of the second heart sound (S_2)
- Presence of LVH can be used as an indication for treatment of young patients having borderline or labile hypertension. In them, echo is also useful to look for an underlying coarctation of aorta
- Serial echos may be performed periodically (e.g., annually) to monitor the progress of hypertensive heart disease and to assess the regression of LVH with antihypertensive drugs.

33
CHAPTER

Elastography

INTRODUCTION

Ultrasonography is being used in clinical practice for decades for its ease of use, portability, real-time assessment, and low cost. However, it lacked fundamental and quantitative information on tissue elastic properties. With the advent of elastography since two decades, and its on-going advancements, this limitation has taken a back foot now.

Ultrasonographic elastography (sonoelastography) is a noninvasive imaging technique which can be used to depict relative tissue stiffness in response to a given force. Stiff tissues deform less and exhibit less strain than compliant tissues in response to the same force applied. Thus, the basis of elastography stands analogous to manual palpation. Compared to manual palpation, sonoelatography has the advantage of evaluating deeper tissues and is also semi-quantifiable.

TECHNIQUES

Several sonoelastographic techniques have been devised, including compression strain imaging, vibration sonoelastography, acoustic radiation force generated by the ultrasound pulse, and real-time shear velocity. Among these techniques, compression sonoelastography and vibration sonoelastography currently have the most prominent role. As the name implies, in compression technique, there is an externally applied force on the region of interest and on the other hand, vibration technique generates tissue displacement through the use of an independent external vibration source.

These techniques mainly use two methods which can measure strain of the tissue. One uses visual-scale score; another uses strain ratios and compares the strain of a region with that of the surrounding tissue.

The strain of a tissue is defined by the change in length during compression divided by the length before compression. The relationship between the compression, or the stress, and the strain is calculated in the Young's modulus.

Strain elastography measures axial displacement of tissue caused by mechanical stress in real-time. The stress is either applied externally with the transducer by the operator or by physiological shifts inside the patient. Transducer stress is applied by continuously compressing and decompressing the skin of the patient a few millimeters.

The elastogram is derived from data of the change of radio frequency signals before and after compression and is displayed in a split-screen mode with the conventional B-mode image and the elastogram on the monitor. Most strain elastography display tissue stiffness in a continuum of colors from red to green to blue, designating soft (high strain), intermediate (equal strain) and hard (no strain) tissue, depending upon the settings done by the operator.

The visual scoring system compares the strain (elastographic color of the lesion), with the strain of the surrounding tissue and is applied in other anatomic areas as well. The elastograms are categorized according to the likelihood of malignancy and range from benign (I), probably benign (II), uncertain (III), probably malignant (IV) to malignant (V).

There is another way of semi-quantifying the stiffness of a tissue by using strain-ratios. A strain-ratio measurement compares the strain in two manually selected regions of interest on the elastograms. One region of interest is placed in the focal lesion, and the reference region of interest is placed in the surrounding normal tissue, preferably in the same depth as the lesion. The strain-ratio is automatically calculated by the inbuilt elastography software and yields the fraction of the average strain in the reference area divided by the average strain in the lesion. Higher the strain-ratio, higher is the likelihood of malignancy. Various studies have defined Cut-off values of the strain-ratio depending upon the tissue.

CLINICAL APPLICATIONS

With advancement in the techniques of sonoelastography, there has been a significant rise in its clinical application and decision making.

Apart from its use in breast and prostate, it is being indicated in thyroid, liver, and skin lesions in many institutions after their numerous publications in literature.

Breast

Sonoelastography have a role for further evaluating abnormal findings on conventional breast ultrasonography and differentiating benign from malignant breast lesions **(Figs. 33.1 and 33.2)**. Thus, the eventual goal of incorporating elastography into routine practice is to reduce

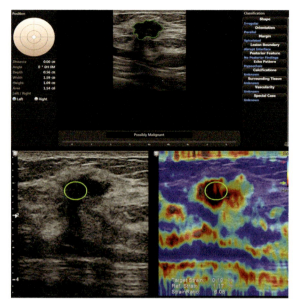

Fig. 33.1: Gray scale shows an ill-defined lesion in the breast with irregular margins which appears hard on elastography having a higher strain ratio(>3) suggesting malignant lesion.

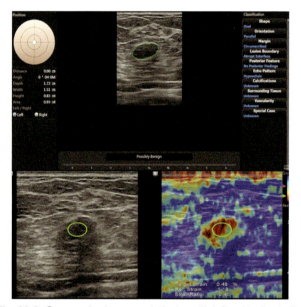

Fig. 33.2: Gray scale shows a relatively well-defined lesion in the breast with lobulated margins which appears soft on elastography and having a lower (<3) strain ratio suggesting benign lesion.

the biopsy rate of benign lesions. Normal fibroglandular breast tissue is markedly stiffer than normal fatty breast tissue. Therefore, at elastography, fatty tissue appears bright with respect to the adjacent glandular tissue, and normal fibrous parenchyma appears darker.

Simple cyst, complex cyst, and fibrocystic change are apparent on elatography showing presence benign cystic component. The typical manifestation of a simple cyst at elastography is a "target" or "bull's-eye" appearance, in which central bright compressible material is surrounded by a dark concentric rim.

Fibroadenomas could be differentiated from malignant tumors on the basis of elastographic size and brightness criteria. However, those which are larger than 2 cm in size and contain calcifications, give false positive results of malignancy.

Invasive ductal carcinoma typically is appreciably darker than normal tissues or benign lesions and is substantially larger on the elastogram than on B-mode US images.

Lymph nodes that contain metastases tend to appear stiffer and disproportionately larger at elastography.

Prostate

Prostate cancers have a higher stiffness than that of surrounding normal prostate tissue. Consequently, prostate cancers appear dark on elastograms. Often, intermediate-grade and high-grade malignant lesions that are subtle or even unapparent on B-mode US images are prominent on elastograms as dark areas of low strain.

Benign prostatic hyperplasia have stiffness that is greater than those of normal prostate tissues but are less than those of prostate carcinomas. As a result, on elastograms, benign prostatic hyperplasia will appear darker than normal prostate tissue. However, the difference between benign prostatic hyperplasia and prostate carcinoma can be difficult because benign prostatic hyperplasia also appears darker than the background tissues. Consequently, benign prostatic hyperplasia can represent a false-positive finding for cancer.

Thyroid

Elastography is capable of differentiating between benign cystic lesions showing less of stiffness than surrounding tissue from solid malignant lesions which appear darker. However, the presence of calcification may add to false positive results towards malignancy.

Liver

The main clinical indication for liver elastography is fibrosis staging of chronic liver disease, with a main objective of determining the presence or absence of advanced fibrosis.

Skin

Most useful clinical implication of skin sonoelastography is in patients of scleroderma where there is invariable cutaneous involvement in form of increased stiffness. Elastography is able to assess subclinical skin involvement and thus helps in early management.

CONCLUSION

Sonoelastography is widely available and easy to use in a clinical setting. The fact that sonoelastography is real-time and can be done bedside along with the B-mode examination makes its use feasible in a lot of different anatomic areas. However, the major drawback is its operator dependence and inter-observer variability.

34
CHAPTER

Musculoskeletal Ultrasonography

SKIN AND SUBCUTANEOUS TISSUE

The normal layers of the skin from without inwards include the epidermis, dermis, and subcutaneous fat. The superficial fascia separates the skin from muscles. The epidermis appears as an echogenic band like structure measuring 1–3 mm in thickness. The dermis is homogeneously, relatively hypoechoic and measures 1–3.5 mm in thickness according to the site. The dermis is poorly separated from the subcutaneous fat, this layer is also relatively hypoechoic. It often contains thin echogenic strand due to connective to tissue fibers and measures 5 mm to 1 cm in thickness. The superficial fascia forms a linear echogenic, layer parallel to the skin surface sharply delineating the subcutaneous fat/muscle interface **(Fig. 34.1)**.

While scanning, the axis of the probe should be strictly perpendicular to the skin surface. A 7.5 MHz probe with a 2 cm stand-off pad should be used and plenty of gel helps to maintain a good contact especially while scanning lesions with irregular surface. Excessively hairy skin ought to be shaved prior to examination. Comparative scans of normal skin areas are very useful.

Muscles

Normal muscles have a stripped pattern on longitudinal scans and the plane of striations varies with the orientation of the fibers. Sections at 90° to this alignment show speckled or uniformly mottled pattern. Adjacent muscles may demonstrate a confusing variation in reflectivity. Comparison with the opposite side of the body can avoid errors. Each muscle is surrounded by an echogenic capsule, sometimes adjacent to layers of reflective fat. Vessels may be seen within the muscles as echo-free stripes. On contraction the striations become more prominent and the muscle widens and shortens with moderate increase in echogenicity. Small veins are temporarily obliterated.

Tendons

Linear array electronic transducers of 7.5–10 MHz provide exquisite results because of their wider field of view and better near-field resolution, for tendon sonography.

The combination of longitudinal and transverse scans provides a three-dimensional approach to the tendon.

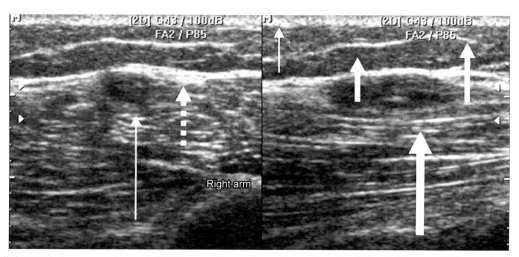

Fig. 34.1: High resolution scan through thigh revealing echogenic epidermis (thin white arrow), hypoechoic dermis and subcutaneous fat containing lipoma (thick white arrows), deep fascia (broken white arrow) and muscle (thick large arrow). Incidental note is made of healed cysticercus (thin long arrow).

Scanning the contralateral normal region can be available reference for normal anatomy. Tendons should be examined at rest and during active and passive flexion/extension. Performing palpation under real-time sonography can also be useful.

If the transducer is not parallel to the surface of the tendon, obliquity of the ultrasound beam can cause an artifactual hypoechogenicity of the tendon. Changing the position of the probe or suppressing the curvature of the tendon through muscle contraction, clears this artifact.

Tendons are made of densely packed parallel bundles of collagen fibers separated by ground substance and fibroblasts. The peritoneum, a layer of loose connective tissue wraps around the tendon and sends intratendinous septae between the bundles of collagen fibers. In areas of mechanical constraint and tendons are associated with additional structures that provide mechanical support or protection. These include fibrous sheaths, sesamoid bones, synovial sheaths and synovial bursae. High frequency 7.5–10 MHz linear array electronic probes are used to visualize the tendons at rest and during active and passive movements through flexion and extension maneuvers. A stand-off pad is used to visualize very superficial tendons and for evaluating tendons in regions with uneven surface. Care should be taken to always maintain the ultrasound beam perpendicular to surface of the tendon being examined to avoid unnecessary artifacts like false hypoechogenicity. The contralateral extremity or region should always be examined for comparison.

On ultrasound examination, all tendons appear moderately echogenic and display a fibrillar texture on longitudinal scan and a finely punctate appearance on transverse scanning with high frequency transducers. Transverse scans are essential for measurement of maximum width thickness of tendons **(Fig. 34.2)**. Sesamoid bones are seen as echogenic structures with posterior acoustic shadowing. Synovial sheaths when seen with very high frequency (15 MHz) transducer, appear as hypoechoic area around the tendon. The large synovial bursae appear as flattened, fluid filled structures 2–3 mm thick.

Synovium

The normal synovium appears as thin linear echogenic structure without any vascularity. In synovial proliferation there is thickening of the synovial layer with occasional vascularity on power Doppler suggesting active disease process. The synovial proliferation is echogenic in gout **(Figs. 34.3 to 34.5)**.

Bone

Ultrasonography can be used to assess the bony cortex very effectively. Small erosions can be picked up easily and earlier than X-ray. Small fractures can also be diagnosed if assessed properly. For labeling it as bone erosion, the irregularity in the cortical margins should be seen in long as well as short axis.

Shoulder

High resolution linear array transducer of 7.5 MHz frequency is used to visualize the rotator cuff tendon which is made of tendon of four muscles—the subscapularis, the supraspinatous, the infraspinatous and the teres minor. The rotator cuff tendons are echogenic relative to the deltoid muscle belly and are surrounded by a thin hypoechoic synovial layer, less than 1.5 mm thick. The subacromial subdeltoid bursa shows as a hypoechoic stripe thinner than the thickness of the hypoechoic hyaline coartilage over the humeral head. The bursa is loaf-shaped in cross-section and extends from the coracoid anteriorly around the lateral shoulder and posterior part of the glenoid. The bursa is a potential space, and contains small amount of synovial fluid, not visualized on routine ultrasonography. The echogenic peribursal fat separates the bursa from the deltoid muscle **(Fig. 34.2)**.

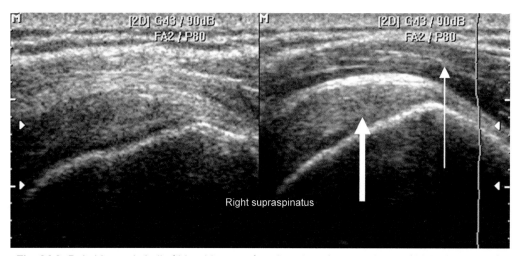

Fig. 34.2: Deltoid muscle belly (thin white arrow) and tendon of supraspinatus (thick white arrow).

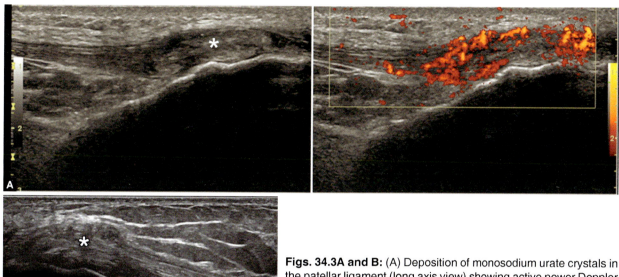

Figs. 34.3A and B: (A) Deposition of monosodium urate crystals in the patellar ligament (long axis view) showing active power Doppler signal suggestive of neovascularity; (B) Long axis view of triceps tendon near its insertion, showing similar tophaceous deposits seen as inhomogeneous echogenicity with loss of the normal fibrillar pattern.

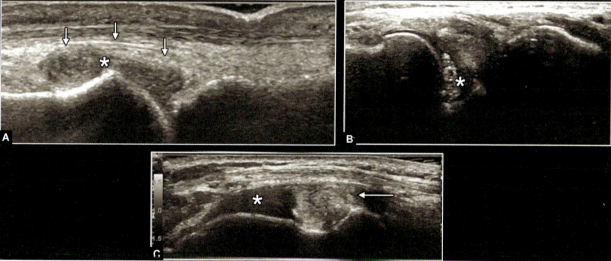

Figs. 34.4A to C: (A) Longitudinal view of right 1st metatarsophalyngeal joint showing echogenic synovial proliferation* distending the joint capsule (arrows); (B) Longitudinal section through right wrist joint of a different patient showing multiple hyperechoic punctate foci* within the joint suggestive of monosodium urate crystal deposits; (C) Longitudinal view of lateral aspect of knee showing anechoic synovial effusion* with large echogenic monosodium urate aggregate within the lateral joint recess (arrow).

The patient is scanned while sitting on a stool without armrests, and the examiner sits 5 cm above the patient, on another stool **(Figs. 34.6 to 34.11)**. To begin with the patient sits with his forearm on his thigh, hand palm pronated. Transverse images are taken through the proximal long biceps tendon, which appears as an echogenic oval structure in the bicipital groove. The bicipital groove is an important landmark over the anterior surface of the proximal humerus and is seen as a concave echogenic line. The long biceps tendon courses through the rotator cuff interval and divides the subscapularis from the supraspinatus tendon. As the transducer is moved superiorly above the bicipital groove the intracapsular portion of the tendon is seen obliquely in the shoulder capsule. Inferiorly the transverse scanning should be done up to the musculotendinous junction of the biceps to allow detection of the smallest fluid collection in the medial triangular recess at the distal end of the biceps tendon sheath. The transducer is rotated by 90° and aligned along the biceps groove to visualize the biceps tendon longitudinally. The transducer position is then returned to the transverse plane and moved proximally along the humerus to visualize subscapularis tendon which is viewed

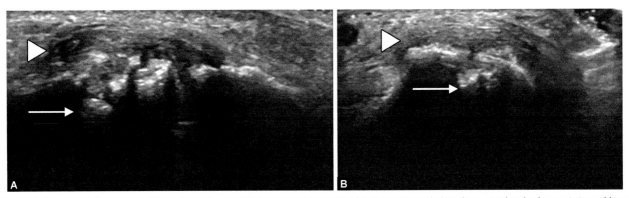

Figs. 34.5A and B: Long axis (A) and short axis (B) ultrasound images of 1st metatarsal showing erosion in the metatarsal head as focal breaks in cortical hyperechoic outline seen in two perpendicular planes, with overhanging edge in subarticular location (arrows) with adjacent synovitis (arrowheads).

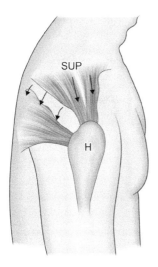

Fig. 34.6: General anatomic landmarks. Lateral photograph shows the bony structure, which limits the acoustic window for the examination of the cuff. SUP—Supraspinatus muscle and tendon; infraspinatus muscle and tendon; (arrowheads), scapular spine. (arrows), acromion.

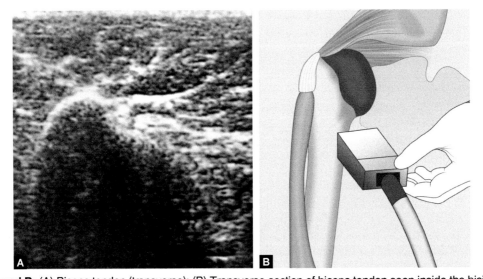

Figs. 34.7A and B: (A) Biceps tendon (transverse); (B) Transverse section of biceps tendon seen inside the bicipital groove.

parallel to its axis and appears as a band of medium level echoes, deep to the subdeltoid fat and bursa. Scanning is also done during passive and external rotation to assess the integrity of the subscapularis tendon. Longitudinal scans of the tendon are obtained by rotating the transducer head by 90°. The normal subdeltoid bursa is recognized between the deltoid muscle on one side of the rotator cuff tendons and biceps tendon on the deep side. Next, the supraspinatous

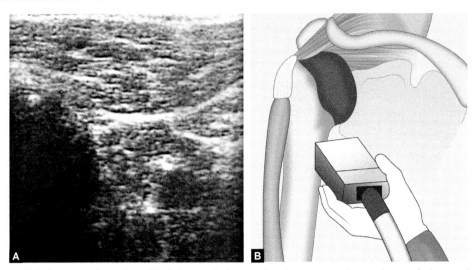

Figs. 34.8A and B: (A) Subscapularis tendon; (B) Subscapularis muscle in transverse plane subscapularis muscle in sagittal plane.

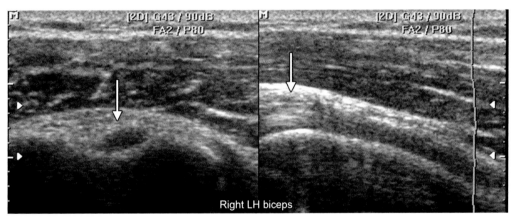

Fig. 34.9: High resolution scan through long head of biceps in transverse scan at the most dependant part of shoulder cavity and longitudinal scan in the upper part (white arrows).

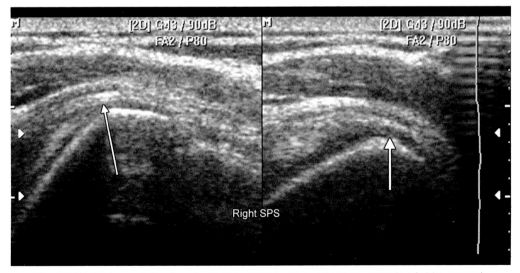

Fig. 34.10: High resolution longitudinal scan through supraspinatus tendon (white arrows).

tendon is scanned, perpendicular to its axis, by moving the transducer posteriorly, over the humeral head, such that the probe head is directed downwards and slightly medially. The tendon is visualized as a band of medium level echoes deep to the subdeltoid bursa and superficial to the echogenic bony surface of the greater tuberosity.

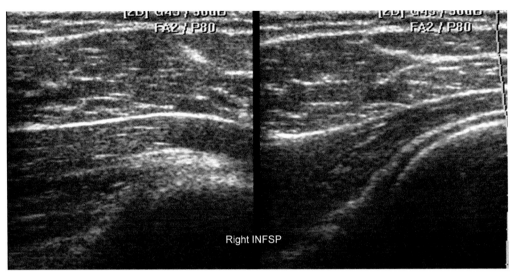

Fig. 34.11: High resolution longitudinal scan through infraspinatus tendon (white arrows).

The rest of the examination is done with the arm adducted and hyperextended and the should be in moderate internal rotation, as if the patient is reaching the opposite back pocket, longitudinal and transverse views of the supraspinatus tendon are obtained. During longitudinal scanning, the transducer overlays the acromion medially and lateral aspect of the greater tuberosity laterally. The transducer sweeps around the femoral head circumferentially starting anteriorly next to large biceps tendon and covering an area of 2.5 cm laterally. The infraspinatous tendon is scanned beyond this point. The musculotendinous junction shows as hypoechoic muscle surrounding the echogenic infraspinatous tendon. The transverse scanning of the supraspinatous tendon begins just lateral to the acromion and translates downward over the tendon and the greater tuberosity.

The transducer is then moved posteriorly, in the plane parallel to the scapular spine. The infraspinatous tendon appears as a beak shaped soft tissue structure as it attaches to the posterior surface of the greater tuberosity. The tendon is examined during internal and external rotation of the shoulder that relaxes and contracts the tendon respectively. At this level a portion of the posterior glenoid labrum is seen as an echogenic triangular structure surrounded by the hypoechoic fluid of the infraspinatous recess. The hypoechoic articular cartilage of the humeral head appears lateral to the labrum. Scanning is extended medially to visualize the suprascapular vessels and nerve in the spinoglenoid notch. The transversely oriented transducer is moved distally and trapezoid shaped teres minor is visualized. It is differentiated from the infraspinatious tendon by its broad and more muscular attachment. At the end of the examination, coronal images through the acromioclavicular joint are obtained. The superior glenoid labrum is shown with the transducer aligned posterior to the acromioclavicular joint and oriented perpendicular to the superior glenoid. Right and left sides are compared.

Elbow (Figs. 34.12 and 34.13)

With the elbow flexed at 90°, the tendon of triceps brachii is readily identified on coronal and transverse scans. The common tendons of the flexor and extensor muscles of forearm arising from medial and lateral epicondyle respectively are also best demonstrated with the elbow flexed at this angle.

Hand and Wrist (Fig. 34.14)

When the wrist is moderately flexed, the echogenic flexor tendons of the fingers are seen surrounded by the hypoechoic ulnar bursa, in the carpal tunnel. The median nerve which is slightly less echogenic than the tendons, courses anterior to the flexor tendons of the second finger outside the ulnar bursa. In the palm, the pairs of superficial and deep flexor tendons of the fingers are seen adjacent to the corresponding hypoechoic lumbrical muscles. At the fingers the flexor tendons lie in the concavity of the phalanges and this appear falsely echopoor along most of their course. Visualization of external tendon of the fingers requires the use of stand off pads.

Pediatric Hip

A 7.5 MHz linear transducer and a 5 MHz linear transducer is used for an infant up to 3 months and between 3–7 months respectively. All scanning is performed from the lateral or posterolateral aspect of the hip from the neutral position at rest to one in which the hip is flexed, and four standard views are obtained (Fig. 34.15). Dynamic hip assessment is done to determine the position and stability of the femoral head and to assess the development of the acetabulum (Fig. 34.16). With the hip flexed at 90°, the femur is moved through a range of abduction and adduction with stress views performed in the flexed position. The stress maneuvers are the imaging counterparts of the clinical Barlow and Ortolani

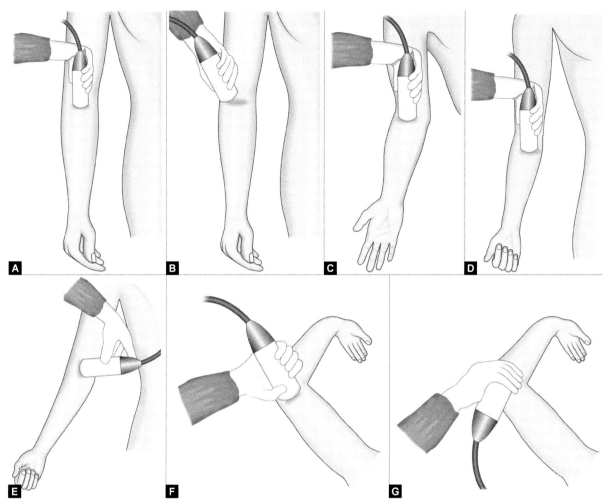

Figs. 34.12A to G: (A) Anterior longitudinal view—lateral aspect of elbow. This plane allows the visualization of radiohumeral articulation and capitulum. Diagram shows neutral position of hand and transducer is aligned with radiohumeral articulation along lateral aspects of elbow; (B) Shows slight obliquity necessary to align transducer a long axis of common extensor muscle group of forearm. Note that hand remains neutrally positioned to show tendinous origin of common forearm extensor muscle group from lateral epicondyle; (C) This plane is useful for evaluation of radioulnar articulation and for watching supination and pronation of proximal radius. Drawing shows transverse orientation of transducer so that side of image on viewer left is assigned for lateral aspect of elbow joint. Hand is supinated; (D) Anterior longitudinal view used for visualization of ulnohumeral articulation and coronoid process of ulna. Drawing shows transducer aligned longitudinally along long axis of ulna to visualize ulnohumeral articulation. Hand is supinated; (E) Anterior anteromedial longitudinal sonogram. This view is designed to visualize common tendon from which forearm flexor muscle group arise. Drawing shows that with hand in supination, transducer is slightly oblique to match long axis of common forearm flexor muscle group arising from common tendon attached to medial epicondyle; (F) Posterior midline longitudinal sonogram. This plane is useful in evaluating distal humerus and displacement of post fat-pad indicating fluid in joint. Drawing shows that for posterior scanning, arm is elevated 180° next to patient's head and elbow flexed 90° transducer should be oriented so that proximal portion of arm is oriented to viewers left on image; (G) Posterior superior transducer with sonogram. This view is useful in identifying fluid in joint and displacement of fat pad. Epicondylar injuries may also be detected. Drawing shows that arm remains in same position and transducer is oriented transversely at level of post-fat pad in olecranon fossae of distal humerus.

maneuvers and which are used clinically to determine hip abnormality. The Barlow test determines whether the hip can be dislocated. The hip is flexed, thigh adducted and a gentle push applied posteriorly. An unstable femoral head moves out of the acetabulum. The Ortolani test determines if the dislocated hip can be reduced. As the flexed, dislocated hip is abducted the examiner feels a vibration of click that results when the femoral head returns to the acetabulum at rest, with abduction and adduction motions when the hip is flexed and during the application of stress.

At birth the proximal femur and much of the acetabulum are composed of cartilage, which is hypoechoic compared with soft tissue and easy to distinguish. The cartilaginous femoral head has low ultrasound attenuation and provides a window into the acetabulum, allowing a detailed examination of the joint. Ossification begins between

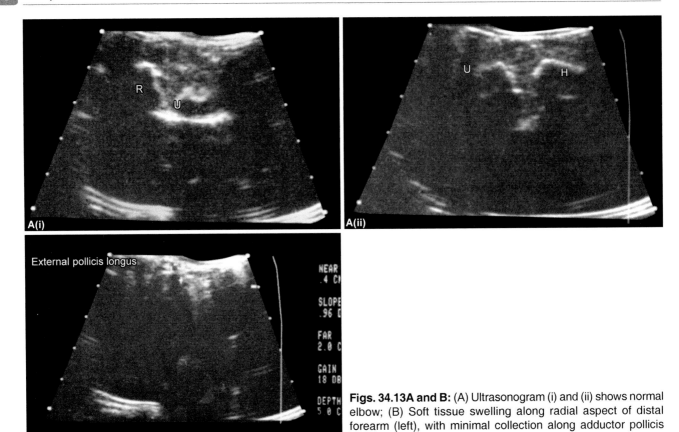

Figs. 34.13A and B: (A) Ultrasonogram (i) and (ii) shows normal elbow; (B) Soft tissue swelling along radial aspect of distal forearm (left), with minimal collection along adductor pollicis longus tendon-synovitis.

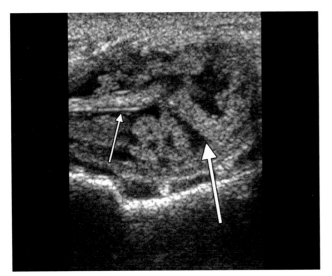

Fig. 34.14: Shows a high resolution longitudinal scan through wrist showing tendon (thin white arrow) with proliferative synovial thickening surrounding it (thick white arrow) in a case of tenosynovitis.

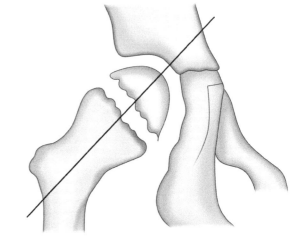

Fig. 34.15: Sonographic scan plane along with neck of femur for detecting joint effusion in hip joint.

6 weeks and 8 months in the femoral head which blocks further transmission of sound and makes hip sonography practical only up to one year of age.

The acetabulum is composed of both bone and cartilage. At birth the bony ossification centers in the ilium, ischium and pubis are separated by a Y-shaped triradiate cartilage. The acetabular labrum is a rim of hyaline cartilage extending outwards from the acetabular margin and it form the cup that normally contains the femoral head. The labrum is poorly reflective and has echogenic fibrocartilage at its lateral margin. The joint space may be identified as a line between the femoral and acetabular cartilage. The echogenic hip capsule, composed of fibrous tissue is seen lateral to the femoral head **(Figs. 34.17 to 34.19)**.

- *Coronal/neutral view* with the patient supine the linear transducer is placed vertically on the lateral aspect of the hip and the hip is scanned until a standard plane of section is obtained. This plane demonstrates the mid-portion of the acetabulum, with the straight iliac line superiorly and the inferior tip of the os ilium seen medially within the acetabulum. The echogenic tip of the labrum is also visualized. In the normal hip, the acetabular roof has a concave configuration and covers at least half of the femoral head. The acetabulum can be assessed visually or with alpha and beta angles, noting the depth and angulation of the acetabular roof as well as the appearance of the labrum. The alpha angle measures the inclination of superior osseous acetabular rim with respect to the lateral margin of the iliac bone. The beta angle is formed by the baseline iliac bone and the inclination of the cartilaginous acetabular roof for which the tip of the labrum is the key landmark.
- *Coronal/flexon view:* With the same transducer position as in coronal neutral view, the hip is flexed at 90° and the transducer moved in an anteroposterior direction to visualize the entire hip. The curvilinear margin of the bony femoral shaft is identified anteriorly to the femoral head. In the mid-portion of the acetabulum, the normally positioned femoral head is surrounded by echoes from the long acetabular components. The transducer position should be so adjusted that superiorly the lateral margin of the iliac bone is seen as a straight horizontal line. This plane ensures that the mid-acetabulum is accurately visualized and the maximum acetabular depth obtained. A normal hip gives the appearance of "a ball on a spoon" in the mid-acetabulum. The femoral head represents the ball, the acetabulum forms the bowl of the spoon and the iliac line form the handle. When the transducer is moved posteriorly the posterior lip of the triradiate cartilage is visualized. The bone above and below the cartilage notch is flat and the normal femoral head is never seen over the posterior lip of the acetabulum, while the push and pin maneuvers are used during dynamic scanning. Also with the plane of scan comprising the mid-acetabulum, a Barlow type maneuver is performed

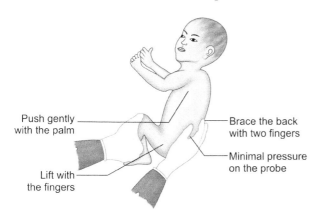

Fig. 34.16: Dynamic study of the infant hip. Direction of pressure exerted during the dynamic study of an infant's hip.

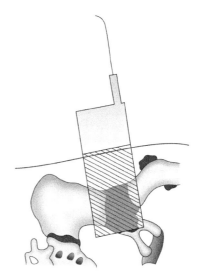

Fig. 34.17: The coronal plane of hip joint. Diagram to show the main anatomical structures.

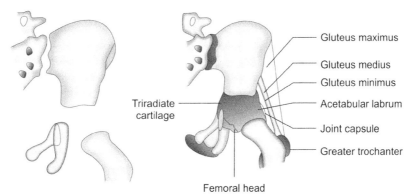

Fig. 34.18: Comparison of the X-ray and ultrasound anatomy. Anatomy as seen on a radiograph compared to the ultrasound coronal section of an infant's hip.

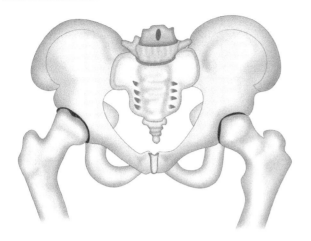

Fig. 34.19: Plane of the routine examination of irritable hip.

TABLE 34.1: Classification of hip dysplasia on the basis of ultrasonographic measurements.

Character	Type I (normal)	Type II (dysplasia)	Type III (subluxation)
Alpha angle	>60°	44°–60°	<34°
Beta angle	<55°	55°–77°	>77°
Percentage coverage	>58%	58–33%	<33%

with adduction and gentle pushing against the knee, a normal hip remains in place against the acetabulum.

- *Transverse/flexion view:* The transducer is rotated through 90° and moved posteriorly, so that it is posterolateral to the joint. The bony shaft and metaphysis of the femur produce a bright echogenic line anteriorly adjacent to the sonolucent femoral head. The echoes from the bony acetabulum are posterior to the femoral head and produce a U shape configuration in the normal hip. The flexed hip is moved from maximum adduction to wide abduction and the deep U configuration of the acetabulum seen in maximum abduction, changes to a shallower V appearance in adduction. In adduction the hip is stressed with a gentle push (a Barlow test), in the normal hip the femoral head remains deeply in the acetabulum, in contact with the ischium.
- *Transverse/neutral view:* The leg is brought down and transducer directed horizontally into the acetabulum from the lateral aspect of hip. The plane of interest passes through the femoral head into the acetabulum at the center of the triradiate cartilage. In the normal hip the sonolucent femoral head is positioned against the bony acetabulum over the triradiate cartilage. The elements of the sonogram resemble the components of a flower. The femoral head represent the flower, echoes from the ischium posteriorly and pubis anteriorly forms the leaves at its base. The stem is formed by echoes that pass through the triradiate cartilage into the area of acoustic shadowing created by osseous structures. The presence and size of the ossific nucleus are evaluated in this view.

Congenital Dislocation of the Hip (CDH)

In neonates, sonography has become the technique of choice to examine hips.

Graf in 1980 developed a set of measurements on coronal scanning for diagnosis of CDH **(Table 34.1)**. These lines are drawn about the acetabulum. The first, baseline, connects the osseous acetabulum convexity to the point of insertion of joint capsule to perichondrium. A second inclination line joins osseous convexity to labrum acetabulare. The third, acetabular roof line connects lower edge of acetabular roof medially to osseous convexity.

Two angles are then measured; one between acetabular roof line and baseline (alpha) measures "osseous acetabular convexity." A small acetabular angle indicates a shallow bony acetabulum. The second angle (Beta) is measured between baseline and line of inclination and gives an indication of additional coverage of femoral head by cartilaginous coverage.

In normal hip   α is more than 60° and
                 β is less than 55°.
In subluxation   α is less than 44°
                 β is more than 77°.

Coronal images are used to evaluate the position of femoral head within the acetabulum. If acetabular cup accommodates less than one-third of femoral head then acetabular dysplasia is definitely present. If one-half to one-third of head is accommodated, acetabular dysplasia must be suspected.

In addition, shape of acetabular rim and roof is assessed. In all pathological hips, the lateral bony rim is rounded or has bony defects.

In complete dislocation, position of limbic cartilage is important since it may be interposed between femoral head and acetabulum.

Hip Joint Effusion (Figs. 34.20 to 34.22)

The hip is commonly evaluated for joint effusion in children, the causes may be septic arthritis, transient synovitis, traumatic hemarthrosis, Perthes' disease, rheumatoid arthritis. Ultrasonography can delineate clearly the presence and the nature of fluid. Anterior approach along the plane of neck is used. The joint capsule is lifted and becomes convex. Comparison with the opposite hip is always useful. If the fluid is completely hypoechoic, it is likely to be transudate. If the fluid is dense and echogenic, it is an exudate or hematoma. Increased echogenicity of fluid and thick capsule (more than 2 mm) suggest septic arthritis. An anterior synovial space of more than 3 mm with asymmetry of more than 2 mm with opposite side is taken as abnormal (effusion). It is idiopathic (more common) or secondary to number of conditions. Among them sickle cell anemia, gout, renal osteodystrophy, exogenous steroid use, Cushing syndrome, Gaucher's disease and rarely repeated pregnancy.

Perthes' disease: It is a self limiting osteonecrosis of the femoral head epiphysis and commonly occurs between

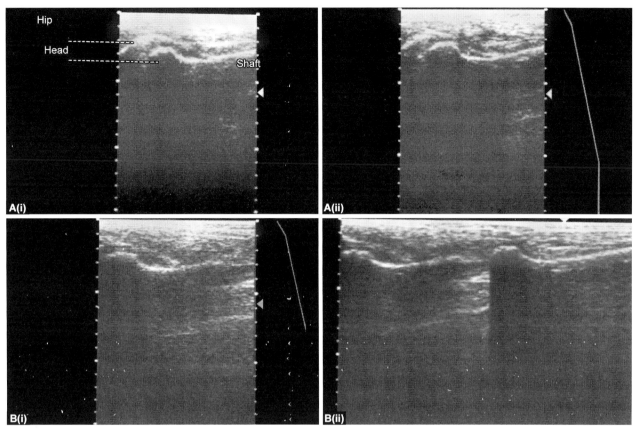

Figs. 34.20A and B: (A) Right hip shows hypoechoic collection—TB hip. Left hip is normal, (B) right hip septic arthritis. Left hip normal.

3 and 10 years in boys. Ultrasound assessment shows widening of anterior joint space, and fragmentation. It not only helps in measuring the growth and development, i.e., size of femoral head but also helps in detecting progress of lesions.

Trauma: Trauma in a growing child may involve growth plate and result in growth disturbances. Ultrasound examination may show fluid (blood) within the joint **(Figs. 23A to E)**.

Transient Synovitis of Hip (Fig. 34.24)

Transient synovitis of the hip refers to a self-limiting acute inflammatory condition affecting the synovial lining of the hip. It is considered one of the most common causes of hip pain and limping in young children. Ultrasonography is useful at demonstrating a joint effusion which is often seen in the anterior recess. Herniation of the synovial membrane through a joint capsular defect (pseudodiverticulum) between the iliopsoas muscle and the anterior border of the joint capsule may be seen in very small proportion of patients.

Adult Hip

Bone obscures, the majority of the joint space in the mature hip. Fortunately the vertical recess of the joint capsule and the anterior extension of the joint space are readily seen on ultrasound images and so joint effusion or synovial thickening are easily diagnosed.

The iliofemoral ligament is applied closely to the anterior surface of the joint and provides an important landmark. The adjacent muscles are divided by distinct facial planes. The articular cartilage is thin 1-2 mm hypoechoic rim on the femora. In children the immature femoral head has a layer of unossified cartilage deep to the articular cartilage and both merge to form a thick hypoechoic band on ultrasound images.

Knee (Figs. 34.25 to 34.30)

As both the quadriceps and patellar tendons are slightly concave anteriorly when the knee is extended and at rest, scans should be obtained during active extension of the knee, or with the knee flexed, which straightens the tendons and eliminates the hypoechoic artefact. The quadriceps tendon lies under the subcutaneous fat and anterior to a fat pad and to the collapsed suprapatellar bursa. On transverse scans, the quadriceps tendon is oval, while the patellar tendon shows a convex anterior and flat posterior surface. The patellar tendon is a flat band extending from the patella to the tibial tuberosity over a length of 5-6 cm. It is 2-2.5 cm wide and 4-5 mm thick. The subcutaneous prepatellar and

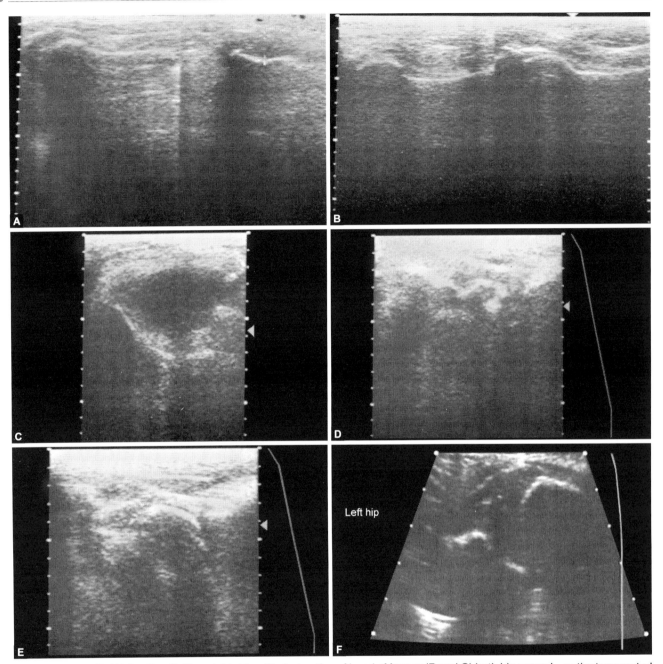

Figs. 34.21A to F: (A) Septic arthritis—right side with destruction of head of femur; (B and C) both hip normal—patient presented as right flexion deformity abscess in right iliac fossae; (D and E) Right hip normal. Left hip shows avascular necrosis (Perthes' disease); (F) Ultrasound left hip shows dislocation of left hip.

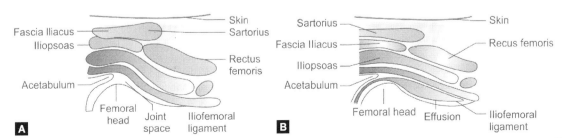

Figs. 34.22A and B: (A) Anatomy of the hip seen in the oblique sagittal plane; (B) Diagram of a hip containing an effusion.

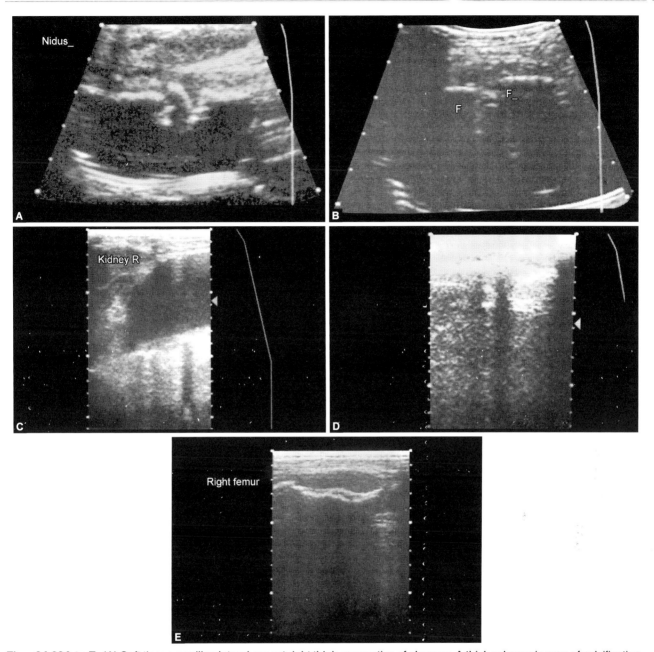

Figs. 34.23A to E: (A) Soft tissue swelling lateral aspect right thigh suggestive of abscess. A thick echogenic area of calcification-chronic osteomyelitis; (B) Ultrasonogram shows fracture right femur; (C) A hypoechoic collection is seen medial, posterior and inferior to right kidney in paravertebral gutterpsoas abscess; (D) A hypoechoic lesion seen in mid thigh anteriorly with c/o calcification-cysticercosis; (E) Longitudinal scan of right thigh showing hypoechoic area adjacent to bone with cortical irregularity-osteomyelitis.

infrapatellar bursae are not visible. The deep infrapatellar bursa appears as a flattened anechoic structure 2–3 mm thick. Prepatellar fibers connect quadriceps tendon with the patellar tendon.

The collateral ligaments of the knee blend with the articular capsule and are poorly differentiated from the surrounding subcutaneous tissues. Because of their deep location and limited ultrasound window the cruciate ligaments cannot be reliably visualized with ultrasound.

Foot and Ankle

The Achilles tendon inserts into the posterior surface of the calcaneum. The echogenic, fatty Kager's triangle lies anterior to the distal half of the tendon. More anteriorly lies the hypoechoic flexor hallucis longus muscle and the echogenic posterior surface of the tibia. The flattened hypoechoic subtendinous calcaneal bursa is sometimes seen in the angle formed by the tendon and calcaneum.

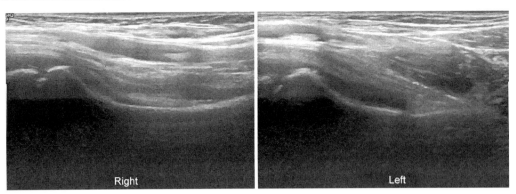

Fig. 34.24: Transient synovitis of left hip. Longitudinal section along the anterior recess of hip joint in a child shows fluid on the left side which is not seen on the right side.

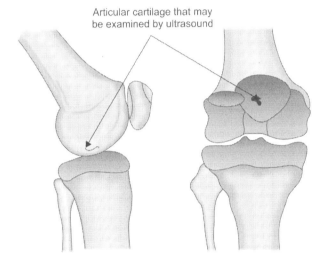

Fig. 34.25: Areas of the knee that may be examined by ultrasound.

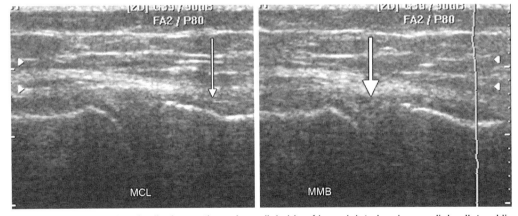

Fig. 34.26: Shows high resolution longitudinal scan through medial side of knee joint showing medial collateral ligament (MCL) (thin white arrow) and medial meniscus (thick white arrow).

The tendon fibers have an oblique course forward and medially and in cross section the tendon appears elliptical, tapering medially. At 2-3 cm above its insertion, the tendon is 5-7 mm thick and 12-15 mm wide. The tendons of peroneus longus and brevis muscles are readily demonstrated posteriorly and that of tibialis posterior muscle medially. The tendons of the flexor digitorum longus and flexor hallucis longus muscles are also identified behind the medial malleolus, whereas the tendon of the tibialis anterior, extensor hallucis longus, and extensor digitorum longus are seen at the anterior aspect of the ankle, all enveloped in synovial sheaths. In the foot, the flexor and extensor tendons of the toes are evaluated similar to tendon of the fingers.

CHAPTER 34: Musculoskeletal Ultrasonography   437

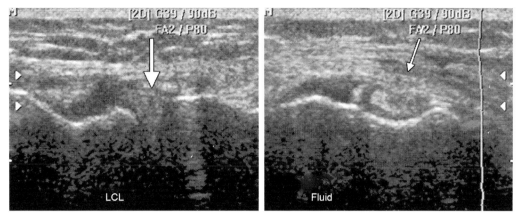

Fig. 34.27: Shows high resolution longitudinal scan through lateral side of knee joint showing lateral collateral ligament (thin white arrow) and lateral meniscus (thick white arrow) associated with some anechoic joint fluid.

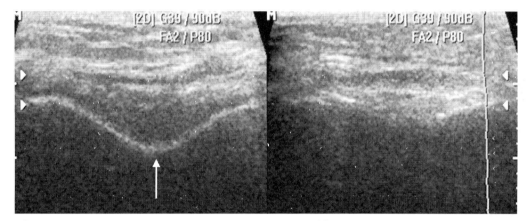

Fig. 34.28: Shows high resolution scan through intercondylar region of femur showing no evidence of any joint collection (thin white arrow).

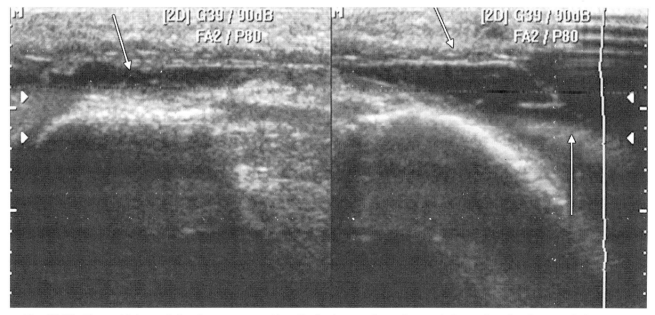

Fig. 34.29: Shows high resolution transverse and longitudinal scans through prepatellar region showing anechoic septate collection (thin white arrows).

Commonly Detected Musculoskeletal Lesions on Ultrasound

Tendon tears: In complete tears, the two tendon fragments are separated by a gap of variable length and echogenicity. This corresponds to the hematoma which is subsequently replaced by granulomatous tissue. A bone avulsion may also be visualized as a brightly echogenic focus with acoustic shadowing.

Rotator cuff lesions **(Figs. 34.31A to E)***:* The diagnostic criteria for rotator cuff is the nonvisualization of the rotator cuff retracted under the acromion process. Focal thinning

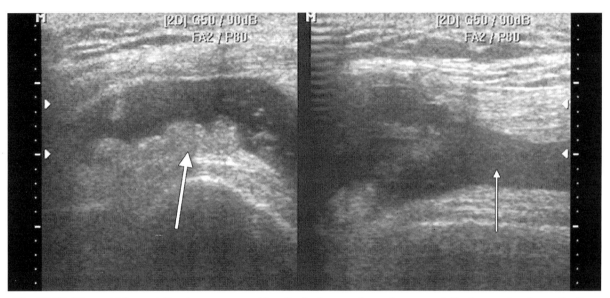

Fig. 34.30: Shows high resolution transverse and longitudinal scans through suprapatellar bursa showing collection (thin white arrow) with thickened nodular synovium (thick white arrow).

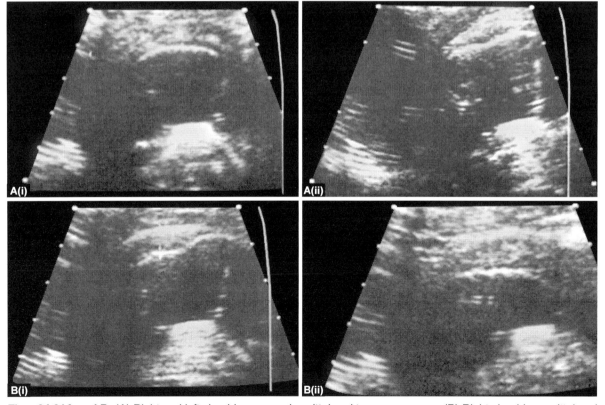

Figs. 34.31A and B: (A) Right and left shoulder—normal sagittal and transverse scan; (B) Right shoulder sagittal and transverse scans show swelling and edema of rotator cuff.

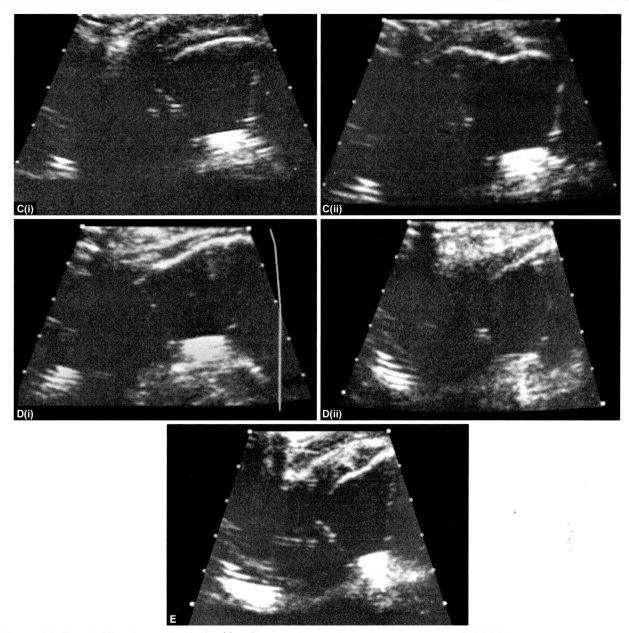

Figs. 34.31C to E: (C) RT normal, left shoulder shows evidence of partial tear of rotator cuff; (D) Right shoulder sagittal scan shows complete tear of rotator cuff; (E) Right shoulder shows partial atrophy of rotator cuff.

and discontinuity are the other two criteria. The presence of foci of increased echogenicity in the cuff is the least reliable indicator of rotator cuff tear.

Meniscal tear **(Figs. 34.32A to C)** are one of the most common lesions of the knee joint. Tears are more common in the medial than lateral. The menisci are well evaluated of USG. The normal menisci are seen as homogeneously echogenic triangular structure with apex of triangle pointed towards middle of the joint. The tear is seen as an irregular hypoechoic area in the echogenic menisci.

Patellar tendon tears: This result in a small well-defined, hypoechoic hematoma which is located in the midline (best seen on transverse scans).

Achilles tendon tears: Mostly it ruptures in the midportion of the tendon, about 2 to 3 cm from calcaneal attachment. In complete tears, the gap between the two fragments is variable, and the hematoma may extend along the tendon over a long distance. The tendon fragments show jagged margins, resembling a frayed loupe.

Tendinitis: In acute tendinitis, the tendon is swollen, its echogenicity is decreased, and its contours are blurred. Minute calcifications can be demonstrated on sonography.

Bursitis: This may be isolated or associated tendinitis. Subdeltoid, olecranoid, patellar, and calcaneal bursae are involved most frequently. Sonography demonstrates a

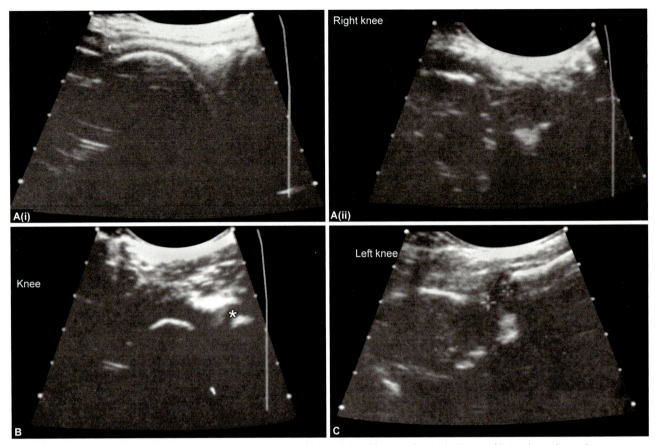

Figs. 34.32A to C: (A) (i) Ultrasonogram shows normal knee joint, (ii) tear of anterior horn of lateral meniscus is seen; (B) Right knee shows synovial effusion as shown by arrow; (C) Tear of posterior horn of medial meniscus is as asterisk.

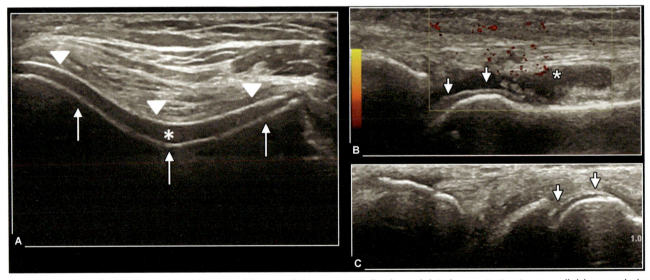

Figs. 34.33A to C: (A) Transverse ultrasound image of the suprapatellar knee joint demonstrates two parallel hyperechoic contours on either side of the hypoechoic hyaline cartilage*. The deep echogenic contour (long arrows) represents the femoral cortex, while the superficial echogenic contour (arrowheads) represents uric acid crystals accumulating on the surface of the hypoechoic hyaline cartilage. Longitudinal ultrasound image of 1st metatarsophalyngeal joint (B) and wrist joint (C) showing the double contour (arrows) around hyaline cartilage. Note the anechoic synovial effusion with hyperechoic crystal deposits in the 1st metatarsophalyngeal joint (* in B).

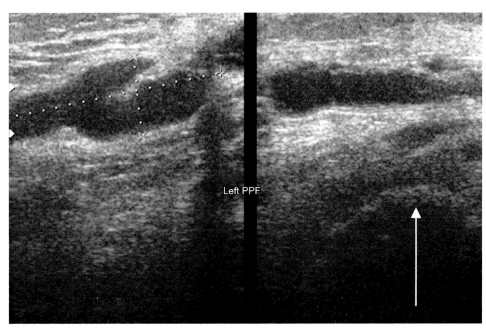

Fig. 34.34: Irregular anechoic popliteal cyst, femoral condyle is indicated by white arrow.

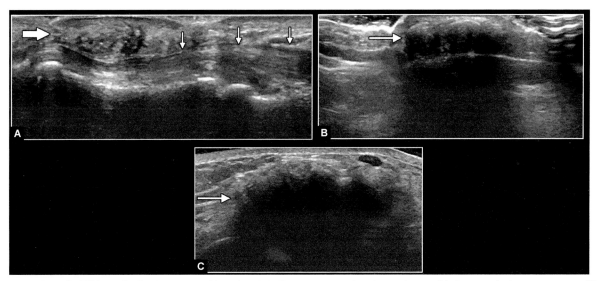

Figs. 34.35A to C: (A) Longitudinal section of hand digit in flexor aspect showing polymorphic hyperechoic aggregates of MSU crystals with a hypoechoic surrounding rim without any posterior acoustic shadowing suggestive of a soft tophus (notched arrow) in subcutaneous tissue superficial to the flexor digitorum tendon (arrows); (B) Longitudinal ultrasound image of dorsal aspect of hand digit shows compact tophaceous material with posterior acoustic shadowing seen in the subcutaneous tissue suggestive of hard tophus (arrow); (C) Axial section of wrist joint showing hard tophaceous deposit within the joint (arrow) with posterior acoustic shadowing.

swollen rounded, fluid-filled bursa with ill-defined margins. In chronic bursitis, the bursa may exhibit a complex appearance, while calcification gives rise to hyperechoic foci with shadowing.

Joint effusions **(Figs. 34.33A to C):** Sonography demonstrates intra-articular fluid collections. Septic effusion may contain debris. Sonography is ideal for guiding aspiration of small effusions.

Synovial cysts: These develop from joint spaces/adjacent bursae. Popliteal cysts **(Fig. 34.34)** typically appear as fluid filled collections, often wrapping around the gastronemius-semimembranous bursa. Inflamed cysts may contain echogenic fibrinous debris. In patients with rheumatoid arthritis., the cysts may be filled with pannus and mimic solid masses. A ruptured cyst may be diagnosed as fluid dissecting into the calf.

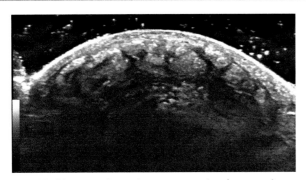

Fig. 34.36: Olecranon bursa in transverse view (seen under a gel standoff to minimise the compression), showing multiple polygonal echogenic crystal deposits within, suggestive of bursitis.

Trauma: In neonates and children, sonography can demonstrate fractures and dislocations of unossified epiphysis. Bone formation at fracture site can be visualized and monitored easily on sonography.

Osteomyelitis: Sonographically, it is visualized as fluid collection abutting the bone. It can also be seen as a detached sequestrum (brightly echogenic with acoustic shadowing) lying at a variable distance from the bone. It can also distinguish osteomyelitis born cellulitis and abscess **(Figs. 34.33A to E)**.

Gout

Ultrasonography is a highly sensitive modality for diagnosing gout. The constellation of findings in gout includes soft tissue crystal deposition (tophus), synovitis, bursitis, bone erosions, double contour sign, and soft tissue edema **(Figs. 34.35 and 34.36)**.

Index

Page numbers followed by *f* refer to figure and *t* refer to table.

A

Abdomen 38, 51, 82*f*
   acute 167
   adrenal glands 193
   adult 51
   cause of acute 169
   cyst in 359
   fascial planes of 81*f*
   gastrointestinal tract 164
   hepatobiliary system 130
   laparoscopic sonography of 295
   pancreas 158
   part of 204
   pediatric 60, 224
   peritoneum 202
   retroperitoneum 196
   right side of 225
   spleen 130
   urinary tract 172
   uterus and adnexa 209
Abdominal aorta 55, 55*f*, 319, 389
   aneurysm of 390
   dilated 196*f*
   upper 79
Abdominal aortic aneurysm 390
Abdominal area, posterior 79
Abdominal cavity 361*f*
Abdominal circumference 338, 339*f*
Abdominal injury 2
Abdominal pregnancy 337
Abdominal tuberculosis 167*f*, 208*f*
Abdominal vessels, great 82
Abdominal wall 55, 77
   multiple anterior 395*f*
Abortion 46
   complete spontaneous 334
   incomplete 333, 335*f*
   inevitable 335
   threatened 333
Abscess 132, 144, 177, 198, 204, 240, 241, 256, 435*f*
   drainage 379*f*
   intrahepatic 132
   parietal 171*f*
   perinephric 177
   periorbital 249
   pyogenic 132
   subphrenic 206*f*
   testicular 256
   tubo-ovarian 223
Acalculous cholecystitis, acute 150
Acardiac parabiotic twin 353
Acetabulum 127, 430
   development of 126

Achilles tendon 113, 435
   tears 268, 439
Achondrogenesis 365
Achondroplasia 366
Acoustic cavitation 45
Acoustic field small bubbles 46
Acoustic gel 101
Acoustic impedance 8, 16
Acoustic lens 18*f*
Acoustic mirror 18*f*
Acoustic shadowing 41
Acquire information 30
Acquired renal cystic disease 185
Adductor pollicis longus tendon-synovitis 430*f*
Adenocarcinoma 160, 162*f*, 166, 182, 183*f*
   colon 145*f*, 199*f*
Adenomyomas 211*f*, 212
Adenomyosis 210
Adrenal adenoma 193*f*
Adrenal cystic lesions 193
Adrenal gland 55, 55*f*, 83, 124, 319
   anatomy of 85*f*
   normal right 125*f*
Adrenal hyperplasia, congenital 229
Adrenal metastases 195, 195*f*
Adrenal tumors 193
Adventitia 75
Air 6, 8, 11
   molecules 4
Airless contact 4
Air-tissue interface 9
Albumen, cardiac applications of 315
Alcohol
   chronic 160
   consumption 137
Alcoholic hepatitis, acute 137
Alfatoxins 140
Aliasing 43
Alobar holoprosencephaly 364
Amebic abscess, large 134*f*
Amebic liver abscess 133, 134*f*
Amnionicity and chorionicity, sonographic determination of 352
Amniotic fluid 350
Ampulla 224
Amyloidosis 186
Analog scan converter 28, 28*f*
   advantage of 29
   disadvantage of 29
Anechoic cyst, large 181*f*
Anechoic follicles 97
Anechoic joint fluid 437*f*
Anechoic popliteal cyst, irregular 272*f*, 441*f*

Anechoic retroperitoneal cyst 199*f*
Anechoic structure 41
Anechoic urinary bladder 40*f*
Anemia 372
Aneurysm 196, 303, 403
   diagnosis of 403
   ostium 308
Angioma 298*f*
Angiomyolipoma 86, 180, 181
Annular array 35*f*
Anophthalmia 243
Anterior abdominal wall 38, 69, 79*f*, 93, 268*f*
   defects 368*t*
   hernia 268*f*
Antibioma 171*f*
Antibiotic therapy 170
Antrum 70
Aorta 41, 80, 82*f*, 196, 389, 389*f*, 405*f*
   anterior to 77*f*
   bifurcation of 82*f*
   location and anatomy of 84*f*
   sagittal scan of 83*f*
Aortic aneurysm 197*f*
Aortic arch 128*f*
   branches of 128*f*
Aortic bifurcation 200*f*
Aortic branches 80, 389
Aortic dissection 196
Aortic occlusions 196
Aortic pathology 390
Aortic rupture, chronic 196
Aortic transection 304
Aortic valve 405*f*
Aortoarteritis, nonspecific 303
Aortocaval fistula 307*f*
Appendicitis 167
Appendicular lump 168*f*
Appendix 77
   mucocele of 171
   normal 79*f*
   testis with hydrocele 259*f*
Aqueous emulsions 316
Arachnoiditis 240
Arnold–Chiari malformation 363, 363*f*
Artefact, color mirror image 45
Arterial system 385
   laminar flow 385
   pulsatile flow 386
Arterial wall, normal 302
Arteriosclerosis 403
Arteriovenous fistula 381, 404
Arteriovenous malformation 401*f*
Articulate arm scanners 27

Artifactual displacement 43
Ascaris 156f
Ascites 148f, 202
Asepsis, complete 378
Aspiration 253
Asplenia 75
Asteroid hyalosis 243
Asymmetrical septal hypertrophy 420
Atelectasis 234
Atherectomy 304, 305
Atheroma 196
Atheromatous disease 390
Atherosclerotic plaque 197f
Atrial septal defect 412f
Automatic pull back device 302f

B

B mode
    display 26f
        grayscale imaging 30
        scanner, conventional 30
B scan image 27
Barlow type maneuver 431
Basic Doppler systems 383
Battledore placenta 376
Beam energy, fraction of 31
Beam width artifacts 43
Bezoar 169, 171, 230
Biceps tendon 59, 111f, 426f
Bicornuate uterus 209f, 333f
Bilateral echogenic
    basal ganglia 239f
    large kidneys 369
Bile duct 51
    benign lesions of 156
    common 52, 68f, 70, 310, 380
    measurement of extrahepatic 320t
    neoplasm 156
    pathology 152
    spontaneous perforation of 224
    stones 152
    syndrome, inspissated 224
    tumor obstructing 157
Biliary ascariasis 155
Biliary atresia 224, 225
Biliary cirrhosis 137
Biliary duct 70, 318
Biliary enteric fistulas 167
Biliary hamartomas 130
Biliary sludge 146
Biliary system 224
Biliary tract 311, 321t
    anatomy of 69f
    dilatation, cause of 155
Biliary tree 311
    lumen of 155f
Biliopancreatic pathology 313
Bilomas 204
Biologic materials, absorption coefficients of 11t
Biological effects, evaluation of 1
Biophysical scoring 349
Biopsy 253
    techniques 378
Biparietal diameter 337
Bladder 89, 367
    diverticulum 187
    outlet obstruction 227
    tumors 188
    wall thickness 322t
Blood 6, 8, 11
    absorbs 238
    pressure, normal 348
Blood flow
    demonstration of 395
    direction of 406f
    dynamics 385
Blood vessels
    anatomy of major 285f
    veins and arteries 128
Blunt abdominal trauma 135f
Body wall defect syndrome 366
Bone 424
    obscures 108
    tissue 10, 271
Bowel gas 83
Bowel obstruction 169
Brain 6, 8, 11, 51
    and spine, pathologies of infant 236
    congenital anomalies of 239
    pediatric 60
    scan 117f
        sagittal 116
    supplying 285
    vascular supply of 285
Breast 58, 106, 253, 401, 421
    abscess 256f
    anatomy 106f
    carcinoma 195, 256f
    cryptorchidism 261
    cyst 253
    disease, evaluation of 253
    extratesticular lesions 258
    glandular part of 107f
    lesion 254
        benign from malignant 421
    lump, benign 254f
    malignant
        neoplasms 255
        tumors 257
    masses, malignant 255
    miscellaneous conditions 255
    neoplasm, benign 254f
    normal 107f
    scrotal ultrasound 256
    specific conditions 253
    testicular torsion 260
    trauma 261
    ultrasound 253
Brenner tumor 222
Breu's mole 375
Brevis muscles 113
Bronchogenic carcinoma 195f
Budd–Chiari syndrome 138, 395
Buerger's disease 280f, 403f
Bull's eye 75, 142f
Bursitis 271, 439

C

Cable conducting signal 32
Calcified hydatid transverse 132f
Calcified plaque 303f
Calcium 302
    disodium edetic acid 316
Calculus cholecystitis, acute 149f
Candida albicans 180
Candidiasis 133
Carcinoma colon 166f
Cardiac injury 2
Cardiac malpositions 225
Cardiovascular anomalies 371
Caroli's disease 155
Caroticocavernous sinus fistula 402
Carotid artery 104f
    anatomy 128
    common 128f, 286f, 287, 288f, 292f
    disease, role of duplex ultrasonography in 285
    external 122f, 128f, 286f, 287, 287f, 289t, 392f
    internal 122f, 128f, 286, 287, 287f, 393f
        external 289t
    left internal 288f
    normal 287
    right internal 286f
Carotid dissection 393
Carotid Doppler signals, assessment of 288
Carotid examination technique, step in 286
Carotid occlusion 393
Carotid plaques 287
Carotid stenosis, assessment of 288
Castor oil 8
    soft tissue 9
Cataract, congenital 243
Catheter angiography, limitations of 301
Cathode ray tube 23, 24f
Caudal pancreatic artery 74f
Caudate lobe, sagittal scan of 67f
Caudate nucleus 116f, 117f
Caudothalamic groove 118f
Cavernous hemangioma 134, 135, 135f, 402
Cavum septi pellucidi 117f
Celiac axis 72
Cellular damage, severe 46
Central hematoma 135
Central nervous system 46
Central placenta previa 375f
Cephalad direction 62
Cerebellar vermis 236

Cerebellum 118f
　banana shaped 363f
Cerebral arteries
　anterior 60
　middle 404
Cerebral ventricular, measurement of 321t
Cerebrospinal fluid 295
　production of 236
Cerebrovascular sonography, limitations of 289
Cervical
　bruits 286
　carcinoma 215
　incompetence 376f
　nerve, seventh 122
　polyp 215
　pregnancy 337
　spine 338
　subcutaneous tissue 320
Cervix 94, 96f, 97f, 376
　abnormalities of 215
　carcinoma 216f
　normal 94f, 377
Charcot's triad 152
Chemoembolization 381
Chest
　cyst in 362
　pediatric 125
　sonography, indications for 102, 125
Chiari malformation 239
Chiari syndrome 394
Chlamydia 223, 260
Cholangiocarcinoma 155, 156f
Cholangitis 155
Cholecystitis
　acute 150
　chronic 147f, 148, 150, 151
　glandularis proliferans 151
　with cholelithiasis, chronic 149f
Cholecystokinin 150
Cholecystosonography 52
Choledochal cyst 154f, 155, 155f, 224, 361f
　diagnosis of 155
Choledocholithiasis 152, 155, 153f, 159
Cholelithiasis 146, 147f
Cholesterol 151
Choriocarcinoma 214f, 258
Choroid 246
　plexus 117f, 118f, 338
Choroidal detachment 246, 246f
Choroidal melanomas 402
Choroidal metastases 247
Cirrhosis 137, 139, 225
　causes of 137
Clear cell tumor 219
Cloacal exstrophy 367
Clostridium difficile 170
Cluster sign 132
Coincidence master synchronizers 25

Collapsed suprapatellar bursa 113
Collateral ligaments 113, 435
Colloid adenoma 252f
Colloid goiter 250
Colloidal suspensions 315
Colon carcinoma 166
Color Doppler 383
　advantages of 410
　applications of 410
　limitations of 410
　principles of 409
　techniques of 409
Color flow imaging 45, 387
　advantages of 387
　artifacts in 45
　limitation of 388
　principles of 387
Common femoral vein, thrombosis of 281f
Composite biparietal diameter 323t
Compound B mode scanning 26
Conception, retained products of 214
Congenital abnormality 170, 225
Congenital anomalies 75, 158, 186, 196
Congenital aqueductal stenosis 239f
Congenital cytomegalovirus infection 241f
Congenital diseases 243
Congenital disorders 231
Congenital duodenal obstruction 230
Congenital exophthalmos 243
Congenital extrahepatic biliary atresia 224
Congenital mega calyces 174
Congenital megaureter 174
Connective tissue septa 108f
Contrast echocardiography 316
Convex transducers 331
Convex volume probe with cable 38f
Cooper's ligaments 108
Cork coat, acoustic insulator of 12
Coronal brain scans 116
Coronary artery
　anomalies 418
　disease 412
　　multi-vessel 420
　right 415f
　stenting 306f
　supply 415f
Corpora amylacea 90
　calcification of 191f
Corpora cavernosa 101
Corpus callosum 117f, 121
　agenesis of 239, 365
Corpus cavernosum 101
Corpus luteal cyst 215
Cortical adenomas 193
Cortical cysts 183
　complex 184
Cortical echotexture 124f
Cortical necrosis, acute 186

Cortical nephrocalcinosis 227
Cortical renal cyst 184f
Corticosteroids 136
Couinaud's anatomy 64
Coupling agents 47
Craniofacial abnormalities 370
Craniofacial malformations 369
Cremasteric fascia 98
Crohn's disease 166
Cryptorchidism, complications of 261
Crystal
　surfaces of 12
　tissue 9
Crystalline bile 41
Curie temperature 12, 14
Cyst 253, 256
　and tumors 145
　bronchogenic 362
　complex 184, 422
　congenital 158
　diagnosis of 254
　functional 215
　multiple 130, 132
　peribiliary 130
Cystadenocarcinoma 219, 220f
Cystic adenomatoid malformation 362
Cystic duct calculus 153f
Cystic endometrial hyperplasia 213f
Cystic fibrosis 158, 231
Cystic follicles 97
Cystic hygroma 298f, 366
Cystic lesions 145, 206
Cystic masses 235
Cystic neoplasm 133, 162
Cystic peritoneal
　lesions 206
　masses 206
Cystic renal diseases 228
Cystic teratoma 222, 222f
Cystitis 188, 188f

D

Dandy-Walker cyst 240, 364
Dandy-Walker syndrome 240, 364f
Dartos muscle 98
Date pregnancy, clinically small for 347
Daughter cysts 132
Deep infrapatellar bursa 113
Deep vein thrombosis 283
Deep venous system 280, 281
Deltoid muscle 110
Deltoid muscle belly 110f, 424f
Demonstrate pelvic mass 37
Dermoid cyst 232f, 241, 249
Detrusor areflexia 188
Detrusor hyperreflexia 188
Diabetes mellitus 186
Diabetic retinopathy 245
Diaphragm 56, 79
　abdominal wall 51

Diaphragmatic crura 80
Diaphragmatic hernia 362, 369
Diastematomyelia 242
Diffuse parenchymal liver disease 225
Diffuse pleural thickening 234
Digastric muscle, posterior belly of 122*f*
Digestive carcinomas 312
Digestive pathology 312
Digestive wall, stages of tumoral infiltration of 312
Digital subtraction angiography 308
Digitization techniques 49
Dipolar molecules 13
Dipoles, random arrangement of 13*f*
Distal reverberation artifacts 214
Diverticular disease 169
Diverticulitis, acute 169
Doppler cerebral vascular examination, indications for 285
Doppler characteristics 287
Doppler effect 383
Doppler imaging
  artifacts in 43
  diagnosis on 403
Doppler information, display of 387
Doppler systems 383
  limitation of 384
Doppler ultrasound analysis 348
Doppler waveforms 402
Double decidual
  sac sign 332
  sign 333*f*
Double liver 75
Down's syndrome 358, 369
Drainage techniques 379
Duct ectasia 256
Ductus deferens, distal part of 92*f*
Duodenal atresia 359, 360
Duodenal wall 164*f*
Duodenum 70, 71, 81*f*, 131, 171, 230, 311
  parts of 79
Duplex collecting system 173
Duplex Doppler systems 385
Duplication cyst 231
Dysgerminoma 232
Dysraphic spinal defect 367
Dystrophic calcification 176

E

Early B mode scanner 27
Early pregnancy, complication of 333
Ebstein-Barr virus 225
Eccentric fibrofatty plaque 303*f*
Echinococcus granulosus, eggs of 131
ECHO
  amplitude information 28
  amplitude, digitalization of 25
  applications of 408
  basics of 405
  indications for 412, 419
  strikes 25

Echoendoscope, types of 310
Echogenic bile 146
Echogenic dermoid plug 222*f*
Echogenic epidermis 115*f*
Echogenic foci 131
Echogenic foreign body 246*f*
Echogenic glandular breast 107*f*
Echogenic infraspinatous tendon 112
Echogenic kidney 184*f*
Echogenic medulla 97
Echogenic membrane, thin 352*f*
Echogenic nerve roots 122
Echogenic parenchyma, abnormal 241
Echogenic stroma 219*f*
Echovist 317
Ectopia 172
Ectopic kidney 172*f*
Ectopic pregnancy 213*f*, 214, 336*f*
  in adnexa 215*f*
  role of Doppler sonography in 337
Edetic acid 47
Elastography 421
  clinical applications 421
  techniques 421
Elbow 60, 113, 428
  normal 272*f*
Electric field 14
Electric pulse 15
Electrodes on crystal, alignment of 13*f*
Electromagnetic radiation 4
Electron beam 23, 28
Electronic focusing 34
  principle of 35*f*
  technique 35
Electronic scanner 32
Embolization, complications of 381
Embryo 46, 332*f*
  development of 46
Embryonal carcinoma 232
Embryonal cell carcinoma 257
Embryonic gestational sac 335*f*
Emphysematous cholecystitis 150, 167
Emphysematous cystitis 188
Emphysematous pyelonephritis 179
Empyema 150, 234
Encapsulated gas bubbles 315
Encephalocele, large 366*f*
Encephalomalacia 240
Endocyst 131
Endometrial adhesions 214
Endometrial atrophy 212
Endometrial carcinoma 213
Endometrial cavity 95*f*
  normal 94
Endometrial ECHO 210
Endometrial hyperplasia 212
Endometrial polyp 213, 213*f*
Endometrioma 213*f*
Endometriosis 218
Endometriotic cyst 219*f*
Endometritis 213

Endometrium 96*f*, 320
  abnormalities of 212
Endometroid tumor 219
Endophthalmitis 247
Endoscopic retrograde cholangiopancreatography 313
Endoscopic ultrasonography 310
Endosonographic anatomy 311
Endoultrasonography 310
Endovascular graft procedures 306
Energy returning, amount of 40
Entamoeba histolytica 133
Epidermoid cyst 241, 249*f*, 256
Epididymis 98, 101*f*, 260
  head of 100*f*
Epididymo-orchitis 260
Epigastrium 43, 66*f*
Epiphyseal cartilages 339
Epithelial glandular cysts 193
Epithelial stromal tumors 222
Epithelial tumors 232
Epoxy resin propagate sound 19
Equipment 293, 331
  and documentation 277
Erectile dysfunction, evaluation of 399
Escherichia coli 260
Esophagus 76, 230, 311, 312
  carcinoma 141*f*
Estrogen production, clinical signs of 222
Ethylene oxide 293
Ewing's sarcoma 249
Exophytic mass, small 151*f*
Exstrophy 187
Extensor hallucis longus 436
Extra-adrenal pheochromocytoma 199*f*
Extracranial cerebral arteries 128*f*
Extrahepatic bile duct 52
Extrahepatic obstruction 225
Extrahepatic portal hypertension 284
Extratesticular lesions 258
Extremity veins, upper 129, 280
Eye
  agenesis of 243
  and orbit 58, 243, 300
  lens of 8
Eyeball 103, 249*f*
  and orbit 103
  anterior curvature of 103
  axial length of 105*f*
  transverse section of 105*f*

F

Face and upper neck 122
Facial vein, posterior 122*f*
Falciform ligament 69, 79*f*, 84
Fallopian tube 93*f*, 218, 222, 223*f*
Fascia, superficial 115
Fast fourier transform 384
Fasting, advantage of 37
Fat 6, 8
  necrosis 255

Fat-liver 9
Fat-soft tissue 9
Fatty infiltration 136
Fatty tissue, caused by 108
Femoral artery
   common 277
   left superficial 279f
   right 278f
   superficial 277, 305f, 404f
Femoral vein 278f, 282f
   common 277, 283f
Femoral venous system 281
Femur
   intercondylar region of 114f
   lesser trochanter of 80
Femur length 338, 371
   measurement of 340f
   predicted menstrual age for 325t
Fetal abdomen 357, 359f, 361f
Fetal anomalies 353
   major 358
Fetal ascites 369
Fetal breathing movements 350
Fetal chromosomal abnormalities 369
Fetal death, sonographic appearances of 350
Fetal growth abnormalities 340
Fetal hand 358f
Fetal head 6, 356
   anatomy of 355f
Fetal heart 358
   rate 350
Fetal hydrops 371
Fetal lobulation 172
Fetal movements 350
Fetal spine 356
Fetal teratoma 361f
Fetal thorax 357
Fetal tone 350
Fetus 300
Fever 136
Fibroadenoma 254, 254f, 422
Fibroblasts 109
Fibroid
   multiple 211f
   uterus 210f
Fibrolamellar carcinoma 226
Fibrosis and scarring 250
Fibrous histiocytoma 201
Fibrous tissue 303
   composed of 127
Fine needle aspiration 378
   cytology 313
First trimester pregnancy
   evaluation of 332
   loss 352
First-trimester sonography, guidelines for 331
Flexion deformity abscess, right 275f
Flowing blood 302
Fluid enema 53

Fluoroscopy 378
Focal caliectasis 180f
Focal fatty
   change 134
   infiltration 135f, 136
Focal hypoechoic lesions 143
Focal liver lesions, benign 130
Focal nodular hyperplasia 135
Focal pancreatitis 158
Focusing transducer 18f
Foley's catheter 190f
Follicular carcinoma 252
Follicular cyst 215
Foot and ankle 113, 435
Foramen of monro 116f, 117f
Foregut duplication cyst 361f
Foreign body 246
   in uterus 214f
Fossa cyst, large posterior 364f
Fourth lumbar arteries 80
Fracture right femur 273f
Frame rate artifact 45
Free gas bubbles 314
Frog's eye appearance 365f
Frontal horn 118f
Functioning tumors 163
Fungal abscess 133, 144f
Fungal infection 180f

G

Galactoceles 256
Galen aneurysm, vein of 364
Gallbladder 39, 51, 52, 70f, 136, 145, 204, 204f, 224, 318
   adenomyomatosis of 151, 151f
   anatomy of 69f
   and bile ducts 69
   anterior wall of 151f
   ascaris in 149f
   carcinoma 151, 396
   cholesterolosis of 151, 151f
   consists 69
   contracted 146
   distended 224
   empyema of 150
   examination of 52
   lumen 148f
   mucocele of 152f
   neck of 71f, 147f, 156
   normal pediatric 321t
   polyps 150
   primary disease of 224
   septations 145
   stones 146
   transverse scan of 150f
Gallbladder wall 146, 150, 152f
   anterior 148f
   causes of 147
   edema of 148
   thickened 149f

Gallstones 159
   diagnosis of 146
Ganglioneuromas 312
Gas bodies 46
Gas-filled duodenum 52
Gastric diaphragms 230
Gastric masses
   intraluminal 53
   intramural 53
Gastrinomas 163
Gastroesophageal junction 66f, 77f, 312
Gastroesophageal reflux 230
Gastrointestinal anomalies 372
Gastrointestinal bleeding, management of acute 381
Gastrointestinal cystic processes 360
Gastrointestinal infections 170
Gastrointestinal masses 231
Gastrointestinal system 357
Gastrointestinal tract 51, 53, 75, 125, 230
   anomalies 370
   malformation 370
   neoplasms 166
   obstruction of 159, 169
Gastroschisis 367
Gaucher's disease 225, 226, 276, 432
G-cell tumors 163
Gelatin encapsulated nitrogen microspheres 315
Genetic disorders 372
Genitalia 357
Genitourinary
   abnormalities 370
   system 356
   tract abnormalities 370
Germ cell tumor 222, 257
Gestation sac 332f
Gestational age 348f
   estimation by
      biparietal diameter 338t
      crown-rump length 334t
      femur length 339t
      head circumference 339t
Gestational sac 37
   measurement 322t, 333t
Gland enlargement 103
Glenoid
   labrum, superior 112
   posterior part of 110
Gliding sign 102
Glisson's capsule 63
Globus major 98
Glomerulonephritis 186
Glycogen storage disease 225
Goiter 250
Gonococcus 260
Gonorrhea 223
Gout 442
Graft dysfunction, cause of 403
Granulomatous hepatitis 137
Granulomatous infection 187

Granulosa cell tumors 212
Graves' disease 248, 250
Gross fetal ascites 369f
Gut edema 171
Gut signature 76f, 77, 164
Gut wall
    histologic layers of 76f
    intrinsic causes of 169
    pathology 164
Gynecology and obstetrics, role of color Doppler in 404

H

Hand 358
    and wrist 113, 428
Hashimoto's thyroiditis 250, 251f
Head
    and abdominal circumference, measurement of 348f
    and brain malformations 365
    and neck, pediatric 122
    circumference, measurement of 338f
    cyst in 362
Healed granuloma 138f
Heart 30, 311
    and vascular system 300
Hemangioma 133, 135, 204, 225, 233, 400, 401f
Hematoma, marginal 375, 375f
Hematometra 212
Hemidiaphragm, right 81f
Hemoptysis, management of 381
Hemorrhage 133
    adrenal 229
    intracranial 236
    intraparenchymal 238
    intraventricular 238
Hemorrhagic cyst 217f
Hemorrhagic infarction, periventricular 239
Hemorrhagic thyroid cyst 251f
Hemothorax 234
Hepatic abscess 225
Hepatic adenoma 135
Hepatic and splenic artery 83f
Hepatic artery, branches of 70
Hepatic calcification 225
Hepatic candidiasis 133
Hepatic duct
    common 70, 156
    right and left 70
Hepatic lesions, color Doppler in 395
Hepatic lipoma 135
Hepatic malformation, benign developmental 130
Hepatic masses 225
Hepatic neoplasm 225
    benign 225
    malignant 226
Hepatic portal hypertension 284

Hepatic veins 63, 67f, 134, 284f, 318, 391
    Doppler tracing of 392f
    left 67f
    major 63
    middle 65f, 67f, 68f
    obstruction of 138
    right 63, 67f
Hepatitis 136, 140, 148
    A 225
    acute 136f, 225
    alcoholic 140
    B 225
    chronic 137
        viral 137
    postchronic 140
Hepatobiliary drainage techniques 380
Hepatobiliary surgery 71
Hepatobiliary system 295
    and spleen, pediatric 126
Hepatoblastoma 225, 226
Hepatocellular carcinoma 140, 141f, 226
Hepatocellular tumor 140
Hepatoduodenal ligament 63
Hepatorenal pouch 78f
Hepatorenal recess 86
Hereditary pancreatitis 231
Heterogeneous echotexture 183f
Hip
    adult 108, 433
    anatomy of 109f, 434f
    congenital dislocation of 271, 432
    dysplasia, classification of 276t, 432t
    normal, both 275f
    pediatric 62, 428
    septic arthritis, right 274f, 433f
    transient synovitis of 433
Hip joint 51
    coronal plane of 108f, 431f
    effusion 432
    joint effusion in 430f
Hirschsprung's disease 361
Hodgkin's disease 186
Hodgkin's lymphoma 201
Homogeneous echotexture 63, 97, 99f
Horn, anterior 116f
Horseshoe kidney 172, 173f
Human fetus 46
Human soft tissue 6
Hydatid cyst 145, 207f, 248
    diagnosis of 131
    infected 131f
Hydatid disease 131, 133, 180, 206
Hydatidiform mole 335, 335f, 373, 373f
Hydrocele 258, 259f
    gross 259f
    with epididymitis 259f
Hydrocephalus 362f
Hydrocolpos 232
Hydrometra 212
Hydrometrocolpos 232, 362
Hydromyelia 242

Hydronephrosis 174, 226
    mild 175f
    moderate 175
Hydronephrotic kidney 226
Hydrops 152
    causes of 371
    fetalis 340
Hydroureter, bilateral 187f
Hyperbilirubinemia 224
Hyperechoic plaque 288f
Hyperplastic endometrium 212
Hypertension 348
Hyperthermia 46
Hypertrophic cardiomyopathy 420
Hypertrophic pyloric stenosis 230
Hypertrophy prostate, benign 190
Hyphema, posterior 245
Hypochondrium pain, right 155
Hypoechoic articular cartilage 112
Hypoechoic cerebellar hemispheres 116
Hypoechoic collection 274f
Hypoechoic lesion 182f
    multiple 144f
    small 200f
Hypoechoic mass 182f
    lesion, large 194f
Hypoechoic muscle 112
Hypoechoic parenchyma 108, 177
Hypoechoic renal medullary pyramids 86
Hypoechoic thrombus 279f
Hypoechoic ulnar bursa 60
Hypoglycemic symptoms 163
Hypoplastic cervix 215f
Hypoplastic kidney 172
Hypoplastic uterus 232f
Hypoxic-ischemic encephalopathy 238, 239, 239f

I

Idiopathic megaureter 360
Iliac artery
    common 80, 82f
    internal 83f
    leg-common 277f
    right common 83f
Iliac fossa, right 169, 275f, 434f
Iliac vein 281
Iliofemoral ligament 108
Ill-defined echogenic adenomyomatous lesion 212f
Immune hydrops 371
Imperforate anus 359
In utero fetal sonographic weight standards 340t
Infant spine 121
Infant's hip 109f, 431f
Infantile hypertrophic pyloric stenosis 230f
Infantile polycystic renal disease 359
Infarction 257
Infected hydrocephalus 238f

Infection 133
Infectious cystitis 187
Infectious diseases 193
Inferior vena cava 63, 67f, 81f, 83, 196, 226, 281, 319, 391, 391f
  branches 391
Infertile females 404
Infertility, cause of 219
Inflammatory bowel disease 76, 166, 313
Inflammatory disease 148, 158, 192
Inflammatory lymph node 296f
Infraspinatus muscle and tendon 426f
Infraspinatus tendon 112f, 428f
Innominate artery 128f
Interhemispheric fissure 121
Interstitial pregnancy 337
Interventional techniques 382
Interventricular septum 413f
  motion of 413t
Intestinal atresia 361
Intestinal tuberculosis 170
Intra-arterial thrombolysis 381
Intracardiac shunts 411
Intracavitary probes 50
Intracerebral bleed 238f
Intracoronary injections 315
Intracranial infections 240
Intracranial sonography 236
  axial sections 236
  normal anatomy 236
  sonographic appearance 238
Intragastric gas 71
Intrahepatic bile duct 152, 152f
Intrahepatic gallbladder, small 149f
Intrahepatic obstruction 225
Intraluminal air 310
Intraocular tumors 247
Intraoperative biliary sonography, indications for 295
Intraoperative cranial sonography 294
Intrapancreatic bile duct 52
Intraperitoneal cystic processes 361
Intraplacental hematomas 375
Intrascrotal anatomy, normal 99f
Intraspinal lipoma 242
Intrasplenic pseudoaneurysms 396
Intratesticular lesions, benign 256
Intrathoracic masses, evaluation of 265
Intrauterine contraceptive device 214
Intrauterine gestational sac 215f
Intrauterine growth retardation 347, 353
  fetus 349f
  types of 347
Intravascular ultrasound
  recent advances of 308
  technical consideration of 301
Intussusception 169, 230
Irritable hip
  examination of 432f
    routine 109f

Ischemic bowel disease 170
Ischemic cardiomyopathy 415f
Islet cell tumors 163
Isoechoic lesions 138
Isthmus 104f

J

Jaundice
  mild physiological 224
  neonatal 224
  obstructive 155, 157, 159
Jejunal loops 165f
Joint 126
  and tendons 51
  effusion 271, 276, 441
  lesions, ultrasound of 271
  neonatal hips 126
  soldered 40
Jugular vein, internal 123, 129f

K

Kidney 6, 8, 11, 81f, 83, 172, 228, 319
  abnormally located 369
  absent 172, 172f
  anatomical relations of 81f
  anatomy of 86f
  and liver 300
  congenital 172
  eight 70f, 87f, 88f, 124f, 181f, 183f
  enlarged 177f
  intraoperative sonography of 295
  midpolar region of 181f
  neonatal 124, 124f
  normal 89
  small 369
  transplanted 399f
Klatskin tumors 157
Knee 60, 113, 113f, 433
  right 271f
Knee joint 114f, 437f
  medial side of 436f
  normal 89f, 270f, 440f

L

Lacrimal gland 106
Lactobezoars 230
Lamina propria 75
Laparoscopic sonography 295
Laparoscopic ultrasound, goals of 296
Lead zirconate titanate 14
Left atrium 405f
Left circumflex artery 415f
Left common femoral artery 279f
Left dome 80f, 81f
Left hip
  dislocation of 275f
  transient synovitis of 436f
Left kidney
  dilated pelvis of 360f
  sagittal scan of 87f, 88f
  transverse section of 89f

Left ovary, cystic lesion in 213f
Left pleural cavity 264f
Left ventricle
  cavity 419f
  systolic wall motion score 412t
Left ventricular aneurysm 416
Left ventricular dysfunction 413
Left ventricular hypertrophy 419, 420
  differential diagnosis of 420
Left ventricular mass, calculation of 420f
Left ventricular posterior wall 413f
Leiomyoma 210, 312
Leiomyosarcoma 199, 210
Lesion 134
  ablation 380
    technique of 380
  benign solid 254
  multiple 59
Lesser saphenous vein 129
Leukemia 133, 183, 184f, 226, 249
Leukocytosis 224
Leukomalacia, periventricular 239
Ligamentum teres acts 64
Limb shortening 365
Limb-body wall complex 367
Linear array transducer, development of 2
Lipid emulsions 316
Lipoma 312
  containing 423f
Liposarcoma 199
Liquid bath transducers 32
Liver 6, 8, 11, 51, 63, 87f, 124f, 126, 225, 318, 394, 422
  anterior part of 40f
  calcification 135
  cirrhosis of 395f
  congenital cysts of 225
  cyst 130
    secondary 130
    simple 130, 130f
  disease
    benign diffuse 136
    chronic 225
    malignant 140
  enlargement 143
  hypoechoic mass in 136f
  left lobe of 66f, 67f, 77f
  malignant lesions of 140
  parenchyma 63
  posterior surfaces of 63f
  right lobe of 65f, 66f, 69, 131f, 133f, 135f, 181f
  sonography, applications of intraoperative 295
  surface, irregular 138, 138f
  transplantation 396
  visualization of 39
Lobar fissure 71f
Lobar variet 364
Logarithmic amplification 25

Low pressure 4
Lower extremity veins, anatomy of 129f, 281
Lower gastrointestinal tract 311, 313
Lower limb 403
Lower lumbar canal regions 122
Lumbosacral meningomyelocele 363f
Lung 6, 11
　abscess 235, 265f
　normal 126f
　parenchyma 234
　tumors 234
Lymph node 201, 252, 310, 319
　normal 108
Lymphadenopathy 233, 235
Lymphangioma 233, 248
Lymphocele 204
Lymphoma 133, 144, 166, 183, 190, 226, 228, 233

M

Macrocystic neoplasms 163
Malakoplakia 187
Male genitalia, normal 357f
Male pelvis 99f
Mammary ducts 107
Manufacturer's instructions 55
Maple syrup 11
Marfan's syndrome 304
Marginal placenta 374
Marginal previa 374
Massa intermedia 116f
Massive splenomegaly 143f, 144f
Massive subchorial thrombosis 375
Matted bowel loop 167f
Mechanical energy 4
Mechanical obstruction 169
Mechanical scanner 31
　type of 32
Mechanical vibration 32
Meconium cyst 361
Meconium peritonitis 231
Meconium plug syndrome 361
Medial hyoglossus muscle 123
Mediastinal masses, posterior 57
Mediastinum 56, 235, 311
　testis 98, 100f
Medical imaging equipment, types of 24
Medical renal diseases 227
Medullary carcinoma 252
Medullary cystic disease 184, 228
Medullary cysts 184
Medullary nephrocalcinosis 176
Medullary sponge kidney 176, 184, 227
Melanoma, malignant 166
Memory device 28
Meningitis 240
Meningocele 241, 242f
Meniscal tear 268
Menopause uterus atrophies 94

Mesenchymal hamartoma 225
Mesenchymal tumors 166
Mesenchymoma 226
Mesenteric artery, superior 72, 73f, 80, 81f, 169, 197, 199, 319
Mesenteric cyst 168f, 231
Mesenteric Doppler 390
Mesenteric vein, superior 72, 81f
Mesoblastic nephroma 228
Metabolic disorders 224
Metabolic liver disease 225
Metastases 145, 145f, 190, 195f, 226
Metastatic lesions, large 141f
Metastatic tumors 140, 166, 198, 222
Metatarsophalangeal joint 425f
Mid gut malrotation 169
Mirizzi syndrome 156
Missed abortion 334, 335f
Mitral regurgitation, acute 415, 416
Mitral valve, normal 409f
M-mode ECHO 409
Monoamniotic twinning 353
Monochorionicity 353
Morrison's pouch 86
Mucinous cystadenoma 219
Mucocele 249
Multicystic dysplastic kidney 185, 228, 359, 359f
Multifetal pregnancies, complications of 352
Multifocal carcinoma 190f
Multilocular cystic nephroma 180, 228
Multilocular nephroma 181f
Multinodular goiter 250, 251f
Multiple color Doppler 401f
Multiple echogenic nodules 255f
Multiple follicles, ovaries with 97f
Multiple gestations 351f
　ultrasound evaluation in 351
Multiple glands, dysfunction of 158
Multiple peritoneal ligaments 84
Multiple varicoceles 400f
Mural nodularity 180
Muscle 6, 8, 11, 115, 423
　hypertrophy 248
　relaxation 38
Muscularis mucosa 75
Muscularis propria 75
Musculoskeletal system 108, 358, 400
Musculoskeletal ultrasonography 423
Musculoskeletal ultrasound 268
Mycobacterium tuberculosis 170, 180
Myelolipoma 193
Myelomeningocele 121, 241, 242f, 367
Myeloschisis 121
Mylohyoid muscle 123
Myocardial infarction 412
Myocardial ischemia 412
Myometrial abnormalities 210
Myometrium, posterior 212

N

Nabothian cyst 215, 216f
Narrow neck diverticulum 188f
Nausea 136
Neck 102, 356
　lymph nodes 252
Neonatal ovaries 125
Neonatal spine, sonographic imaging of 241
Neonate cortex and medulla of kidney 124f
Neoplasms 160, 219
　malignant 255
Nephroblastoma 228
Nephrocalcinosis 176, 227
Nephrocalcinosis-stippled calcification 177f
Nephrotic syndrome 227
Neuroblastoma 194f, 226, 229, 229f, 233
Neuroenteric cysts 362
Neurogenic bladder 188, 227
　types 188
Nipple-areolar complex 58, 108f
Nodular surface 138
Nodular synovium, thickened 115f, 438f
Non-fasting gallbladder, normal 127f
Nonfunctioning islet-cell tumors 163
Non-glandular fibromuscular stroma 90
Non-Hodgkin's lymphoma 166, 195, 248
Nonimmune hydrops 371
Non-neoplastic cysts 215
Nonstress test 350
Nonvascular procedures 378
Non-viable pregnancy, early diagnosis of 334t
Normal sonographic anatomy 75, 86
Normal triphasic pattern, loss of 280f
Nose 356
　and lips 356f
Nuchal skin fold thickness 371
Nuchal translucency 371
Nulliparous uterus 94

O

Obstetric ultrasound 38, 56, 331
Obstruction, absence of 387
Occipital horn 117f
Occipital lobe 118f
Ocular melanoma 247, 248f
Ocular tumors 402
Olecranon bursa 442f
Oligohydramnios 354, 354f, 357
Omental cyst 231
Omentum, thickened 167f
Ommon iliac veins 83
Omohyoid muscles 103
Omphalocele 366, 367f
Oncocytomas 181
Ophthalmic scanning 43
Optic nerve 105f
　tumors 249

Optic neuritis 249
Oral fluid 53
Orbital cysticercosis 248, 248f
Orbital diseases 248
Orbital lymphoma 248
Orbital metastases 249
Orbital trauma 248
Orbital vessels, normal 402
Orthogonal beam 43
    width artifact 43
Oscillating contact
    scanner touches 31
    transducer 31f
Oscillating nonreflecting transducer 32f
Oscillating transducer 31
Oscilloscopes 28
Osteomyelitis 271, 442
    calcification-chronic 273f, 435f
Ovarian cyst 218f
    functional 216f
Ovarian ectopic pregnancy 337
Ovarian mass 232
    malignant 221f
Ovarian neoplasm, primary malignant 219
Ovarian veins 391
Ovarian volume 98
Ovary 37, 97, 125, 215, 218, 320
    right 98f
Ovum, blighted 334

P

Palpable nontender gallbladder 160
Pancake kidney 180f
Pancreas 39, 51, 53, 71, 81f, 126f, 158f, 231, 311, 391, 396
    anatomy of 72f
    body of 72
    evaluation of 295
    examination of 53
    head of 73f
    normal 159
    pediatric 126
    transverse section of 73f
Pancreatic ascites 160
Pancreatic carcinoma 140
Pancreatic head, normal dimension of 73f
Pancreatic masses 231
Pancreatic necrosis 159
Pancreatic pseudocyst 160f, 231
Pancreatic tail, region of 161f
Pancreatic transplantation 396
Pancreatic tumor 162f
Pancreatic visualization 53
Pancreatitis 208
    acute 158, 158f, 159f
        on chronic 159f
    chronic 140, 160, 161f
        calcific 161f
    complications of 159
    diagnosis of acute 158
    diffuse 158
Papillary carcinoma 252f
Papillary necrosis 176, 179
Paralytic ileus 76, 170
Parapelvic cysts 184
Parasagittal scan 53f
Parathyroid
    adenoma 401
    glands 102, 103, 123, 401
Parenchyma 9, 397
    atrophy 179f
    echogenicity, abnormal 240
Parietal lobe 118f
Parotid gland 58, 122, 123f
    normal 122f
Parovarian cysts 218
Particle interaction 5f
Patellar ligament, monosodium urate crystals in 425f
Patellar tendon tears 268, 439
Peak end diastolic velocity 289
Peak systolic velocity 289
Pectoralis muscle 107f
Pediatric hip, sonographic evaluation of 271
Pelvic abscess 205f
Pelvic anatomy 37
Pelvic collection 314
Pelvic cystic processes 361
Pelvic hematoma 206f
Pelvic inflammatory disease 222, 336
Pelvic masses 232
Pelvic organs 56
Pelvic scanning 37
Pelvis 204
    female 90f,
    low in 38
    pediatric 125
Pelviureteric junction obstruction 173, 174f
Penis 59, 98
    anatomy of 102f
    exhibits 101
Peptic ulcer 171
Percent stenosis 288
Percutaneous insertion techniques 379
Percutaneous nephrostomy 380
Percutaneous stenting 380
Percutaneous transluminal angioplasty 305
Perendoscopic ultrasound 310
Perfluoroctyl bromide 315
    advantages of 316
Periampullary carcinoma 162f
Pericardial effusion, acute 417
Perinatal meningitis 240
Peripheral arteries 128, 278f, 392f, 403f
    ultrasound examination of 277
Peripheral vascular system 402
Peripheral veins 129
Perirenal fascia, posterior 79
Perisac bleeds 335
Peritoneal cavity 202
    anatomy of 80f
Peritoneal inclusion cysts 218
Peritoneal lesions 204, 206
Peritoneal mesothelioma 206
Peritoneal metastases 204, 206f
Peritoneum 55, 84, 231
Periurethral glands urethra 90
Persistent hyperplastic primary vitreous 243, 243f
Perthes' disease 275f, 276, 432
Phantom 21
Pharmacopenile duplex ultrasonography 399
Pheochromocytoma 194f, 195
Phocomelia 366
Piezoelectric crystal 14, 14f
    causes 16f
    construction 12
    element 12
Piezoelectric effect 1, 14, 21
Piezoelectric material 13, 14
Piezoelectric polymers 8
Placenta 372
    abruption of 336f
    creta 374
    low lying 374
    normal 373f
    previa
        partial 374
        types of 374f
    shape of 373
    sonographic evaluation of 372
Placental abruption 374
Placental grading 350, 368f
Placental previa 374
Placental tumors 373
Plaque composition 288
Plaque extent and thickness 287
Plaque morphology 302
Plasma cell mastitis 256
Pleural effusion 160, 261, 362
    bilateral 262f
Pleural masses 234
Pleural mesothelioma 234
Pleural metastases 234
Pleural plaques 234
Pleural space 56
Pleural thickening 234
Pneumobilia 155
    echogenic foci 155f
Pneumothorax 234
Polyarteritis nodosa 257
Polycystic kidney disease 130f, 184
    adult 185f, 359
    autosomal recessive 228
Polycystic liver disease 130, 130f
Polycystic ovarian disease 219

Polycystic ovaries, vascular stroma of 404
Polyhydramnios 357
Polymorphic hyperechoic aggregates 441f
Polyps 312
Polysplenia 75
Polystyrene 19
Popliteal and calf veins 281
Popliteal fossa 129
Popliteal vein 282
Porta hepatis 68f, 70, 157
Portal cavernoma 395f
Portal hypertension 139, 225, 394, 396
    collaterals 143f
    sonographic findings in 394
Portal vein 319
    thrombosis 140, 140f
        causes of 140
Portal venous system 72f, 283, 283f
Portal-splenic confluence 71
Portocaval shunts 140
Portosplenic vein thrombosis 160
Postabortal uterus 215f
Post-abortion complication 223
Posterior fossa cyst, small 364f
Postmenopausal ovaries, normal 98
Postmenopausal uterus, shape of 94
Poststenotic flow changes 386
Post-traumatic cataract 246f
Post-traumatic cysts 145
Potential cardiac applications 315
Pouch of Douglas 37, 78f, 169f
Power Doppler flow imaging 388
Power Doppler mode, inferior vena cava in 394f
Pre-aortic lymph node 200f
Precutaneous transluminal angioplasty 304
Predicted menstrual age 324t
Prehepatic portal hypertension 284
Preplacental hematomas 375
Propagation speed 4
Propylene glycol 47
Prostate 51, 92f, 125, 190, 192f, 300, 422
    abnormality of 54
    and seminal vesicles 89
    carcinomas 192f, 422
    enlarged 191f
    gland 54, 319
        normal 89
Prostatic abscess 192
Prostatic carcinoma 89, 192
Prostatic urethra 89, 190f
Prostatism, acute 192f
Prostatitis 192
Prourokinase 381
Proximal pelvicaliectasis 182
Prune belly syndrome 227
Pseudoaneurysm 159, 390, 404, 417t
Pseudocysts 193
Pseudokidney 164
    sign 166f, 170f
Pseudomembranous colitis 170
Pseudomonas 260
Pseudomyxoma peritonei 204
Pseudopancreatic cyst 159, 206
Pseudotumor 183f
Psoas abscess 198f, 233
Pulmonary AV fistula 381
Pulsatile neck masses 393
Pulse dimension affects 17
Pulse ECHO 21
    distance ranging technique 1
Pulse generator 20
Pulse repetition frequency 30
Pulsed Doppler technique 279
Pulsed wave Doppler 384, 408, 409
Pyelonephritis 176, 397f
    acute 177f
    chronic 176, 179, 179f
Pylorus, sagittal scan of 78f
Pyonephrosis 41, 177, 179f
Pyriform shape, normal 71f

Q
Q factor 15
Q transducer 17

R
Radiofrequency digitization 49
Radiofrequency signal 22
Rapid systolic upstroke 287f
Real-time ultrasound 30
    scanning systems 19
Reception and amplification 21
Rectangular array 34
Rectovesical pouch 37
Rectum 311
Rectus abdominis 79
    originates 79
Recurrent ischemic neurological deficit 285
Red blood cell 383
Reflection 8
    amount of 8, 9
    angle of 9
    refraction
        and absorption 8
        and scattering 11
Reflects sound waves 55
Refraction 10
Regional lymph nodes 182
Regurgitant aortic valve 408f, 410f
Regurgitant lesions 411
Regurgitant mitral valve 411f
Reidel's lobe 66
Relaxation time 11
Relevant fetal anatomy 355
Remote localizers 299
Renal abnormality, congenital 209
Renal abscess 177, 179f
Renal anatomy, pediatric 124
Renal arterial occlusion and infarction 185
Renal artery 285f, 391, 398f
    Doppler 284
    left 82f
    normal 285
    right 83f
    stenosis 185, 398
        diagnosis of 398
    thrombosis 398
Renal calculus 176f
Renal cell carcinoma 181, 181f, 398
Renal cortex 63, 89
Renal cortical echogenicity 86
Renal cystic
    disease 183, 225
    processes 359
Renal duplication 226
Renal dysplasia 228
Renal ectopia, crossed 172
Renal fossa, right 173f
Renal hilum 86
Renal hydatid disease 180
Renal hypertension 285f
Renal masses 398
Renal medical disorders 185
Renal moieties, fused 173f
Renal parenchyma 86
Renal pyramid 89
    region of 177f
Renal sinus 42, 86, 177
Renal stones/calculi 174
Renal transplant 398
Renal trauma 178f
Renal tubular acidosis 176
Renal tumors 180
    malignant 181
    secondary 182
Renal ultrasonography, contrast media in 316
Renal ultrasound beam 43
Renal vein
    occlusion 185
    thrombosis 227
        acute 398
Respiration 387
    venous effect of 387
Respiratory variations 283f
Rete testis 98
Retina 105f, 245
    section of 43
Retinal detachment 244f, 245
Retinal tears 245
Retinal vessel abnormalities 402
Retinoblastoma 247, 247f
Retinoschisis 246
Retrobulbar region 105f
Retrofascial space 80
Retromammary fat 107f

Retroperitoneal cysts 199, 233
Retroperitoneal fibrosis 198
Retroperitoneal fluid collections 198, 233
Retroperitoneal sarcoma 199f
Retroperitoneal tumors 199
Retroperitoneal vessels 389
Retroperitoneum 55, 79, 232, 311
Retroplacental clot, resolving 375f
Retroplacental hematoma 374, 375f
    large 336f
Reverberation artifacts 42
Reye's syndrome 225
Rhabdomyosarcoma 199, 224, 232, 233, 248
Rheumatoid arthritis 186
Ribs, scan between 57f
Riedel's lobe 137f
Right adrenal gland 83, 125f, 195f
Right atrium 197f, 416f
Right dome 80f, 81, 81f
Right kidney
    hilum of 83f
    lower pole of 228f
    pelvicalyceal system of 177f
    pelvis of 182f
    sagittal scan of 88f
    transverse section of 87f
Rokitansky-Aschoff sinuses 151
Rotating contact transducer 32f
Rotating wheel transducer 32
Rotator cuff 59, 110, 438f
    complete tear of 270f
    lesions 438
    partial atrophy of 270f, 439f
    tear of 268, 439f
    tendons 426
Rubber coat, acoustic insulator of 12

S

Sacral theca 121
Salivary gland 58, 122, 401
Scan converter 28
Scan protocol and technique 284
Scanning spleen, technique for 52f
Scar tissue 250
Schwannoma, malignant 201
Scleral rupture, posterior 246
Scrotal blood supply 99f
Scrotal hematoma 261f
Scrotal sac, right 259f
Scrotal ultrasound 256
Scrotum 59, 98, 125, 399
    anatomy 99f
Semilobar holoprosencephaly 364
Seminal vesicles 91f, 93f
Seminoma 261
Sepsis 391
Septate uterus 209f, 298f, 351f
Septic abortion 335
Septic arthritis 434f
Septicaemia 140

Septula 98
Septum
    and mitral leaflets 411f
    pellucidum 237f
Serosa 75
Serous cystadenoma 219
Sertoli-leydig cell tumor 222
Severe stenosis evaluation, quantitative Doppler for 289
Sex cord-stromal tumors 222
Shorter spatial pulse length 16
Shoulder 424
    capsule 110
    right and left 269f
Sickle cell anemia 224
Silicon oxide element 28
Simple cortical cysts 183, 184f
Simple cyst 130, 133, 422
Sinus ECHO 174
Situs ambiguous 75
Skeletal dysplasia 372
Skin 98, 422
    and subcutaneous tissue 114, 423, 400
    benign lipomatosis of 268f, 400f
    overlying breast 107f
    thickening 369
Skull
    adult 6
    lemon shaped 363f
    wall, lateral 1
Skull-bone 8, 11
Sludge balls 147
Small bowel obstruction 230
Snell's law 10, 10f
    of optics 10
Snow storm 232
Soft tissues 271
    air 9
    bone 9
    fat 9
    findings 368
    half value for 11
    lung 9
    swelling 272f, 273f, 435f
Solid masses 233, 235
Solid renal cell carcinoma 182f
Solid-state realtime transducer 33f
Sonoelastographic techniques 421
Sonographic anatomy, basic 63
Sonographic milestones 334t
Sonography 250
    mucinous cystadenomas 219
    pediatric 116
    scanning techniques in 51
Sound
    beam 11
        path of 28
    frequency and speed of 4
    pulse 27
    speed of 4
    velocity of 4, 6
    wave, direction of 4

Spalding sign 351f
Spectral information 44
Specular ECHO 8f
Specular interfaces 40
Spermatic cord 98
Spermatic fascia
    external 98
    internal 98
Spina bifida 367
Spinal canal 51, 62, 121
    content of 121
    pediatric 61
Spinal deformity, severe 121
Spinal dysraphism 241
Spinal sonography 121
Spinal ultrasound, intraoperative 294
Splanchnic aneurysms 391
Spleen 51, 72, 83, 126, 127f, 143, 226, 318, 396
    accessory 75
    anatomy of 74f
    and water distended stomach 74f
    diffuse diseases of 143
    focal diseases of 144
    longitudinal scan of 74f
    sagittal scan of 74f
    size of 126
    tuberculosis of 143
    upper pole of 74f
    with bright echogenic diaphragm 42f
Splenectomy 140
Splenic abscess 144f
Splenic artery 72
    aneurysm 381
    embolization 381
Splenic enlargement 144
Splenic hilum 74f, 143, 143f
Splenic hydatid 146f
Splenic infarction 396
Splenic masses 226
Splenic parenchyma 144f
Splenic trauma 145f
Splenic vein 319
    cavernous transformation of 143f
Splenomegaly, mild 143f
Splenorenal ligament 144f
Splenunculus 146f
Squamous cell carcinoma 182, 190
Starry sky appearance 136
Stenosis
    aqueduct 363f
    percentage of 287t
    severe 288f
Stenotic aortic valve 407f, 408f, 411f
Stenotic lesion 289, 410
Stenson's duct, mildly dilated 123f
Stent deployment 305
Stent grafts 306
Sternocleidomastoid muscle 123
Sternohyoid muscles 103
Stomach 77, 171, 230, 311

and duodenum, region of 165f
carcinoma of 164f, 312
pediatric 125
wall, thickened 164f
Strain elastography 421
Strawberry gallbladder 151
Streptokinase 381
Stress echocardiography 418
   indications 418
   limitations 419
   negative test 419
   positive test 418
   principle 418
   technique 418
Stress, application of 127
Stromal tumors 258
Styloid process 122f
Subacromial subdeltoid bursa 110
Subchorionic hemorrhage 375f
Subclavian artery 128, 128f
Subcutaneous lipomatous lesion 268f
Subdeltoid bursa, normal 110
Sublingual glands 58, 123
Submandibular gland 58, 102f, 122, 123, 123f
Submucosa 75
Subscapularis from supraspinatus 59
Subscapularis tendon 111f, 427f
Subxiphoid region 38
Succenturiate lobes 373
Supramesocolic spaces, right and left 84
Suprapatellar knee joint 440f
Supraspinatus muscle and tendon 426f
Supraspinatus tendon 112, 112f, 424f, 427f
Suspensory ligament 106
Sylvian fissure 118f
Sylvius, aqueduct of 116f
Synovial cysts 271, 441
Synovial effusion 271f
Synovial sheaths 109
Synovium 424
Systemic arterial hypertension 419
Systolic wall
   motion, abnormal 412
   thickening
      abnormal 412
      lack of 412

T

Tardus parvus waveform 403f
Target lesion 165f
Technological development 1
Temporal horn 117f, 118f
Temporal lobes 121
Tendinitis 269, 439
Tendon 60, 108, 423
   fibers 436
   tears 268, 438
Tenon's capsule 103
Tenosynovitis 113f, 430f
Teratoma 231, 257, 233
Terminal duct lobular units 108
Testicular artery 399f
Testicular cyst 256, 257f
Testicular malignancy 258
Testicular metastases 258
Testicular torsion 260, 399
Testis 98
   anteroposterior dimension of 100f
   hypoechoic to 98
   isoechoic to 98
   ruptured 261
   substance of 98
   superior pole of 101f
Tethered spinal cord 242
Thalamus, normal 117f
Thanatophoric dwarfism 365
Theca luteal cyst 218
Theolamine 47
Therapeutic procedures, real time monitoring of 306
Therapeutic ultrasound 45
Thermal effects 45
Thick walled cystic adenomyotic lesions 211f
Thorax 51, 56, 82f, 102, 233, 261
Thrombus 196, 303
Thymus, echogenicity of 126
Thyroglossal cyst 251f
Thyroid 58, 126, 250, 422
   adenoma 252, 252f
   cartilage 102
   classical follicular adenoma of 252f
   cyst 250
   enlarged 251f
   follicular adenoma of 402f
   gland 58, 102, 103f, 123, 320, 401
      anatomy of 103f
      normal 103, 103f
   left lobe of 104f
   lesions 250
   lobe, left 251f
   malignancies 252
   nodule 296f
   right lobe of 104f
Thyroiditis 250
Tibial artery
   and vein, posterior 291f
   posterior 129
Tibioperoneal trunk 128
Tissue
   acoustic impedance 8
   air interfaces 9
   bone-tissue phantom 10f
   boundary 11
   plane 43
Todani's classification 155
Tracheoesophageal atresia 369
Tractional retinal detachment 245
Transabdominal sonography 56
Transabdominal technique 89
Transcranial Doppler ultrasound 393
Transducer 9f
   construction 12
   crystal element 21
   focusing 17
   technology, advances in 30
   types of 39f, 302f
Transesophageal transverse sections 311
Transfontanellar scan, technique for 116f
Transient ischemic attack 285
Transitional cell
   carcinoma 182, 182f, 188, 189f
   tumor 222
Transluminal angioplasty 382
Transmitter 25
Transplant dysfunction 398
Transrectal ultrasound 54
Transvaginal sonography 56, 317, 331
   disadvantage of 56
Transvaginal transducers 331
Trauma 140, 145, 246, 271, 276, 433, 442
   anterior segment 246
   dehydration 391
   posterior segment 246
Trichobezoar 171
Tricuspid valve 410f
Triethanolamine 47
Triphasic waveform, normal 280f, 403
Trophoblastic tumors 373
Tuberculosis 137, 180, 186, 223
Tubular necrosis, acute 185, 227
Tumefactive sludge 147
Tumor 228, 233
   benign 180, 223t
   malignant 223t, 257
   types of 222t
Tunica vaginalis 98
Twin
   embolization syndrome 353
   transfusion syndrome 353
Two-dimensional ECHO 405
Typhilitis 168f

U

Ulcerative colitis 166
Ulnar veins 280
Ultrasonic beam 30, 34
Ultrasonic information 24
Ultrasonic system, components of 24f
Ultrasound 8
   artifacts 37
   contrast agents for 314
   diagnostic 7
   ECHO, portions of 28
   equipment 30
   gastroesophageal junction 230
   identified fetal abnormality 371
   imaging, artifact in 40
   instrumentation 20
   reflection of 9
   safety, biological effect of 45

small part 253
therapeutic 7
transducer 12
types of 20
units 22
velocity of 6t
Ultrasound beam 9, 30, 34
　characteristics of 17
　direction of 27
　generation of 20
Ultrasound contrast agents
　classification of 314
　mode of action 314
Ultrasound machine
　control panel of 39f
　part of 39f
Ultrasound pulse 50
　reflection of 8
Umbilical cord 297f, 376
Umbilical cyst 231f
Umbilical granuloma 231f
Umbilical herniation, normal 296f
Unfocused transducer 17
Unicollis 209
Unicornuate uterus 209
Upper abdomen, preparation for 37
Upper extremity veins, anatomy of 129f
Upper limb 403
　arteries 403
Urachal anomalies 187
Ureter 89
　dilated lower 186f
　left lower 187f
Ureteral obstruction 227
Ureterocele 173, 187f
Ureteropelvic junction obstruction 226
Ureterovesical junction obstruction 360
Ureters
　proximal ureters 54
　sonography of 186
Urethra
　bulbar part of 192f
　posterior 361f
Urethral lumen 102
Urethral valve, posterior 227, 360f
Urinary bladder 54, 90f, 93f, 95f, 96f, 180f, 186, 189f, 320, 361f
　anterior portion of 42f
　inflammatory pathology of 187
　pediatric 124
　posterior wall of 188f
　urine-filled 54
　wall of 188f

Urinary system 397
　location of 86f
Urinary tract 51, 53, 86, 174, 226
　anomalies 372
　congenital anomalies of 226
Urinoma 177f
Urokinase 381
Uterine abnormalities, congenital 209
Uterine bleeding 210
Uterine cavity 212f
　multiple synechia in 214f
Uterine fibroids 222
Uterine fundus 37
Uterine malformation 317
Uterine musculature 209f
Uterine secretions 46
Uterine septum, thin 351f
Uterine wall, anterior 373f
Uterorectal pouch 204f
Uterovesical pouch 204f
Uterus 95f, 96f, 125, 320
　anatomy of 93f
　and adnexa 56, 90, 93, 209
　anteverted 96f
　didelphys 209, 209f
　hyperplastic endometrium in 213f
　neoplasms of 210
　transvaginal scan of 216f
　unicornis 209
　varies 94

V

Vagina 94, 96f
　normal 94f
Vancomycin 170
Varices 312
Varicocele 258, 259f
Vascular interventional techniques 378
Vascular lesions 235, 400
Vascular masses 248
Vascular procedures 380
Vascular system 128
Vascular therapy 381
Velamentous insertion 376
Velocity calculation 44
Vena cava, anatomy of inferior 84f
Venous embolization 381
Venous hemodynamics 386
Venous obstruction 387
Venous system, anatomy of 280
Ventricular mural thrombus 417

Ventricular septal
　defect 416, 417f
　motion 413
Vertebral artery 128f, 393
　anatomy 128
Vesical calculus 188
Vesicoureteric junction
　right 188f
　and left 90f
Vesicoureteric reflux 227
Video amplifier 26
Viral hepatitis, acute 136
Viscosity 11
Vitamin D 176
Vitreal cyst 243f
Vitreous detachment, posterior 243, 245
Vitreous examination 243
Vitreous hemorrhage 243, 245
Vomiting 136
von Hippel-Lindau disease 185
von Meyenburg complexes 130

W

Wall-ECHO-shadow sign 147f
Water 11
　distended stomach 77f
Waterlily sign 132
Wave propagation 5f
Wharton's duct 123
Wilms' tumor 226, 228, 228f, 249
Wilson's disease 137, 225
Wobbler
　advantage of 32
　disadvantage of 32
　transducer 31
Wolman's disease 230
Wrist 60
　joint, right 425f

X

X deflection plates 23
Xanthogranulomatous 179
Xiphoid 71

Y

Ying-Yang sign 404f
Yolk sac 320, 332f
　and embryo, detection of 334t

Z

Zygomatic arch 122